Prostate Cancer

A Multidisciplinary Approach to Diagnosis and Management

Current Multidisciplinary Oncology Series

Charles R. Thomas, Jr., MD
Series Editor

Breast Cancer
A Multidisciplinary Approach to Diagnosis and Management
Alphonse G. Taghian, Barbara L. Smith, and John K. Erban

Lung Cancer
A Multidisciplinary Approach to Diagnosis and Management
Kemp H. Kernstine and Karen L. Reckamp

Cancers of the Colon and Rectum
A Multidisciplinary Approach to Diagnosis and Management
Al B. Benson III, A. Bapsi Chakravarthy, Stanley R. Hamilton, and Elin R. Sigurdson

Gynecologic Cancers
A Multidisciplinary Approach to Diagnosis and Management
Kunle Odunsi and Tanja Pejovic

Prostate Cancer
A Multidisciplinary Approach to Diagnosis and Management
Adam P. Dicker, William Kevin Kelly, Nicholas G. Zaorsky, and Edouard J. Trabulsi

Current Multidisciplinary Oncology

Prostate Cancer

A Multidisciplinary Approach to Diagnosis and Management

Edited by

Adam P. Dicker, MD, PhD

Professor and Chairman
Department of Radiation Oncology
Sidney Kimmel Medical College at Thomas Jefferson University
Sidney Kimmel Cancer Center
Philadelphia, PA

William Kevin Kelly, DO

Professor
Department of Medical Oncology and Urology
Sidney Kimmel Medical College at Thomas Jefferson University
Sidney Kimmel Cancer Center
Philadelphia, PA

Nicholas G. Zaorsky, MD

Department of Radiation Oncology
Fox Chase Cancer Center
Sidney Kimmel Medical College at Thomas Jefferson University
Philadelphia, PA

Edouard J. Trabulsi, MD

Associate Professor
Department of Urology
Sidney Kimmel Medical College at Thomas Jefferson University
Sidney Kimmel Cancer Center
Philadelphia, PA

Illustrations by Nicholas G. Zaorsky, MD

demosMEDICAL
New York

Visit our website at www.demosmedical.com

ISBN: 9781936287598
e-book ISBN: 9781617051067

Acquisitions Editor: Rich Winters
Compositor: diacriTech

Library of Congress Cataloging-in-Publication Data

Prostate cancer (Dicker)
Prostate cancer : a multidisciplinary approach to diagnosis and management / edited by Adam P. Dicker, William Kevin Kelly, Nicholas G. Zaorsky, Edouard J. Trabulsi.
p. ; cm. — (Current multidisciplinary oncology)
Includes bibliographical references and index.
ISBN 978-1-936287-59-8—ISBN 978-1-61705-106-7 (e-book)
I. Dicker, Adam P., editor. II. Kelly, Wm. Kevin (William Kevin), editor. III. Zaorsky, Nicholas G., editor. IV. Trabulsi, Edouard J., editor. V. Title. VI. Series: Current multidisciplinary oncology.
[DNLM: 1. Prostatic Neoplasms—diagnosis. 2. Early Detection of Cancer. 3. Patient Care Team. 4. Prognosis. 5. Prostate-Specific Antigen. 6. Prostatic Neoplasms—therapy. WJ 762]

RC280.P7
616.99'463—dc23

2014033133

Printed in the United States of America by Edwards Brothers.
14 15 16 17 / 5 4 3 2 1

To my parents, Zachary and Roslyn Dicker, who encouraged me to pursue my passion of science forty-years ago.
Fred and Judith Hochstadter, who later in my life were supportive of my career in medicine, research and oncology.

Carolyn, Michal, Shimshon and Yehuda. Thank you, love you, you're the best!!!!!

Adam P. Dicker

To Pam, Ryan and Liam Kelly who continue to support my career in medical oncology—Thank you!. With Love.

William Kevin Kelly

To my mentors who have guided me down the path of Medicine.

Nicholas G. Zaorsky

To my supportive family, Karen, John, Marc and Michael, and my parents who pushed me to medicine.

Ed Trabulsi

Contents

Contributors

Neeraj Agarwal, MD
Assistant Professor of Medicine
Director, GU Medical Oncology, Division of Medical Oncology
Co-leader, Urologic Oncology Multidisciplinary Program
Huntsman Cancer Institute
University of Utah
Salt Lake City, Utah

Ayal A. Aizer, MD
Clinical Fellow
Department of Radiation Oncology
Massachusetts General Hospital
Boston, Massachusetts

Naveed H. Akhtar, MD
Division of Hematology and Medical Oncology
Weill Cornell Cancer Center
New York, New York

Emma H. Allott, PhD
Postdoctoral Associate
Department of Surgery
Duke University
Durham, North Carolina;
Postdoctoral Associate
Department of Epidemiology
University of North Carolina at Chapel Hill
Chapel Hill, North Carolina

Abdel Hai Alqwasmi, MD
Clinical Ventures Group
Medical College of Wisconsin
Milwaukee, Wisconsin

Ajjai Alva, MD, MS
Assistant Professor
Division of Hematology/Oncology
Department of Internal Medicine
University of Michigan
Ann Arbor, Michigan

Gerald L. Andriole, MD
Robert Killian Royce Distinguished Professor
Department of Surgery
Chief, Division of Urologic Surgery
Director, Men's Health Center
Washington University
Saint Louis, Missouri

Leslie Ballas, MD
Assistant Professor of Radiation Oncology
Department of Radiation Oncology
Keck School of Medicine
University of Southern California
Los Angeles, California

Julia Batten, MSN, MPH
Nurse Practioner
Department of Internal Medicine
Huntsman Cancer Institute
University of Utah
Salt Lake City, Utah

Nathan Bittner, MD, MS
Radiation Oncologist
Radiation Oncology
Tacoma/Valley Radiation Oncology Centers
Tacoma, Washington

Otis W. Brawley, MD, FACP, FASCO
Chief Medical Officer
American Cancer Society;
Professor of Hematology, Medical Oncology, Medicine and Epidemiology
Emory University
Atlanta, Georgia

Peter R. Carroll, MD, MPH
Professor and Chair
Department of Urology
University of California San Francisco Medical Center
San Francisco, California

Sameer Chopra, MD
Urologic Oncology, Research Fellow
Department of Urology
University of Southern California
Los Angeles, California

Peter L. Choyke, MD
Molecular Imaging Program
National Cancer Institute
National Institutes of Health
Bethesda, Maryland

Joshua A. Cohn, MD
Section of Urology
University of Chicago
Chicago, Illinois

Jonathan A. Coleman, MD
Associate Professor of Urology
Department of Surgery, Division of Urology
Memorial Sloan Kettering Cancer Center
New York, New York

Matthew R. Cooperberg, MD
Associate Professor of Urology
Epidemiology and Biostatistics
Helen Diller Family Chair in Urology
University of California San Francisco Medical Center
San Francisco, California

Carlos Cordon-Cardo, MD, PhD
Professor and Chair
Department of Pathology, Genetics and Genomic Sciences
Icahn School of Medicine at Mount Sinai
New York, New York

Annie Darves–Bornoz, MD
Resident Physician
Department of Urology
Vanderbilt University Hospital
Nashville, Tennessee

Elai Davicioni, PhD
President and Chief Scientific Officer
GenomeDx Biosciences Inc.
San Diego, California

Johann S. de Bono, MB, ChB, FRCP, MSc, PhD, FMedSci
Professor
Prostate Targeted Therapy Group
The Royal Marsden NHS Trust
The Institute of Cancer Research
London, United Kingdom

Angelo M. DeMarzo, MD, PhD
Sidney Kimmel Comprehensive Cancer Center
James Buchanan Urological Institute
Department of Pathology
Johns Hopkins University School of Medicine
Baltimore, Maryland

Robert B. Den, MD
Assistant Professor
Department of Radiation Oncology
Sidney Kimmel Medical College at Thomas Jefferson University
Sidney Kimmel Cancer Center
Philadelphia, Pennsylvania

Michael J. Donovan, MD, PhD
Research Professor
Experimental Pathology and Precise Medicine
Director of the Biorepository and Pathology Core
Department of Pathology
Icahn School of Medicine at Mount Sinai
New York, New York

Charles Drake, MD, PhD
Assistant Professor
Oncology, Immunology and Urology
Johns Hopkins Sidney Kimmel Comprehensive Cancer Center
Baltimore, Maryland

James A. Eastham, MD, FACS
Chief, Urology Service
Florence and Theodore Baumritter/Enid Ancell Chair of Urologic Oncology
Memorial Sloan Kettering Cancer Center
New York, New York

Jason A. Efstathiou, MD, DPhil
Associate Professor
Department of Radiation Oncology
Massachusetts General Hospital
Boston, Massachusetts

Scott E. Eggener, MD
Associate Professor of Surgery
Co-director, Prostate Cancer Program
Director of Translational and Outcomes Research
Section of Urology
University of Chicago
Chicago, Illinois

Gerardo Fernandez, MD
Senior Faculty
Department of Pathology and Precise Medicine
Icahn School of Medicine at Mount Sinai
New York, New York

Stephen J. Freedland, MD
Department of Surgery
Durham VA Medical Center;
Departments of Surgery and Pathology
Division of Urology
Duke University Medical Center
Durham, North Carolina

Leonard G. Gomella, MD, FACS
Bernard W. Godwin Professor of Prostate Cancer
Chairman, Department of Urology
Associate Director of Clinical Affairs, Jefferson Sidney Kimmel Cancer Center
Clinical Director, Jefferson Sidney Kimmel Cancer Center Network
Sidney Kimmel Medical College at Thomas Jefferson University
Philadelphia, Pennsylvania

Phillip J. Gray, MD
Harvard Radiation Oncology Program
Department of Radiation Oncology
Massachusetts General Hospital
Boston, Massachusetts

David E Greene, MD
LCDR, MC, USN
Radiation Oncologist
Naval Medical Center San Diego
San Diego, California;
Assistant Professor
Department of Radiology
Uniformed Services University of the Health Sciences
Bethesda, Maryland

Peter Grimm, DO
Director
Prostate Cancer Center of Seattle
Seattle, Washington

Robert L. Grubb III, MD
Herbert Lourie Professor of Neurological Surgery
Professor, Radiation Services
Washington University
Saint Louis, Missouri

Thomas J. Guzzo, MD, MPH
Vice-Chief of Urology
Assistant Professor of Urology
Division of Urology
The University of Pennsylvania
Perelman Center for Advanced Medicine
Philadelphia, Pennsylvania

Ethan J. Halpern, MD
Department of Radiology
Jefferson Prostate Diagnostic Center
Sidney Kimmel Medical College at Thomas Jefferson University
Philadelphia, Pennsylvania

Waleed A. Hassen, MD
Staff Physician
Glickman Urological and Kidney Institute
Cleveland Clinic
Cleveland, Ohio;
Consultant Physician
Surgical Subspecialties Institute
Cleveland Clinic Abu Dhabi
Abu Dhabi, UAE

Elisabeth I. Heath, MD, FACP
Director
Prostate Cancer Research
Karmanos Cancer Institute;
Professor of Oncology and Medicine
Wayne State University School of Medicine
Detroit, Michigan

Jean Hoffman-Censits, MD
Assistant Professor
Department of Medical Oncology
Sidney Kimmel Medical College at Thomas Jefferson University
Philadelphia, Pennsylvania

Mark Hurwitz, MD
Professor
Vice Chair for Quality, Safety and Performance Excellence
Director of Thermal Oncology
Department of Radiation Oncology
Sidney Kimmel Medical College at Thomas Jefferson University
Philadelphia, Pennsylvania

Clara Hwang, MD
Senior Staff Physician
Department of Internal Medicine
Henry Ford Medical Group;
Clinical Assistant Professor
Department of Internal Medicine
Wayne State University School of Medicine
Detroit, Michigan

Charles M. Intenzo, MD
Director, Nuclear Medicine
Professor, Department of Radiology
Sidney Kimmel Medical College at Thomas Jefferson University
Philadelphia, Pennsylvania

Hossein Jadvar, MD, PhD, MPH, MBA
Associate Professor of Radiology and Vice Chair of Research
Department of Radiology
Keck School of Medicine
University of Southern California
Los Angeles, California

Ryan T. Jones, MD
Department of Radiation Oncology
University of Texas Southwestern Medical Center
Dallas, Texas

Sanjay Kasturi, MD
Department of Urology
Sidney Kimmel Medical College at Thomas Jefferson University
Sidney Kimmel Cancer Center
Philadelphia, Pennsylvania

Michael W. Kattan, PhD
Department of Quantitative Health Sciences
Cleveland Clinic Foundation
Cleveland, Ohio

Aaron Katz, MD
Chairman
Department of Urology
Winthrop University Hospital
Mineola, New York;
Professor
Department of Urology
Stony Brook Medical Center
Stony Brook, New York

Gurveen Kaur, MD
Division of Hematology and Medical Oncology
Weill Cornell Cancer Center
New York, New York

William Kevin Kelly, DO
Professor
Department of Medical Oncology and Urology
Sidney Kimmel Medical College at Thomas Jefferson University
Sidney Kimmel Cancer Center
Philadelphia, Pennsylvania

Faisal M. Khan, BA
Director, Biostatistical Operations
Department of Pathology and Precise Medicine
Icahn School of Medicine at Mount Sinai
New York, New York

Sung M. Kim, MD
Professor
Department of Radiology
Sidney Kimmel Medical College at Thomas Jefferson University
Philadelphia, Pennsylvania

Eric A. Klein, MD
Chairman
Glickman Urological and Kidney Institute
Cleveland Clinic
Cleveland, Ohio

Laurence Klotz, MD, FRCS(C)
Professor of Surgery
Division of Urology
Sunnybrook Health Sciences Centre
University of Toronto
Toronto, Ontario, Canada

Ibrahim Kulac, MD
Sidney Kimmel Comprehensive Cancer Center
James Buchanan Brady Urological Institute
Department of Pathology
Johns Hopkins University School of Medicine
Baltimore, Maryland

Costas D. Lallas, MD, FACS
Associate Professor
Department of Urology
Sidney Kimmel Medical College at Thomas Jefferson University
Philadelphia, Pennsylvania

Jianqing Lin, MD
Department of Medical Oncology
Sidney Kimmel Medical College at Thomas Jefferson University
Philadelphia, Pennsylvania

Liza Lindenberg, MD
Molecular Imaging Program
National Cancer Institute
National Institutes of Health
Bethesda, Maryland

James R. Marshall, PhD
Chair, Department of Cancer Prevention and Population Sciences
Roswell Park Cancer Institute
Buffalo, New York

Joaquin Mateo, MD, MSc
Clinical Research Fellow
Prostate Targeted Therapy Group
The Royal Marsden NHS Trust
The Institute of Cancer Research
London, United Kingdom

Mark V. Mishra, MD
Department of Radiation Oncology
Greenebaum Cancer Center
University of Maryland School of Medicine
Baltimore, Maryland

Anirban P. Mitra, MD, PhD
Senior Research Associate
Department of Pathology and Center for Personalized Medicine
University of Southern California
Los Angeles, California

Judd W. Moul, MD, FACS
James H. Semans MD Professor of Surgery
Director, Duke Prostate Center
Division of Urologic Surgery
Duke University Medical Center
Durham, North Carolina

Lorelei A. Mucci, ScD, MPH
Associate Professor of Epidemiology
Department of Epidemiology
Harvard School of Public Health
Boston, Massachusetts

Alana M. Murphy, MD
Assistant Professor
Department of Urology
Sidney Kimmel Medical College at Thomas Jefferson University
Philadelphia, Pennsylvania

Hao G. Nguyen, MD, PhD
Clinical Fellow
Department of Urology
University of California San Francisco School of Medicine
San Francisco, California

Janine L. Oliver, MD
Division of Urologic Surgery
Washington University
Saint Louis, Missouri

Peter Orio, DO, MS
Dana Farber Cancer Institute
Brigham and Women's Hospital;
Department of Radiation Oncology
Harvard Medical School
Boston, Massachusetts

Aytekin Oto, MD
Professor of Radiology and Surgery
Section Chief, Abdominal Imaging
Director, Body MR Imaging
University of Chicago
Chicago, Illinois

Peter A. Pinto, MD
Urologic Oncology Branch
National Cancer Institute
National Institutes of Health
Bethesda, Maryland

Austin Poole, MD
Resident
Department of Internal Medicine
Huntsman Cancer Institute
University of Utah
Salt Lake City, Utah

Thomas J. Pugh, MD
Assistant Professor
Department of Radiation Oncology
University of Texas MD Anderson Cancer Center
Houston, Texas

David I. Quinn, MBBS (Hons. I), PhD, FRACP, FACP
Associate Professor of Medicine
Division of Medical Oncology
Keck School of Medicine
University of Southern California
Los Angeles, California

Farhang Rabbani, MD
Associate Professor
Department of Urology
Montefiore Medical Center
Albert Einstein College of Medicine of Yeshiva University
Bronx, New York

Dima Raskolnikov, BS
Urologic Oncology Branch
National Cancer Institute
National Institutes of Health
Bethesda, Maryland

Chad A. Reichard, MD
Glickman Urological and Kidney Institute
Cleveland Clinic
Cleveland, Ohio

Victor Sai, MD
Assistant Clinical Professor
Department of Radiology
David Geffen School of Medicine at UCLA
University of California, Los Angeles
Los Angeles, California

Gurdarshan S. Sandhu, MD
Division of Urologic Surgery
Washington University
Saint Louis, Missouri

Jillian Scambia, DO
Resident Physician
Department of Urology
Cook County Hospital
Chicago, Illinois

Richard Scott, PhD
Biomedical Software Developer
Department of Pathology and Precise Medicine
Icahn School of Medicine at Mount Sinai
New York, New York

Fernando Pablo Secin, MD, PhD
Assistant Professor
Urology Section, Department of Surgery
CEMIC University Hospital and San Lazaro Foundation
Buenos Aires, Argentina

Andrew Sharabi, MD, PhD
Resident Physician
Department of Radiation Oncology and Molecular Radiation Sciences
Johns Hopkins University School of Medicine
Baltimore, Maryland

Patrick J. Shenot, MD
Associate Professor
Department of Urology
Sidney Kimmel Medical College at Thomas Jefferson University
Philadelphia, Pennsylvania

Heesun Shin, PhD
Manager
Scientific and Clinical Communications
GenomeDx Biosciences Inc.
San Diego, California

Timothy N. Showalter, MD, MPH
Associate Professor
Department of Radiation Oncology
University of Virginia School of Medicine
Charlottesville, Virginia

Jonathan L. Silberstein, MD
Department of Urology
Tulane School of Medicine
New Orleans, Louisiana

Beerinder K. Singh, MD
Division of Hematology and Medical Oncology
Weill Cornell Cancer Center
New York, New York

Susan F. Slovin, MD, PhD
Attending Physician
Genitourinary Oncology Service
Sidney Kimmel Center for Prostate and Urologic Cancers
Memorial Sloan Kettering Cancer Center;
Professor
Department of Medicine
Weill Cornell College of Medicine
New York, New York

Alan D. Smith, MD
Clinical Research Fellow
Prostate Targeted Therapy Group
The Royal Marsden NHS Trust
The Institute of Cancer Research
London, United Kingdom

Zachary L. Smith, MD
Resident Physician
Division of Urology
The University of Pennsylvania
Perelman Center for Advanced Medicine
Philadelphia, Pennsylvania

Toru Sugihara, MD, MPH
Assistant Professor
Department of Urology
Tokyo Medical University
Tokyo, Japan

Scott T. Tagawa, MD, MS
Division of Hematology and Medical Oncology
Weill Cornell Cancer Center
New York, New York

Mathew L. Thakur, PhD
Director, Laboratories of Radiopharmaceutical Research and Molecular Imaging
Professor of Radiology and Radiation Oncology
Sidney Kimmel Medical College at Thomas Jefferson University
Philadelphia, Pennsylvania

Karim Touijer, MD
Department of Urology
Memorial Sloan Kettering Cancer Center
New York, New York

Edouard J. Trabulsi, MD
Associate Professor
Department of Urology
Sidney Kimmel Medical College at Thomas Jefferson University
Sidney Kimmel Cancer Center
Philadelphia, Pennsylvania

Timothy J. Triche, MD, PhD
Professor, Pathology and Pediatrics
University of Southern California;
Director, Center for Personalized Medicine
Children's Hospital Los Angeles
Los Angeles, California

Baris Turkbey, MD
Molecular Imaging Program
National Cancer Institute
National Institutes of Health
Bethesda, Maryland

Ulka Vaishampayan, MD
Professor of Oncology
Karmanos Cancer Institute
Wayne State University School of Medicine
Detroit, Michigan

Richard K. Valicenti, MD, MA
Professor and Chairman
Department of Radiation Oncology
University of California Davis
Sacramento, California

Ismael A. Vergara, PhD
Bioinformatician
GenomeDx Biosciences Inc.
San Diego, California

Antonio C. Westphalen, MD, PhD
Associate Professor
Department of Radiology and Biomedical Imaging
Department of Urology
UCSF School of Medicine
University of California, San Francisco
San Francisco, California

Steve K. Williams
Urologist
Department of Urology
Florida Hospital
Orlando, Florida

Kathryn M. Wilson, ScD
Research Scientist
Department of Epidemiology
Harvard School of Public Health
Boston, Massachusetts

Ashley G. Winter, MD
Department of Urology
New York Presbyterian Hospital
Weill Cornell Medical Center
New York, New York

Nicholas G. Zaorsky, MD
Resident Physician
Department of Radiation Oncology
Fox Chase Cancer Center;
Radiation Oncology
Sidney Kimmel Medical College at Thomas Jefferson University
Philadelphia, Pennsylvania

Series Foreword

In this fifth volume of the series, Current Multidisciplinary Oncology, devoted to prostate cancer, it brings me great pleasure to introduce practicing clinicians to a new resource that will aid in the multidisciplinary approach of solid tumors.

Drs. Adam Dicker, William Kelly, Nicholas Zaorsky, and Edouard Trabulsi have put together a cadre of highly respected thought leaders as contributors on the multidisciplinary approach to prostate cancer.

Over the past two decades, a myriad of advances in the diagnosis and treatment of prostate cancer have occurred. These advances include, but are not unlimited to, diagnostic molecular tools that may aid in predicting a response to certain treatment approaches and/or providing a guide of a prognostic outcome for certain patients.

Our distinguished co-editors have compiled more than 50 chapters on this disease, authored by an international contingent of leading-edge investigators, into well-defined sections.

Prostate cancer is one of the most common malignancies in the world affecting men and hence warrants intense efforts to find a cure. In recent years, investment of resources to help further understand the nature of this malignancy has increased.

It is clear that Drs. Dicker, Kelly, Zaorsky, and Trabulsi represent some of the best academic, forward-thinking oncologists to commit their careers to eradicating prostate cancer. Their collective vision and ability to assemble an outstanding group of investigators in the field have provided a very high-quality product that will be a useful resource to busy clinicians as well as those along various stages of the learning spectrum. I'm sure that you will enjoy this innovative and easy-to-read volume and as you look for guidance in the multidisciplinary approach of your patients with prostate cancer.

Charles R. Thomas, Jr., MD
Series Editor
Department of Radiation Medicine
Oregon Health and Science University
Knight Cancer Institute
Portland, Oregon

Preface

Prostate cancer is the second most commonly diagnosed cancer among men globally, with more than 1.1 million new cases each year. In the United States, 233,000 men are expected to be diagnosed in 2014, and an American man's lifetime risk of prostate cancer is 1 in 6. With the introduction of genomic diagnostics and novel therapeutics, the past 5 years have seen an explosion in the amount of new data and opportunities for clinical benefit to prostate cancer patients. This book, a volume in the series Current Multidisciplinary Oncology, is designed to provide a comprehensive view of the entire spectrum of multidisciplinary management of prostate cancer.

The chapters in this book are arranged in a logical progression from screening and prevention to diagnosis, treatment and surveillance, similar to other books in the series. Dr. Leonard Gomella, a urologist who was the first to advocate multidisciplinary care for prostate cancer patients over two decades ago, has contributed an introduction that provides a macro view of the field over the past 50 years and puts into perspective where the treatment of prostate cancer has been, what has been accomplished, and where future challenges remain. The subchapters comprising Chapter 2 cover the epidemiology of prostate cancer, with in-depth analysis of the global burden, incidence, mortality, risk factors, physical activity, smoking, antioxidants, and the impact of diet and obesity. The controversial area of screening is covered in depth, with Drs. Gerald Andriole et al and Dr. Otis Brawley providing opposing views. There are also discussions of improving the accuracy of PSA screening and an update on the International Society of Urological Pathology (ISUP) Modified Gleason Score and its controversies. Advances in molecular pathology using cancer genomics have now entered the clinical realm with at least three companies offering diagnostic genomic tests and are addressed in the subchapters comprising Chapter 5, covering novel molecular and genotype profiling in prostate cancer, including morphometric and systems pathology. The current uses of radiographic imaging for diagnosis and staging are also discussed including detailed information on MRI, ultrasound, and nuclear medicine.

The treatment sections of the book correspond to the staging of disease. For low-risk localized disease, the use of active surveillance—*the concept of less is more*—is covered in Chapter 7. Other chapters cover the surgical treatment of prostate cancer from different perspectives—radical prostatectomy, laparoscopic radical prostatectomy, robotic radical prostatectomy, and surgical training. Radiation therapy using external beam radiation therapy for the treatment of low risk adenocarcinoma of the prostate is covered in Chapter 10, with additional discussions of hypofractionated radiation therapy, stereotactic body radiation therapy, protons and brachytherapy, either low dose rate (LDR) or high dose rate (HDR). Also included is coverage of the general principles of ablative focal therapies, vascular-targeted photodynamic therapy, laser, irreversible electroporation, and hyperthermia, a field that has grown considerably. An appreciation that quality of life (QoL) is a critical component of any therapeutic option is addressed in separate chapters that evaluate QoL for surgery, androgen deprivation, external beam radiation therapy, and brachytherapy.

Full coverage of the options and optimal treatment of patients with metastatic disease including hormone sensitive and metastatic castrate resistant prostate cancer. The full array of treatment options for metastatic patients includes an understanding of hormone escape, the use of androgen synthesis blockade, immunotherapy and chemotherapy. As prostate cancer frequently metastasizes to the bone, special emphasis for these patients is given to provide awareness of pharmaceuticals to reduce skeletal-related events, a major advance and novel radiopharmaceutical that provides for the first time a survival advantage.

A number of chapters incorporate models of care delivery, patient navigation for the multidisciplinary care of prostate cancer patients, genomics and risk assessment and comparative effectives research in treatment decision-making.

This book reflects the editors Drs. Dicker, Kelly, Zaorsky, and Trabulsi who work together at Thomas Jefferson University in a truly multidisciplinary manner. The book is designed as a management text for all health care professionals who provide care for prostate cancer patients including medical oncologists, radiation oncologists, surgeons, radiologists, pathologists, nurses and other allied health professionals, students, residents and fellows in training, prostate cancer researchers, as well as patients, families and advocates. The prostate cancer thought leaders who have contributed to this volume have offered their considerable expertise to provide the most current evidence-based approach, including extensive references, to provide a valuable tool designed to enhance evaluation and management of prostate cancer patients.

Acknowledgments

The editors would like to thank the leadership at Thomas Jefferson University (*Health is all we do*) who helped us combine a sophisticated patient-first, multidisciplinary care of genitourinary cancer patients with high-impact science.

The editors are grateful to Dr. Charles Thomas, Jr. for his scholarly vision and encouragement, and Mr. Rich Winters and Ms. Lee Oglesby of Demos Medical Publishing for editorial guidance and timeliness. Finally we are indebted to our patients and colleagues who contributed their time and knowledge toward this effort.

Prostate Cancer

A Multidisciplinary Approach to Diagnosis and Management

Epidemiology, Screening, and Diagnosis

I

1 Introduction: The Multidisciplinary Approach to Prostate Cancer

LEONARD G. GOMELLA

One only needs to scan the table of contents of this book to appreciate the inherently complex nature of counseling and treating a patient with prostate cancer today. As recently as the late 1970s if a patient was believed to have prostate cancer, a simple prostate biopsy, often performed transperineally, was the diagnostic procedure of choice. No blood test existed to help detect early disease. Treatment was only based on the clinical stage. This simple treatment approach was due to the limited options available. If the prostate cancer was localized, radiation or surgery was the monotherapy choice with only orchiectomy or estrogen therapy available for advanced disease.

Today there are many more factors to consider in the prostate cancer decision-making process. This starts with an informed decision around screening an asymptomatic man for prostate cancer. If prostate cancer is diagnosed, should it even be treated? Patients who are appropriate candidates for active surveillance (AS) need a detailed discussion concerning the risks and benefits of that relatively new approach. If a decision is made for active treatment (AT), many additional factors need to be considered. These include the cancer characteristics (grade, prostate-specific antigen [PSA], histologic characteristics, clinical stage), imaging results, overall health and age of the patient, the beliefs and desired outcomes of the patient, family, and provider, and a decision between all competing treatment options. The evergrowing array of surgical, minimally invasive, and radiation-based therapies all have advantages and disadvantages with the long-term implications of some of these newer therapies unknown. In a relatively short period of time, basic science discoveries, completed clinical trials, new technologies, clinical observations, and advances in drug development have forever changed the nature of diagnosing and managing all phases of the prostate cancer care continuum.

■ PROSTATE CANCER IN THE 20TH CENTURY

Until the 1980s, prostate cancer was a relatively ignored disease that seemed to only gain interest when it afflicted a family member or a close friend. Some of this was due to societal values that were about to change. In addition, the work by Huggins and Hodges in the 1940s that identified prostate cancer as being hormonally responsive had been the last major breakthrough in prostate cancer (1). The field of prostate cancer was about to enter the mainstream and move ahead. This came about due to the evolution of our collective impressions of cancer and thanks to a series of key scientific discoveries in the early 1980s. Dr. Patrick Walsh's pioneering work on refining the radical prostatectomy, the discovery and development of PSA as a marker for prostate cancer, the expansion of prostate brachytherapy, the introduction of injectable luteinizing hormone–releasing hormone analogs, and the transrectal ultrasound-directed biopsy are some of the more prominent discoveries that began to change the face of prostate cancer.

About 20 years ago, I was fortunate to work with *Philadelphia Inquirer* science writer John Fried to produce the first book written for the lay public that specifically addressed the issue of prostate cancer. *Recovering From Prostate Cancer*, published by Harper Collins in 1993, led the way for dozens of other books that took prostate cancer from the back pages of men's health publications to the prominence on their covers (2). Since our first publication that focused on the topic, the greatly expanded portfolio of prostate cancer books for the general public has been authored by prominent physicians and surgeons as well as celebrities and ordinary citizens.

Beyond the important scientific discoveries noted, there is more to the story of how prostate cancer came into the public eye. To gain perspective on how society's perception of cancer in general and prostate cancer specifically changed by the 1990s, the following excerpt from *Recovering From Prostate Cancer* provides some insight:

There was a time when cancer was a taboo topic. When prominent people died of it, their obituaries invariably said that they had passed on "after a long illness." As recently as twenty years ago, many doctors did not tell their cancer patients that they had the illness. When one family member was afflicted by the disease, the relatives talked of it in whispers.

In the 1970s cancer began to come out of the closet, no longer kept there by a lingering feeling that it was a "dirty" disease, something to be ashamed of. That emergence, though, was not a complete one. Cancers of the reproductive tract or of parts of the body associated with sex, even into the late seventies, were talked about only reluctantly. It was not until prominent women began to make it known that they had fought breast cancer that this touchy topic was found fit for talk shows and magazine articles. But Betty Ford, the former first lady, and others like her did not go public for the sake of seeking sympathy. They did it to help make women aware that breast cancer was a leading killer of women and that regular checkups, including mammograms, could help save lives.

Despite the example set by women, another major killer, prostate cancer, eluded public (and even private) discussion until the 1990s, this even though the male cancer takes a toll that is not far behind the one breast cancer takes on women. One result of this reluctance to bring prostate cancer out into the open has been that research aimed at curing it has received relatively little financial support. Federal funding for breast-cancer research exceeded $70 million in 1989. Money for prostate cancer investigation came to a paltry $9.5 million. Another consequence of the hush-hush way in which prostate cancer has been approached is that many men still do not understand that once they reach fifty, they should have regular physical exams that include checkups for the presence of prostate cancer. Appallingly, some studies have shown that many doctors, because men are embarrassed by the prospect of submitting to the rectal exam that will give the physician access to the prostate gland, don't press them to undergo the procedure.

But change is in the air. In May 1992, the news that Linus Pauling had prostate cancer made the front pages of many newspapers. In fact, by 1992 a host of other prominent men had also let it be known that they had prostate cancer: Robert Dole, the senator from Kansas; Frank Zappa, the musician; Robert Penn Warren, the nation's first poet laureate; Joseph Papp, the eminent theater producer; and several United States Supreme Court justices, including John Paul Stevens, Harry A. Blackmun, William J. Brennan, and Lewis F. Powell (2).

A review of the table of contents of *Recovering From Prostate Cancer* reveals how much progress we have made in this cancer the last 20 years. The concept of screening asymptomatic men for prostate cancer using PSA and rectal exam was just beginning. The same year our book was published (1993), the American Cancer Society made its first recommendations on the use of PSA to detect prostate cancer (3). The digitally directed ("digital" referring to the index finger) prostate biopsy was still commonly used with transrectal ultrasound, something that all urologists were increasingly incorporating into daily practice. Only the most basic surgery and radiation comprised our armamentarium for localized disease. However, now injectable daily and monthly agents with or without oral androgen receptor blockers could be used for androgen ablation in metastatic disease. Chemotherapy was hit or miss and was not even considered a viable option except in the most extreme end-of-life situations. It was also around that time that the alarm bells began to sound as deaths from prostate cancer began to peak.

During the 1990s, intense debate raged in the medical community as to the superiority of one treatment modality over the other for localized prostate cancer. No one debated the use of hormonal ablation for cases of metastatic disease although there were minor skirmishes (early vs. late, monotherapy vs. combined androgen blockade) that are still with us today. However, for localized cancer, it was radical prostatectomy versus standard radiation (external beam or brachytherapy) with surgeons and radiation oncologists locked in a dogmatic battle (4). Often it was only patients not considered to be surgical candidates and those with significantly bulky locally advanced disease that surgeons would refer for radiation. Some of the earliest randomized clinical trials were just beginning to take shape in the early 1990s involving radiation oncology, the hormonal treatment of advanced disease, and the earliest attempts to study prostate cancer chemoprevention and screening.

■ PROSTATE CANCER IN THE 21ST CENTURY

Fast forward to 2014; what was once fairly simply in the diagnosis and treatment of prostate cancer has become incredibly complex for both the patient and the practitioner as evidenced by the numerous topics covered in this book. In some respects, those of us who work in the field of prostate cancer have become victims of our own success. We have developed our screening techniques to the point where we are diagnosing more and more small and clinically unimportant cancers. This has contributed in part to the backlash against routine population-based screening for prostate cancer (5). The recent unprecedented development of new drugs, molecular diagnostics, and surgical and radiation advances are becoming commonplace in the treatment of prostate cancer. Newer tests such as genomic assays and specialized imaging have proven useful although the experiences are still very early and insurance coverage can be problematic.

The cost issues surrounding these advances in the management of prostate cancer are also often subject to debate and often criticism. Are we getting our money's worth for prostate cancer care? Philipson et al. reviewed per capita spending in European countries for different cancers including prostate cancer over a 16-year period (6). They noted that U.S. cancer patients experienced greater survival gains than their European counterparts even after considering higher U.S. costs. The additional survival gain was highest for prostate cancer, estimated to be $627 billion, with the findings not driven solely by earlier diagnosis.

What is clear is that throughout the last 20 years, the death rate has declined and the quality of life of men with all stages of prostate cancer has dramatically improved. Much of the improvement can be readily attributed to the medical advances noted earlier. What may not be readily apparent is the new emphasis on improved communication and coordination of care of men with prostate cancer that appears to play a role in improving outcomes.

Medical oncology as a discipline has more to offer men with advanced prostate cancer than ever before with at least five new therapeutic agents specifically approved for metastatic castration-resistant prostate cancer since 2010 (7). Many of these new and pending prostate cancer therapies are based on sophisticated investigations by basic scientists who appreciate the clinical implications of their translational research efforts. So-called "Dream Teams" embody this forward thinking concept (8). Surgeons and radiation oncologists are working more closely together to present the best treatment options to men with localized disease, with each field increasingly recognizing the advantages and disadvantages of their specific modalities. The rigidly held beliefs of each specialty in the superiority of their modality have given way to numerous collaborative efforts. This coordination often combines the skills of each practitioner such as in the use of prostate brachytherapy or recommending adjuvant radiation therapy following radical prostatectomy. Joint investigations and publications focusing on important questions in prostate cancer have begun to appear, such as the American Urologic Association and American Society for Therapeutic Radiation Oncology soliciting the input from all specialties and publishing joint papers and issuing recommendations on the treatment of localized prostate cancer and on the use of postoperative radiation therapy (9, 10). Groups such as the National Comprehensive Cancer Network (NCCN) meet several times a year to update treatment guidelines of all stages of prostate cancer with multidisciplinary input into all recommendations (11). Combining therapies to improve prostate cancer outcomes is perhaps best illustrated by the numerous clinical trials that support the use of neoadjuvant and adjuvant androgen ablation in combination with external beam radiation therapy (12).

Now more than ever there is a significant need for urologic surgeons, medical oncologists, and radiation oncologists to join forces and provide coordinated counseling and care for men with all stages of prostate cancer. This multidisciplinary approach has its origins in the advances made in the diagnosis and treatment of prostate cancer that have evolved over the past quarter century.

■ PROSTATE CANCER PATIENT DESCISION MAKING

Options for our patients to receive information about prostate cancer and most other medical conditions have been dramatically transformed in the 21st century. The physician as the sole source of information on a disease is a historic concept. Because of all the differing treatment options available for prostate cancer, patients can become overwhelmed when seeking information from resources such as the web. A Google search in April of 2014 yielded over 49 million page hits for prostate cancer, overwhelming for anyone, to say the least.

A recent Cochrane review evaluated a group of patients with a diversity of diseases who used a variety of decision aids such as pamphlets, videos, and web-based tools to assist with medical decision making (13). These tools were useful at improving knowledge of the treatment options. They also provided objective information on the benefits and harms and allowed patients to make choices consistent with personal values. Although these decision tools have value in areas such as prostate cancer, the unique needs of the individual patient must also be taken into consideration. Decision making for multimodality treatment plans in men with high-risk disease often requires the input of all specialists and consideration for clinical trials. Treatment regret can be minimized if patients are given the opportunity to openly discuss treatment options with different specialists (14).

Warren et al. studied information comprehensiveness on a variety of websites for breast and prostate cancer. Web-based information can provide useful cancer information online and enable patients to be more proactive regarding their information needs. However, multiple deficiencies were noted, and also that more comprehensive information needs to be provided on breast and prostate cancer websites in areas such as decision making (15). Another study indicated that although web-based information is useful, physicians remain a key information source for medical advice and the face-to-face interaction is critical (16). Taking all of these unique patient and disease factors together, prostate cancer therapeutic options appear to be best determined through close and coordinated face to face multidisciplinary collaboration.

■ THE MULTIDISCIPLINARY APPROACH TO PROSTATE CANCER

How do we define "multidisciplinary prostate cancer care"? In its simplest form, it encompasses collaborative patient care by a team of different specialists where all treatment options are discussed and individualized for each patient. One definition of a true multidisciplinary care model is described as encompassing "collaborative patient care by a team of individuals where all diagnostic and treatment options are discussed and tailored for each patient. Although the team composition may vary by disease site and institution, independent contributors may include representatives from medical oncology, radiation oncology, surgery/surgical oncology, pathology, diagnostic imaging, palliative care, nursing, nutrition, and social work" (17). Although this is a generally applicable definition in the field of oncology, the existing models of prostate cancer multidisciplinary clinic (MDC) care can be different. In its purest and possibly most effective form, a true multidisciplinary clinical setting involves real-time interaction between the various medical specialists, the patient, and the patient's family. Other models do exist such as the agreement to follow defined clinical care pathways or a discussion of cases at tumor boards. There is a paucity of literature studying these other models at present.

There is increasing interest in both academic and community cancer programs to develop some version of a patient centric genitourinary (GU) or prostate cancer MDC. The specific design of each multidisciplinary prostate clinic in the United States can vary greatly as there are no specific guidelines or recommendations for such activity. The centers that have published on their GU MDC suggest that simultaneous provider and patient encounters in a real-time clinic setting are a common feature (18, 19).

An important concept in the GU MDC approach to prostate cancer involves the education of patients and involving them in "shared decision making." The U.S. Institute of Medicine has noted that this shared decision making is at the heart of patient-centered care and is "responsive to individual patient preferences, needs and values" (20). The traditional medical "paternalistic" approach to patient care with physicians making the treatment decision that they thought was best is no longer considered to be the standard of care. In the field of prostate cancer, the overwhelming number of treatment options makes shared decision making a core value in providing the best patient care possible.

■ EXPERIENCE WITH THE MULTIDISCIPLINARY APPROACH TO PROSTATE CANCER

A variety of groups have reported on the MDC approach to prostate cancer care. The majority have focused on the decision-making process for those with newly diagnosed localized disease, often the most controversial aspect of management. In 1996, we established a GU MDC at the Kimmel Cancer Center of Thomas Jefferson University in Philadelphia. We believe that this is the longest continually operating MDC at any National Cancer Institute-designated cancer center in the United States. Since we originally described the structure and operation of the clinic, there have been only minor modifications to its operational structure (18, 21). Having all specialists present during the visit (urologic surgery, radiation oncology, and medical oncology) with pathology and radiology support remains a core feature. Although all GU tumor types are seen in the weekly clinic, the majority of patients (historically more than 80%) have prostate cancer, and we recently reported our 15-year experience focusing on prostate cancer (18). Other groups such as the Prostate Cancer Programme of Milans Istituto Nazionale dei Tumori have adapted and validated our model of multidisciplinary care (22).

The current operational structure of our Kimmel Cancer Center GU MDC is shown in Figure 1.1. The only major change we have made over the last 15 years was in 2008 when we moved to a preclinic conference instead of a postclinic conference. This important preclinic conference includes second-opinion pathologic review, imaging review (if necessary), and a brief case presentation and discussion. General treatment recommendations based on available data are made, and potential confounders are identified. This preclinic conference also offers the opportunity to identify patients who might be eligible for clinical trial participation.

In the clinical patient care area, social service support is on site. Genetic counselors, integrative medicine, and nutritional and pain management are made available to our patients at the Kimmel Cancer Center outside of the GU MDC[**]. Support groups and the opportunity to participate in the "Buddy System," matching demographically similar patients, are also encouraged as part of the program and coordinated by our on-site social worker. A critical element is a dedicated patient navigator who conducts a telephone interview before the appointment is scheduled, gathers all necessary information including pathology slides if available, and pre-assigns the providers whom the patient will see based on their clinical needs. It cannot be stressed enough that the assignment of a dedicated MDC navigator is essential for this type of program to optimize patient care and the time constraints of the providers. All stages of disease are evaluated by appropriate specialists as needed. Although the majority of patients remain with us for their longitudinal care, second opinions are also provided. Treatment recommendations are shared with the patient and the referring physician. In cases where the treatment pathway is not clear, follow-up visits and testing might be scheduled. Finally, patients are

[**] Effective September 2014 a genetic counselor is available during each MDC session.

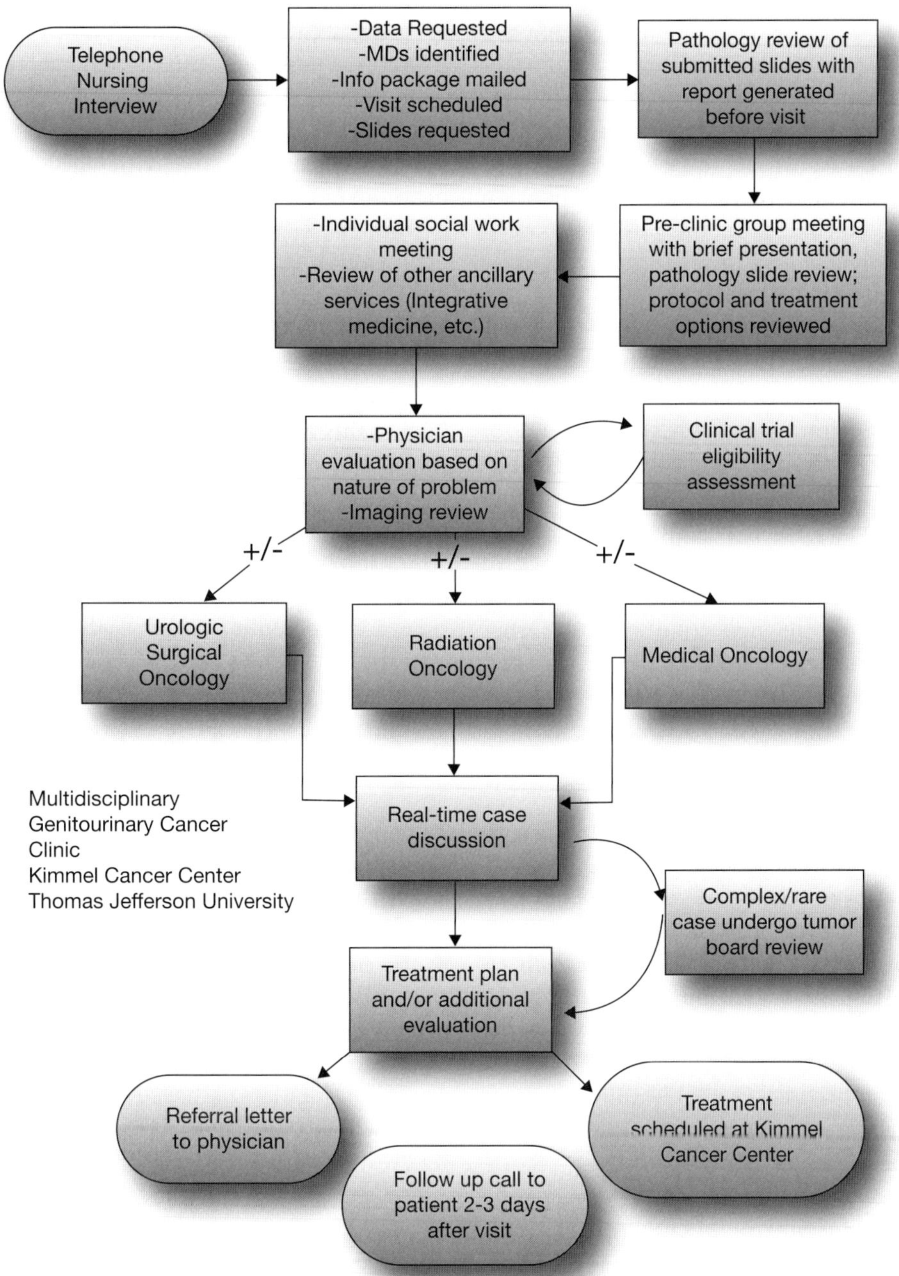

FIGURE 1.1 Organization of the Jefferson Kimmel Cancer Center GU Multidisciplinary Clinic. Courtesy of the Kimmel Cancer Center GU MDC, Thomas Jefferson University.

often given several treatment options to consider, most often related to localized prostate cancer. We believe that an objective review of the risks and benefits of these multiple options provides the patients with as unbiased an opinion as possible.

In 2010, we reported for the first time in prostate cancer that patient survival outcomes for high-risk men are improved by our GU MDC approach (18). When reviewing survival data in men with locally advanced disease, the enhanced outcome was most pronounced for T3 prostate cancer with a statistically significant improvement in 5-year survival of almost 90% compared to Surveillance, Epidemiology and End Results (SEER) with a 78% survival probability (18). As expected, in localized T2 disease, our 5-year survival data approached 100% based on SEER benchmarks. Consistent with other contemporary reports, we noted a dramatic increase in robotically assisted radical prostatectomy with a relative decrease in the utilization of brachytherapy.

International interest in the multidisciplinary approach to cancer care in general has increased. Numerous centers in the United States, Europe, and other nations have reported on their design and implementation of the MDC approach to cancer care including prostate cancer (23). The European School of Oncology has discussed the design, implementation, and certification of Prostate Cancer Units based on the positive experience of specialists involved with European Breast Cancer multidisciplinary care (24). These Prostate Cancer Units are more commonly referred to as Genitourinary Cancer or Prostate Cancer Multidisciplinary Clinics in the United States. This MDC model has been successfully implemented in Europe for breast care. A network of certified multidisciplinary breast cancer units was established based on a 2003 policy enacted by the European Parliament (25). The German Oncology Society (Deutsche Krebsgesellschaft) has created a network of Prostate Cancer Units that manages prostate cancer in a multidisciplinary manner in their country (24). Other organizations in the United States, United Kingdom, Asia, and Australia have had discussions to promote and establish multidisciplinary programs as a tenet of routine cancer care for most disease sites including prostate cancer (17).

Magnani et al. reviewed their 6-year experience with their multidisciplinary prostate cancer clinic in Italy (22). Their experience has proved successful for both physicians and patients. The team agrees on basic treatment strategies. More complex cases are managed by a multidisciplinary team. Their unit also incorporates a dedicated psychologist, which is uncommon in GU MDC in the United States.

As new information becomes available and guidelines are updated, these patient-centric programs must be flexible not only in their structure but also in their recommendations. In March 2010, a GU MDC was created at William Beaumont Hospital in Michigan to provide patients with a comprehensive multidisciplinary evaluation and consensus treatment recommendations in a single visit. The authors noted that their GU MDC improved the quality of care for patients as demonstrated by improved adherence to NCCN guidelines, and a broadening of treatment choices made available (26).

Researchers at the Duke Prostate Center in Durham, North Carolina, have reviewed their utilization trends for the first 5 years of their multidisciplinary prostate cancer clinic (27). The factors predictive of pursuing treatment at the Duke Prostate Center included high-risk disease and specific physician referral. The factors predictive of not receiving care at their unit included a distance traveled of greater than 100 miles. These data suggest that having a multidisciplinary prostate cancer at a remote location may not allow patients to take full advantage of the treatment expertise offered in this specialized setting.

One other unique contribution that MDC can make is in the area of active surveillance (AS). It appears that decision counseling and adherence to this approach is enhanced by this type of MDC structure. Available data suggest that low-risk patients who are seen at an MDC for prostate cancer appear to select AS in a greater proportion (28). The Prostate Cancer Programme of Milan's Istituto Nazionale dei Tumori data on AS shows significant growth in choosing this option in low-risk patients. Their AS roles increased from 40% to greater than 70% between 2006 and 2010 (22). Since AS is also a focus of a clinical trial at their Prostate Cancer Programme, demonstrating enhanced recruitment to trials is another advantage to this MDC model of care.

We have used our Kimmel Cancer Center GU MDC to develop a decision counseling program for AS (29). Men with previously identified low-risk prostate cancer who present to our GU MDC are met by a research assistant, who consents participants and administers a baseline survey. A nurse then meets each participant to conduct a decision counseling session. In the session, the nurse and participant review information on treatment options of AS versus AT. The nurse elicits the participant's pro and con decision factors that influence treatment preference, determines specific and relative decision factor weights, and enters these data into an online Decision Counseling Program available at www.jefferson.edu/university/jmc/departments/medical_oncology/divisions/population_science/center_for_health_decisions/decision_counseling.html. From baseline to endpoint, participants were better informed, felt less decisional conflict about treatment decision making, and moved from being undecided about AS versus AT to favoring AS.

U.S. population–based studies of prostate cancer localized disease suggest that oncology specialist visits relate strongly to prostate cancer treatment choices (30). These studies also suggest that that specialists tend to prefer and recommend the modality they themselves deliver. It is recognized that there is a paucity of comparative studies demonstrating superiority of one standard treatment modality, surgery, or radiation over another in regard to localized prostate cancer. The inherent physician bias may be minimized in such an MDC environment with improved patient satisfaction rates (28). The potential benefits of providing prostate cancer patient care in the GU MDC setting are summarized in Table 1.1.

A major challenge in establishing such a clinic is securing a genuine commitment from all parties to the success of the operation. This includes commitments of the institution, support staff, medical specialists, nurses, social workers, and other health care professionals who must share in the core principles of the center. The Kimmel Cancer Center GU MDC has had the commitment necessary for success with our ability to demonstrate many benefits: high levels of patient satisfaction, enhanced learning

Table 1.1 Potential benefits of the multidisciplinary clinic approach to prostate cancer

- Improve treatment outcomes through collaborative management
- Reduce time from diagnosis to treatment
- Reduce or eliminate treatment regret
- Improve adherence to NCCN or other treatment guidelines
- Minimize unfounded provider treatment bias
- Enhance patient satisfaction
- Increase clinical trial accruals
- Centralize research data management
- Provide educational opportunities and enhanced support for patients and their families
- Provide educational opportunities for students, residents, and fellows to interact with other disciplines
- Provide educational opportunities for nursing and other health care providers
- Disseminate information about support groups and other ancillary cancer care services
- Coordinated communication with outside providers may improve referrals

opportunities, and perhaps most important, a defined oncologic outcome benefit to many high-risk men. To quote Dr. Magnani, "the multidisciplinary approach needs to be adaptable to meet new needs and improve quality," which should be a take-home message for those currently operating or considering starting a multidisciplinary program (22). It should be noted that clinicians who work in this environment do lose some autonomy. Clinicians appear to recognize the value of the MDC in terms of effective communication with patients but may feel that other aspects of relationship building are hindered in a multidisciplinary setting. Organizational and teamwork issues need to be addressed to optimize the implementation of a multidisciplinary approach and can be easily overcome by a commitment of all parties (31).

CONCLUSIONS

Significant progress has been made in the diagnosis and management of prostate cancer over what might be considered a relatively short period of time. However, significant challenges remain. A top priority is to define the optimum prostate cancer screening paradigm. Chemoprevention strategies and their randomized trials have been uniformly disappointing, some from an outcome standpoint and others from an agent approval standpoint. How to best prevent prostate cancer will need to be seriously reconsidered based on the past investment of multiple long-term trials that raised more questions than answers (32). AS and AT decision making will become more sophisticated courtesy of improved biomarkers. AS as a "treatment" option needs to be increased in acceptance as an appropriate standard of care by both patients and providers including those in primary care. Primary care providers are very influential in prostate cancer–related decision making from screening to treatment options and should be informed of the dramatic changes in the field. Treatments for localized disease must better address the side-effect profiles now that many are demonstrating improved long-term cancer control. Novel strategies to convert high-risk prostate cancer from a life-threatening disease state to a manageable chronic disease state will require a more in-depth understanding of the biology of the disease. As with all scientific and technical advances, costs will continue to increase and will need to be balanced in terms of their relative effectiveness.

The extent of treatment options in prostate cancer can be overwhelming to the patient and his family. Decision making can be further complicated by the potential for poor outcomes and treatment regret due to not being adequately informed about the various options available. It is here that the MDC approach to prostate cancer can have a major impact. Cooperation of all stakeholders including patients, providers, researchers, industrial partners, insurers, and governmental agencies must work together in the spirit of multidisciplinary care to reduce the burden of prostate cancer for our current patients and future generations.

REFERENCES

1. Elder JS, Scott WW, Nyberg LM. Overview of past and current philosophy of prostatic cancer. *Prostate.* 1980;1(3):287–301. Review.
2. Gomella LG, Fried JJ. *Recovering From Prostate Cancer.* 1st ed. New York, NY: Harper Paperbacks a Division of Harper Collins; 1993.
3. Mettlin C, Jones G, Averette H, Gusberg SB, Murphy GP. Defining and updating the American Cancer Society guidelines for the cancer-related checkup: prostate and endometrial cancers. *CA Cancer J Clin.* 1993;43(1):42–46.
4. Hanks GE. Radiotherapy or surgery for prostate cancer? Ten and fifteen-year results of external beam therapy. *Acta Oncol.* 1991;30(2):231–237. Review.
5. Chou R, Croswell JM, Dana T, et al. Screening for prostate cancer: a review of the evidence for the U.S. Preventive Services Task Force. *Ann Intern Med.* 2011;155(11):762–771.
6. Philipson T, Eber M, Lakdawalla DN, Corral M, Conti R, Goldman DP. An analysis of whether higher health care spending in the United States versus Europe is 'worth it' in the case of cancer. *Health Affairs.* 2012;31(4):667–675.
7. Gomella LG, Petrylak D, Shayegan B. Current management of advanced and castration resistant prostate cancer. *Can J Urol.* 2014;21(supp 1):1–6.
8. SU2C Scientific Research Teams. http://www.standup2cancer.org/dream_teams/view/precision_therapy_for_advanced_pros tate_cancer. Accessed April 19, 2014.
9. Thompson IM, Valicenti RK, Albertsen P, et al. Adjuvant and salvage radiotherapy after prostatectomy: AUA/ASTRO Guideline. *J Urol.* 2013;190(2):441–449.

10. Thompson I, Thrasher JB, Aus G, et al.; AUA Prostate Cancer Clinical Guideline Update Panel. Guideline for the management of clinically localized prostate cancer: 2007 update. *J Urol.* 2007;177(6):2106–2131.
11. Mohler JL, Kantoff PW, Armstrong AJ, et al. Prostate cancer, version 1.2014. *J Natl Compr Canc Netw.* 2013;11(12):1471–1479.
12. Lam ET, Glodé LM. Neoadjuvant and adjuvant hormonal and chemotherapy for prostate cancer. *Hematol Oncol Clin North Am.* 2013;27(6):1189–1204.
13. Stacey D, Bennett CL, Barry MJ, et al. Decision aids for people facing health treatment or screening decisions. *Cochrane Database Syst Rev.* 2011;(10):CD001431.
14. Diefenbach MA, Mohamed NE. Regret of treatment decision and its association with disease-specific quality of life following prostate cancer treatment. *Cancer Invest.* 2007;25(6):449–457.
15. Warren E, Footman K, Tinelli M, McKee M, Knai C. Do cancer-specific websites meet patient's information needs? *Patient Educ Couns.* 2014;95(1):126–136.
16. Silk KJ, Perrault EK, Nazione S, Pace K, Hager P, Springer S. Localized prostate cancer treatment decision-making information online: improving its effectiveness and dissemination for non-profit and government-supported organizations. *J Cancer Educ.* 2013;28(4):709–716.
17. Hong NJ, Wright FC, Gagliardi AR, Paszat LF. Examining the potential relationship between multidisciplinary cancer care and patient survival: an international literature review. *J Surg Oncol.* 2010;102:125–134.
18. Gomella LG, Lin J, Hoffman-Censits J, et al. Enhancing prostate cancer care through the multidisciplinary clinic approach: a 15-year experience. *J Oncol Pract.* 2010;6(6):e5–e10.
19. Hudak JL, McLeod DG, Brassell SA, et al. The design and implementation of a multidisciplinary prostate cancer clinic. *Urol Nurs.* 2007;27(6):491–498.
20. Paget L, Han P, Nedza S, et al. *Patient-Clinician Communication: Basic Principles and Expectations* [discussion paper]. Institute of Medicine. http://www.iom.edu/Activities/Quality/~/media/Files/Activity%20Files/Quality/VSRT/Discussion%20Papers/PCCwLogos.pdf. Updated June 2011.
21. Valicenti RK, Gomella LG, El-Gabry EA, et al. The multidisciplinary clinic approach to prostate cancer counseling and treatment. *Semin Urol Oncol.* 2000;18(3):188–191.
22. Magnani T, Valdagni R, Salvioni R, et al. The 6-year attendance of a multidisciplinary prostate cancer clinic in Italy: incidence of management changes. *BJU Int.* 2012;110(7):998–1003.
23. Gomella LG. The prostate cancer unit: a multidisciplinary approach for which the time has arrived. *Eur Urol.* 2011;60(6):1197–1199.
24. Valdagni R, Albers P, Bangma C, et al. The requirements of a specialist prostate cancer unit: a discussion paper from the European School of Oncology. *Eur J Cancer.* 2011;47(1):1–7.
25. EUSOMA. The requirements of a specialist breast unit. *Eur J Cancer.* 2000;36:2288.
26. Korman H, Lanni T Jr, Shah C, et al. Impact of a prostate multidisciplinary clinic program on patient treatment decisions and on adherence to NCCN guidelines: the William Beaumont Hospital experience. *Am J Clin Oncol.* 2013;36(2):121–125.
27. Stewart SB, Bañez LL, Robertson CN, et al. Utilization trends at a multidisciplinary prostate cancer clinic: initial 5-year experience from the Duke Prostate Center. *J Urol.* 2012;187(1):103–108.
28. Aizer AA, Paly JJ, Efstathiou JA. Multidisciplinary care and management selection in prostate cancer. *Semin Radiat Oncol.* 2013;23(3):157–164.
29. Petrich A, Quinn AM, Leader A, et al. Decision counseling about active surveillance and active treatment for early stage low risk prostate cancer patients. 35th Annual Meeting of the Society for Medical Decision Making; October 23, 2013; Baltimore, MD.
30. Jang TL, Bekelman JE, Liu Y, et al. Physician visits prior to treatment for clinically localized prostate cancer. *Arch Intern Med.* 2010;170(5):440–450.
31. Bellardita L, Donegani S, Spatuzzi AL, Valdagni R. Multidisciplinary versus one-on-one setting: a qualitative study of clinicians' perceptions of their relationship with patients with prostate cancer. *J Oncol Pract.* 2011;7(1):e1–e5.
32. Thompson IM Jr, Cabang AB, Wargovich MJ. Future directions in the prevention of prostate cancer. *Nat Rev Clin Oncol.* 2014;11(1):49–60.

2.1 Epidemiology of Prostate Cancer

KATHRYN M. WILSON

LORELEI A. MUCCI

INTRODUCTION

The prevention of prostate cancer is a key public health challenge that would improve health and reduce suffering from this disease. Prostate cancer contributes substantially to cancer incidence and mortality among men globally, particularly in westernized countries (1). The disease is notable in its biologic heterogeneity in metastatic potential over a man's lifetime. This heterogeneity is an important feature of the disease, and efforts to understand risk factors of lethal prostate cancer are paramount in epidemiological research and prevention efforts. In this chapter, we discuss the evidence surrounding specific lifestyle and dietary factors in the prevention of prostate cancer, with a focus on prevention of lethal disease. We provide global descriptive data around prostate cancer incidence and mortality, and summarize evidence for the following selected behavioral risk factors: genetics, obesity and weight change, physical activity, smoking, antioxidant intake, vitamin D and calcium, and statins.

GLOBAL BURDEN OF PROSTATE CANCER

Descriptive epidemiology sets the framework for understanding the global burden of prostate cancer from a public health perspective. A comparison of incidence and mortality across populations as well as trends over time and by other characteristics can provide clues about the role of lifestyle factors or screening patterns.

Incidence

Prostate cancer is the second most commonly diagnosed cancer among men globally, with more than 1.1 million new cases each year (2). In the United States, 233,000 men are expected to be diagnosed in 2014, and an American man's lifetime risk of prostate cancer is 1 in 6 (3).

Prostate cancer incidence shows remarkable worldwide variation (Figure 2.1.1), with a 60-fold difference in age-adjusted incidence rates between population groups with the highest (African American men in the United States) and lowest (Japanese and Chinese men living in their native countries) incidence. Part of the variation in incidence rates across populations can be explained by differences in diagnostic intensity, primarily due to prostate-specific antigen (PSA) screening. However, geographic differences in prostate cancer incidence were evident before the introduction of PSA screening in the early 1990s, highlighting a potential role of environmental factors in disease etiology. Results from migrant studies lend additional support to a role of lifestyle factors in prostate cancer incidence. Prostate cancer incidence and mortality rates increase among men moving from low-risk (e.g., Asia) to high-risk (e.g., United States) countries compared with those in their native countries (4, 5).

There have been significant increases in prostate cancer incidence rates over time across the globe (**Figure 2.1.2**). In the United States, Europe, and Australia, this is likely due in part to uptake of PSA testing which is noted by a sharp peak in incidence due to the detection of prevalent subclinical disease. However, incidence rates have also increased in Japan and some other Asian and Eastern European countries where PSA testing has to date not been widely used (6). PSA screening has also led to a shift in stage presentation, with increases in the ratio of localized to advanced disease cases and a decrease in the age at diagnosis (7). Screening has also led to the detection of a significant number of latent lesions that may never have come to light clinically nor harmed a man during his lifetime (8, 9).

The introduction of PSA screening has likely resulted in changes in the observed associations between specific lifestyle factors and risk of total prostate cancer over time. First, different factors may impact prostate cancer at various stages from initiation to progression to metastases, and therefore the associations may differ according to disease clinical characteristics, such as those defined by cancer stage or tumor grade (10). Indeed, it seems unlikely that the factors associated with development of indolent

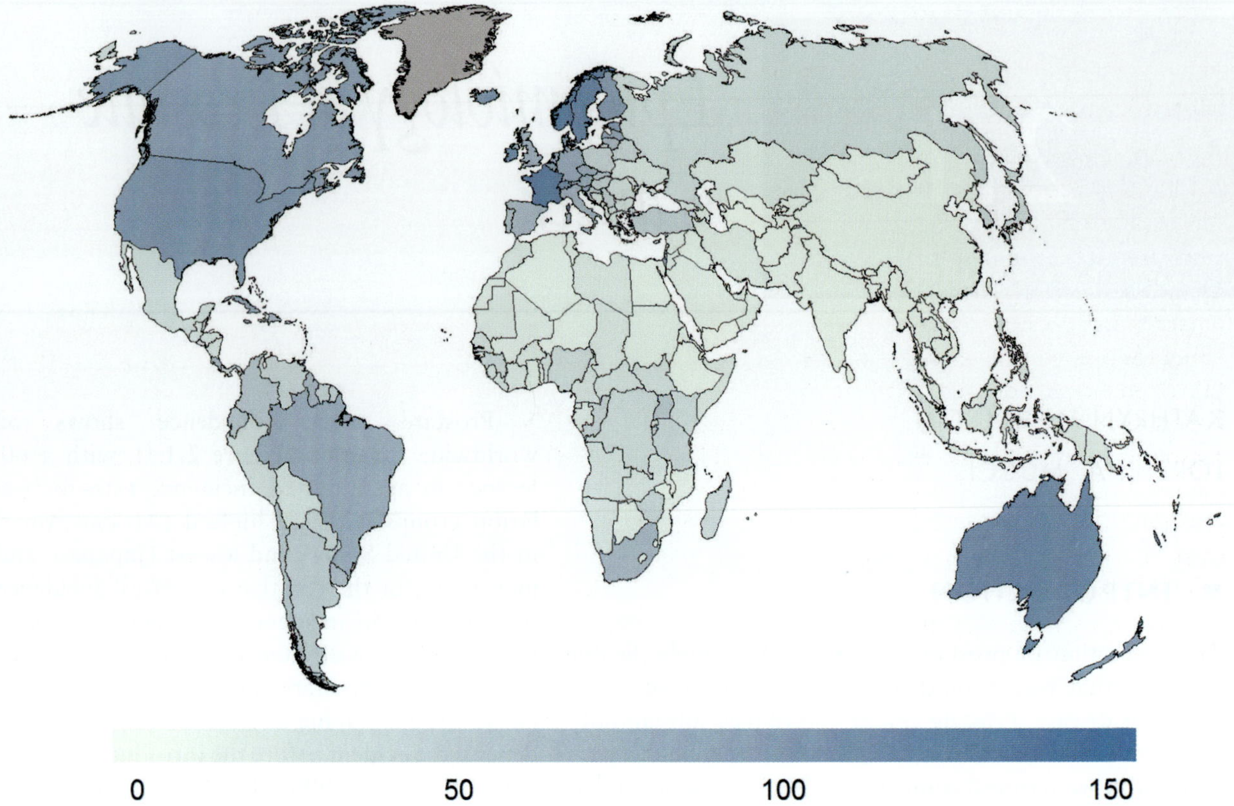

FIGURE 2.1.1 Comparison of prostate cancer incidence rates globally. Rates are age-adjusted for comparisons across countries and are presented per 100,000 in the population. Globocan 2012.
Source: From Ref. (2). IARC. *Globocan 2008 Cancer Fact Sheet: Prostate Cancer Incidence and Mortality Worldwide in 2008 Summary.* Lyon, France: IARC Press; 2008.

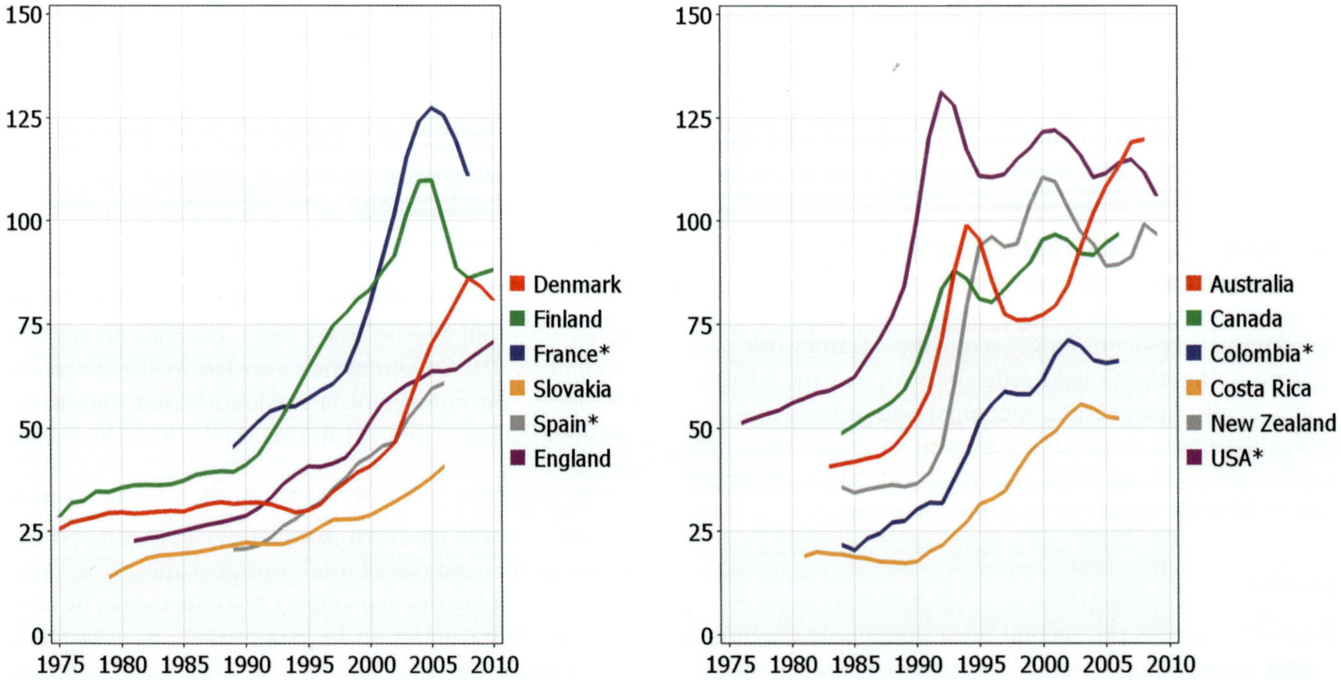

FIGURE 2.1.2 Trends in age-adjusted prostate cancer incidence rates over time in selected populations. Rates are presented per 100,000 in the population. Globocan 2012. http://globocan.iarc.fr/factsheets/cancers/prostate.asp. Updated 2008. Accessed August 2014.
Source: From Ref. (2). IARC. *Globocan 2008 Cancer Fact Sheet: Prostate Cancer Incidence and Mortality Worldwide in 2008 Summary.* Lyon, France: IARC Press; 2008.

cancers would be similar to those associated with cancers demonstrating malignant potential.

Mortality

An estimated 307,000 men died of prostate cancer worldwide (2), with a 10-fold variation in mortality rates among countries (Figure 2.1.3). Notably, mortality rates are highest among men in the Caribbean countries as well as parts of Africa. Prostate cancer is the second most common cause of cancer death among men in the United States, with 29,480 cancer deaths expected in 2014 (3). Over the past decade, prostate cancer mortality rates have shown declines in many westernized countries. The reasons for this decline remain controversial, but may be attributable in part to earlier detection through PSA screening and subsequent earlier treatment (11). In contrast, mortality rates from prostate cancer are rising, for example, in Africa.

Mortality rates are estimated as the number of cancer deaths per 100,000 in the population, and these rates are influenced as a function of both the incidence of the disease and survival among prostate cancer patients. The ratio of incidence to mortality rates ranges from 10:1 in North America and Australia to 2:1 in Central America and Caribbean to 1.2:1 in parts of Africa. Part of these differences can attributed on the one hand to the slow growing cancers diagnosed as a result of PSA screening (12, 13) and on the other due to later presentation of disease in countries with little diagnostic intensity.

Globally, 4 million men are prostate cancer survivors living with a cancer diagnosis, of whom 2.4 million are in the United States (3).

■ ESTABLISHED RISK FACTORS FOR TOTAL PROSTATE CANCER INCIDENCE

There are few established risk factors for the incidence of total prostate cancer: older age, African American race, and positive family history. Moreover, there are now more than 77 genetic risk loci that have been identified and confirmed in genome wide association studies (14) in ethnically diverse populations. It is noteworthy that none of these factors are modifiable.

Older age is one of the strongest risk factors for prostate cancer. Prostate cancer rarely is diagnosed among men before the age of 40 years. As with other epithelial cancers, incidence rates of prostate cancer increase exponentially from around age 55 years, a pattern observed across multiple populations. Screening with PSA, with an

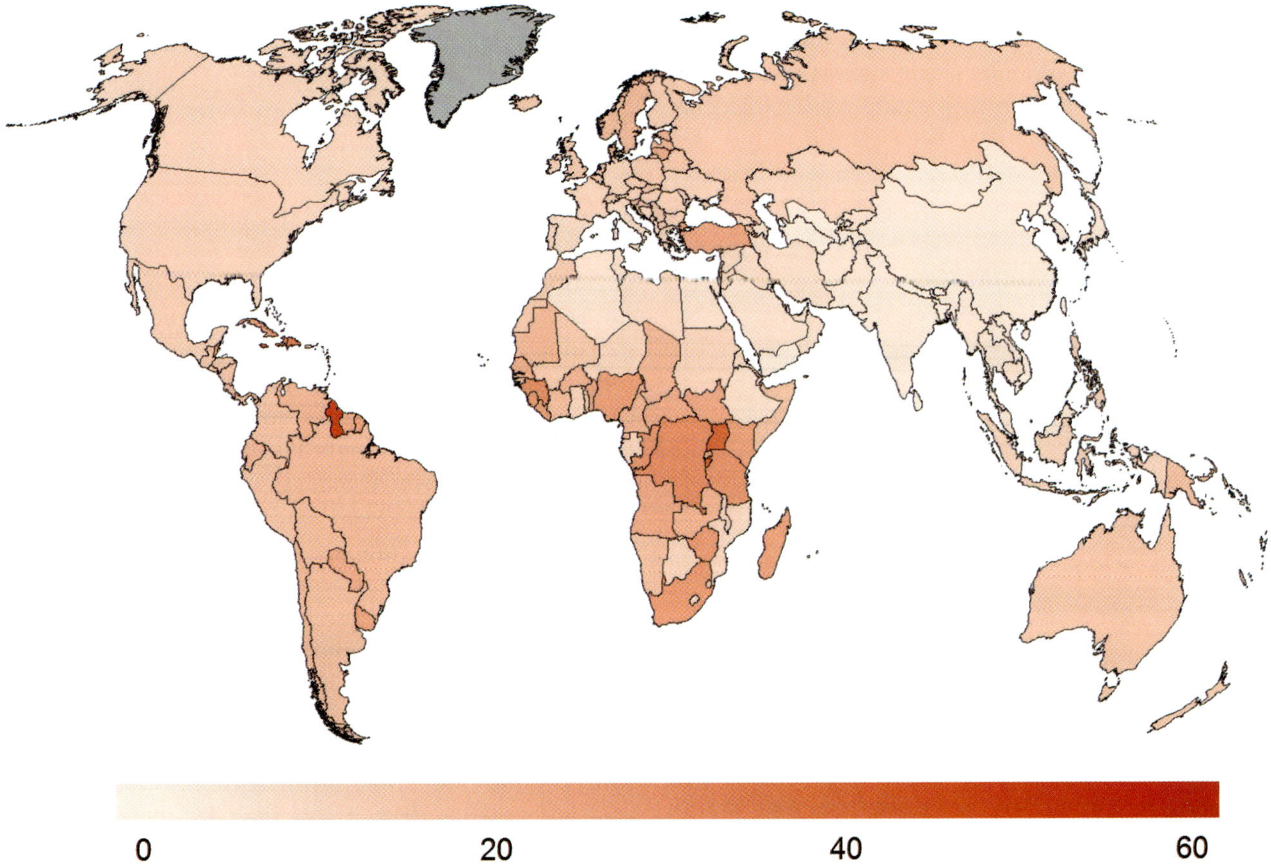

FIGURE 2.1.3 Comparison of prostate cancer mortality rates globally. Rates are age-adjusted for comparisons across countries and are presented per 100,000 in the population. Globocan 2012.
Source: From Ref. (2). IARC. *Globocan 2008 Cancer Fact Sheet: Prostate Cancer Incidence and Mortality Worldwide in 2008 Summary.* Lyon, France: IARC Press; 2008.

estimated 10-year lead time, has led to a shift to an earlier average age of cancer diagnosis.

Prostate cancer incidence and mortality rates differ by race/ethnicity. In the United States, incidence and mortality rates are highest among black men (Figure 2.1.4), with mortality 2.4 times greater than that of white men. There are considerable efforts ongoing to identify the causes of the disparity in prostate cancer rates among black men, although of note, the prevalence of PSA screening is similar among white and black men in the United States. Both incidence and mortality rates are lower among Asian/Pacific-Islanders, Native Americans, and Hispanic men than among non-Hispanic whites (3).

Results from family and twin studies support a strong familial component to prostate cancer. Men whose father or brother was diagnosed with prostate cancer have a two- to threefold higher risk than men without a family history. A family history in both the father and a brother increases risk of diagnosis almost ninefold (15). Family history is also associated with lethal prostate cancer. The risk of death from prostate cancer is approximately twofold higher for men with a father or a brother who died of prostate cancer compared with men with prostate cancer who do not have a positive family history (16).

Data from twin studies suggest that the familial aggregation of prostate cancer incidence is in large part due to genetic factors (17), with an estimated heritability of 56% (18). Multiple genome-wide association studies have been conducted to identify common single nucleotide polymorphisms (SNPs) associated with prostate cancer incidence (19). To date, 77 risk loci have been identified and confirmed across multiple studies (14), and these loci explain about one-third of the heritability. The heritability of prostate cancer appears to be the result of small associations of low penetrant genetic variants, rather than large associations with high penetrance alleles. The majority of the identified germline risk loci do not appear to be more strongly associated with lethal or nonlethal prostate cancer (20, 21), suggesting that inherited factors may play a role quite early in the pathogenesis of the disease. There are marked differences in the prevalence of several of the genetic risk loci among black and white (22) men, which could account for at least part of the difference in incidence rates.

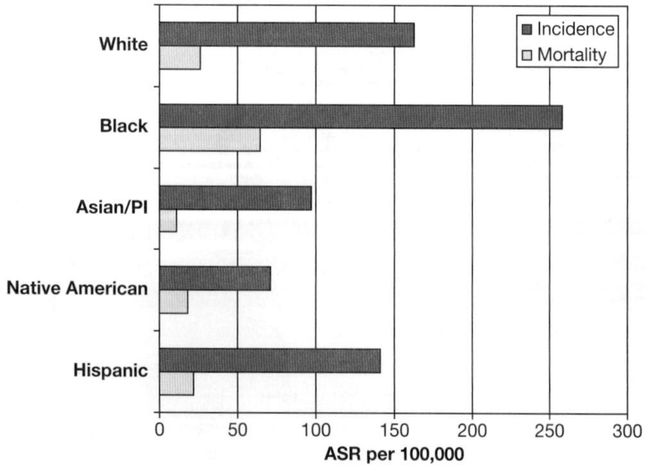

FIGURE 2.1.4 Incidence and mortality of prostate cancer by race/ethnicity in the United States. Rates are age-standardized for comparisons and presented per 100,000 in the population. Howlader N, Noone A, Krapcho M, et al. *SEER Cancer Statistics Review 1975-2008*. Bethesda, MD: National Cancer Institute; 2011. http://seer.cancer.gov/csr/1975–2008/, based on http://seer.cancer.gov/registries/ November 2010 SEER data submission, posted to the SEER web site.

■ OVERVIEW OF POTENTIAL RISK FACTORS FOR LETHAL PROSTATE CANCER

Prostate cancer progression to lethal disease likely involves the activation of a number of different biological pathways. Risk factors for lethal prostate cancer and opportunities for prevention act through these pathways. In this paper, we focus on obesity and weight change, physical activity, smoking, antioxidants, vitamin D and calcium, and statins.

Obesity and Weight Change

The obesity epidemic looms large globally, with 1.5 billion adults estimated in 2008 to be overweight or obese (23). The increase in overweight and obesity in the United States in recent decades has been well documented. In the United States, one-third of adults were obese, which is defined as having a body mass index (BMI) ≥ 30.0 kg/m^2 (24). The proportion of adults classified as overweight, with a BMI of 25.0 to 29.9 kg/m^2, has been fairly constant over this time, at approximately one-third of the adult population (25).

Obesity dysregulates multiple hormonal pathways, including higher levels of insulin, lower levels of adiponectin, lower levels of testosterone and sex hormone binding globulin, higher estradiol, and higher levels of inflammatory cytokines, all of which may be factors in prostate cancer progression (26–29). From a prevention perspective, it is notable that weight loss and physical activity are associated with positive changes in these biomarkers.

The relation between body size and incidence of prostate cancer is complex (10, 26, 30–33). However, obesity in adulthood has been associated with worse outcomes among prostate cancer patients in most studies (33, 34). Obese men are at higher risk of developing advanced stage prostate cancer and have higher rates of recurrence and cancer-specific mortality after diagnosis. A meta-analysis of six cohort studies among men with prostate cancer found that a 5 kg/m^2 increase in BMI was associated with a 20% (95% CI: 0.99–1.46) increased risk of prostate cancer–specific mortality (33). The association between obesity and poor prostate cancer outcomes does not appear to reflect solely differences in screening, as similar associations are seen after adjusting for stage and grade at diagnosis.

In a study of men diagnosed with prostate cancer, higher prediagnosis levels of C-peptide, a circulating marker of insulin secretion, were associated with increased cancer-specific mortality, independent of BMI (164). Men who were both overweight and who had high insulin levels had a fourfold greater risk of death. It is possible that men who are obese and have higher C-peptide levels have a more metabolically active obesity than obese men with lower C-peptide measures, making the combined measure of BMI and C-peptide levels more predictive of prognosis. However, two prospective studies found no association between prediagnosis C-peptide and risk of aggressive or advanced disease (35). Understanding drivers of the association with obesity are critical to understand mechanisms and guide prevention.

Abdominal obesity, as measured by waist circumference, may indicate a more metabolically active obesity, and in many parts of the world central obesity has been rapidly increasing. In the European Prospective Investigation into Cancer and Nutrition (EPIC) of 150,000 European men, waist circumference was positively associated with risk of advanced prostate cancer with a 1.06 times greater risk with a 5 cm increase in circumference (36). Waist circumference was also significantly associated with more aggressive disease in the Melbourne Collaborative Cohort Study (37), but not in the Health Professionals Follow-Up Study (38). The EPIC study found that the waist circumference associations were stronger among men with lower BMI, suggesting a possible interaction between overall and abdominal obesity; however, the number of men in opposite extreme categories of BMI and waist was low.

Weight Change

Weight change before or after prostate cancer diagnosis is a possible modifiable risk factor. Several cohort studies have examined adult weight change and the risk of prostate cancer. Overall, weight gain from early adulthood (age 18 or 21) to mid-life was not associated with prostate cancer incidence in all (39–47) but one study (48). However, the AARP-NIH Diet and Health Study (49) found that weight gain from age 18 to baseline at ages 50 to 71 years was significantly associated with an increased risk of prostate cancer mortality. Only one study has examined weight change in the period shortly before and after prostate cancer diagnosis and the risk of recurrence, measured by posttreatment PSA increase (50). This retrospective cohort study found that weight gain from 5 years before treatment by prostatectomy to 1 year after treatment was associated with statistically significant increase in recurrence, while weight loss was nonstatistically significantly associated with lower risk of recurrence. This study found no indication that physical activity modified the association between weight change and recurrence.

Physical Activity

Physical activity has not been associated with overall prostate cancer risk. However, several studies report an inverse association between recreational physical activity and the risk of advanced prostate cancer. The Health Professionals Follow-Up Cohort (51) and the Cancer Prevention Study (CPS) II (52) both reported lower risks of more advanced disease with increasing physical activity, independent of BMI. For example, in the CPS II, men reporting > 35 met-hours activity per week had a relative risk for aggressive cancer (high stage and/or grade) of 0.69 (95% CI: 0.52–0.92). The EPIC cohort found no association between recreational physical activity and advanced or high-stage disease; however, activity levels were substantially higher in this cohort, and the reference group included men with up to 25 met-hours per week (53). On the other hand, the National Institutes of Health-American Association of Retired Persons (NIH-AARP) Diet and Health Study found no association between vigorous exercise and risk of advanced or fatal prostate cancer (54).

The association between physical activity after diagnosis and risk of prostate cancer mortality or recurrence among men with prostate cancer has been examined. Among 2,705 men with prostate cancer, those who exercised vigorously for 3 or more hours per week had a 61% lower risk of prostate cancer–specific mortality than those with less than 1 hour per week of vigorous activity (RR 0.4, 95% CI: 0.2–0.8) (55). Both vigorous and nonvigorous activities were associated with lower risk of all-cause mortality among these men with prostate cancer. Similarly, brisk walking was associated with a lower risk of recurrence (RR 0.4, 95% CI: 0.2–0.9) for those walking 3 or more hours per week versus easy walking for less than 3 hours per week (56). Physical activity also has been shown in observational studies to improve some aspects of quality of life. Taken together, physical activity may represent a potential intervention for men after prostate cancer diagnosis that may improve overall health of prostate cancer patients.

Smoking

As with other factors, smoking is not associated with prostate cancer incidence. However, the latest review of evidence by the United States Surgeon General concluded that smoking is a "probable" contributor to higher rates of prostate cancer mortality (57). In the Health Professionals Follow-Up Study, greater pack-years of smoking in the 10 years prior to prostate cancer diagnosis were associated with an increased risk of lethal disease, whereas total lifetime smoking was not associated with risk (58). However, current smokers report less PSA testing than nonsmokers (59), and the positive associations between smoking and prostate cancer mortality may be due in part to later diagnosis and treatment of these cancers among smokers.

Smoking may also influence cancer-specific outcomes by influencing response to treatment. Studies in specific treatment populations have consistently reported worse outcomes for smokers than nonsmokers among prostate cancer patients treated with radiation, androgen deprivation therapy, and radical prostatectomy (60–64).

To date, one prospective study of smoking and cancer-specific mortality among men with prostate cancer has been published (65). Among 5,366 men diagnosed with prostate cancer between 1986 and 2006 in the Health Professionals Follow-Up Study, there were 524 prostate cancer deaths. The relative risk of prostate cancer–specific mortality was 60% higher (95% CI: 1.1–2.3) among current versus never smokers after adjusting for potential confounders. The relative risk was attenuated, although still elevated, when models were further adjusted for stage and grade, which may suggest that part of the relationship between smoking and prostate cancer mortality is through its influence on these clinical parameters. The apparent increased risk of prostate cancer–specific mortality was restricted to men diagnosed with localized or locally advanced cancer (stages T1–T3). Former smokers who quit 10 or more years before diagnosis or who had smoked less than 20 pack-years had the same risk as never smokers.

The possible biological basis for an association between smoking and risk of fatal prostate cancer or survival among men with prostate cancer is not clear, but several mechanisms have been proposed (65). Tumor promotion through carcinogens from tobacco smoke is a possibility, with several studies finding prostate cancer–specific mechanisms in animal and in vitro studies. In addition, nicotine may have epigenetic effects such as on gene methylation patterns and effects on angiogenesis and tumor cell proliferation that contribute to initiation or progression of disease.

Antioxidants

Several dietary antioxidants, including selenium, vitamin E, and lycopene/tomato sauce have been investigated with respect to prostate cancer incidence. Antioxidants are compounds that inhibit the oxidation of other species, thereby limiting the damaging effects of oxidation in animal tissues. Oxidative stress may damage molecules including proteins and DNA, and has been implicated in carcinogenesis.

Vitamin E and Selenium

Vitamin E generally refers to a group of fat-soluble compounds that include tocopherols and tocotrienols. Alpha-tocopherol is the biologically most active form, and current dietary recommendations in the United States are based on alpha-tocopherol alone. Gamma-tocopherol is the most common tocopherol in the U.S. diet. Possible anticarcinogenic actions of vitamin E include its ability to reduce DNA damage and inhibit malignant cellular transformation (66, 67). In experimental models, derivatives of vitamin E inhibit growth, induce apoptosis (68), and enhance therapeutic effects in human prostate cancer cells (69).

Secondary results of the Alpha-Tocopherol Beta-Carotene Cancer Prevention (ATBC) Study (70) showed a 32% reduction in prostate cancer risk among men assigned to alpha-tocopherol supplementation compared with placebo (71). Another large trial of a variety of nutrients found that vitamin E (in combination with selenium and beta-carotene) reduced overall cancer mortality (72). These results, along with laboratory evidence and some epidemiologic support, motivated two trials of vitamin E supplementation on the risk of prostate cancer.

The Selenium and Vitamin E Cancer Prevention Trial (SELECT), planned for 7 to 12 years, was stopped early because of lack of efficacy for risk reduction. The initial report based on an average of 5.5 years of treatment, found a nonsignificant suggestion of *increased* prostate cancer risk among men receiving 400 IU/d of alpha-tocopherol (73). With additional follow-up, the vitamin E group was found to have a significant increase in prostate cancer risk (RR 1.17; 99% CI: 1.004–1.36, $P = .008$, among 1,149 cases) (74). Interestingly, there was not a statistically significant increased risk of prostate cancer in the vitamin E and selenium combination group (HR 1.05; $P = .46$), suggesting the two may interact. The Physicians Health Study II (PHS II), conducted contemporaneously with SELECT, found no effect on the incidence of prostate cancer (HR, 0.97; 95% CI: 0.85–1.09; $P = .58$), with a dose of 400 IU/d for a median of 8 years of follow-up (75).

Of note, all men in the ATBC trial were smokers, and the prostate cancers were diagnosed outside the context of PSA screening, and thus, were generally aggressive. Interestingly, epidemiological studies of vitamin E and prostate cancer risk have had mixed results, generally pointing toward no overall association, but observed associations have generally been for advanced cancers and among smokers. In the VITamins And Lifestyle (VITAL) study, a cohort study specifically designed to examine supplement use and future cancer risk, a 10-year average intake of supplemental vitamin E was not associated with a reduced prostate cancer risk overall but it was associated with a reduced risk for advanced prostate cancer (regionally invasive or distant metastatic, n = 123) (HR 0.43, 95% CI: 0.19–1.0 for 10-year average intake > or =400 IU/d vs. nonuse) (76). In a prospective study of plasma vitamin E and prostate cancer mortality, there was a reduced risk associated with higher circulating levels limited to smokers, although the number of cases in the subgroup was small (<30) (77). Other epidemiological studies have similarly found a protective association limited to ever smokers, including prospective studies of dietary vitamin E (78), vitamin E through supplementation on lethal prostate cancer (79), and plasma alpha-tocopherol levels and aggressive prostate cancer (80).

The SELECT and PHS II trials were done in the PSA screening era, and had small numbers of current smokers. Thus, neither trial could address the effect of alpha-tocopherol specifically on advanced or fatal prostate cancers, or among current smokers. However, the results overall do not support the use of supplemental vitamin E for prostate cancer prevention.

The trace element selenium is not an antioxidant per se, but plays an important role as an essential element for the antioxidant enzyme glutathione peroxidase (81) as well as other selenoproteins involved in exerting antitumor effects, including apoptosis and inhibition of cellular proliferation (82, 83). Dietary intake of selenium depends on the selenium content of soil in which foods are grown, which varies greatly by geographic area. Ecologic studies have suggested an inverse association between selenium soil content and prostate cancer incidence (84). Because selenium contents in specific foods vary as a function of the selenium content of the soil, epidemiological studies of selenium require biological sampling, primarily measuring levels in blood or toenails. Since the activity of some selenoenzymes plateau with higher selenium level (85), the chemopreventive effect of selenium may be greatest in populations with low selenium exposure (86).

Like vitamin E, selenium was tested in the SELECT trial based on secondary results of other randomized trials. The Nutritional Prevention of Cancer Trial found a 63% reduction in prostate cancer risk among men taking selenium supplements (87); with additional follow-up time, the protective effect was limited to those with low baseline levels of PSA or selenium (86). Another trial of selenium (with vitamin E and beta-carotene) found a reduction in total cancer mortality in China (72). As discussed above, the SELECT trial was stopped early due to lack of efficacy of the supplements. With additional follow-up, there was still no association between selenium and prostate cancer risk (RR 1.09; 99% CI: 0.93–1.27; P = .18). In addition, baseline selenium status (measured in toenails) was not associated with prostate cancer risk among men in the trial, and baseline status did not modify the association between selenium supplementation and risk (88).

Six prospective biomarker studies have reported significant associations between higher levels of selenium and reduced prostate cancer risk (89–95), particularly for advanced disease (89, 90, 93). Not all epidemiological studies have reported a protective association of selenium, however (96–98). Two recent randomized studies found no effect of selenium supplementation, alone or in combination, in reducing progression of high-grade PIN to invasive cancer (99, 100).

In conclusion, there is some evidence that selenium may play a role in prostate cancer biology; however, there is no evidence to support the use of selenium supplements to prevent prostate cancer.

Lycopene and Tomato-Based Products

The carotenoid lycopene is found in high quantities in tomato and tomato-based products, as well as pink grapefruit and watermelon (3). Lycopene accumulates in high levels in prostate tissue, and given its role as a potent antioxidant, is plausible as a potential protective factor for prostate cancer. This hypothesis has been tested in multiple studies that have investigated lycopene, or lycopene-rich food, such as tomato and tomato-based products, in relation to prostate cancer risk (4–21). In a meta-analysis of studies published up to 2003 (30), high intakes of tomato or tomato-based products was associated with a 10% to 20% reduction in prostate cancer risk. For the serum- or plasma-based studies, high concentrations of lycopene conferred a 25% reduction in prostate cancer risk. Recent epidemiological studies of lycopene and prostate cancer showed mixed results. Some support an inverse association (20, 21, 31, 32), while others present null findings (8, 9, 19, 24, 26, 33). The association between tomatoes and prostate cancer has been studied extensively in the epidemiological literature, with evidence suggesting a significant benefit associated with higher intake of tomatoes, particularly cooked tomatoes, or lycopene, the major antioxidant in tomatoes.

In a meta-analysis of studies on tomatoes and prostate cancer risk among 10 prospective cohort or nested case-control studies, the relative risk of prostate cancer among consumers of higher amounts of raw tomato (5th quantile of intake) was 0.89 (95% CI: 0.80–1.00) (101). For cooked tomato products, which are more bioavailable sources of lycopene than fresh tomatoes (102), the summary RR was 0.81 (95% CI: 0.71–0.92) comparing extreme categories of intake. The results from cohort studies generally indicate a 25% to 30% reduction in risk of prostate cancer, whereas dietary-based case-control studies are not supportive of an association. For example, the summary RR of prostate cancer from the meta-analysis related to an intake of one serving/day of raw tomato (200 g) was 0.97 (95% CI: 0.85–1.10) for the case-control studies and 0.78 (95% CI: 0.66–0.92) for cohort studies (101).

The 2004 meta-analysis found an inverse association in studies of plasma lycopene and prostate cancer risk, with corresponding summary relative risks of 0.55 (95% CI: 0.32–0.94) for case-control studies and 0.78 (95% CI: 0.61–1.00) for cohort studies (101). An additional nested case-control study not included in the meta-analysis found a modest, not statistically significant, inverse association overall, and a significantly reduced risk with higher levels among men over 65 years old and among those without a family history of prostate cancer (103). However, several more recent studies have found no associations for serum lycopene (104–108). It is possible that these conflicting results are due, in part, to the changing mix of prostate cancer cases diagnosed in the United States with the advent of PSA screening (109). As a result of PSA screening, many more prostate cancers are being diagnosed, including a pool of biologically indolent cancers which would have gone undiagnosed in previous decades and in older studies.

Indeed, epidemiological studies generally point to a stronger reduction in risk of advanced stage or lethal prostate cancer, suggesting that tomato products and lycopene may play a role in prostate cancer progression. For example, in the Health Professionals Follow-Up Study, the associations comparing high and low quintiles of lycopene intake were 0.91 (0.84–1.00) for total prostate cancer and 0.72 (0.56–0.94) for fatal or metastatic disease (110). This study also found that higher lycopene intake was associated with biomarkers indicating lower angiogenic potential in tumor specimens. In the European Prospective Investigation into Cancer and Nutrition study based on 966 total cases and 205 advanced stage cases of prostate cancer, there was no association between plasma lycopene and overall risk, but men in the top quintile of plasma lycopene had a significantly reduced risk of advanced stage prostate cancer (RR = 0.40, 95% CI: 0.19–0.88) (108).

Although not definitive, the available data suggest that increased consumption of tomato and tomato-based products is associated with lower prostate cancer risk and progression. Whether the effect is driven through lycopene or other aspects of tomatoes remains undetermined. The relationship appears to be stronger for advanced prostate cancer than indolent disease.

Calcium, Dairy Products, and Vitamin D

Calcium intake has been associated with an increased risk of prostate cancer in many but not all epidemiological studies. A meta-analysis of studies in 2005 found an increased risk of 1.39 (95% CI: 1.09–1.77), for extreme categories of intake (111). Since the meta-analysis, four prospective cohort studies found some suggestion of an increased risk of prostate cancer with higher calcium intakes (3, 8, 9, 112), while five studies found no associations (2, 3, 12, 13, 15, 16). Total calcium intakes varied widely across study populations; the highest category of intake was less than 1,000 mg/d in three studies, whereas the highest category was greater than 2,000 mg/d in three other studies (2, 3, 9, 12, 15). Some, but not all, studies have reported stronger associations between high intake of calcium and risks of aggressive forms of prostate cancer, defined by high-grade, or advanced or lethal prostate cancer (10, 113, 114).

The association between serum calcium and risk of prostate cancer has been studied in several prospective studies. Serum levels of calcium were associated with an increased risk of fatal disease in NHANES I and NHANES III (National Health and Nutrition Examination Survey) (115, 116). The adjusted relative risk of fatal prostate cancer was 2.68 (95% CI: 1.02–6.99; $P = .04$) for the top versus bottom tertile of total serum calcium in NHANES. In NHANES III, similar increases in risk were seen for both total serum calcium and ionized serum calcium, the biologically active component. Two studies nested in prospective cohorts of Swedish men found no association between serum calcium and overall risk of prostate cancer (117, 118); in fact, there was a weak inverse association with overall risk in one study (118). This study also found no indication of an association between serum calcium and risk of fatal prostate cancer. Circulating calcium levels are tightly regulated and are related to diet only at very high levels of intake, so it is unclear how this finding related to dietary calcium intake, if at all. However, it suggests a role for calcium, vitamin D, and perhaps related factors, such as parathyroid hormone, in the etiology of lethal prostate cancer.

Dairy foods, a major dietary source of calcium, have also been associated with risk, with the 2005 meta-analysis reporting a summary relative risk of 1.11 (95% CI: 1.03–1.19) for total dairy, 1.06 (0.91–1.23) for milk, and 1.11 (0.99–1.25) per serving for cheese (111). Most (119–121), but not all (122) studies published since this meta-analysis have tended to support an association between higher milk or dairy consumption and total prostate cancer risk. However, findings specifically for advanced or lethal cancer are mixed (123). The correlation between dairy foods and calcium and other nutrients creates challenges in trying to disentangle the independent effects of these compounds; however, studies that have tried to separate effects generally suggest calcium may be the predominant player in explaining positive associations with prostate cancer. As a result, the WCRF/AICR 2007 Expert Report on Diet and Cancer concluded that calcium is a "probable" risk factor for prostate cancer, while the evidence for dairy was weak/inconclusive (124). Since then, however, the large EPIC study found that dairy calcium, but not nondairy calcium, was associated with total and high-grade prostate cancer risk (119).

One proposed mechanism of calcium and prostate cancer is by suppressing circulating levels of dihydroxyvitamin D (1,25$(OH)_2$D), the bioactive metabolite of vitamin D.

It is involved in regulating cellular differentiation and proliferation of many cell types, including prostate epithelia. The main source of vitamin D is endogenous production in the skin resulting from sun exposure, and diet is a secondary source. $1,25(OH)_2D$ is the most biologically active form, whereas 25(OH)D is found in much higher concentrations and better reflects sun and dietary exposure (125). An alternate hypothesis is that dairy protein increases levels of insulin-like growth factor (126), which may thus influence risk of advanced or lethal prostate cancer (127).

None of the studies of dietary or supplemental vitamin D have reported protective effects for prostate cancer incidence (128–131). Results of studies using prediagnostic circulating vitamin D metabolites have reported mainly null results (132–144), in addition to significant positive (145–147), inverse (148), and U-shaped (149, 150) associations. There is, however, a suggestion that vitamin D plays a role in prostate cancer progression. Genetic variants in the vitamin D receptor (VDR) are associated with Gleason score (151) and genetic variants in the vitamin D pathway are associated with risk of recurrence or progression and prostate cancer–specific mortality (152). In addition, high expression of the VDR protein in prostate cancer tissue has been associated with lower risk of lethal cancer among men with prostate cancer in the Health Professionals Follow-Up Study and Physicians' Health Study. Men in the highest versus lowest quartile of VDR expression had a relative risk of 0.37 (95% CI: 0.14–0.94), with adjustment for PSA at diagnosis, Gleason grade, and stage (153). Another recent study of prostate cancer mortality nested in the HPFS and PHS found that prostate cancer patients with the lowest levels of prediagnostic 25(OH)D had significantly greater risk of prostate cancer–specific mortality, with an RR of 1.59 (95% CI: 1.06–2.39) for the highest versus lowest quartiles (154). Prediagnostic vitamin D levels were significantly associated with both stage and grade in this study. Thus, while vitamin D exposure does not seem to be associated with lower risk of incident prostate cancer, several lines of evidence suggest that the vitamin D pathway may play a role in prostate cancer progression.

Coffee

There are several potential mechanisms by which coffee could be associated with a lower risk of lethal prostate cancer. Coffee is rich in several biologically active compounds including caffeine, minerals, and phytochemicals. In observational and animal studies, long-term coffee drinking has been associated with improved glucose metabolism and insulin secretion in observational and animal studies (155). Moreover, coffee is a potent antioxidant (156, 157) and intake may be associated with levels of different sex steroid hormones (158, 159).

Most prior epidemiological studies of coffee and prostate cancer have focused on total incidence of disease, with generally null results. However, several recent meta-analyses support an inverse association with fatal or advanced disease (160–163). Combining four studies with a fatal prostate cancer outcome, Discacciati et al. (163) found a relative risk of 0.89 (95% CI: 0.82–0.97) per three cups/d increment in coffee intake. There was also an inverse association with high-grade (Gleason 8–10) disease. These intriguing data, while biologically plausible, need to be confirmed in additional study populations with large numbers of fatal or advanced disease.

Statins

The class of lipid-lowering medications known as statins has been proposed to have antitumor effects in prostate by influencing cell proliferation, inflammation, and steroidogenesis. The first study to look at the association between statins and the risk of lethal prostate cancer was by Platz et al. who found a relative risk of 0.39 (95% CI: 0.19–0.77) among men who were statin users compared with nonusers (165). In a 2012 meta-analysis of 27 observational studies, the pooled relative risk of statins of 0.93 (95% CI: 0.87–0.99) for total incident prostate cancer and a more pronounced inverse association for advanced disease, with a relative risk of 0.80 (95% CI: 0.70–0.90) based on seven studies (166). Since publication of the 2012 meta-analysis, five additional epidemiological studies have reported on associations between statin use and lethal prostate cancer, all suggesting inverse associations (167–171). The largest to date was by Yu and colleagues, who studied more than 11,000 prostate cancer patients in the United Kingdom and studied both prediagnostic and postdiagnostic statin use (171). They found that postdiagnostic statins were associated with 34% (95% CI: 0.66–0.88) lower risk of prostate cancer death, and that most of the apparent benefit was from earlier use of statins before diagnosis. These findings are consistent with those of previous studies and nicely illustrate the need to identify the specific window of timing for the effect of a chemopreventive agent.

■ SUMMARY

From a public health perspective, the prevention of lethal prostate cancer is a paramount issue to improve the health of men in the United States and globally. Moreover, the identification of lifestyle factors after cancer diagnosis that could improve outcomes is appealing for the 4 million men currently living with a prostate cancer diagnosis. Research is in the early stages on both fronts, and research prerequisites include large, prospective cohort studies with long-term follow-up for cancer outcomes, detailed and updated questionnaire data, and consideration of the potential biases associated with epidemiological research. Still, there is now intriguing evidence that several behavioral risk factors may play a role in the prevention of lethal prostate cancer.

■ REFERENCES

1. Ferlay J, Bray F, Pisani P, et al. *GLOBOCAN 2002: Cancer Incidence, Mortality and Prevalence Worldwide*. Lyon, France: IARC Press; 2004.
2. IARC. *Globocan 2008 Cancer Fact Sheet: Prostate Cancer Incidence and Mortality Worldwide in 2008 Summary*. Lyon, France: IARC Press; 2008.
3. Howlader N, Noone A, Krapcho M, et al. *SEER Cancer Statistics Review 1975-2008*. Bethesda, MD: National Cancer Institute; 2011. http://seer.cancer.gov/csr/1975–2008/, based on http://seer.cancer.gov/registries/ November 2010 SEER data submission, posted to the SEER web site.
4. Shimizu H, Ross RK, Bernstein L, Yatani R, Henderson BE, Mack TM. Cancers of the prostate and breast among Japanese and white immigrants in Los Angeles County. *Br J Cancer*. 1991;63:963.
5. Yu H, Harris RE, Gao YT, Gao R, Wynder EL. Comparative epidemiology of cancers of the colon, rectum, prostate and breast in Shanghai, China versus the United States. *Int J Epidemiol*. 1991;20:76.
6. Jemal A, Center MM, DeSantis C, Ward EM. Global patterns of cancer incidence and mortality rates and trends. *Cancer Epidemiol Biomarkers Prev*. 2010;19:1893.
7. Etzioni R, Gulati R, Falcon S, Penson DF. Impact of PSA screening on the incidence of advanced stage prostate cancer in the United States: a surveillance modeling approach. *Med Decis Making*. 2008;28:323.
8. Ciatto S, Gervasi G, Bonardi R, et al. Determining overdiagnosis by screening with DRE/TRUS or PSA (Florence pilot studies, 1991–1994). *Eur J Cancer*. 2005;41:411.
9. Etzioni R, Penson DF, Legler JM, et al. Overdiagnosis due to prostate-specific antigen screening: lessons from U.S. prostate cancer incidence trends. *J Natl Cancer Inst*. 2002;94:981.
10. Giovannucci E, Liu Y, Platz EA, et al. Risk factors for prostate cancer incidence and progression in the health professionals follow-up study. *Int J Cancer*. 2007;121:1571.
11. Etzioni R, Tsodikov A, Mariotto A, et al. Quantifying the role of PSA screening in the US prostate cancer mortality decline. *Cancer Causes Control*. 2008;19:175.
12. Albertsen PC, Hanley JA, Fine J. 20-year outcomes following conservative management of clinically localized prostate cancer. *JAMA*. 2005;293:2095.
13. Johansson JE, Andren O, Andersson SO, et al. Natural history of early, localized prostate cancer. *JAMA*. 2004;291:2713.
14. Eles, RA, Olama, AA, Benlloch, S, et al. Identification of 23 new prostate cancer susceptibility loci using the iCOGS custom genotyping array. *Natural Genetics*. 2013. Apr;45(4):385-91, 391e1-2.
15. Hemminki K, Czene K. Attributable risks of familial cancer from the Family-Cancer Database. *Cancer Epidemiol Biomarkers Prev*. 2002;11:1638.
16. Brandt A, Sundquist J, Hemminki K. Risk for incident and fatal prostate cancer in men with a family history of any incident and fatal cancer. *Ann Oncol*. 2012;23:251–256.
17. Lichtenstein P, Holm NV, Verkasalo PK, et al. Environmental and heritable factors in the causation of cancer–analyses of cohorts of twins from Sweden, Denmark, and Finland. *N Engl J Med*. 2000;343:78.
18. Hjelmborg, JB, Scheike, T, Holst,K, et al. The heritability of prostate cancer in the Nordic Twin Study of Cancer. *Cancer Epi Biomarkers Prevention*. 2014 (Epub ahead of Print). *CEBP*. 2014.
19. Thomas G, Jacobs KB, Yeager M, et al. Multiple loci identified in a genome-wide association study of prostate cancer. *Nat Genet*. 2008;40:310.
20. Pomerantz MM, Freedman ML. Genetics of prostate cancer risk. *Mt Sinai J Med*. 2010;77:643.
21. Shui, IM, Lindstrom, S, Kibel, AS, et al. Prostate cancer (PCa) risk variants and risk of fatal PCa in the National Cancer Institute Breast and Prostate Cancer Cohort Consortium. *European Urology*. 2014. Jun;65(6):1069-1075.
22. Haiman, CA, Chen, GK, Blot, WJ. Characterizing genetic risk at known prostate cancer susceptibility loci in African-Americans. *PLoS Genetics*. 2011. May;7(5):e1001387.
23. Finucane MM, Stevens GA, Cowan MJ, et al. National, regional, and global trends in body-mass index since 1980: systematic analysis of health examination surveys and epidemiological studies with 960 country-years and 9.1 million participants. *Lancet*. 2011;377:557.
24. Flegal KM, Carroll MD, Ogden CL, Curtin LR. Prevalence and trends in obesity among US adults, 1999–2008. *JAMA*. 2010;303:235.
25. Ogden CL, Carroll MD. *CDC/NCHS 2010: Prevalence of Overweight, Obesity, and Extreme Obesity Among Adults: United States, Trends 1960–1962 Through 2007–2008*; Hyattsville, MD: National Center for Health Statistics; 2010
26. Ma J, Li H, Giovannucci E, et al. Prediagnostic body-mass index, plasma C-peptide concentration, and prostate cancer-specific mortality in men with prostate cancer: a long-term survival analysis. *Lancet Oncol*. 2008;9:1039.
27. Li H, Stampfer M J, Mucci L, et al. A 25-year prospective study of plasma adiponectin and leptin concentrations and prostate cancer risk and survival. *Clin Chem*. 2010;56:34.
28. Platz EA, Giovannucci E. The epidemiology of sex steroid hormones and their signaling and metabolic pathways in the etiology of prostate cancer. *J Steroid Biochem Mol Biol*. 2004;92:237.
29. De Marzo AM, Platz EA, Sutcliffe S, et al. Inflammation in prostate carcinogenesis. *Nat Rev Cancer*. 2007;7:256.
30. Discacciati A, Orsini N, Andersson SO, Andrén O, Johansson JE, Wolk A. Body mass index in early and middle-late adulthood and risk of localised, advanced and fatal prostate cancer: a population-based prospective study. *Br J Cancer*. 2011;105:1061.
31. MacInnis RJ, English DR. Body size and composition and prostate cancer risk: systematic review and meta-regression analysis. *Cancer Causes Control*. 2006;17:989.
32. Robinson WR, Poole C, Godley PA. Systematic review of prostate cancer's association with body size in childhood and young adulthood. *Cancer Causes Control*. 2008;19:793.
33. Cao Y, Ma J. Body mass index, prostate cancer-specific mortality, and biochemical recurrence: a systematic review and meta-analysis. *Cancer Prev Res (Phila)*. 2011;4:486.
34. Allott EH, Masko EM, Freedland SJ. Obesity and prostate cancer: weighing the evidence. *Eur Urol*. 2013. 63(5):800–809.
35. Lai, GY, Giovannucci, EL, Pollak, MN, et al. Association of C-peptide and leptin with prostate cancer incidence in the Health Professionals Follow-Up Study. *Cancer Causes Control*. 2014;25(5):625–632; Stevens, VL, Jacobs, EJ, Sun, J, Gapstur, SM. No association of plasma levels of adiponectin and c-peptide with risk of aggressive prostate cancer in the Cancer Prevention Study II Nutrition Cohort. *Can Epi Bio Prev*. 2014; 23(5):890–892.
36. Pischon R, Boeing H, Weikert S, et al. Body size and risk of prostate cancer in the European Prospective Investigation into Cancer and Nutrition. *Cancer Epidemiol Biomarkers Prev*. 2008;17;3252.
37. MacInnis RJ, English DR, Gertig DM, Hopper JL, Giles GG. Body size and composition and prostate cancer risk. *Cancer Epidemiol Biomarkers Prev*. 2003;12:1417–1421.
38. Giovannucci E, Rimm EB, Stampfer MJ, Colditz GA, Willett WC. Height, body weight, and risk of prostate cancer. *Cancer Epidemiol Biomarkers Prev*. 1997;6:557–563.
39. Nomura A, Heilbrun LK, Stemmermann GN. Body mass index as a predictor of cancer in men. *J Natl Cancer Inst*. 1985;74:319.

40. Cerhan JR, Torner JC, Lynch CF, et al. Association of smoking, body mass, and physical activity with risk of prostate cancer in the Iowa 65+ Rural Health Study (United States). *Cancer Causes Control.* 1997;8:229.
41. Giovannucci E, Rimm EB, Stampfer MJ, Colditz GA, Willett WC. Height, body weight, and risk of prostate cancer. *Cancer Epidemiol Biomarkers Prev.* 1997;6:557.
42. Putnam SD, Cerhan JR, Parker AS, et al. Lifestyle and anthropometric risk factors for prostate cancer in a cohort of Iowa men. *Ann Epidemiol.* 2000;10:361.
43. Schuurman AG, Goldbohm RA, Dorant E, van den Brandt PA. Anthropometry in relation to prostate cancer risk in the Netherlands Cohort Study. *Am J Epidemiol.* 2000;151:541.
44. Spitz MR, Strom SS, Yamamura Y, et al. Epidemiologic determinants of clinically relevant prostate cancer. *Int J Cancer.* 2000;89:259.
45. Jonsson F, Wolk A, Pedersen NL, et al. Obesity and hormone-dependent tumors: cohort and co-twin control studies based on the Swedish Twin Registry. *Int J Cancer.* 2003;106:594.
46. Friedenreich CM, McGregor SE, Courneya KS, Angyalfi SJ, Elliott FG. Case-control study of anthropometric measures and prostate cancer risk. *Int J Cancer.* 2004;110:278.
47. Littman AJ, White E, Kristal AR. Anthropometrics and prostate cancer risk. *Am J Epidemiol.* 2007;165:1271.
48. Hernandez BY, Park SY, Wilkens LR, Henderson BE, Kolonel LN. Relationship of ody mass, height, and weight gain to prostate cancer risk in the multiethnic cohort. *Cancer Epidemiol Biomarkers Prev.* 2009;18:2413.
49. Wright ME, Chang SC, Schatzkin A, et al. Prospective study of adiposity and weight change in relation to prostate cancer incidence and mortality. *Cancer.* 2007;109:675.
50. Joshu CE, Mondul AM, Menke A, et al. Weight gain is associated with an increased risk of prostate cancer recurrence after prostatectomy in the PSA era. *Cancer Prev Res (Phila).* 2011;4:544.
51. Giovannucci EL, Liu Y, Leitzmann MF, Stampfer MJ, Willett WC. A prospective study of physical activity and incident and fatal prostate cancer. *Arch Intern Med.* 2005;165:1005.
52. Patel AV, Rodriguez C, Jacobs EJ, Solomon L, Thun MJ, Calle EE. Recreational physical activity and risk of prostate cancer in a large cohort of U.S. men. *Cancer Epidemiol Biomarkers Prev.* 2005;14:275.
53. Johnsen NF, Tjonneland A, Thomsen BL, et al. Physical activity and risk of prostate cancer in the European Prospective Investigation into Cancer and Nutrition (EPIC) cohort. *Int J Cancer.* 2009;125:902.
54. Moore SC, Peters TM, Ahn J, et al. Physical activity in relation to total, advanced, and fatal prostate cancer. *Cancer Epidemiol Biomarkers Prev.* 2008;17:2458.
55. Kenfield SA, Stampfer MJ, Giovannucci E, Chan JM. Physical activity and survival after prostate cancer diagnosis in the health professionals follow-up study. *J Clin Oncol.* 2011;29:726.
56. Richman EL, Kenfield SA, Stampfer MJ, Paciorek A, Carroll PR, Chan JM. Physical activity after diagnosis and risk of prostate cancer progression: data from the cancer of the prostate strategic urologic research endeavor. *Cancer Res.* 2011;71:3889.
57. US Department of Health and Human Services. *The Health Consequences of Smoking. A Report of the Surgeon General.* Washington, DC: US Dept of Health and Human Services; 2004.
58. Giovannucci E, Rimm EB, Ascherio A, et al. Smoking and risk of total and fatal prostate cancer in United States health professionals. *Cancer Epidemiol Biomarkers Prev.* 1999;8:277.
59. Byrne MM, Davila EP, Zhao W, et al. Cancer screening behaviors among smokers and non-smokers. *Cancer Epidemiol.* 2010;34:611.
60. Pickles T, Liu M, Berthelet E, et al. The effect of smoking on outcome following external radiation for localized prostate cancer. *J Urol.* 2004;171:1543.
61. Moreira DM, Antonelli JA, Presti JC Jr, et al. Association of cigarette smoking with interval to biochemical recurrence after radical prostatectomy: results from the SEARCH database. *Urology.* 2010;76:1218.
62. Joshu CE, Mondul AM, Meinhold CL, et al. Cigarette smoking and prostate cancer recurrence after prostatectomy. *J Natl Cancer Inst.* 2011;103:835.
63. Pantarotto J, Malone S, Dahrouge S, et al. Smoking is associated with worse outcomes in patients with prostate cancer treated by radical radiotherapy. *BJU Int.* 2007;99:564.
64. Oefelein MG, Resnick MI. Association of tobacco use with hormone refractory disease and survival of patients with prostate cancer. *J Urol.* 2004;171:2281.
65. Kenfield SA, Stampfer MJ, Chan JM, Giovannucci E. Smoking and prostate cancer survival and recurrence. *JAMA.* 2011;305: 2548.
66. Meydani M. Vitamin E. *Lancet.* 1995;345:170–175.
67. Meydani SN, Hayek MG. Vitamin E and aging immune response. *Clin Geriatr Med.* 1995;11:567.
68. Gunawardena K, Murray DK, Meikle AW. Vitamin E and other antioxidants inhibit human prostate cancer cells through apoptosis. *Prostate.* 2000;44:287.
69. Ripoll EA, Rama BN, Webber MM. Vitamin E enhances the chemotherapeutic effects of adriamycin on human prostatic carcinoma cells in vitro. *J Urol.* 1986;136:529.
70. The effect of vitamin E and beta carotene on the incidence of lung cancer and other cancers in male smokers. The Alpha-Tocopherol, Beta Carotene Cancer Prevention Study Group. *N Engl J Med.* 1994;330:1029.
71. Heinonen OP, Albanes D, Virtamo J, et al. Prostate cancer and supplementation with alpha-tocopherol and beta-carotene: incidence and mortality in a controlled trial. *J Natl Cancer Inst.* 1998;90:440.
72. Blot WJ, Li JY, Taylor PR, et al. Nutrition intervention trials in Linxian, China: supplementation with specific vitamin mineral combinations, cancer incidence, and disease-specific mortality in the general population. *J Natl Cancer Inst.* 1993;85:1483.
73. Lippman SM, Klein EA, Goodman PJ, et al. Effect of selenium and vitamin E on risk of prostate cancer and other cancers: the Selenium and Vitamin E Cancer Prevention Trial (SELECT). *JAMA.* 2009;301:39.
74. Klein EA, Thompson IM Jr, Tangen CM, et al. Vitamin E and the risk of prostate cancer: the Selenium and Vitamin E Cancer Prevention Trial (SELECT). *JAMA.* 2011;306:1549.
75. Gaziano JM, Glynn RJ, Christen WG, et al. Vitamins E and C in the prevention of prostate and total cancer in men: the Physicians' Health Study II randomized controlled trial. *JAMA.* 2009;301:52.
76. Peters U, Littman AJ, Kristal AR, Patterson RE, Potter JD, White E. Vitamin E and selenium supplementation and risk of prostate cancer in the Vitamins and lifestyle (VITAL) study cohort. *Cancer Causes Control.* 2008;19:75.
77. Eichholzer M, Stahelin HB, Gey KF, Lüdin E, Bernasconi F. Prediction of male cancer mortality by plasma levels of interacting vitamins: 17-year follow-up of the prospective Basel study. *Int J Cancer.* 1996;66:145.
78. Kirsh VA, Hayes RB, Mayne ST, et al. Supplemental and dietary vitamin E, beta-carotene, and vitamin C intakes and prostate cancer risk. *J Natl Cancer Inst.* 2006;98:245.
79. Chan JM, Stampfer MJ, Ma J, Rimm EB, Willett WC, Giovannucci EL. Supplemental vitamin E intake and prostate cancer risk in a large cohort of men in the United States. *Cancer Epidemiol Biomarkers Prev.* 1999;8:893.
80. Gann PH, Ma J, Giovannucci E, et al. Lower prostate cancer risk in men with elevated plasma lycopene levels: results of a prospective analysis. *Cancer Res.* 1999;59:1225.
81. Combs GF Jr, Combs SB. The nutritional biochemistry of selenium. *Annu Rev Nutr.* 1984;4:257.
82. Menter DG, Sabichi AL, Lippman SM. Selenium effects on prostate cell growth. *Cancer Epidemiol Biomarkers Prev.* 2000;9:1171.

83. Redman C, Scott JA, Baines AT, et al. Inhibitory effect of selenomethionine on the growth of three selected human tumor cell lines. *Cancer Lett.* 1998;125:103.
84. Rayman MP. The importance of selenium to human health. *Lancet.* 2000;356:233.
85. Neve J. Human selenium supplementation as assessed by changes in blood selenium concentration and glutathione peroxidase activity. *J Trace Elem Med Biol.* 1995;9:65.
86. Duffield-Lillico AJ, Dalkin BL, Reid ME, et al. Selenium supplementation, baseline plasma selenium status and incidence of prostate cancer: an analysis of the complete treatment period of the Nutritional Prevention of Cancer Trial. *BJU Int.* 2003;91:608.
87. Clark LC, Combs GF Jr, Turnbull BW, et al. Effects of selenium supplementation for cancer prevention in patients with carcinoma of the skin. A randomized controlled trial. Nutritional Prevention of Cancer Study Group. *JAMA.* 1996;276:1957.
88. Kristal AR, Darke AK, Morris JS, et al. Baseline selenium status and effects of selenium and vitamin e supplementation on prostate cancer risk. *J Natl Cancer Inst.* 2014;106(3):djt456. 24563519.
89. Li H, Stampfer MJ, Giovannucci EL, et al. A prospective study of plasma selenium levels and prostate cancer risk. *J Natl Cancer Inst.* 2004;96:696.
90. Yoshizawa K, Willett WC, Morris SJ, et al. Study of prediagnostic selenium level in toenails and the risk of advanced prostate cancer. *J Natl Cancer Inst.* 1998;90:1219.
91. Brooks JD, Metter EJ, Chan DW, et al. Plasma selenium level before diagnosis and the risk of prostate cancer development. *J Urol.* 2001;166:2034.
92. Helzlsouer KJ, Huang HY, Alberg AJ, et al. Association between alpha-tocopherol, gamma-tocopherol, selenium, and subsequent prostate cancer. *J Natl Cancer Inst.* 2000;92:2018.
93. Nomura AM, Lee J, Stemmermann GN, Combs GF Jr. Serum selenium and subsequent risk of prostate cancer. *Cancer Epidemiol Biomarkers Prev.* 2000;9:883.
94. van den Brandt PA, Zeegers MP, Bode P, Goldbohm RA. Toenail selenium levels and the subsequent risk of prostate cancer: a prospective cohort study. *Cancer Epidemiol Biomarkers Prev.* 2003;12:866.
95. Geybels, MS, van den Brandt, PA, Schouten, LJ, et al. Selenoprotein gene variants, toenail selenium levels, and risk for advanced prostate cancer. *J Natl Cancer Institute.* 2014 Mar; 106(3): dju003.
96. Goodman GE, Schaffer S, Bankson DD, et al. Predictors of serum selenium in cigarette smokers and the lack of association with lung and prostate cancer risk. *Cancer Epidemiol Biomarkers Prev.* 2001;10:1069.
97. Hartman TJ, Albanes D, Pietinen P, et al. The association between baseline vitamin E, selenium, and prostate cancer in the alpha-tocopherol, beta-carotene cancer prevention study. *Cancer Epidemiol Biomarkers Prev.* 1998;7:335.
98. Peters U, Takata Y. Selenium and the prevention of prostate and colorectal cancer. *Mol Nutr Food Res.* 2008;52:1261.
99. Fleshner NE, Kapusta L, Donnelly B, et al. Progression from high-grade prostatic intraepithelial neoplasia to cancer: a randomized trial of combination vitamin-E, soy, and selenium. *J Clin Oncol.* 2011;29:2386.
100. Marshall JR, Tangen CM, Sakr WA, et al. Phase III trial of selenium to prevent prostate cancer in men with high-grade prostatic intraepithelial neoplasia: SWOG S9917. *Cancer Prev Res (Phila).* 2011;4:1761.
101. Etminan M, Takkouche B, Caamano-Isorna F. The role of tomato products and lycopene in the prevention of prostate cancer: a meta-analysis of observational studies. *Cancer Epidemiol Biomarkers Prev.* 2004;13:340.
102. Maiani G, Caston MJ, Catasta G, et al. Carotenoids: actual knowledge on food sources, intakes, stability and bioavailability and their protective role in humans. *Mol Nutr Food Res.* 2009;53 (suppl 2):S194.
103. Wu K, Erdman JW Jr, Schwartz SJ, et al. Plasma and dietary carotenoids, and the risk of prostate cancer: a nested case-control study. *Cancer Epidemiol Biomarkers Prev.* 2004;13:260.
104. Beilby J, Ambrosini GL, Rossi E, de Klerk NH, Musk AW. Serum levels of folate, lycopene, beta-carotene, retinol and vitamin E and prostate cancer risk. *Eur J Clin Nutr.* 2010;64:1235.
105. Karppi J, Kurl S, Nurmi T, Rissanen TH, Pukkala E, Nyyssönen K. Serum lycopene and the risk of cancer: the Kuopio Ischaemic Heart Disease Risk Factor (KIHD) study. *Ann Epidemiol.* 2009;19:512.
106. Peters U, Leitzmann MF, Chatterjee N, et al. Serum lycopene, other carotenoids, and prostate cancer risk: a nested case-control study in the prostate, lung, colorectal, and ovarian cancer screening trial. *Cancer Epidemiol Biomarkers Prev.* 2007;16:962.
107. Kristal AR, Till C, Platz EA, et al. Serum lycopene concentration and prostate cancer risk: results from the Prostate Cancer Prevention Trial. *Cancer Epidemiol Biomarkers Prev.* 2011;20:638.
108. Key TJ, Appleby PN, Allen NE, et al. Plasma carotenoids, retinol, and tocopherols and the risk of prostate cancer in the European Prospective Investigation into Cancer and Nutrition study. *Am J Clin Nutr.* 2007;86:672.
109. Giovannucci E. Commentary: serum lycopene and prostate cancer progression: a re-consideration of findings from the prostate cancer prevention trial. *Cancer Causes Control.* 2011;22:1055.
110. Zu K, Mucci L, Rosner BA, et al. Dietary lycopene, angiogenesis, and prostate cancer: a prospective study in the prostate-specific antigen era. *J Natl Cancer Inst.* 2014;106(2):djt430. PMID: 24463248.
111. Gao X, LaValley MP, Tucker KL. Prospective studies of dairy product and calcium intakes and prostate cancer risk: a meta-analysis. *J Natl Cancer Inst.* 2005;97:1768.
112. Steineck G, Helgesen F, Adolfsson J, et al. Quality of life after radical prostatectomy or watchful waiting. *N Engl J Med.* 2002;347:790.
113. Giovannucci E, Liu Y, Stampfer MJ, Willett WC. A prospective study of calcium intake and incident and fatal prostate cancer. *Cancer Epidemiol Biomarkers Prev.* 2006;15:203.
114. Tseng M, Breslow RA, Graubard BI, Ziegler RG. Dairy, calcium, and vitamin D intakes and prostate cancer risk in the National Health and Nutrition Examination Epidemiologic Follow-up Study cohort. *Am J Clin Nutr.* 2005;81:1147.
115. Skinner HG, Schwartz GG. Serum calcium and incident and fatal prostate cancer in the National Health and Nutrition Examination Survey. *Cancer Epidemiol Biomarkers Prev.* 2008;17:2302.
116. Skinner HG, Schwartz GG. A prospective study of total and ionized serum calcium and fatal prostate cancer. *Cancer Epidemiol Biomarkers Prev.* 2009;18(2):575–578.
117. Halthur C, Johansson AL, Almquist M, et al. Serum calcium and the risk of prostate cancer. *Cancer Causes Control.* 2009;20(7):1205–1214.
118. Van Hemelrijck M, Hermans R, Michaelsson K, et al. Serum calcium and incident and fatal prostate cancer in the Swedish AMORIS study. *Cancer Causes Control.* 2012;23(8):1349–1358. PMID: 22710746.
119. Allen NE, Key TJ, Appleby PN, et al. Animal foods, protein, calcium and prostate cancer risk: the European Prospective Investigation into Cancer and Nutrition. *Br J Cancer.* 2008;98:1574.
120. Rohrmann S, Platz EA, Kavanaugh CJ, Thuita L, Hoffman SC, Helzlsouer KJ. Meat and dairy consumption and subsequent risk of prostate cancer in a US cohort study. *Cancer Causes Control.* 2007;18:41.

121. Park Y, Leitzmann MF, Subar AF, Hollenbeck A, Schatzkin A. Dairy food, calcium, and risk of cancer in the NIH-AARP Diet and Health Study. *Arch Intern Med*. 2009;169(4):391–401. doi:10.1001/archinternmed.2008.578.
122. Koh KA, Sesso HD, Paffenbarger RS Jr, Lee IM. Dairy products, calcium and prostate cancer risk. *Br J Cancer*. 2006;95:1582.
123. Park Y, Mitrou PN, Kipnis V, Hollenbeck A, Schatzkin A, Leitzmann MF. Calcium, dairy foods, and risk of incident and fatal prostate cancer: the NIH-AARP Diet and Health Study. *Am J Epidemiol*. 2007;166:1270.
124. WCRF report WCRF/AICR. *Food, Nutrition, Physical Activity, and the Prevention of Cancer: A Global Perspective*. Washington, DC: WCRF/AICR; 2007.
125. Ali MM, Vaidya V. Vitamin D and cancer. *J Cancer Res Ther*. 2007;3:225.
126. Giovannucci, E, Pollak, M, Liu, Y, et al. Nutritional predictors of insulin-like growth factor I and their relationships to cancer in men. *Can Epi Bio Prev*. 2003. Feb;12(2):84–89.
127. Chan, JM, Stampfer, MJ, Ma, J, et al. Insulin-Like Growth Factor-I (IGF-I) and IGF Binding Protein-3 as Predictors of Advanced-Stage Prostate Cancer. *JNCI*. 2002. Jul 18;94(14): 1099–1106.
128. Giovannucci E. Dietary influences of 1,25(OH)2 vitamin D in relation to prostate cancer: a hypothesis. *Cancer Causes Control*. 1998;9:567.
129. Chan JM, Giovannucci E, Andersson SO, Yuen J, Adami HO, Wolk A. Dairy products, calcium, phosphorous, vitamin D, and risk of prostate cancer (Sweden). *Cancer Causes Control*. 1998;9:559.
130. Chan JM, Pietinen P, Virtanen M, et al. Diet and prostate cancer risk in a cohort of smokers, with a specific focus on calcium and phosphorus (Finland). *Cancer Causes Control*. 2000;11:859.
131. Kristal AR, Cohen JH, Qu P, Stanford JL. Associations of energy, fat, calcium, and vitamin D with prostate cancer risk. *Cancer Epidemiol Biomarkers Prev*. 2002;11:719.
132. Corder EH, Guess HA, Hulka BS, et al. Vitamin D and prostate cancer: a prediagnostic study with stored sera. *Cancer Epidemiol Biomarkers Prev*. 1993;2:467.
133. Travis RC, Crowe FL, Allen NE, et al. Serum vitamin D and risk of prostate cancer in a case-control analysis nested within the European Prospective Investigation into Cancer and Nutrition (EPIC). *Am J Epidemiol*. 2009;169:1223–1232.
134. Li H, Stampfer MJ, Hollis JB, et al. A prospective study of plasma vitamin D metabolites, vitamin D receptor polymorphisms, and prostate cancer. *PLoS Med*. 2007;4:e103.
135. Barnett CM, Nielson CM, Shannon J, et al. Serum 25-OH vitamin D levels and risk of developing prostate cancer in older men. *Cancer Causes Control*. 2010;21:1297–1303.
136. Faupel-Badger JM, Diaw L, Albanes D, Virtamo J, Woodson K, Tangrea JA. Lack of association between serum levels of 25-hydroxyvitamin D and the subsequent risk of prostate cancer in Finnish men. *Cancer Epidemiol Biomarkers Prev*. 2007;16:2784–2786.
137. Park SY, Cooney RV, Wilkens LR, Murphy SP, Henderson BE, Kolonel LN. Plasma 25-hydroxyvitamin D and prostate cancer risk: the multiethnic cohort. *Eur J Cancer*. 2010;46:932–936.
138. Gilbert R, Metcalfe C, Fraser WD, et al. Associations of circulating 25-hydroxyvitamin D with prostate cancer diagnosis, stage and grade. *Int J Cancer*. 2012;131:1187–1196.
139. Ahn J, Peters U, Albanes D, et al. Serum vitamin D concentration and prostate cancer risk: a nested case-control study. *J Natl Cancer Inst*. 2008;11:796–804.
140. Braun MM, Helzlsouer KJ, Hollis BW, et al. Prostate cancer and prediagnostic levels of serum vitamin D metabolites (Maryland, United States). *Cancer Causes Control*. 1995;6:235.
141. Gann PH, Ma J, Hennekens CH, Hollis BW, Haddad JG, Stampfer MJ. Circulating vitamin D metabolites in relation to subsequent development of prostate cancer. *Cancer Epidemiol Biomarkers Prev*. 1996;5:121.
142. Nomura AM, Stemmermann GN, Lee J, et al. Serum vitamin D metabolite levels and the subsequent development of prostate cancer (Hawaii, United States). *Cancer Causes Control*. 1998;9:425.
143. Platz EA, Leitzmann MF, Hollis BW, Willett WC, Giovannucci E. Plasma 1,25-dihydroxy- and 25-hydroxyvitamin D and subsequent risk of prostate cancer. *Cancer Causes Control*. 2004;15:255.
144. Jacobs ET, Giuliano AR, Martinez ME, Hollis BW, Reid ME, Marshall JR. Plasma levels of 25-hydroxyvitamin D, 1,25-dihydroxyvitamin D and the risk of prostate cancer. *J Steroid Biochem Mol Biol*. 2004;89–90:533.
145. Albanes D, Mondul AM, Yu K, et al. Serum 25-hydroxy vitamin D and prostate cancer risk in a large nested case-control study. *Cancer Epidemiol Biomarkers Prev*. 2011;20:1850.
146. Albanes D, Mondul AM, Yu K, et al. Serum 25-hydroxy vitamin D and prostate cancer risk in a large nested case-control study. *Cancer Epidemiol Biomarkers Prev*. 2011;20:1850–1860.
147. Meyer HE, Robsahm TE, Bjorge T, Brustad M, Blomhoff R. Vitamin D, season, and risk of prostate cancer: a nested case-control study within Norwegian health studies. *Am J Clin Nutr*. 2013;97:147–154.
148. Ahonen MH, Tenkanen L, Teppo L, Hakama M, Tuohimaa P. Prostate cancer risk and prediagnostic serum 25-hydroxyvitamin D levels (Finland). *Cancer Causes Control*. 2000; 11:847.
149. Tuohimaa P, Tenkanen L, Ahonen M, et al. Both high and low levels of blood vitamin D are associated with a higher prostate cancer risk: a longitudinal, nested case-control study in the Nordic countries. *Int J Cancer*. 2004;108:104.
150. Kristal AR, Till CA, Song X, et al. Plasma Vitamin D and prostate cancer risk; results from the selenium and vitamin e cancer prevention trial. *Cancer Epidemiol Biomarkers Prev*. 2014. [Epub ahead of print]. Published OnlineFirst April 14, 2014; doi: 10.1158/1055-9965.EPI-14-0115
151. Chen L, Davey Smith G, Evans DM, et al. Genetic variants in the vitamin d receptor are associated with advanced prostate cancer at diagnosis: findings from the prostate testing for cancer and treatment study and a systematic review. *Cancer Epidemiol Biomarkers Prev*. 2009;18:2874.
152. Holt SK, Kwon EM, Koopmeiners JS, et al. Vitamin D pathway gene variants and prostate cancer prognosis. *Prostate*. 2010;70:1448.
153. Hendrickson WK, Flavin R, Kasperzyk JL, et al. Vitamin D receptor protein expression in tumor tissue and prostate cancer progression. *J Clin Oncol*. 2011;29:2378.
154. Fang F, Kasperzyk JL, Shui I, et al. Prediagnostic plasma vitamin D metabolites and mortality among patients with prostate cancer. *PLoS One*. 2011;6:e18625.
155. Tunnicliffe JM, Shearer J. Coffee, glucose homeostasis, and insulin resistance: physiological mechanisms and mediators. *Appl Physiol Nutr Metab*. 2008;33(6):1290–1300.
156. Svilaas A, Sakhi AK, Andersen LF, et al. Intakes of antioxidants in coffee, wine, and vegetables are correlated with plasma carotenoids in humans. *J Nutr*. 2004;134(3):562–567.
157. Pulido R, Hernandez-Garcia M, Saura-Calixto F. Contribution of beverages to the intake of lipophilic and hydrophilic antioxidants in the Spanish diet. *Eur J Clin Nutr*. 2003;57(10):1275–1282.
158. Kempf K, Herder C, Erlund I, et al. Effects of coffee consumption on subclinical inflammation and other risk factors for type 2 diabetes: a clinical trial. *Am J Clin Nutr*. 2010;91(4):950–957.
159. Svartberg J, Midtby M, Bonaa KH, Sundsfjord J, Joakimsen RM, Jorde R. The associations of age, lifestyle factors and chronic disease with testosterone in men: the Tromsø study. *Eur J Endocrinol*. 2003;149(2):145–152.

160. Lu Y, Zhai L, Zeng J, et al. Coffee consumption and prostate cancer risk: an updated meta-analysis. *Cancer Causes Control.* 2014;25(5):591–604.
161. Cao S, Liu L, Yin X, Wang Y, Liu J, Lu Z. Coffee consumption and risk of prostate cancer: a meta-analysis of prospective cohort studies. *Carcinogenesis.* 2014;35(2):256–261.
162. Zhong S, Chen W, Yu X, Chen Z, Hu Q, Zhao J. Coffee consumption and risk of prostate cancer: an up-to-date meta-analysis. *Eur J Clin Nutr.* 2014;68(3):330–337.
163. Discacciati A, Orsini N, Wolk A. Coffee consumption and risk of nonaggressive, aggressive and fatal prostate cancer—a dose-response meta-analysis. *Ann Oncol.* 2014;25(3):584–591.
164. Ma, Jing, Haojie, Li, Giovannucci, E, et al. Prediagnostic body-mass index, plasma C-peptide concentration, and prostate cancer—specific mortality in men with prostate cancer: a long-term survival analysis. *Lancet Oncology.* 2008 Nov;9(11):1039–1047.
165. Platz EA, Leitzmann MF, Visvanathan K, et al. Statin drugs and risk of advanced prostate cancer. J Natl Cancer Inst. 2006;98(24): 1819–1825.
166. Bansal D, Undela K, D'Cruz S, Schifano F. Statin use and risk of prostate cancer: a meta-analysis of observational studies. *PLoS One.* 2012;7(10):e46691.
167. Geybels MS, Wright JL, Holt SK, et al. Statin use in relation to prostate cancer outcomes in a population-based patient cohort study. *Prostate* 2013;73(11):1214–1222.
168. Nielsen SF, Nordestgaard BG, Bojesen SE. Statin use and reduced cancer-related mortality. *N Engl J Med.* 2012;367(19):1792–1802.
169. Grytli HH, Fagerland MW, Fosså SD, Taskén KA. Association between use of beta-blockers and prostate cancer—specific survival: a cohort study of 3561 prostate cancer patients with high-risk or metastatic disease. *Eur Urol.* 2014;65(3): 635–641.
170. Margel D, Urbach DR, Lipscombe LL et al. Metformin use and all-cause and prostate cancer-specific mortality among men with diabetes. *J Clin Oncol.* 2013;31(25):3069–3075.
171. Yu O, Eberg M, Benayoun S, et al. Use of statins and the risk of death in patients with prostate cancer. *J Clin Oncol.* 2014;32(1):5–11.

2.2 Diet and Prostate Cancer

JAMES R. MARSHALL

■ INTRODUCTION

An important goal of the dietary epidemiology of any cancer is to identify a diet predictive of risk; that information could be used to help individuals at risk to modify their diets, to adopt one predictive of diminished risk. Alternatively, if components of the diet that are protective could be identified, those components might be used as chemopreventive agents. One of the attractions of focusing on agents found in the diet is that these agents might be widely consumed; their being a part of the diet might mean that they are unlikely to induce toxicity.

International variation in prostate cancer risk, with incidence significantly higher in the western industrial world than that in the developing world, has helped to fuel suspicion that diet is related to risk (1). The diets that dominate the western world are characterized by higher levels of fat and protein, with animal products a major food source; the diets within the developing world, based to a greater extent on plant products, tend also to deliver fewer calories and fewer simple carbohydrates. Obesity is a much greater problem in the western industrialized world than in the developing world (1).

Animal experimentation has suggested a number of promising leads to the dietary etiology of prostate cancer. The result of attempts to test these leads among human beings, however, has been highly disappointing. Agents that slow the growth of cancer cell lines, or that retard the growth of cancer in laboratory animals, do not appear to prevent the development of cancer among human populations (2, 3).

Ecologic studies, in which countries or political entities are the units of analysis, suggest strongly that diet is a factor in prostate cancer risk (2). However, it has proven difficult to validate the findings of ecologic studies by individual-based human-based studies; a major complication of such studies is that the risk of prostate cancer does not become substantial until males reach their sixth decade (3). The lag between exposure to carcinogenic agents and the appearance of risk is not known; the lag could extend over decades. Etiologic studies attempt to effect some telescoping of time, so that studies can be completed within years, rather than in decades (4). Thus, for example, in case-control studies of diet and prostate cancer, such as those reported by Graham et al. (5) and by Hayes et al. (6), subjects were asked about the frequency with which they consumed various foodstuffs in a period specified for cases as the several years prior to the onset of disease symptoms; controls were asked to describe this period up to a year, or more than 2 years, prior to the date of interview. In the prospective study reported by Gann et al. (7), blood samples from a large number of healthy subjects were collected, frozen, and stored; blood levels of nutrients in samples from individuals who later became cases were compared with those of individuals who remained prostate cancer free. Cohort studies of diet and prostate cancer in which subjects report their dietary practice (8, 9) and are then followed often require decades to complete.

A critical limitation of our understanding of diet and prostate cancer is the difficulty of diet measurement. Descriptions of dietary practice have to be based in large part on self-report. A number of techniques have been devised for measurement of diet: short-term diet diaries, long-term diet history, short-term dietary recall (10). Each of these techniques brings specific advantages to diet measurement, and each measures a domain of diet; the precision with which they measure it, however, is more problematic (11–13). One approach to this problem might be to collect additional data from subjects. Unfortunately, however, the ability of researchers to induce research subjects to provide additional data is limited. Diet history questionnaires often take two to three hours to complete, and diet diaries and recent diet recalls require repeated contacts. Attempts to gather additional data by the use of more extensive questioning have proven disappointing. It is likely that half or more of the variance observed in dietary data is random, not related to actual dietary practice (11, 12), and there are not any promising candidates on the horizon that promise to lessen the extent of measurement imprecision. This inability to precisely characterize diet means first that observed associations between dietary practice and prostate cancer risk will be biased, generally underestimated. In addition, this imprecision lessens the ability of the investigator to separate the effects of nutrient intakes that are correlated (11, 12).

■ THE VARIABLE COURSE OF PROSTATE CANCER

Although prostate cancer in 2012 in the United States was responsible for some 30,000 deaths, nearly 240,000 cases of prostate cancer were diagnosed. Clearly, the vast majority of patients diagnosed with prostate cancer do not die of their disease. The number of men who carry a probably indolent form of prostate cancer is in all likelihood even higher than the above figure indicates. The diagnosis of prostate cancer is in part due to the aggressiveness with which screening is conducted. Thompson et al. found, in a large sample of men who were by most indicators believed to be at low risk of prostate cancer, that the prevalence of biopsy-confirmed prostate cancer was nearly 25% (14). Only about 3% of men in the United States die of prostate cancer, so that as many as 8 times as many American men may develop prostate cancer as die of it. Prostate cancer may be a heterogeneous disease: some cases are very aggressive and likely to be lethal, while some appear to be quite indolent and not likely to induce symptoms or shorten life. These different forms could well have distinct dietary or nutritional etiologies. It has been observed that, although the incidence of aggressive prostate cancer varies substantially over the world, the prevalence of what is in all likelihood a very indolent form is quite consistent in different cultures and regions (4).

The likely presence of undiagnosed prostate cancer among men believed not to have cancer substantially complicates the ability to link dietary practice to risk. As noted, among men believed to be at substantially low risk, the prevalence of undiagnosed prostate cancer was approximately 24%; among men only regarded as average risk, the prevalence of undiagnosed prostate cancer could be higher yet (14, 15). Thus, a study understood to be comparing prostate cancer patients with nonpatients could actually be comparing patients to a group comprised of nonpatients and substantial numbers of patients. This would clearly lessen the difference between patients and nonpatients with respect to any etiologic factors.

Aggressive cancer may be more affected than indolent cancer by environmental exposures. As noted, the difference among countries in the incidence of diagnosed and treated cancers is much larger than that of prevalent, more indolent cancers discovered only at postmortem examination of men who have died of other causes (4). The rate at which the huge reservoir of indolent prostate cancer is transformed to an aggressive phenotype is not well understood, but, apparently, much of it in that reservoir never becomes aggressive or life threatening within the life course. There is apparently a large difference between the more indolent and more aggressive forms of prostate cancer, and there is evidence that the etiologies of these two forms are distinct. Attempts to decrease the human cost of prostate cancer by diet may be more effective if they are targeted at preventing the development of a more lethal phenotype than to attempt to prevent the development of early cancer by focusing on the healthy population.

■ NUTRITIONAL COMPONENTS OF THE DIET

Fat

It has been widely suspected that fat is a risk factor for many cancers (2). Fat is a potent source of energy: Each gram of fat contributes 9 cal, while each gram of carbohydrate contributes 4 cal, and each gram of protein contributes 4 cal. This greater caloric density could lead to obesity, although the evidence that it does is limited. Fat intake in the more industrialized countries is greater than in the developing countries, so that it is correlated with the greater prostate cancer risk seen in those industrialized countries (2). Nonetheless, the inconsistency of the evidence (2, 3, 5, 9, 16, 17) suggests that overall fat intake is not likely to be a risk factor for prostate cancer.

Although fat is often described as one compound, fat as a macronutritional category is highly heterogeneous; hydrogen bonding within the fat molecule creates saturated, monounsaturated, and unsaturated fats with distinct properties and likely effects on prostate cancer risk (18). In one small case control study, the plasma level of alpha-linolenic acid was a strong, statistically significant predictor of prostate cancer risk (17). It is important, however, that this fatty acid is a very minor component of the total fat content of any one person's diet. A prospective study based upon diet history found only weak evidence of an alpha-linolenic acid association; the strongest predictor of prostate cancer risk among fats in that study was monounsaturated fatty acid (9). Several forms of vegetable fat have been chemically processed to make them soluble at room temperature and to preserve their shelf life; the impact of this processing upon cancer risk in general has not been adequately studied (2). There may, in addition, be differences of note in the composition of animal-source as opposed to vegetable-source fats. It has been suspected that the processing of vegetable fat, so that it in several dimensions resembles animal fat, may cause its effects on disease risk to mimic those of animal fats. Data from a large cohort study (9) and from a large case-control study

(6) suggested that fat derived from meat is strongly associated with prostate cancer risk.

Vitamin D/Calcium

Vitamin D and calcium's effects are closely linked, as they act synergistically. Thus, in one major supplementation study (13), calcium and vitamin D were administered together. Basic science strongly suggests that vitamin D, which induces cellular differentiation and apoptosis, has strong antiproliferative effects and inhibits invasiveness, angiogenesis, and metastasis of tumor cells, and should be protective against cancer (19); there is only very limited epidemiologic evidence that vitamin D intake is associated with altered risk of prostate cancer. It is important, however, that sunlight exposure has a massive effect on vitamin D stores. Thus, in many regions of the United States, sunlight exposure is a more important determinant than diet of vitamin D levels. In these regions, vitamin D from the diet is a minor component of total vitamin D exposure. The importance of dietary vitamin D exposure may be greater in the Northeastern United States than it is in the rest of the country (20). Giovannucci et al. suggested that the dietary vitamin D level required to achieve protection against cancer could be as high as 1,500 mcg/d; this level is well above what can be achieved with dietary practice alone.

On the other hand, calcium intake has been associated with increased risk of advanced or high-grade prostate cancer (19). In the study that linked vitamin D to diminished risk of prostate cancer, calcium intake was associated with insignificantly decreased risk of low-grade prostate cancer. This finding held up with adjustment for the major dietary factor in vitamin D, dairy product intake (19). It is possible that the intake of calcium interferes with the uptake of vitamin D, and that this diminished uptake of vitamin D is responsible for the risk enhancement observed with calcium (19).

Vitamin E and Carotenoids

Vitamin E, understood to be an antioxidant, has received a good deal of epidemiologic attention (8, 10). The strongest evidence that vitamin E is protective against prostate cancer came not from an observational epidemiologic study but from a clinical prevention trial in which prostate cancer was an unanticipated endpoint (21). The 29,000-subject Alpha-Tocopherol Beta-Carotene (ATBC) trial was designed to test the protective effects of vitamin E against coronary heart disease and beta-carotene against lung cancer among smokers. Neither agent proved to be protective against its target. However, among subjects assigned to vitamin E, there was a 30% decrease in the incidence of prostate cancer.

The ATBC finding provided a major impetus to the formulation of an even larger chemoprevention trial involving vitamin E: the Selenium and Vitamin E Cancer Prevention Trial (SELECT). In that study of over 35,000 men at average risk of prostate cancer, subjects were randomized, in a factorial design framework, to selenium 200 mcg/d or placebo, and to vitamin E 400 IU/d or placebo. The trial was stopped early, on the basis of a statistical futility analysis, as it had become clear that assignment to neither supplement decreased the risk of prostate or any other cancer. Nor did it decrease the risk of any other chronic disease or mortality (22). Subsequent analysis of the impact of vitamin E, based on extended follow-up, indicated that vitamin E supplementation actually increased the risk of prostate cancer (23); the increase in risk was approximately 17%. Thus, research in vitamin E–based chemoprevention is faced with the dilemma of one extremely large clinical trial indicating that vitamin E decreased the risk of an unanticipated endpoint, prostate cancer, while an even larger trial, in which prostate cancer was an anticipated endpoint, indicates that a larger dose of vitamin E actually increases the risk of prostate cancer.

Carotenoids are pigments found in foods. Nutritionally active, their powerful antioxidant capability could enable them to reduce free radical damage (5, 6, 8). A number of the more common carotenoids have received the bulk of nutritional attention: alpha- and beta-carotene, lycopene, luteine, cryptoxanthin, and zeaxanthine (7, 16, 24, 25). Lycopene, found mainly in tomato products, was shown in one large cohort study to be associated with substantially decreased risk of prostate cancer. Foods that contain substantial amounts of tomato products, including tomato sauce, tomatoes, and pizza, appeared to be strongly associated with decreased risk.

Selenium

Interest in selenium stemmed first from ecologic analyses that showed increased cancer risk in regions with low soil selenium. Foods grown in such areas have low selenium content, so that it is reasonably suspected that the diets of those in these regions would have low selenium stores (26). Clark's rationale for a trial of selenium supplementation, based largely on this ecologic observation, along with a number of observational studies (27–31), contributed strongly to the impetus for an even larger trial of selenium as a chemopreventive agent. Clark first designed a placebo-controlled trial, with some 1,200 subjects assigned to placebo or to 200 mcg/d selenium, to focus on nonmelanoma skin cancer. Clark had observed an excess of nonmelanoma skin cancer among residents of the southeastern and eastern United States, in a region marked by low soil selenium levels (26). After the trial had opened, Clark added prostate and several other cancers as trial endpoints; the final analysis of the trial indicated that selenium supplementation was associated a 50% decrease in the risk of prostate cancer (32). The study also showed significant effect modification by baseline blood selenium; among men with blood selenium in the lowest tertile (<105.2 ng/mL), selenium supplementation was associated with a substantial decrease in prostate cancer; among men with blood selenium in the middle tertile (105.3–121.6 ng/mL), it was associated with a less marked decrease in risk; among those with blood selenium in the highest tertile (>121.6 ng/mL), it was associated with an increase in risk of prostate cancer (32). As noted, the SELECT study, designed to build on the Clark results, recruited men from the entire United States population. The average baseline blood selenium level of these subjects was over 135 ng/mL. Thus, the finding that 200 mcg/d selenium supplementation had no effect on prostate cancer risk was consistent with what had been observed among comparable subjects in the Clark trial (32). A smaller trial, conducted among men with a condition believed to be premalignant, high-grade prostatic intraepithelial neoplasia (HGPIN), randomized 450 subjects to selenium 200 mcg/d or to placebo; this trial also found no alteration of prostate cancer risk with selenium supplementation (33). A similar trial, also conducted among men with HGPIN, tested the effect of assignment to a three-agent regimen consisting of soy protein 40 g, vitamin E 800 IU, and selenium 200 mcg, and showed no protection against progression from HGPIN to prostate cancer (34). Thus, the epidemiologic studies that have observed selenium exposure to be associated with decreased cancer risk have not been supported by randomized, placebo-controlled trials that tested the effect of selenium supplementation.

One possible explanation of the discrepancy between the observational and experimental research on selenium has to do with the form of selenium used in the supplementation trials. The earliest trial (26) administered selenium in yeast that had been cultured in a seleniferous medium. It was believed at the time of the trial that most of the selenium was in the form of selenomethionine (26), although careful speciation of the yeast Clark used raised questions about this understanding (35). The other trials (22, 23, 33, 34) used selenomethionine. It is possible, however, that selenomethionine is a poor vehicle for generating the bioactive compounds in selenium that were shown to be protective against prostate cancer in observational studies (36). A single-dose pharmacokinetics trial has suggested that selenomethionine may have a different profile than some other selenium species; a multiple-dose pharmacokinetics and pharmacokinetics trial is under way (36).

Folate

It is widely recognized that folate has important metabolic effects. It plays important roles in cell replication and repair (1), enabling nucleotide formation, and dietary folate has been shown to be associated with diminished risk of a number of cancers. Nonetheless, studies of folate supplementation have shown surprising and disappointing results; in one large and well-controlled study, randomization to folate supplementation 1 mg/d led to increased risk of prostate cancer (37). That same study also had shown that folate supplementation was associated with the formation of advanced colorectal cancer. Folate intake at study baseline was associated with slightly diminished risk of prostate cancer, but supplementation resulted in a near tripling of risk. The authors noted the assumption that folic acid, the agent used to deliver folate, has effects equal to those of dietary folate; they suggested that the assumption may be incorrect (37). They also recognized the possibility that folate in cell replication and repair could support the growth of cancer cells as well as those of normal cells. Thus, given the extremely long duration of premalignant lesions and early cancers of the prostate, an agent that supports cellular growth could confer an advantage to cells with disturbed growth patterns, such as prostatic intraepithelial neoplasia or early cancer.

Plant and Animal Products

As noted, a large cohort study (9) and two large case-control studies (5, 6) found that the consumption of fat from red meat was associated with increased risk of prostate cancer. In general, this animal fat was more linked to risk than was fat from plant products. As already noted, fat from meat and animal products could have significantly different effects than fat from plant products. Plant products, for example, do not contain cholesterol, and their fat is more likely than that from animal products to contain unsaturated, as opposed to saturated, fat. An evaluation of the relative impact of vegetable as opposed to animal products, including fats and proteins, is needed. The limitations of observational studies of plant as opposed to animal product consumption, however, are daunting (38–42). It is simply very difficult to accurately measure the intake of plant as opposed to animal products.

An effort currently underway in the Alliance for Clinical Trials in Oncology, the Men's Eating and Living (MEAL) study, will address the need for additional data. The MEAL study is a randomized-control trial of diet change for men with low-grade, low-volume prostate cancer. It is actually a trial meant to forestall the development of higher grade, aggressive prostate cancer. Men who have low-grade, low-volume prostate cancer are increasingly assigned to expectant management, also known as watchful waiting. Approximately 20% of patients on expectant management proceed to develop higher grade, potentially lethal prostate cancer. The MEAL study will be distinct in an important dimension that is critical; it will be a study of objectively measured dietary *change*, not only of dietary constituents, nutrients, or a dietary pattern.

Patients assigned to diet intervention work with a lifestyle coach, with the intervention delivered over the telephone. The extent of change in experimental as opposed to control patients, however, is monitored by self-report and by an objective measure: change in the blood levels of several carotenoids. Patients will be closely monitored for the prostate-specific antigen (PSA). Any patient who experiences a rapid rise in the PSA will be referred for additional follow-up and biopsy, according to clinical judgment. Progression will be marked by an increase in the PSA above a concentration of 10 ng/mL, an increase in the rate of rise of the PSA, an increase in the Gleason grade of the cancer, or in the size of the tumor. Preliminary pilot data have shown that the dietary intervention leads to significantly changed dietary reports, as well as to noteworthy changes in blood levels of biomarker nutrients that are only found in plant products (43–45).

■ OBESITY AS A MARKER OF ENERGY IMBALANCE

An often overlooked but potentially critical biomarker of the balance between energy intake and energy expenditure is obesity. It can be argued that, in the Western industrialized countries, obesity, which is associated with altered insulin levels (46, 47), elevated oxidative stress, and genetic damage, is a significant public health problem (1). The etiology of obesity and its significance for prostate cancer risk, however, are complex. Energy and nutrient intake at critical points of the life cycle are associated with greater height, while intakes at other points are associated with obesity (48). Height has been associated with increased risk of prostate cancer, while obesity during childhood has also been linked to risk (48). However, the association of obesity, generally measured by the body mass index (weight in kg/(height in meters)^2), has not been consistently linked to increased risk of prostate cancer (49, 50). It has been claimed that the strongest association is of obesity with more aggressive prostate cancer, although not even that observation is entirely consistent (50–52). Part of the complexity may be because the total body mass may affect the diagnosis of prostate cancer (50). The type of obesity, especially the distribution of body fat, may be critical (53).

■ ISSUES FOR FUTURE RESEARCH

Inconsistency

A troubling characteristic of epidemiologic studies of diet and prostate cancer—indeed, of diet and each of the major cancers—is the inconsistency of findings. One study may find an association between diet and prostate cancer, while others do not see it. It is highly uncommon for dietary epidemiologic findings not to find one or more risk factors for prostate cancer; the problem is that these findings are rarely replicated in repeated studies. Thus, a series of epidemiologic studies and a small prevention trial found selenium and vitamin E deficiencies to be risk factors for prostate cancer; replication by trials showed that neither selenium supplementation nor vitamin E supplementation was linked to diminished risk. Inconsistency of this sort suggests that the methods used for study do not provide reliable results; also troubling is that this inconsistency reduces public trust in prevention research.

The sources of this inconsistency may be multiple. One impediment to progress may be reliance among prevention researchers on small case-control studies. These are relatively inexpensive and easy to execute; they can be undertaken by researchers with relatively few resources. They are, unfortunately, susceptible to a number of complications that confound attempts to interpret them. For example, in case-control studies of diet and prostate cancer, subjects may be asked to recall their dietary practice from years to decades prior to interview. Studies have suggested that recall of prior diet has some validity; whether the validity is adequate to reveal moderate-to-weak associations between diet and cancer risk, however, is less clear. A more appropriate means of assessing the diet may be to use biologic markers of diet: blood markers of carotenoids, lipids, or minerals in animal as opposed to plant products. Research in diet and prostate cancer may necessarily need to rely more on prospective studies and prevention trials, and less on small case-control studies. Unfortunately, however, biomarkers cannot be readily used in a case-control context: in a comparison of cases and controls, especially in a comparison of cases with aggressive cancer, as opposed to controls, it is possible that differences in nutritional levels may be a consequence of, rather than a source of, differences.

Given the inconsistency in findings regarding diet and prostate cancer, it is difficult to escape the suspicion that diet has a relatively minor role in prostate cancer risk. One of the challenges for the future may be distinguishing the different types and grades of prostate cancer. As noted, prostate cancer in epidemiologic studies has been treated as a unitary, homogeneous cancer category; this may, as already noted, be an oversimplification (4). It may be that future research on dietary effects on prostate needs to focus less on the development of prostate cancer per se than on the progression of prostate cancer from indolent to aggressive disease. The MEAL study may be a prototype of the research that is needed: a randomized trial in which subjects are assigned to a dietary intervention, or to receive no intervention. The focus of this study is dietary change, rather than dietary practice.

Finally, there may be need for substantially increased investment in the pharmacokinetics of dietary elements. It has often been assumed that, if a nutrient or compound is useful and protective against cancer, then more of that nutrient can only be more useful and more protective. This has, however, been shown to be incorrect in a number of cases. In one study addressed to prevention of colorectal cancer, 81 mg of aspirin was protective, but 325 mg conferred absolutely no protection (54). Beta carotene was associated with decreased lung cancer risk in a large number of epidemiologic studies, but it was shown to increase the risk of lung cancer in supplementation studies (55, 56): it became clear, after the studies were completed, that the dose of beta-carotene used was far in excess of the amount usually ingested in epidemiologic studies (57). Thus, the impact of diet on prostate cancer risk will require a good deal more attention to the metabolic and pharmacokinetic behavior of the elements of diet among humans.

■ REFERENCES

1. Thompson IM, Goodman PJ, Tangen CM, et al. The influence of finasteride on the development of prostate cancer. *N Engl J Med.* 2003;349(3):215–224.
2. Thompson IM, Pauler DK, Goodman PJ, et al. Prevalence of prostate cancer among men with a prostate-specific antigen level <4.0 ng per Milliliter. *N Engl J Med.* 2004;350(22):2239–2246.
3. Andriole GL, Bostwick DG, Brawley OW, et al. Effect of dutasteride on the risk of prostate cancer. *N Engl J Med.* 2010;362(13):1192–1202.
4. GLOBOCAN. *Prostate Cancer Incidence and Mortality Worldwide in 2008 Summary.* http://globocan.iarc.fr/factsheets/cancers/prostate.asp. Updated 2008. Accessed September 2011.
5. Hayes RB, Ziegler RG, Gridley G, et al. Dietary factors and risks for prostate cancer among blacks and whites in the United States. *Cancer Epidemiol Biomarkers Prev.* 1999;8(1):25–34.
6. Freedland SJ, Platz EA. Obesity and prostate cancer: making sense out of apparently conflicting data. *Epidemiol Rev.* 2007;29:88–97.
7. Freeman VL, Meydani M, Yong S, et al. Assessing the effect of fatty acids on prostate carcinogenesis in humans: does self-reported dietary intake rank prostatic exposure correctly? *Am J Clin Nutr.* 2001;73:815–820.
8. Kolonel LN, Wilkens LR. Migrant studies. In: Schottenfeld D, Fraumeni JF, eds. *Cancer Epidemiology and Prevention.* New York, NY: Oxford University Press; 2006:189–201.
9. Gronberg H, Damber L, Damber JE. Total food consumption and body mass index in relation to prostate cancer risk: a case-control study in Sweden with prospectively collected exposure data. *J Urol.* 1996;155(3):969–974.
10. Willett W. *Nutritional epidemiology.* New York, NY: Oxford University Press; 1998.
11. Marshall JR, Hastrup JL. Mismeasurement and the resonance of strong confounders: uncorrelated errors. *Am J Epidemiol.* 1996;143(10):1069–1078.
12. Marshall JR, Hastrup JL, Ross JS. Mismeasurement and the resonance of strong confounders: correlated errors. *Am J Epidemiol.* 1999;150(1):88–96.
13. Wactawski-Wende J, Kotchen JM, Anderson GL, et al. Calcium plus vitamin D supplementation and the risk of colorectal cancer. *N Engl J Med.* 2006;354(7):684–696.
14. Breslow N, Chan CW, Dhom G, et al. Latent carcinoma of prostate at autopsy in seven areas. Collaborative Study organized by the International Agency for Research on Cancer, Lyons, France. *Int J Cancer.* 1977;20:680–688.
15. Allen NE, Key TJ, Appleby PN, et al. Serum insulin-like growth factor (IGF)-I and IGF-binding protein-3 concentrations and prostate cancer risk: results from the European prospective investigation into cancer and nutrition. *Cancer Epidemiol Biomarkers Prev.* 2007;16(6):1121–1127.
16. Giovannucci E, Rimm EB, Colditz GA, et al. A prospective study of dietary fat and risk of prostate cancer. *J Natl Cancer Inst.* 1993;85(19):1571–1579.
17. Augustsson K, Michaud DS, Rimm EB, et al. A prospective study of intake of fish and marine fatty acids and prostate cancer. *Cancer Epidemiol Biomarkers Prev.* 2003;12:64–67.
18. Gann PH, Hennekens CH, Sacks FM, et al. Prospective study of plasma fatty acids and risk of prostate cancer. *J Natl Cancer Inst.* 1994;86(4):281–286.
19. Gong Z, Neuhouser ML, Goodman PJ, et al. Obesity, diabetes, and risk of prostate cancer: results from the Prostate Cancer Prevention Trial. *Cancer Epidemiol Biomarkers Prev.* 2006;15(10):1977–1983.
20. Giovannucci E. The epidemiology of vitamin D and cancer incidence and mortality: a review (United States). *Cancer Causes Control.* 2005;16:83–95.
21. Hsing AW, Sakoda LC, Chua SC. Obesity, metabolic syndrome, and prostate cancer. *Am J Clin Nutr.* 2007;86(suppl):843S–857S.
22. Kane CJ, Bassett WW, Sadetsky N, et al. Obesity and prostate cancer clinical risk factors at presentation: data from CaPsure. *J Urol.* 2005;173(3):732–736.
23. Chen C, Freeman R, Voigt LF, et al. Prostate cancer risk in relation to selected genetic polymorphisms in insulin-like growth factor-1, insulin-like growth factor binding protein-3, and insulin-like growth factor-1 receptor. *Cancer Epidemiol Biomarkers Prev.* 2006;15(12):2461–2466.
24. Schuurman AG, Goldbohm RA, Dorant E, et al. Vegetable and fruit consumption and prostate cancer risk: a cohort study in the Netherlands. *Cancer Epidemiol Biomarkers Prev.* 1998;7(8):673–680.
25. Marshall JR, Chen Z. Diet and health risk: risk patterns and disease-specific associations. *Am J Clin Nutr.* 1999;69(6):1351S–1356S.
26. Giovannucci E, Liu Y, Stampfer MJ, et al. A prospective study of calcium intake and incident and fatal prostate cancer. *Cancer Epidemiol Biomarkers Prev.* 2006;15(2):203–210.
27. Heinonen OP, Albanes D, Virtamo J, et al. Prostate cancer and supplementation with a-tocopherol and B-carotene: incidence and mortality in a controlled trial. *J Natl Cancer Inst.* 1998;90(6):440–446.
28. Lippman SM, Klein EA, Goodman PJ, et al. Effect of selenium and vitamin E on risk of prostate cancer and other cancers the selenium and vitamin E cancer prevention trial (SELECT). *JAMA.* 2009;301(1):E1–E13.
29. Clark LC, Combs GF, Turnbull BW, et al. Effects of selenium supplementation for cancer prevention in patients with carcinoma of the skin a randomized controlled trial. *J AMA.* 1996;276(24):1957–1963.
30. Brooks JD, Jeffrey ME, Chan DW, et al. Plasma selenium level before diagnosis and the risk of prostate cancer development. *J Urol.* 2001;166(6):2034–2038.
31. Ghadirian P, Maisonneuve P, Perret C, et al. A case-control study of toenail selenium and cancer of the breast, colon, and prostate. *Cancer Detect Prev.* 2000;24(4), 305–313.
32. Goodman GE, Schaffer S, Bankson DD, et al. Predictors of serum selenium in cigarette smokers and the lack of association with lung and prostate cancer risk. *Cancer Epidemiol Biomarkers Prev.* 2001;10(10):1069–1076.
33. Vogt TM, Ziegler RG, Graubard BI, et al. Serum selenium and risk of prostate cancer in U.S. blacks and whites. *Int J Cancer.* 2003;103:664–670.

34. Fleshner NE, Kapusta L, Donnelly B, et al. Progression from high-grade prostatic intraepithelial neoplasia to cancer: a randomized trial of combination vitamin-E, soy, and selenium. *J Clin Oncol.* 2011;29(17):2386–2390.
35. Uden PC, Boakye HT, Kahakachchi C, et al. Element selective characterization of stability and reactivity of selenium species in selenized yeast. *J Anal At Spectrom.* 2004;19(1):65–73.
36. Marshall JR, Clement I, Romano K, et al. Methyl selenocysteine: single-dose pharmacokinetics in men. *Cancer Prev Res.* 2011;4(11):1938–1944.
37. Figueiredo JC, Grau MV, Haile RW, et al. Folic acid and risk of prostate cancer: results from a randomized clinical trial. *J Natl Cancer Inst.* 2009;101(6):432–435.
38. Allen NE, Appleby PN, Roddam AW, et al. Plasma selenium concentration and prostate cancer risk: results from the European Prospective Investigation into cancer and nutrition (EPIC)1-3. *Am J Clin Nutr.* 2008;88:1567–1575.
39. Duffield-Lillico AJ, Dalkin BL, Reid ME, et al. Selenium supplementation, baseline plasma selenium status and incidence of prostate cancer: an analysis of the complete treatment period of the nutritional prevention of cancer trial. *BJU Int.* 2003;91:608–612.
40. Helzlsouer KJ, Huang HY, Alberg AJ, et al. Association between a-Tocopherol, y-Tocopherol, Selenium, and subsequent prostate cancer. *J Natl Cancer Inst.* 2000;92(24):2018–2023.
41. Marshall JR, Tangen CM, Sakr WA, et al. Phase III trial of selenium to prevent prostate cancer in men with high-grade prostatic intraepithelial neoplasia: SWOG S9917. *Cancer Prev Res.* 2011;4(11):1761–1769.
42. Graham S. Diet and cancer. *Am J Epidemiol.* 1980;112(2):247–252.
43. Khan MA, Carter HB, Epstein JI, et al. Cancer prostate specific antigen derivatives and pathological parameters predict significant change in expectant management criteria for prostate cancer? *J Urol.* 2003;170(6):2274–2278.
44. Warlick C, Trock BJ, Landis P, et al. Delayed versus immediate surgical intervention and prostate cancer outcome. *J Natl Cancer Inst.* 2006;98(5):355–357.
45. Carter HB, Kettermann A, Warlick C, et al. Expectant management of prostate cancer with curative intent: an update of the Johns Hopkins experience. *J Urol.* 2007;178(6):2359–2365.
46. Andersson SO, Wolk A, Bergstrom R, et al. Energy, nutrient intake and prostate cancer risk: a population-based case-control study in Sweden. *Int J Cancer.* 1996;68:716–722.
47. Kristal AR, Stanford JL. Cruciferous vegetables and prostate cancer risk: confounding by PSA screening. *Cancer Epidemiol Biomarkers Prev.* 2004;13(7):1265.
48. Giovannucci E, Rimm EB, Stampfer MJ, et al. Height, body weight, and risk of prostate cancer. *Cancer Epidemiol Biomarkers Prev.* 1997;6(8):557–563.
49. Graham S. Epidemiolgic studies of diet and cancer (42420). *Proc Soc Exp Biol Med.* 1986;183:281–286.
50. Kolonel LN, Hinds MW, Nomura AMY, et al. Relationship of dietary vitamin A and ascorbic acid intake to the risk for cancers of the lung, bladder, and prostate in Hawaii. *Monogr Natl Cancer Inst.* 1985;69:137–142.
51. Gann PH, Ma J, Giovannucci E, et al. Lower prostate cancer risk in men with elevated plasma lycopene levels: results of a prospective analysis. *Cancer Res.* 1999;59(6):1225–1230.
52. Schuurman AG, Goldbohm RA, Brants HA, et al. A prospective cohort study on intake of retinol, vitamins C and E, and carotenoids and prostate cancer risk (Netherlands). *Cancer Causes Control.* 2002;13(6):573–582.
53. Huang HY, Alberg AJ, Norkus EP, et al. Prospective study of antioxidant micronutrients in the blood and the risk of developing prostate cancer. *Am J Epidemiol.* 2003;157(4):335–344.
54. Baron JA, Cole BF, Sandler RS, et al. A randomized trial of aspirin to prevent colorectal adenomas. *N Engl J Med.* 2003;348(10):891–899.
55. Omenn GS, Goodman GE, Thornquist MD, et al. Effects of a combination of beta carotene and vitamin A on lung cancer and cardiovascular disease. *N Engl J Med.* 1996;334(18):1150–1155.
56. Heinonen OP, Albanes D. The effect of vitamin E and beta carotene on the incidence of lung cancer and other cancers in male smokers. *N Engl J Med.* 1994;330(15):1029–1035.
57. Institute of Medicine (IOM). *Dietary Reference Intakes for Vitamin C, Vitamin E, Selenium, and Carotenoids.* Washington, DC: National Academy Press; 2000.

2.3 Epidemiology: Obesity as a Risk Factor

EMMA H. ALLOTT

STEPHEN J. FREEDLAND

INTRODUCTION

Obesity is associated with increased risk of incidence of and mortality from numerous tumor types, including prostate cancer (PC) (1–3). An improved understanding of the role of this modifiable risk factor in PC etiology, especially aggressive PC, is imperative to optimize screening, treatment, and prevention of PC. This chapter focuses on the epidemiologic association between obesity and PC incidence, treatment, and mortality.

OBESITY AND PC INCIDENCE

Meta-analyses have consistently reported modest positive associations between obesity and total PC incidence (3–5). Of note, a meta-analysis that separated localized from advanced PC revealed that while there was a null or slightly protective effect for localized disease, obesity was more strongly associated with increased incidence of advanced PC (6). This dichotomous effect of obesity on PC incidence is multifactorial: attributable in part to detection biases associated with obesity (leading to delayed diagnosis and more advanced disease at diagnosis) and also to underlying biological mechanisms. Numerous factors contribute toward difficulty detecting PC in obese men. First, obese men have lower prostate-specific antigen (PSA) values, resulting in reduced PSA-driven biopsy rates (7–9). Second, obesity may make it more challenging to perform a thorough digital rectal examination (DRE), leading to yet more missed cancers (10). Third, obese men have larger prostates, reducing the likelihood of finding cancer at biopsy (11). These detection biases may allow PC growth to continue unchecked, thus contributing to elevated incidence of advanced disease in obese men (Figure 2.3.1). However, given that obesity was associated with PC mortality even in the pre-PSA, premodern biopsy era (12) (i.e., in the absence of these aforementioned detection biases), detection bias cannot fully explain the link between obesity and aggressive PC; biological mechanisms must also play a role.

OBESITY AND PC TREATMENT

Radical Prostatectomy

A systematic review and meta-analysis reported 21% increased risk of biochemical recurrence (BCR) and a 15% increased risk of PC-specific mortality following RP, per 5 kg/m^2 increase in BMI (13). While some data showed that obesity was associated with capsular incision, reflecting a less-than-ideal operation (14), obesity remained associated with poor outcome even after adjusting for pathological features including margin status (13, 15). This suggested that poor technique alone cannot explain the link between obesity and aggressive PC, but that biological mechanisms also play a part.

Nonsurgical Treatment

Regarding outcomes after radiation, while a meta-analysis found no association between obesity and BCR for brachytherapy-treated patients, obesity was associated with 16% increased risk of BCR for external beam radiation–treated patients, per 5 kg/m^2 increase in BMI (13).

One study found that obesity at the time of androgen deprivation therapy (ADT) increased risk of castrate resistant PC (CRPC), metastases, and PC-specific mortality (16). Another reported elevated testosterone levels in obese relative to normal weight men on ADT, suggesting inadequate testosterone suppression may contribute to these worse outcomes (17). Beyond possibly predicting a poor oncologic outcome, obesity may also increase ADT side effects: one study found that it was associated with almost fivefold increased risk of new-onset type II diabetes (18).

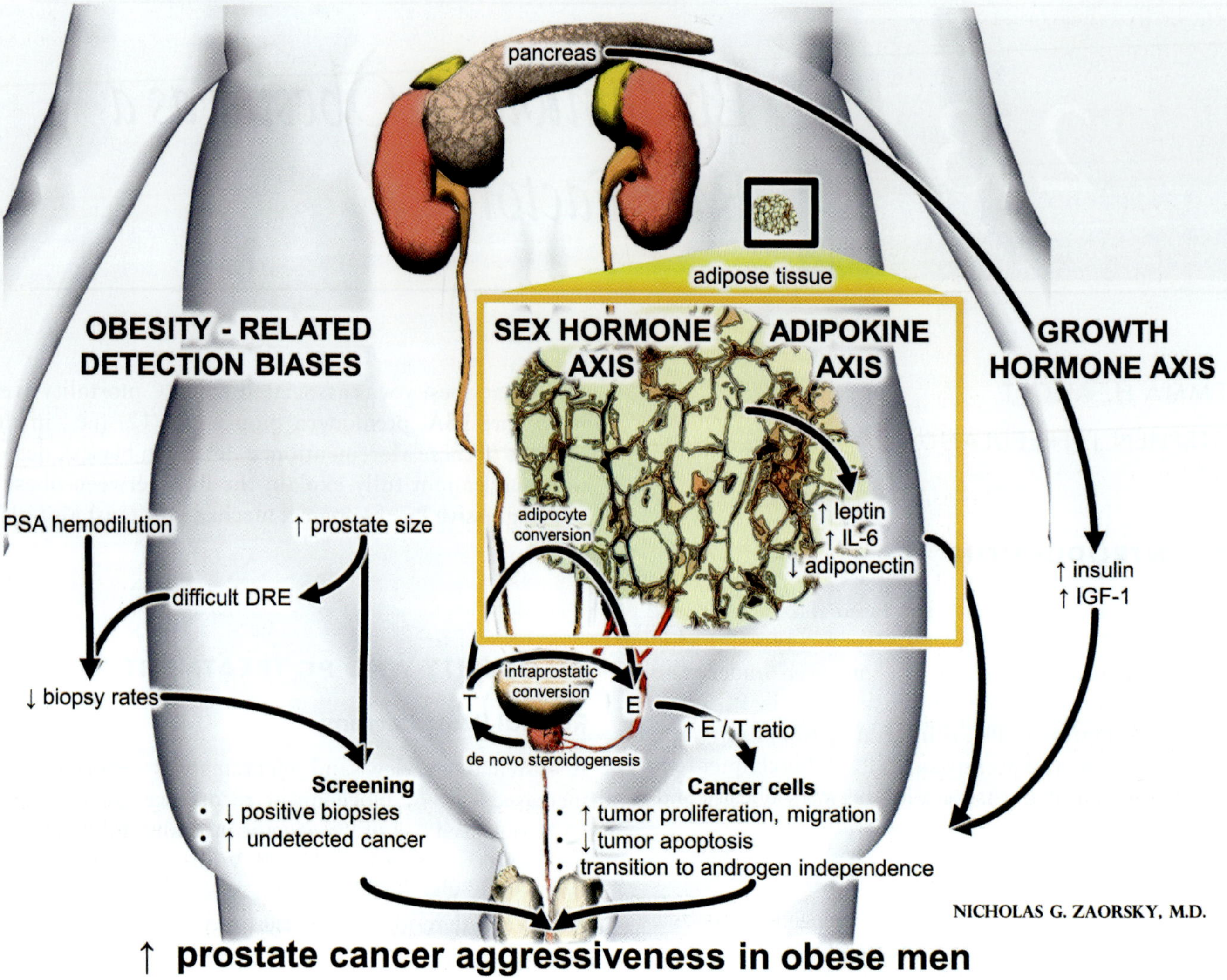

FIGURE 2.3.1 Obesity-related detection biases and biological mechanisms contributing to the epidemiologic association between obesity and aggressive prostate cancer (T = testosterone, E = estrogen).
Source: From Ref. (22). Allott EH, Masko EM, Freedland SJ. Obesity: weighing the evidence. Eur Urol. 2013;63(5):800–809.

Finally, given obesity is associated with upgrading at RP (19), body size should be taken into account when considering patients for active surveillance, highlighting the need for close monitoring of these patients.

■ OBESITY AND PC-SPECIFIC MORTALITY

Multiple large cohort studies have consistently demonstrated a positive, dose-response relationship between increasing BMI and fatal PC (1, 20, 21), with a meta-analysis reporting 15% increased PC-specific mortality, per 5 kg/m^2 increase in BMI (13). While this effect may be attributable in part to delayed PC diagnosis in obese versus normal weight men, obesity was associated with PC mortality even in the pre-PSA era (12, 20), demonstrating that this association cannot be explained by detection bias alone, and that underlying biologic mechanisms play an important role.

■ CONCLUSIONS

Epidemiologic evidence linking obesity and aggressive PC underlines the importance of taking body size into account when screening, treating, and monitoring PC patients, as well as counseling obese patients toward healthier lifestyle choices and weight loss (22). Unfortunately, no clinical trials specifically examining the effects of weight loss in PC patients have been completed, nor are the biologic mechanisms linking obesity and PC fully elucidated, though multiple pathways have been implicated (Figure 2.3.1). Improved understanding of the contributing mechanisms would likely provide valuable information regarding the etiology of aggressive PC, which could in turn be used to develop better approaches for prevention and treatment for all men. Furthermore, it is advisable for all individuals to maintain a healthy weight, especially for those beginning ADT, which can lead to further weight gain and metabolic disturbances. Indeed, given that more men diagnosed with

PC die from heart disease than from the cancer itself, this recommendation more than any other is most likely to have a positive impact on quality and quantity of life.

REFERENCES

1. Calle EE, Rodriguez C, Walker-Thurmond K, Thun MJ. Overweight, obesity, and mortality from cancer in a prospectively studied cohort of U.S. adults. *N Engl J Med*. 2003;348:1625–1638.
2. Reeves GK, Pirie K, Beral V, et al. Cancer incidence and mortality in relation to body mass index in the Million Women Study: cohort study. *BMJ*. 2007;335:1134.
3. Renchan AG, Tyson M, Egger M, Heller RF, Zwahlen M. Body-mass index and incidence of cancer: a systematic review and meta-analysis of prospective observational studies. *Lancet*. 2008;371:569–578.
4. MacInnis RJ, English DR. Body size and composition and prostate cancer risk: systematic review and meta-regression analysis. *Cancer Causes Control*. 2006;17:989–1003.
5. Bergstrom A, Pisani P, Tenet V, Wolk A, Adami HO. Overweight as an avoidable cause of cancer in Europe. *Int J Cancer*. 2001;91:421–430.
6. Discacciati A, Orsini N, Wolk A. Body mass index and incidence of localized and advanced prostate cancer–a dose-response meta-analysis of prospective studies. *Ann Oncol*. 2012;23:1665–1671.
7. Banez LL, Hamilton RJ, Partin AW, et al. Obesity-related plasma hemodilution and PSA concentration among men with prostate cancer. *JAMA*. 2007;298:2275–2280.
8. Hekal IA, Ibrahiem EI. Obesity-PSA relationship: a new formula. *Prostate Cancer Prostatic Dis*. 2010;13:186–190.
9. Grubb RL, Black A, Izmirlian G, et al. Serum prostate-specific antigen hemodilution among obese men undergoing screening in the Prostate, Lung, Colorectal, and Ovarian Cancer Screening Trial. *Cancer Epidemiol Biomarkers Prev*. 2009;18:748–751.
10. Chu DI, De Nunzio C, Gerber L, et al. Predictive value of digital rectal examination for prostate cancer detection is modified by obesity. *Prostate Cancer Prostatic Dis*. 2011;14:346–353.
11. Freedland SJ, Platz EA, Presti JC Jr, et al. Obesity, serum prostate specific antigen and prostate size: implications for prostate cancer detection. *J Urol*. 2006;175:500–504.
12. Rodriguez C, Patel AV, Calle EE, et al. Body mass index, height, and prostate cancer mortality in two large cohorts of adult men in the United States. *Cancer Epidemiol Biomarkers Prev*. 2001;10:345–353.
13. Cao Y, Ma J. Body mass index, prostate cancer-specific mortality, and biochemical recurrence: a systematic review and meta-analysis. *Cancer Prev Res (Phila)*. 2011;4:486–501.
14. Freedland SJ, Grubb KA, Yiu SK, et al. Obesity and capsular incision at the time of open retropubic radical prostatectomy. *J Urol*. 2005;174:1798–1801.
15. Okotie OT, Aronson WJ, Wieder JA, et al. Predictors of metastatic disease in men with biochemical failure following radical prostatectomy. *J Urol*. 2004;171:2260–2264.
16. Keto CJ, Aronson WJ, Terris MK, et al. Obesity is associated with castration-resistant disease and metastasis in men treated with androgen deprivation therapy after radical prostatectomy: results from the SEARCH database. *BJU Int*. 2011;110:492–498.
17. Smith MR. Obesity and sex steroids during gonadotropin-releasing hormone agonist treatment for prostate cancer. *Clin Cancer Res*. 2007;13:241–245.
18. Derweesh IH, Diblasio CJ, Kincade MC, et al. Risk of new-onset diabetes mellitus and worsening glycaemic variables for established diabetes in men undergoing androgen-deprivation therapy for prostate cancer. *BJU Int*. 2007;100:1060–1065.
19. Ploussard G, de la Taille A, Bayoud Y, et al. The risk of upstaged disease increases with body mass index in low-risk prostate cancer patients eligible for active surveillance. *Eur Urol*. 2011;61:356–362.
20. Andersson SO, Wolk A, Bergstrom R, et al. Body size and prostate cancer: a 20-year follow-up study among 135006 Swedish construction workers. *J Natl Cancer Inst*. 1997;89:385–389.
21. Wright ME, Chang SC, Schatzkin A, et al. Prospective study of adiposity and weight change in relation to prostate cancer incidence and mortality. *Cancer*. 2007;109:675–684.
22. Allott EH, Masko EM, Freedland SJ. Obesity: weighing the evidence. *Eur Urol*. 2013;63(5):800–809.

3.1.1 Screening and Diagnosis: The Pros of PSA Screening

JANINE L. OLIVER
GURDARSHAN S. SANDHU
GERALD L. ANDRIOLE
ROBERT L. GRUBB III

Prostate cancer (PCa) is the most common cancer diagnosed in males, accounting for an estimated 238,590 new cases and 29,720 deaths in 2013 (1). This high incidence to mortality ratio is strongly linked to the introduction of prostate-specific antigen (PSA) as a screening test in the 1980s, which facilitated the detection of PCa over pre-existing methods (2, 3). A sustained decrease in PCa mortality has been noted since the early 1990s (4). There have been annual PCa mortality decreases of 4.1% from 1994 to 2005 and 2.6% from 2005 to 2007 (5). The decline in PCa mortality began as PSA testing was beginning to become widespread. Age-adjusted PCa mortality has also decreased more rapidly in the United States (1990–2005), where screening was more prevalent, than in the United Kingdom (6). Although it is notable that advances in PCa treatment, including the increased practice of radical prostatectomy, the introduction of improved forms of radiation therapy, and the increased use of hormonal therapy in the decade prior to the introduction of PSA screening, may have collectively accounted for some of the mortality reduction, we cannot ignore the fact that since the introduction of PSA screening, the incidence of metastatic disease at presentation has declined by approximately three-fourths in the United States (7). PSA screening was rapidly adopted after its introduction and widely promoted in the United States as a public health initiative without evidence of improved mortality (8). Results of recently completed large-scale screening trials with conflicting results have fueled rather than resolved the controversy surrounding PSA screening. These apparently discordant results have left interpretation open for various medical organizations to issue disparate recommendations for PSA-based screening. Herein, we will review the substantial data that suggest that PSA-based screening, although not a perfect screening modality, remains a valuable test in properly selected patients.

Multiple randomized trials have demonstrated a significant reduction in PCa-specific mortality rates attributable to PSA-based screening for PCa (9–12). The largest of these is the European Randomized Study of Screening for Prostate Cancer (ERSPC) trial, which randomized 182,160 men to a screening arm or control group across 7 European countries (9, 13). The screening regimen was not uniform across all centers, but a PSA of 3.0 ng/mL was most commonly used as the threshold for a biopsy. Digital rectal exam was omitted from the screening process. No difference in overall mortality was noted in the entire study population (risk ratio [RR] 0.99, 95% confidence interval [CI] 0.97–1.01) (13), but for a predefined "core group" of men aged 55 to 69 years (n = 162,243), there was a 21% reduction in PCa-specific mortality seen in the screened group (RR 0.79, 95% CI 0.68–0.91) at 11 years median follow-up. This corresponded to an absolute mortality risk reduction of 1.07 deaths per 1,000 men. Researchers concluded that 1,055 men would need to be screened and 37 cases of PCa would need to be detected to prevent one PCa death. (Notably, the number of women needed to be screened for breast cancer with a mammogram to prevent one death is much larger, approximately 1300–1900 depending on patient's age (14).) Further, based on data from the ERSPC, the cumulative risk of metastatic disease at 9 to 11 years of follow-up was 31% to 33% lower in the screened arm compared to the control arm.

The PCa-specific mortality risk reduction is even greater in the ERSPC trial after adjusting for the effects of noncompliance in the intervention arm as well as contamination in the control group. To adjust for these effects, Roobol et al. extrapolated the contamination seen in the Rotterdam arm (15.2% true contamination) to the entire ERSPC cohort (15). After adjusting only for noncompliance, the PCa mortality risk reduction further increased to 27% (RR 0.73, 95% CI 0.58–0.93). With adjustment for both noncompliance and contamination, the PCa mortality risk reduction increased to 29% to 31% (RR 0.69, 95% CI 0.51–0.92 and RR 0.71, 95% CI 0.55–0.93) (15).

Another significant population-based screening trial was performed in Göteborg, Sweden (16). Although many of the patients were also included in ERSPC, in this trial, 19,904 men aged 50 to 64 years were randomized to screening or a control group. Screening was performed with a PSA every 2 years, with additional evaluation (consisting of digital rectal examination [DRE] and biopsy) performed for an elevated PSA. The PSA cutoff was noted to have changed over the course of the study. (A PSA cutoff of 3.4 was used at the beginning of the study, but this was later lowered to 2.5.) A total of 76% of men in the intervention group attended screening at least once. After a median follow-up of 14 years, a significant 44% decrease in PCa mortality was noted in the screened group (RR 0.56, 95% CI 0.39–0.82), with a 56% risk reduction noted in the group of men actually screened (RR 0.44, 95% CI 0.28–0.68). Based on the observed risk reduction, to prevent one PCa death, the number needed to screen was 293 and the number needed to treat (NNT) was 12.

It is worth noting that even in this strongly positive trial for PSA screening performed in a population at high risk for PCa and PCa mortality, it has been estimated that 1,000 men would need to be screened for 14 years to avert 5 PCa deaths, and with that screening, about 120 men would have been diagnosed and potentially treated (17). An additional important observation stemming from this trial was that this improvement in mortality was seen in a population where about 30% of men in each arm diagnosed with PCa were managed with active surveillance at last follow-up, suggesting that the risks of overtreatment can be minimized by good clinical management (16).

Although not considered as robust due to methodological flaws, the Laval University Prostate Cancer Screening Program trial randomized 46,486 men aged 45 to 80 to screening or no screening in 1988 (12). Screening in this study included serum PSA (with 3.0 ng/mL being the upper limit of normal) and DRE at the first visit, with PSA only on subsequent visits. In the group invited for screening, 23.6% of men were screened compared with 7.3% of controls who received screening. No difference in PCa mortality was observed after a median follow-up of 7.93 years, based on an intention-to-screen analysis (RR 1.085, 95% CI 0.822–1.29). However, based on a per protocol analysis, there was a significant 62% decrease in PCa mortality (RR 0.385, 95% CI 0.207–0.714, $P = .0025$).

The Stockholm trial randomly invited 2,400 men aged 55 to 70 years to a one-time screening for PCa in 1988 (18). These men were subsequently followed up for 15 years and outcomes were compared to the remaining "source" population of 24,804 men who were not invited for screening. Seventy-four percent of men who had been invited attended screening. Participants were screened with a serum PSA, DRE, and transrectal ultrasound (TRUS) with biopsies performed for abnormal findings on DRE or TRUS. If the PSA level was greater than 7 ng/mL, repeat TRUS was performed and if greater than 10 ng/mL, biopsies were performed. On an intention-to-screen analysis, no difference was observed in PCa mortality (RR 0.98, 95% CI 0.92–1.05) or overall mortality (RR 1.10, 95% CI 0.83–1.46). However, improved overall survival was noted when comparing those men who had actually undergone screening with the "source" population (RR 0.82, 95% CI 0.76–0.90).

Sandblom et al. reported on the 20-year follow-up of their screening trial in Nörrkoping, Sweden (19). In 1987, all men aged 50 to 69 were identified, and every sixth man was randomized to screening. There were 1,449 men in the screening group and 7,532 men in the control group. The screening interval was every 3 years from 1987 to 1996. The screening regimen included DRE for the first two occasions and DRE with a PSA (cutoff 4 ng/mL) for the last two. Depending on the screening occasion, 70% to 78% of the invited men were compliant with screening. After a median follow-up of 75 months, no significant difference was observed in PCa mortality between the screened group and controls (RR 1.16, 95% CI 0.78–1.73).

More recently, analysis from the large Prostate, Lung, Colorectal, and Ovarian (PLCO) Cancer Screening Trial showed no overall benefit to PSA-based screening; however, evidence suggesting benefits of PSA screening for selected populations can be gleaned from analysis of the data. In the PLCO trial, 76,685 men were randomized to screening or usual medical care across 10 sites in the United States (10, 20). The screening regimen consisted of an annual PSA for 6 years and an annual DRE for 4 years. All screened men and their caregivers received PSA results, and those with a PSA above 4 ng/mL were advised to seek further diagnostic evaluation. After 13 years of follow-up, no difference in PCa mortality (RR 1.09, 95% CI 0.87–1.36) was observed between the groups. However, criticisms of the PLCO study are well documented, mainly relating to the high rates of screening in the control group (three in four men underwent at least one test) as well as the level of PSA screening prior to trial enrollment (up to 40%) (21). There was a large degree of prescreening among men enrolled in both arms and contamination of up to 52% of men in the usual care group undergoing a PSA test at some point during the study. These circumstances and the fact only 85% of men in the screened arm underwent testing may have affected the power of the trial, resulting in a decreased ability to detect a beneficial effect from screening (22, 23).

Although there was no benefit to screening for the study population as a whole, a post-hoc analysis of men with no or minimal comorbidity in the PLCO trial showed a 44% reduction in the risk of PCa mortality among men in the screening arm (hazard ratio 0.56, 95% CI 0.33–0.95) (24). The median age of this group of men was notably also much lower (61 years). Moreover, NNT to prevent one PCa death at 10 years in this subgroup was five. This analysis is significant because it excluded men with significant comorbidities that were judged by investigators to be likely to shorten a subject's life. The interaction between screening effect and comorbidity was later found to be dependent upon the comorbidity definition used by PLCO investigators (20).

Aside from randomized trials, population level data have provided valuable observations of the influence of PSA screening. Although population level data cannot establish causality, there are epidemiologic data that provide supporting evidence that the introduction of PSA-based screening is generally followed by a decline in rates of advanced disease and, in some cases, by a fall in PCa mortality. Strengths of epidemiologic studies include large sample sizes and a "real-world" experience, which may make these data more generalizable compared with data from a clinical trial. In Olmsted County, Minnesota, for example, age-adjusted PCa mortality rates increased from 25.8 per 100,000 men from 1980 to 1984 to a peak of 34 per 100,000 from 1989 to 1992; rates subsequently decreased to 19.4 per 100,000 from 1993 to 1997 after PSA screening became more commonplace in the United States (25). Similarly, death rates from PCa as reported in the National Cancer Database have declined at the rate of 1% per year since 1990 (26). Improvements in PCa mortality were noted with initiation of population-based screening and treatment in Tyrol, Austria, compared to other regions of Austria where screening was not widely implemented (27). Although some have cautioned that this improvement may result from many additional factors (28) such as the contribution of improved treatments (29, 30) or attribution bias (31), modeling has attributed 45% to 70% of this observed PCa mortality reduction to PSA screening (4).

Prior to the PSA screening era, a majority of men diagnosed with PCa had advanced or metastatic disease (32). With the introduction of screening, a marked increase in the diagnosis of asymptomatic, clinically localized disease has been observed (33, 34). Catalona et al. reported locally advanced tumors in 57% of a comparison group to 29% in a group undergoing serial PSA screening (34). Similarly, the Cancer of the Prostate Strategic Urological Research Endeavor revealed an increase in clinical T1 disease from 23% in 1993 to 1995 to 50% in 2002 (35), and Surveillance, Epidemiology, and End Results data from 2004 to 2005 showed that 94% of newly diagnosed men have localized disease (T1 or T2) (33). A decrease in distant or metastatic disease was seen following the introduction of screening (36, 37). Given this well-described stage migration, and in light of the well-documented competing mortality risks in men diagnosed with PCa, the men expected to benefit the most from a diagnosis and subsequent treatment of PCa would be those who are young with minimal comorbidities (38, 39).

These benefits in a younger population with minimal or no comorbidity are important to consider given the protracted natural history of screen-detected PCa, which can predate a clinical diagnosis by 6 to 14 years (40). The majority of these patients have organ confined and potentially indolent disease (33). Of the men treated with curative intent, up to one-third can be expected to recur (41); however, even following such a recurrence, there can be a prolonged survival before death from PCa (42, 43). Thus, a younger male with a longer life expectancy may be more likely to accept the risk of the potential harms of screening to gain the potential benefits. However, such a patient would also have a longer period of time to live with potential harms of screening and treatment. Currently available data do not allow us to extrapolate in an empirical way beyond 10 to 14 years, which makes it difficult to forecast outcomes beyond that time frame. The large recent studies described earlier will continue to accrue follow-up data and already have hinted that they may show a greater benefit to screening with time.

Although modeling based on ERSPC data showed that PSA-based screening may offer an increase of life-years (76 life-years over 1,000 men undergoing annual PSA screening between 55 and 69 years), 23% of the unadjusted life-years that were gained would be counterbalanced by a loss in quality-adjusted life years (QALYs) (44). A substantial part of the predicted difference between life-years and QALYs gained was caused by overdiagnosed cancers and consequently by short-term and long-term effects of primary (over)treatment. Thus, strategies to reduce overdiagnosis and to distinguish indolent from aggressive cancers are necessary. Several tests are also now available, which may improve the ability of PSA to detect clinically significant PCa and prevent unnecessary biopsies. Rather than reinventing the wheel with a novel biomarker, these tests incorporate existing markers and molecular isoforms of PSA into a single test that, when combined with the standard total PSA (tPSA) test, may improve the performance of PSA-based screening.

The Prostate Health Index (PHI) was approved in the United States in 2012 for use in men 50 years and older with a tPSA between 4.0 and 10 ng/mL and a normal DRE. Based on established findings that a higher proportion of [-2]proPSA (p2PSA) or a lower proportion of free PSA (%fPSA) is associated with PCa, the PHI is calculated ($PHI = (p2PSA/fPSA) \times \sqrt{total\ PSA}$)), which has been shown to improve PSA-based risk stratification. In a tPSA range of approximately 2 to 10 ng/mL, the PHI provides significantly better clinical performance for predicting Gleason ≥ 7 PCa than tPSA or percentage of fPSA or p2PSA (45, 46). This finding was recently confirmed in a study by Lazzeri et al., which showed that the sensitivity and specificity of the PHI exceeds its components in discriminating Gleason ≥ 7 disease from lower grade disease or negative biopsy, resulting in improved decision making for biopsy (47). Further, the data from Lazzeri et al. suggested that in patients with a tPSA between 2.0 and

10 ng/mL, use of the PHI at a sensitivity of 90% would avoid 15.5% of unnecessary biopsies while only missing 1.1% of Gleason ≥ 7 PCa.

A panel of four kallikrein markers (tPSA, fPSA, intact PSA, and kallikrein-related peptidase 2), while not yet commercially available, has also been reported as a highly accurate predictor of biopsy outcome (48). Compared with tPSA and age, the full kallikrein panel enhanced the predictive accuracy for clinically diagnosed PCa (concordance index 0.65 vs. 0.75; $P < .001$) (49). In a statistical model, men with a PSA level of 3 ng/mL or more but defined as low risk by the panel of four kallikrein markers were unlikely to develop advanced PCa (less than 1% of the group).

The role of PSA velocity in improving the sensitivity and specificity of PSA testing is controversial. Initial retrospective observations suggested that PSA velocity improved the ability of testing to identify aggressive disease (50), but analyses of two large prospective trials—the Prostate Cancer Prevention Trial (PCPT) and ERSPC (51, 52)—do not show any advantage to using PSA velocity, perhaps due to the well-recognized biologic variations within individual men when PSA levels are drawn.

Finally, although annual PSA screening has been the standard since its introduction, the optimum screening regimen has never been determined. Current evidence suggests that annual screening is not likely to produce significant incremental benefits when compared with a screening interval of 2 years. In the PLCO trial, a comparison of annual screening with opportunistic screening in the U.S. population, which corresponded to screening on average every 2 years, PCa mortality rates were similar in the two groups through 13 years of follow-up (21). Another analysis of men in the screening arm of the PLCO trial suggested that screening every 5 years for baseline PSA less than 1 ng/mL and every 2 years for PSA 1 to 2 ng/mL could result in a 50% reduction in PSA tests while missing less than 1.5% of men with earlier positive screens (53). A modeling study by Gulati et al. compared 35 screening strategies that differed by ages to start and stop screening, screening intervals, and thresholds for biopsy versus no screening (54). A strategy that screens biennially with longer screening intervals for men with low PSA levels achieves similar risks for PCa death (2.27% vs. 2.15% for the annually screened reference strategy) and overdiagnosis (2.4% vs. 3.3%), but reduces total tests by 59% and false-positive results by 50%. Collectively these data support alternative screening intervals which may improve the tradeoffs of PSA-based screening.

Unfortunately, despite the completion of several large randomized trials and the examination of data from multiple discrete populations, the controversy surrounding PSA screening has not been resolved. We believe that the existing data support continued PSA-based screening for properly selected populations, rather than screening all men based on age alone. Determination of comorbidity status, risk for developing PCa, and life expectancy are important factors that need to be considered in deciding who should undergo testing. The data also suggest that reliance on annual PSA testing for all men likely results in overdiagnosis. It is hoped that in the future, screening will incorporate risk-adapted screening intervals, and adjunct testing such as biomarker panels will result in screening and detecting more significant cancers while avoiding overdiagnosis. Currently, the updated analyses of several large randomized trials, however, do support PSA screening, particularly in a properly selected population. Recently, data from the Malmö Preventive Project demonstrated that men with PSA in the highest 10th percentile at age 45 to 49 years contribute nearly half of PCa deaths over the next 25 to 30 years (52). This finding was reflected in the current strategy of the European Association of Urology, which recommends offering a baseline PSA at 40 to 45 years followed by a risk-adapted follow-up approach to screening in men with a life expectancy ≥10 years (53).

Moving forward with PSA screening at this point mandates careful selection of those men most likely to derive benefit. This population includes patients at higher risk for PCa and PCa mortality with a long-life expectancy due to young age and minimal or no comorbidity who should be offered PSA screening after appropriate counseling.

■ REFERENCES

1. Siegel R, Naishadham D, Jemal A. Cancer statistics, 2013. *CA Cancer J Clin*. 2013;63(1):11–30.
2. Stamey TA, Yang N, Hay AR, McNeal JE, Freiha FS, Redwine E. Prostate-specific antigen as a serum marker for adenocarcinoma of the prostate. *N Engl J Med*. 1987;317(15):909–916.
3. Catalona WJ, Smith DS, Ratliff TL, et al. Measurement of prostate-specific antigen in serum as a screening test for prostate cancer. *N Engl J Med*. 1991;324(17):1156–1161.
4. Etzioni R, Tsodikov A, Mariotto A, et al. Quantifying the role of PSA screening in the US prostate cancer mortality decline. *Cancer Causes Control*. 2008;19(2):175–181.
5. Siegel R, Ward E, Brawley O, Jemal A. Cancer statistics, 2011: the impact of eliminating socioeconomic and racial disparities on premature cancer deaths. *CA Cancer J Clin*. 2011;61(4):212–236.
6. Collin SM, Martin RM, Metcalfe C, et al. Prostate-cancer mortality in the USA and UK in 1975–2004: an ecological study. *Lancet Oncol*. 2008;9(5):445–452.
7. Scosyrev E, Wu G, Mohile S, Messing EM. Prostate-specific antigen screening for prostate cancer and the risk of overt metastatic disease at presentation: analysis of trends over time. *Cancer*. 2012;118(23):5768–5776.
8. Gates TJ. Screening for cancer: evaluating the evidence. *Am Fam Physician*. 2001;63(3):513–522.
9. Schroder FH, Hugosson J, Roobol MJ, et al. Screening and prostate-cancer mortality in a randomized European study. *N Engl J Med*. 2009;360(13):1320–1328.
10. Andriole GL, Crawford ED, Grubb RL III, et al. Mortality results from a randomized prostate-cancer screening trial. *N Engl J Med*. 2009;360(13):1310–1319.
11. Sandblom G, Varenhorst E, Lofman O, Rosell J, Carlsson P. Clinical consequences of screening for prostate cancer: 15 years

follow-up of a randomised controlled trial in Sweden. *Eur Urol.* 2004;46(6):717–723; discussion 724.
12. Labrie F, Candas B, Cusan L, et al. Screening decreases prostate cancer mortality: 11-year follow-up of the 1988 Quebec prospective randomized controlled trial. *Prostate.* 2004;59(3):311–318.
13. Schroder FH, Hugosson J, Roobol MJ, et al. Prostate-cancer mortality at 11 years of follow-up. *N Engl J Med.* 2012;366(11):981–990.
14. Nelson HD, Tyne K, Naik A, et al. Screening for breast cancer: an update for the U.S. Preventive Services Task Force. *Ann Intern Med.* 2009;151(10):727–737, W237–W242.
15. Roobol MJ, Kerkhof M, Schroder FH, et al. Prostate cancer mortality reduction by prostate-specific antigen-based screening adjusted for nonattendance and contamination in the European Randomised Study of Screening for Prostate Cancer (ERSPC). *Eur Urol.* 2009;56(4):584–591.
16. Hugosson J, Carlsson S, Aus G, et al. Mortality results from the Goteborg randomised population-based prostate-cancer screening trial. *Lancet Oncol.* 2010;11(8):725–732.
17. Carroll PR, Whitson JM, Cooperberg MR. Serum prostate-specific antigen for the early detection of prostate cancer: always, never, or only sometimes? *J Clin Oncol.* 2011;29(4):345–347.
18. Kjellman A, Akre O, Norming U, Tornblom M, Gustafsson O. 15-year followup of a population based prostate cancer screening study. *J Urol.* 2009;181(4):1615–1621; discussion 1621.
19. Sandblom G, Varenhorst E, Rosell J, Lofman O, Carlsson P. Randomised prostate cancer screening trial: 20 year follow-up. *BMJ.* 2011;342:d1539.
20. Andriole GL, Crawford ED, Grubb RL III, et al. Prostate cancer screening in the randomized Prostate, Lung, Colorectal, and Ovarian Cancer Screening Trial: mortality results after 13 years of follow-up. *J Natl Cancer Inst.* 2012;104(2):125–132.
21. Pinsky PF, Blacka A, Kramer BS, Miller A, Prorok PC, Berg C. Assessing contamination and compliance in the prostate component of the Prostate, Lung, Colorectal, and Ovarian (PLCO) Cancer Screening Trial. *Clin Trials.* 2010;7(4):303–311.
22. Cuzick J, Edwards R, Segnan N. Adjusting for non-compliance and contamination in randomized clinical trials. *Stat Med.* 1997;16(9):1017–1029.
23. Gulati R, Tsodikov A, Wever EM, et al. The impact of PLCO control arm contamination on perceived PSA screening efficacy. *Cancer Causes Control.* 2012;23(6):827–835.
24. Crawford ED, Grubb R III, Black A, et al. Comorbidity and mortality results from a randomized prostate cancer screening trial. *J Clin Oncol.* 2011;29(4):355–361.
25. Roberts RO, Bergstralh EJ, Katusic SK, Lieber MM, Jacobsen SJ. Decline in prostate cancer mortality from 1980 to 1997, and an update on incidence trends in Olmsted County, Minnesota. *J Urol.* 1999;161(2):529–533.
26. Mettlin CJ, Murphy GP, Rosenthal DS, Menck HR. The National Cancer Data Base report on prostate carcinoma after the peak in incidence rates in the U.S. The American College of Surgeons Commission on Cancer and the American Cancer Society. *Cancer.* 1998;83(8):1679–1684.
27. Bartsch G, Horninger W, Klocker H, et al. Tyrol Prostate Cancer Demonstration Project: early detection, treatment, outcome, incidence and mortality. *BJU Int.* 2008;101(7):809–816.
28. Etzioni R, Feuer E. Studies of prostate-cancer mortality: caution advised. *Lancet Oncol.* 2008;9(5):407–409.
29. Bolla M, Collette L, Blank L, et al. Long-term results with immediate androgen suppression and external irradiation in patients with locally advanced prostate cancer (an EORTC study): a phase III randomised trial. *Lancet.* 2002;360(9327):103–106.
30. Cooperberg MR, Grossfeld GD, Lubeck DP, Carroll PR. National practice patterns and time trends in androgen ablation for localized prostate cancer. *J Natl Cancer Inst.* 2003;95(13):981–989.
31. Lu-Yao G, Stukel TA, Yao SL. Changing patterns in competing causes of death in men with prostate cancer: a population based study. *J Urol.* 2004;171(6 pt 1):2285–2290.
32. Farkas A, Schneider D, Perrotti M, Cummings KB, Ward WS. National trends in the epidemiology of prostate cancer, 1973 to 1994: evidence for the effectiveness of prostate-specific antigen screening. *Urology.* 1998;52(3):444–448; discussion 448–449.
33. Shao YH, Demissie K, Shih W, et al. Contemporary risk profile of prostate cancer in the United States. *J Natl Cancer Inst.* 2009;101(18):1280–1283.
34. Catalona WJ, Smith DS, Ratliff TL, Basler JW. Detection of organ-confined prostate cancer is increased through prostate-specific antigen-based screening. *JAMA.* 1993;270(8):948–954.
35. Cooperberg MR, Lubeck DP, Mehta SS, Carroll PR, CaPsure. Time trends in clinical risk stratification for prostate cancer: implications for outcomes (data from CaPSURE). *J Urol.* 2003;170(6 pt 2):S21–S25; discussion S26–S27.
36. Kopec JA, Goel V, Bunting PS, et al. Screening with prostate specific antigen and metastatic prostate cancer risk: a population based case control study. *J Urol.* 2005;174(2):495–499; discussion 499.
37. Etzioni R, Gulati R, Falcon S, Penson DF. Impact of PSA screening on the incidence of advanced stage prostate cancer in the United States: a surveillance modeling approach. *Med Decis Making.* 2008;28(3):323–331.
38. Albertsen PC, Hanley JA, Fine J. 20-year outcomes following conservative management of clinically localized prostate cancer. *JAMA.* 2005;293(17):2095–2101.
39. Lu-Yao GL, Albertsen PC, Moore DF, et al. Outcomes of localized prostate cancer following conservative management. *JAMA.* 2009;302(11):1202–1209.
40. Draisma G, Etzioni R, Tsodikov A, et al. Lead time and overdiagnosis in prostate-specific antigen screening: importance of methods and context. *J Natl Cancer Inst.* 2009;101(6):374–383.
41. D'Amico AV, Chen MH, Roehl KA, Catalona WJ. Preoperative PSA velocity and the risk of death from prostate cancer after radical prostatectomy. *N Engl J Med.* 2004;351(2):125–135.
42. Freedland SJ, Humphreys EB, Mangold LA, et al. Death in patients with recurrent prostate cancer after radical prostatectomy: prostate-specific antigen doubling time subgroups and their associated contributions to all-cause mortality. *J Clin Oncol.* 2007;25(13):1765–1771.
43. Stephenson AJ, Kattan MW, Eastham JA, et al. Prostate cancer-specific mortality after radical prostatectomy for patients treated in the prostate-specific antigen era. *J Clin Oncol.* 2009;27(26):4300–4305.
44. Heijnsdijk EA, Wever EM, Auvinen A, et al. Quality-of-life effects of prostate-specific antigen screening. *N Engl J Med.* 2012;367(7):595–605.
45. Catalona WJ, Partin AW, Sanda MG, et al. A multicenter study of [-2]pro-prostate specific antigen combined with prostate specific antigen and free prostate specific antigen for prostate cancer detection in the 2.0 to 10.0 ng/ml prostate specific antigen range. *J Urol.* 2011;185(5):1650–1655.
46. Stephan C, Vincendeau S, Houlgatte A, Cammann H, Jung K, Semjonow A. Multicenter evaluation of [-2]proprostate-specific antigen and the prostate health index for detecting prostate cancer. *Clin Chem.* 2013;59(1):306–314.
47. Lazzeri M, Haese A, de la Taille A, et al. Serum isoform [-2] proPSA derivatives significantly improve prediction of prostate cancer at initial biopsy in a total PSA range of 2–10 ng/ml: a multicentric European study. *Eur Urol.* 2013;63(6):986–994.
48. Vickers AJ, Cronin AM, Roobol MJ, et al. A four-kallikrein panel predicts prostate cancer in men with recent screening: data from the European Randomized Study of Screening for Prostate Cancer, Rotterdam. *Clin Cancer Res.* 2010;16(12):3232–3239.
49. Vickers AJ, Gupta A, Savage CJ, et al. A panel of kallikrein marker predicts prostate cancer in a large, population-based cohort followed for 15 years without screening. *Cancer Epidemiol Biomarkers Prev.* 2011;20(2):255–261.
50. Carter HB, Ferrucci L, Kettermann A, et al. Detection of life-threatening prostate cancer with prostate-specific antigen

velocity during a window of curability. *J Natl Cancer Inst.* 2006;98:1521–1527.
51. Vickers AJ, Wolters T, Savage CJ, et al. Prostate specific antigen velocity does not aid prostate cancer detection in men with prior negative biopsy. *J Urol.* 2010;184:907–912.
52. Vickers AJ, Till C, Tangen CM, Lilja H, Thompson IM. An empirical evaluation of guidelines on prostate-specific antigen velocity in prostate cancer detection. *J Natl Cancer Inst.* 2011;103:462–469.
53. Crawford ED, Pinsky PF, Chia D, et al. Prostate specific antigen changes as related to the initial prostate specific antigen: data from the prostate, lung, colorectal and ovarian cancer screening trial. *J Urol.* 2006;175(4):1286–1290; discussion 1290.
54. Gulati R, Gore JL, Etzioni R. Comparative effectiveness of alternative prostate-specific antigen–based prostate cancer screening strategies: model estimates of potential benefits and harms. *Ann Intern Med.* 2013;158(3):145–153.
55. Vickers AJ, Ulmert D, Sjoberg DD, et al. Strategy for detection of prostate cancer based on relation between prostate specific antigen at age 40–55 and long term risk of metastasis: case-control study. *BMJ.* 2013;346:f2023.
56. Heidenreich A, Abrahamsson PA, Artibani W, et al. Early detection of prostate cancer: European Association of Urology recommendation. *Eur Urol.* 2013;64:347–354.

3.1.2 The Argument Against Prostate Cancer Screening

OTIS W. BRAWLEY

The argument against prostate cancer screening is really an argument for caution in its advocacy and use. It is an unfortunate fact that the data to support a benefit to the patient from prostate screening are weak and inconsistent, whereas the data to support harms due to screening are extremely consistent.

Prostate cancer screening has been widespread. It is commonly offered at health fairs. It has even been offered on the floor of political conventions and from vans in supermarket parking lots. It is most concerning that prostate cancer screening is a test that can lead to life-changing and harmful interventions, yet some organizations are offering it with the implication or sometimes even the promise of benefit and with no discussion of the proven risks.

The truth is prostate cancer screening may be a net benefit to the population; but it also may not be. This is an unknown. It might save a small number of men from a prostate cancer death, while causing significant harm to a large number. The benefits may not justify the harms.

A BRIEF HISTORY

The prostate-specific antigen (PSA) was first discovered and converted into a test in the 1970s. Prostate cancer screening using the PSA was first popularized in the early 1990s (1,2). Commonly used arguments in favor of prostate cancer screening include:

- Screening finds lots of disease and it finds localized disease.
- The proportion of men diagnosed through screening and surviving 5 years after diagnosis is substantial and is greater than that of men diagnosed due to symptoms (1,2).

This argument ignores the important fact that the purpose of a screening test is to prevent death (3). Granted an effective test must find localized disease to prevent death, but finding localized disease is only the beginning (3).

There are several examples of cancer screening tests that have found localized disease, increased the amount of disease found, and increased the proportion surviving 5 years without changing the risk of death. This occurred in children with urine vanillylmandelic acid screening for neuroblastoma (4) and in adults with chest x-ray screening for lung cancer (5).

Indeed, the comparison between what occurred in prostate cancer screening in the 1990s and what occurred in lung cancer screening in the 1960s and 1970s is striking (6). Chest x-ray screening was commonly done in the United States for several decades before the completion of well-designed prospective randomized studies to assess it. These studies eventually showed chest x-ray screening not effective. Some even suggested it net harmful (7).

DOES PSA SCREENING FIND LOCALIZED PROSTATE CANCER?

The dramatic increase in prostate cancer incidence after the introduction of screening would seem to suggest that PSA screening is good at finding localized prostate cancer. Studies have shown that about 7.5% of men aged 50 years and older volunteering for screening have a PSA over 4 ng/mL. Of these, 25% have a prostate cancer (8).

The Prostate Cancer Prevention Trial (PCPT) was a randomized prospective study of more than 18,000 men (9). It provides perhaps the best studied screening cohort ever. Participants were median age 62 years at the start and 69 years at the end. They were consented and randomized to treatment with daily finasteride or placebo for a planned 7-year period. Screening with PSA and digital rectal examination (DRE) was done annually. Men with eight normal screens over 7 years at the end of the study were asked to submit to a prostate biopsy.

The findings from the control arm of this study are quite damning of PSA screening (9,10).

- Screening found a lot of prostate cancer; 14% of men in the placebo were diagnosed with prostate cancer during 7 years of screening.
- PSA with a cutoff of 4 ng/mL missed a lot of prostate cancer; 15.2% of men completing eight normal annual screens over 7 years were diagnosed with prostate cancer due to the end-of-study prostate biopsy.
- PSA and DRE also missed a lot of high-grade prostate cancer. Among those completing the trial and diagnosed with prostate cancer, 38% of the high-grade prostate cancers were in men with a PSA less than 4 ng/mL.

It is hard to fathom, but among men completing the study on the placebo arm, more than 28% were diagnosed with prostate cancer. It is estimated that 3% of men, aged 60, will ultimately die of prostate cancer. This suggests that this disease is prone to significant overdiagnosis (11).

With a PSA cutoff of 4 ng/mL, the false-positive rate was 75% during the 7 years of the study. Lowering the PSA cut point for biopsy will increase the false-positive rate and the number of prostate biopsies performed. This would increase the harms associated with screening, as prostate biopsies are associated with a small but significant complication rate (12).

The Prostate Cancer Prevention Trial (PCPT) is the only study in which there was systematic biopsy of men with PSA less than 4 ng/mL. Analysis of the PCPT data has shown that there was no optimal cut point. There were even cancers diagnosed at PSA levels less than 1.0 ng/mL (13).

■ DOES TREATMENT OF LOCALIZED DISEASE SAVE LIVES?

Treatment of localized prostate cancer must be effective, if screening is to be effective. The efficacy of screening has been questioned for more than three decades. It even predates the PSA screening era. The prostate cancer conundrum was best summarized by the distinguished urologist, Willet Whitmore when he said: " Is cure necessary for those in whom it is possible? Is cure possible for those in whom it is necessary?" (14)

This conundrum was illustrated by a landmark analysis of 767 men diagnosed with localized prostate cancer in the 1970s and followed expectantly. A small proportion actually died of prostate cancer: 4% to 7% of men with Gleason 2 to 4 disease, 6% to 11% of those with Gleason 5 disease, and 18% to 30% of men with Gleason 6 cancer (15).

There have been two well-designed prospective randomized trials to assess the efficacy of surgical treatment of localized prostate cancer. They illustrate the limited effect of treatment for localized prostate cancer.

The Scandinavian Prostate Cancer Group-4 prospectively randomized 695 men with clinically localized prostate cancer men (12% diagnosed by PSA testing) to radical prostatectomy or observation (16). Those on the observation arm received hormonal therapy if they became symptomatic. At 15 years follow-up, 15% of the prostatectomy group and 21% of the watchful waiting group had died of prostate cancer. This was statistically significant (risk ratio [RR] 0.62, 95% confidence interval [CI] 0.44–0.87). The absolute risk reduction was 6.1%, meaning the number needed to treat (NNT) to prevent 1 death at 15 years of follow-up was 16. This was not a group detected after PSA screening. If it were, the effect at 12 years would be diminished and the NNT would be higher.

The Prostate Intervention versus Observation Trial study enrolled men with PSA-detected localized disease (17). It randomized subjects to radical prostatectomy or watchful waiting. With a median 12 years follow-up, 48.4% (354 of 731) had died. Radical prostatectomy did not significantly reduce prostate cancer–specific mortality. Prostatectomy was associated with a 2.9% absolute reduction and watchful waiting 2.6%. Subgroup analyses suggested that surgery might cause a small reduction in mortality among men with higher PSA values and possibly among men with higher risk tumors.

■ DOES SCREENING PREVENT DEATH FROM PROSTATE CANCER?

Those of us who are most cautious about screening believe this question is not answered. We note there are studies that suggest yes and studies that suggest no. All these studies have limitations and flaws.

For some time, there has been discussion of prostate cancer demographic data in an effort to demonstrate that screening works or does not work. There are so many variables in ecologic studies such that they can provide some useful information, but they cannot definitively answer the question.

There has been a 40% decline in the U.S. age-adjusted prostate cancer mortality since the late 1980s (11). This would at first glance seem to support prostate cancer screening. Further assessment of the facts shows that the decline in mortality began several years before the popularization of PSA screening. One would expect the effect of screening to be seen at least 6 to 10 years after screening began.

The fact that a decline in prostate cancer mortality began 8 to 10 years before it could be attributed to screening means at least some of the U.S. decline cannot be due to screening. Some have suggested it was an improvement in treatment of regional and metastatic disease diagnosed through symptoms (18). Some have suggested that changes in the World Health Organization definition of death may be responsible for decline in mortality. These changes were put into effect the year that the decline began. They may have caused some deaths that once would have been attributed to prostate cancer to be attributed to infectious diseases, especially pneumonia (19).

Others have theorized that increased use of GNRH analogs to treat prostate cancer might have caused a rise in cardiovascular deaths among men who without early diagnosis and treatment would have died later from prostate cancer (20,21). This is an unproven theory. It is known that GNRH analogs increase risk of cardiovascular disease and cardiovascular death (22). It is known that there was excessive use of these drugs in the United States over the past 20 years (23).

One or all of the four reasons may be the cause of the decline in prostate cancer mortality in the United States. It may be due to screening, more effective treatment, changes in the definition of cause of death, and some cardiovascular deaths due to hormonal treatment.

A COMPARISON OF POPULATIONS

There is the temptation to compare mortality rates in heavily screened populations to mortality rates in populations that are not as heavily screened. Screening was adopted earlier and more intensely in Washington compared to Connecticut. As a result, the National Cancer Institute Surveillance, Epidemiology, and End Results (SEER) region in western Washington reported early increases in the age-adjusted incidence of prostate cancer far greater than seen in Connecticut, which also has a SEER registry. For years, the two populations have had very similar mortality rates including a decline starting in the early 1990s (24).

There were similar findings when comparing age-adjusted incidence and mortality rates in the United States with those in Great Britain (25). Screening in the United States caused the prostate cancer age-adjusted incidence rate to rise dramatically during the 1990s. A dramatic rise was not seen in Great Britain. Age-adjusted mortality rates were near identical over a near 20-year period. Only recently, the U.S. age-adjusted mortality rate has dropped below that in Great Britain. It is not known whether the difference is due to differences in screening or differences in treatment. The treatment of prostate cancer at all stages is less aggressive in Great Britain.

There are many country to country variables, including differences in culture, screening, and treatment, that make it difficult to compare cancer incidence and mortality by country (25). There is also a significant literature to show that the accuracy of death certificate cause of death data can vary (26). Trends in prostate cancer death are likely less affected by this variance than are head-to-head comparisons of the mortality rates in one country versus another.

It is also of note that age-adjusted prostate cancer mortality is declining in 21 countries, and screening is widespread in 3 of the 21 countries (27). Again this is evidence that at least one other factor beyond screening is causing the decline in prostate mortality.

THE PROSPECTIVE RANDOMIZED TRIALS

The most powerful evidence to determine the efficacy of screening is a prospective randomized trial. All published randomized trials to date have flaws. Two suggest screening saves lives and the others do not. All demonstrate the harms and overdiagnosis of screening.

Three published studies show no benefit to screening when analyzed by intention (28–30). Unfortunately, they are considered of poor quality (31).

The Prostate, Lung, Colorectal, and Ovarian (PLCO) randomized 76,700 men aged 55 to 74 years to annual PSA screening with DRE versus usual care (32,33). It is generally considered of fair quality even though there was substantial contamination (screening in the control arm). At 13 years of follow-up, there was a statistically nonsignificant increase in the cumulative prostate cancer mortality among men randomized to the screening arm (RR 1.09, 95% CI 0.87–1.36). Some argue that instead of comparing screening with no screening, the PLCO effectively compared regular screening with opportunistic screening.

The European Randomized Study of Prostate Cancer (ERSPC) was to be a pooling of screening data from nine studies, in nine countries. Eventually the data from seven countries were pooled and published. It is unknown why the trial data from two countries were not included in the eventual publication.

The seven studies making up the published ERSPC study enrolled 182,000 men aged 50 to 74 years. It was a negative study (RR 0.85, 95% CI 0.73–1.0). The analysis of the seven pooled trials failed to demonstrate that PSA screening was associated with a decline in prostate cancer mortality. A planned subset analysis of the 162,243 men aged 55 to 69 at 9 years of follow-up, however, did show a statistically significant difference in prostate cancer death rate in the screened group versus the control group (RR 0.80, 95% CI 0.65–0.98) (34). An update with 11 years of follow-up showed a 21% relative risk reduction (RR 0.79, 95% CI 0.68–0.91).

Analysis of the seven individual studies making up the published ERSPC is telling. Five of the seven studies failed to show that screening saved lives. The ERSPC subset analysis was a positive study because screening saved lives in Sweden and the Netherlands (Table 3.1.2.1).

■ **Table 3.1.2.1** ERSPC 9-year data: relative risk of death for screened versus unscreened by country

Country	Deaths on Screened Arm	Total on Screened Arm	Deaths on Control Arm	Total on Control Arm	Risk Ratio (95% Confidence Interval)
Sweden	39	5,901	70	5,951	0.56 (0.38–0.83)
Belgium	22	4,307	25	4,255	0.86 (0.48–1.52)
Netherlands	69	17,443	97	17,390	0.71 (0.52–0.96)
Italy	19	7,266	22	7,251	0.86 (0.46–1.58)
Finland	139	31,970	237	48,409	0.89 (0.72–1.09)
Spain	2	1,056	1	1,141	2.15 (0.20–23.77)
Switzerland	9	4,948	10	4,955	0.89 (0.36–2.20)
Total subjects	260	66,990	392	83,401	0.80 (0.65–0.98)

The Gotteborg trial was the second positive study (35). It found that PSA was associated with a decreased risk for prostate cancer–specific mortality (RR 0.56, 95% CI 0.39–0.82) at a median of 14 years follow-up. More than 90% of the prostate deaths in the Gotteborg trial are the men dying in the Swedish component of the ERSPC. As such, it does not constitute independent evidence of the efficacy of prostate cancer screening.

The Finnish trial contributed more men to the ERSPC than any other (36). Its data have been published. It demonstrates that screening is associated with a statistically significant decrease in metastatic disease, but it failed to show that screening was associated with a decrease in prostate cancer–specific mortality.

One must wonder why screening saved lives in Sweden and the Netherlands but not in Belgium, Italy, Finland, Spain, or Switzerland. What was different about these seven trials such that only two would be positive? Why was the Swedish study so much more positive than even the Dutch study? These questions have not been completely answered. The Swedish cohort did have younger patients, longer follow-up, more frequent screening, and approximately twice the aggregate prostate cancer mortality rate compared to the other ERSPC trials.

ERSPC had no standard protocol. There were differences in PSA screening schedule, PSA normal values, and other variables. Perhaps most important, there were differences in randomization. In some countries, the men in the control group did not know that they were in the trial. They were followed up through tumor registries. Men on the intervention arms in these countries were more likely to be treated in high-volume specialty centers, whereas men in the control group who were diagnosed with prostate cancer were more likely to be treated in the community.

A screening trial has a serious bias when there is variability between screened and control arms in the initial treatment of patients with similar risk and similar stage disease. These studies may very well have randomized men to screening and U.S. style aggressive treatment versus no screening and more conservative European style treatment if diagnosed (20).

■ APPLYING CLINICAL STUDIES TO THE REAL WORLD

Perhaps the greatest argument for caution in advocating prostate cancer screening is seen when one looks at the ERSPC study finding and applies the data. The NNT to save one life from a prostate cancer death is estimated to be 37 men (37). This means for every 200 men diagnosed and treated, 5 to 6 men would benefit, and 194 or 195 would not. These men have all the risks and side effects associated with diagnosis and treatment but none of the benefits. I note that the death rate associated with radical prostatectomy in the United States is about 1 in 200.

Of those who would not benefit in the aforementioned example, estimates of overdiagnosis range from 40% to 60% (38,39). This is an argument supporting the desperate need for an objective validated test to distinguish the prostate cancers that need to be treated from those cancers that need to be watched.

■ SUMMARY

Every cancer screening test has some harms even if net beneficial. One should have some perspective of the harm–benefit ratio before using a test. The harms of prostate cancer screening are demonstrated in every published randomized prospective clinical trial. The United States is 25 years into an epidemic of prostate cancer screening without adequate understanding of this harm–benefit ratio.

The best way to assess the efficacy of a screening test is a well-designed prospective randomized clinical trial in which subjects volunteer for enrollment and are then randomized to a screening or a control group and followed up over time. This was not done in all of the published prospective randomized studies.

Even if one were to accept as accurate the prospective randomized studies that purport to show screening saves lives, the ERSPC trials suggest that the number of lives saved is low and the number of men receiving unnecessary treatment is high.

Table 3.1.2.2 Prostate cancer screening recommendations of respected organizations

Recommending for informed or shared decision making within the physician–patient relationship
American Cancer Society
National Comprehensive Cancer Network
American Society for Clinical Oncology
European Urology Association
American Urology Association
Recommending against *routine* prostate cancer screening
U.S. Preventive Services Taskforce
Canadian Taskforce on the Periodic Health Examination
American College of Preventive Medicine
American College of Physicians
American Academy of Family Physicians

A man who chooses routine prostate cancer screening from age 50 to 70 definitely doubles his lifelong risk of prostate cancer diagnosis from an absolute risk of about 10% to near 20%. Two studies (ERSPC and Gotteborg) suggest that a man will decrease his relative risk of death from prostate cancer by 20% to 34%. That is an absolute lifetime risk of prostate cancer death going from 3% to a range of 2.4 to 2.0 lifetime risk.

The problem with the data is actually well reflected in the wording of screening statements and recommendations from a number of respected professional organizations. Truth be told, no professional organization that publishes screening guidelines recommends prostate screening without caveat. Indeed of 10 organizations, 5 currently recommend against *routine* screening and 5 recommend some sort of informed or shared decision making between a patient and his physician after a discussion of the proven risks and possible benefits of screening (40–42) (Table 3.1.2.2).

It is the author's belief that the best statement in prostate cancer screening is one that conveys what is known, what is not known, and what is believed and labels them accordingly. Such is the 2009 American Urological Association PSA Best Practice Statement. It recommended against mass screening and stated that a decision must be made within the physician–patient relationship. The statement said:

> Given the uncertainty that PSA testing results in more benefit than harm, a thoughtful and broad approach to PSA is critical. Patients need to be informed of the risks and benefits of testing before it is undertaken. The risks of overdetection and overtreatment should be included in this discussion. (43)

REFERENCES

1. Catalona WJ, Smith DS, Ratliff TL, et al. Measurement of prostate-specific antigen in serum as a screening test for prostate cancer. *N Engl J Med.* 1991;324(17):1156–1161.
2. Mettlin C, Lee F, Drago J, Murphy GP. The American Cancer Society National Prostate Cancer Detection Project. Findings on the detection of early prostate cancer in 2425 men. *Cancer.* 1991;67(12):2949–2958.
3. Croswell JM, Ransohoff DF, Kramer BS. Principles of cancer screening: lessons from history and study design issues. *Semin Oncol.* 2010;37(3):202–215.
4. Woods WG, Gao RN, Shuster JJ, et al. Screening of infants and mortality due to neuroblastoma. *N Engl J Med.* 2002;346(14):1041–1046.
5. Marcus PM, Bergstralh EJ, Zweig MH, Harris A, Offord KP, Fontana RS. Extended lung cancer incidence follow-up in the Mayo Lung Project and overdiagnosis. *J Natl Cancer Inst.* 2006;98(11):748–756.
6. Collins MM, Barry MJ. Controversies in prostate cancer screening. Analogies to the early lung cancer screening debate. *JAMA.* 1996;276(24):1976–1979.
7. Manser R, Wright G, Hart D, Byrnes G, Campbell DA. Surgery for early stage non-small cell lung cancer. *Cochrane Database Syst Rev.* 2005;(1):CD004699.
8. Thompson IM, Ankerst DP, Chi C, et al. Assessing prostate cancer risk: results from the Prostate Cancer Prevention Trial. *J Natl Cancer Inst.* 2006;98(8):529–534.
9. Thompson IM, Goodman PJ, Tangen CM, et al. The influence of finasteride on the development of prostate cancer. *N Engl J Med.* 2003;349(3):215–224.
10. Thompson IM, Pauler DK, Goodman PJ, et al. Prevalence of prostate cancer among men with a prostate-specific antigen level < or =4.0 ng per milliliter. *N Engl J Med.* 2004;350(22): 2239–2246.
11. SEER Cancer Statistics Review, 1975–2009 (Vintage 2009 Populations). http://seer.cancer.gov/csr/1975_2009_pops09. Updated August 20, 2012.
12. Loeb S, Carter HB, Berndt SI, Ricker W, Schaeffer EM. Complications after prostate biopsy: data from SEER-Medicare. *J Urol.* 2011;186(5):1830–1834.
13. Thompson IM, Ankerst DP, Chi C, et al. Operating characteristics of prostate-specific antigen in men with an initial PSA level of 3.0 ng/ml or lower. *JAMA.* 2005;294(1):66–70.
14. Montie JE, Smith JA. Whitmoreisms: memorable quotes from Willet F. Whitmore, Jr, M.D. *Urology.* 2004;63(1):207–209.
15. Albertsen PC, Hanley JA, Fine J. 20-year outcomes following conservative management of clinically localized prostate cancer. *JAMA.* 2005;293(17):2095–2101.
16. Bill-Axelson A, Holmberg L, Ruutu M, et al. Radical prostatectomy versus watchful waiting in early prostate cancer. *N Engl J Med.* 2011;364(18):1708–1717.
17. Wilt TJ, Brawer MK, Jones KM, et al. Radical prostatectomy versus observation for localized prostate cancer. *N Engl J Med.* 2012;367(3):203–213.
18. Boyle P, Brawley OW. Prostate cancer: current evidence weighs against population screening. *CA Cancer J Clin.* 2009;59(4):220–224.
19. Boyle P. Screening for prostate cancer: have you had your cholesterol measured? *BJU Int.* 2003;92(3):191–199.
20. Haines IE, Gabor Miklos GL. PSA screening trials and prostate cancer deaths: the androgen deprivation connection. *J Natl Cancer Inst.* 2013;105:1534–1539.
21. Brawley OW. Prostate cancer screening: biases and the need for consensus. *J Natl Cancer Inst.* 2013;105(20):1522–1524.
22. Levine GN, D'Amico AV, Berger P, et al. Androgen-deprivation therapy in prostate cancer and cardiovascular risk: a science advisory from the American Heart Association, American Cancer Society, and American Urological Association: endorsed by the American Society for Radiation Oncology. *CA Cancer J Clin.* 2010;60(3):194–201.
23. Shahinian VB, Kuo YF, Gilbert SM. Reimbursement policy and androgen-deprivation therapy for prostate cancer. *N Engl J Med.* 2010;363(19):1822–1832.

24. Lu-Yao G, Albertsen PC, Stanford JL, Stukel TA, Walker-Corkery E, Barry MJ. Screening, treatment, and prostate cancer mortality in the Seattle area and Connecticut: fifteen-year follow-up. *J Gen Intern Med*. 2008;23(11):1809–1814.
25. Etzioni R, Feuer E. Studies of prostate-cancer mortality: caution advised. *Lancet Oncol*. 2008;9(5):407–409.
26. Barry MJ, Andriole GL, Culkin DJ, et al. Ascertaining cause of death among men in the Prostate Cancer Intervention Versus Observation Trial. *Clin Trials*. 2013;10(6):907–914.
27. Center MM, Jemal A, Lortet-Tieulent J, et al. International variation in prostate cancer incidence and mortality rates. *Eur Urol*. 2012;61(6):1079–1092.
28. Kjellman A, Akre O, Norming U, Tornblom M, Gustafsson O. 15-year followup of a population based prostate cancer screening study. *J Urol*. 2009;181(4):1615–1621; discussion 1621.
29. Labrie F, Candas B, Cusan L, et al. Screening decreases prostate cancer mortality: 11-year follow-up of the 1988 Quebec prospective randomized controlled trial. *Prostate*. 2004;59(3):311–318.
30. Sandblom G, Varenhorst E, Rosell J, Lofman O, Carlsson P. Randomised prostate cancer screening trial: 20 year follow-up. *BMJ*. 2011;342:d1539.
31. Ilic D, O'Connor D, Green S, Wilt TJ. Screening for prostate cancer: an updated Cochrane systematic review. *BJU Int*. 2011;107(6):882–891.
32. Andriole GL, Crawford ED, Grubb RL III, et al. Mortality results from a randomized prostate-cancer screening trial. *N Engl J Med*. 2009;360(13):1310–1319.
33. Andriole GL, Crawford ED, Grubb RL III, et al. Prostate cancer screening in the randomized Prostate, Lung, Colorectal, and Ovarian Cancer Screening Trial: mortality results after 13 years of follow-up. *J Natl Cancer Inst*. 2012;104(2):125–132.
34. Schroder FH, Hugosson J, Roobol MJ, et al. Screening and prostate-cancer mortality in a randomized European study. *N Engl J Med*. 2009;360(13):1320–1328.
35. Hugosson J, Carlsson S, Aus G, et al. Mortality results from the Goteborg randomised population-based prostate-cancer screening trial. *Lancet Oncol*. 2010;11(8):725–732.
36. Kilpelainen TP, Tammela TL, Malila N, et al. Prostate cancer mortality in the Finnish randomized screening trial. *J Natl Cancer Inst*. 2013;105(10):719–725.
37. Schroder FH, Hugosson J, Roobol MJ, et al. Prostate-cancer mortality at 11 years of follow-up. *N Engl J Med*. 2012;366(11):981–990.
38. Loeb S, Bjurlin MA, Nicholson J, et al. Overdiagnosis and overtreatment of prostate cancer. *Eur Urol*. 2014;65:1046–1055.
39. Draisma G, Etzioni R, Tsodikov A, et al. Lead time and overdiagnosis in prostate-specific antigen screening: importance of methods and context. *J Natl Cancer Inst*. 2009;101(6):374–383.
40. Wolf AM, Wender RC, Etzioni RB, et al. American Cancer Society guideline for the early detection of prostate cancer: update 2010. *CA Cancer J Clin*. 2010;60(2):70–98.
41. Moyer VA. Screening for prostate cancer: U.S. Preventive Services Task Force recommendation statement. *Ann Intern Med*. 2012;157(2):120–134.
42. Carter HB, Albertsen PC, Barry MJ, et al. Early detection of prostate cancer: AUA Guideline. *J Urol*. 2013;190(2):419–426.
43. Greene KL, Albertsen PC, Babaian RJ, et al. Prostate specific antigen best practice statement: 2009 update. *J Urol*. 2009;182(5):2232–2241.

3.1.3 How Do We Improve PSA Accuracy?

TORU SUGIHARA

MICHAEL W. KATTAN

INTRODUCTION

Since the introduction of prostate-specific antigen (PSA) into clinical practice in the 1980s, PSA is recognized as the most reliable biomarker of prostate cancer (PCa) (1). However, worldwide explosive diffusion of PSA screening comes under a criticism for encouraging a large number of unnecessary prostate biopsy, overdiagnoses, and overtreatment. Under the shadow of these current controversies, sophisticated and reasonable decision-making approaches of PCa screening are desired to improve the accuracy of selection of candidates for further thorough examination and to reduce the potential harm, which cancer screenings involve. Today, several tools and algorithms exist for this purpose.

Table 3.1.3.1 Relationship of prostate-specific antigen and prostate cancer detection rate

Serum PSA Level (ng/mL)	DRE	% Prostate Cancer
≤0.5		6.6
0.6–1.0		10.1
1.1–2.0		17
2.1–3.0		23.9
3.1–4.0		26.9
≤4	+	16.6
4–7	+	47.4
	–	31.1
7–10	+	58
	–	34.4
>10	+	90
	–	64.6

DRE, digital rectal examination; PSA, prostate-specific antigen.
"+" means suspicious for cancer; "–" means nonsuspicious for cancer.
Data are derived from contemporary series (2,3).

PSA CUTOFF THRESHOLD

Setting the cutoff point of serum PSA has significant impact on the accuracy of PSA-based screening. In apparently healthy men, serum PSA level remains very low, and elevated levels of PSA can imply the potential presence of PCa (Table 3.1.3.1) (2,3). Traditionally, PSA values more than 4.0 ng/mL were mainly used as cutoff values for further examination of PCa (4). However, recent researches revealed that even at the lower PSA values of less than 4.0 ng/mL, detection of PCa is not a rare event, and optimal upper limit of the normal range for PSA remains a matter of opinion (2,3). For example, the European Randomized Study of Screening for Prostate Cancer (ERSPC) adapted a PSA value of 3.0 ng/mL as a cutoff for a prostate biopsy (5), and other experts proposed age-specific reference range of PSA for subjects younger than 60 years (6).

PERCENT OF FREE PSA (%FPSA)

To improve cancer detection quality by PSA testing, several molecular derivatives of PSA were investigated. In serum, the majority of PSA exists as a complexed form bound with proteins, while some is free form protein and called free PSA. The free PSA accounts for 5% to 35% of total PSA and the proportion diminishes at the coexistence of PCa (7). Therefore, the lower percent of free PSA (%fPSA) suggests the higher likelihood of positive result from prostate biopsy. Scientific research indicates that malignant prostate glands produce PSA that is more likely to bound protein (8). The Food and Drug Administration approved the ratio of free to total PSA (%fPSA) for PCa detection with PSA tests for men with normal result from digital rectal examination and a gray zone range of PSA from 4 to 10 ng/mL.

There is no clear criterion of cutoff value of %fPSA. Catalona et al. performed a prospective multicenter study inclusive of white and black groups of men and revealed that with a %fPSA less than 10%, more than half of men tested positive for PCa with a threshold of 25% of %fPSA and 95% of patients developed PCa with about a 20% reduction in unnecessary biopsies recorded for both races (8).

■ PSA VELOCITY

PSA velocity is the rate at which PSA values elevate from year to year. After the introduction of PSA for PCa screening, some studies noted that PSA levels in men with PCa rises more rapidly than in those without PCa. Carter et al. demonstrated that a PSA velocity greater than 0.75 ng/mL per year as a possible marker for the presence or absence of PCa in men with PSA levels between 4 and 10 ng/mL (9). However, the efficiency of PSA velocity for PCa screening is controversial. A study by ERSPC concluded that PSA velocity was not a significant predictor of a positive biopsy (10), and a recent systematic review does not support the use of PSA velocity as well as PSA doubling time in clinical decision making for detection and treatment of early-stage PCa because of the lack of evidence of its additional predictive information compared with using absolute PSA level alone (11).

■ PSA DENSITY

PSA density (PSAD) is a volume-adjusted PSA level. Consequently, because PSA could elevate with benign prostate enlargement, an index calculated by dividing PSA by prostate volume, determined usually by ultrasonography, is believed to be useful in distinguishing PSA rise caused by PCa (12). A cutoff line, PSAD of 0.15 or greater, is recommended to improve the prediction of the probability of diagnosing PCa in men with PSA levels between 4 and 10 ng/mL and a normal digital rectal examination (13). Similarly, the transition zone PSA density, a value obtained by adjusting PSA by the transition zone volume calculated on transrectal ultrasound, has also been proposed as an additional diagnostic parameter (14).

■ INDIVIDUALIZED PREDICTING TOOLS FOR PROSTATE CANCER

Because PSA is not cancer specific but organ specific, PSA alone results in a high false-positive rate. Among men presenting a PSA of 4 to 10 ng/mL, PCa is presented in only 30% to 40% of them (3). The higher the PSA cutoff point is set as a biopsy indicator, the more its specificity improves, while lessening the opportunity of cancer detection. Inversely, when a lower threshold is used, its sensitivity increases, thus increasing the risk of unnecessary biopsies (15). To compensate for the limitations in the sensitivity and specificity of PSA values alone for prediction, there are various approaches to predict the likelihood of PCa. Currently, dozens of nomograms and artificial neural networks exist for PCa prediction (16); however, even with a wide variety of models, those with external validation and international population heterogeneity are few (17). In addition, users need to be aware that these tools still lack enough evidence of improving the benefit to harm ratio, and generalizability is limited to the population related to their development process. A comprehensive review of these predicting tools by Schroder et al. states that even though various variables are integrated in models with the justification of statistical significances, it often happens that increasing complexity of the model does not afford enough improvement of its predictive quality and ends in making the model less feasible (16). They also pointed out that for men without additional risk factors, including family history, positive digital rectal examination, and history of previous prostate biopsy, PSA value alone provides a sufficiently precise prediction (16). The panel committee of American Urological Association for PCa screening recommended that physicians limit the use of these tests as a complementary reference for decision making regarding the need for a prostate biopsy (18).

■ GUIDELINES BY AMERICAN UROLOGICAL ASSOCIATION

In 2013, the American Urological Association (AUA) released the clinical guideline of "Early Detection of Prostate Cancer" (18). The updated recommendations intended to provide efficient detection of PCa at early and presymptomatic stages while focusing on the merit of early detection and reducing the harm of screening.

The AUA guideline does not support annual routine PSA checks without considering patient risk factors such as family history, race, and information pertinent to benefits and harms associated with PSA screening, especially for people younger than 55 years and older than 70 years. The highest quality evidence for benefit from PSA screening is for the age group 55 to 69 years at intervals of 2 years, which is comparative enough to an annual test and encouraging in terms of reducing and false-positive results (19).

When a man has a family history of PCa with a first-degree relative or is African American, it is advised the health care provider counsel these higher risk patients of the possible and uncertain benefits and risks relating to PSA screening to assist in decision making (20).

The same guideline cautioned against the use of other PSA-related tools such as PSA density, velocity, free PSA, and so on, stating a lack of enough evidence of improving the ratio of benefit to harm in screening and advised to use these as supplementary tools for patients' decision making. Importantly, the AUA guideline recommended against routine PSA screenings for men aged 70 years or older if their estimated life expectancy is less than 10 to 15 years. This is based on the evidence showing that benefit for PSA screening among this group is lacking with the significantly increased incidence of competing risks of mortality in the older patient population (5).

■ CONCLUSIONS

After two decades of PSA screening, the focus of PSA testing has shifted from how to determine when to perform a prostate biopsy to the best way to inform patients and assist them in making an appropriate decision. No perfect tool exists; however, several crystallizations of wisdom including the use of complementary nomograms, the AUA guideline, and the primary recognition of PSA limitations move toward fostering the correct usage of PSA screening.

■ REFERENCES

1. Papsidero LD, Wang MC, Valenzuela LA, et al. A prostate antigen in sera of prostatic cancer patients. *Cancer Res.* 1980;40(7):2428–2432.
2. Thompson IM, Pauler DK, Goodman PJ, et al. Prevalence of prostate cancer among men with a prostate-specific antigen level < or =4.0 ng per milliliter. *N Engl J Med.* 2004;350(22):2239–2246.
3. Andriole GL, Levin DL, Crawford ED, et al. Prostate Cancer Screening in the Prostate, Lung, Colorectal and Ovarian (PLCO) Cancer Screening Trial: findings from the initial screening round of a randomized trial. *J Natl Cancer Inst.* 2005;97(6):433–438.
4. Stamey TA, Yang N, Hay AR, McNeal JE, Freiha FS, Redwine E. Prostate-specific antigen as a serum marker for adenocarcinoma of the prostate. *N Engl J Med.* 1987;317(15):909–916.
5. Schroder FH, Hugosson J, Roobol MJ, et al. Screening and prostate-cancer mortality in a randomized European study. *N Engl J Med.* 2009;360(13):1320–1328.
6. Oesterling JE, Jacobsen SJ, Chute CG, et al. Serum prostate-specific antigen in a community-based population of healthy men. Establishment of age-specific reference ranges. *JAMA.* 1993;270(7):860–864.
7. McCormack RT, Rittenhouse HG, Finlay JA, et al. Molecular forms of prostate-specific antigen and the human kallikrein gene family: a new era. *Urology.* 1995;45(5):729–744.
8. Catalona WJ, Partin AW, Slawin KM, et al. Percentage of free PSA in black versus white men for detection and staging of prostate cancer: a prospective multicenter clinical trial. *Urology.* 2000;55(3):372–376.
9. Carter HB, Pearson JD, Metter EJ, et al. Longitudinal evaluation of prostate-specific antigen levels in men with and without prostate disease. *JAMA.* 1992;267(16):2215–2220.
10. Wolters T, Roobol MJ, Bangma CH, Schröder FH. Is prostate-specific antigen velocity selective for clinically significant prostate cancer in screening? European Randomized Study of Screening for Prostate Cancer (Rotterdam). *Eur Urol.* 2009;55(2):385–392.
11. Vickers AJ, Savage C, O'Brien MF, Lilja H. Systematic review of pretreatment prostate-specific antigen velocity and doubling time as predictors for prostate cancer. *J Clin Oncol.* 2009;27(3):398–403.
12. Benson MC, Whang IS, Olsson CA, McMahon DJ, Cooner WH. The use of prostate specific antigen density to enhance the predictive value of intermediate levels of serum prostate specific antigen. *J Urol.* 1992;147(3 pt 2):817–821.
13. Bazinet M, Meshref AW, Trudel C, et al. Prospective evaluation of prostate-specific antigen density and systematic biopsies for early detection of prostatic carcinoma. *Urology.* 1994;43(1):44–51; discussion 51–52.
14. Djavan B, Zlotta A, Kratzik C, et al. PSA, PSA density, PSA density of transition zone, free/total PSA ratio, and PSA velocity for early detection of prostate cancer in men with serum PSA 2.5 to 4.0 ng/mL. *Urology.* 1999;54(3):517–522.
15. Welch HG, Schwartz LM, Woloshin S. Prostate-specific antigen levels in the United States: implications of various definitions for abnormal. *J Natl Cancer Inst.* 2005;97(15):1132–1137.
16. Schroder F, Kattan MW. The comparability of models for predicting the risk of a positive prostate biopsy with prostate-specific antigen alone: a systematic review. *Eur Urol.* 2008;54(2):274–290.
17. Ouzaid I, Yates DR, Hupertan V, et al. A direct comparison of the diagnostic accuracy of three prostate cancer nomograms designed to predict the likelihood of a positive initial transrectal biopsy. *Prostate.* 2012;72(11):1200–1206.
18. Carter HB, Albertsen PC, Barry MJ, et al. Early detection of prostate cancer: AUA guideline. *J Urol.* 2013;190:419–426.
19. Gulati R, Gore JL, Etzioni R. Comparative effectiveness of alternative prostate-specific antigen–based prostate cancer screening strategies: model estimates of potential benefits and harms. *Ann Intern Med.* 2013;158(3):145–153.
20. Brawley OW. Prostate cancer epidemiology in the United States. *World J Urol.* 2012;30(2):195–200.

3.2 Screening and Diagnosis: An Update on the ISUP-Modified Gleason Score and Its Controversies

IBRAHIM KULAC

ANGELO M. DEMARZO

■ GLEASON SCORING SYSTEM—A BRIEF HISTORY

Donald Gleason developed a histological grading system for prostate cancer during the course of prospective clinical trials studies carried out by the Veterans Administration Cooperative Urological Research Group from 1960 to 1975 (1–4). Since then, Gleason grading has become a widely used and accepted system throughout the world and it still remains one of the most important prognostic factors in prostate cancer. Gleason and others recognized that the morphology of prostate cancer often was heterogeneous (~50% of cases) and the heterogeneity could be captured by a series of patterns of tumor architecture recognizable at relatively low microscopic power. The original nine histologic patterns were grouped into five grades, and these grades were numbered in order of increasing degrees of glandular architectural abnormalities, compared to benign prostatic glands. These grades also corresponded to increasing biological aggressiveness based on mortality data. Unlike many other types of cancers in which the worst grade generally determines overall prognosis, a unique aspect of these prostate cancer studies was that outcomes in patients with two different grades of tumor were intermediate between those with pure tumors of either of those two grades.

The rules of traditional Gleason scoring were based on the sum of the most abundant pattern and the second most abundant pattern. If only a single pattern was present, then it would be multiplied by 2 (e.g., all Gleason pattern 3 results in a Gleason score of 3 + 3 = 6). The inclusion of a simple drawing of the histologic patterns group into the five grades was used as a teaching tool for those seeking to learn the system. The Gleason sum and Gleason score are used interchangeably. The prognostic value of the grading system was validated by a number of other groups using separate datasets in studies in the 1970s and 1980s, and the system gained increasing adoption over time and today it is virtually universally utilized.

■ THE NEED TO UPDATE THE SYSTEM

The studies in the 1970s and 1980s by Gleason and others were performed prior to the era of serum prostate-specific antigen (PSA) screening tests for prostate cancer and were largely carried out using a small number of thick gauge transperineal biopsies of overt palpable lesions in men who often had advanced disease with relatively large tumor foci, or, to a much lesser degree on prostatectomy specimens. In the following years, with the introduction of serum PSA testing and development of thin needle biopsy techniques (e.g., 18 gauge), pathologists were faced with the need to diagnose and grade smaller and smaller tumors that were mostly of clinical stage T1C. These tumors were generally diagnosed using systematic (e.g., sextant) sampling methods that randomly sampled tumor lesions(5). Further, after the widespread introduction of radical prostatectomy in the 1980s, it became clear that in the majority of cases, tumors were multifocal. Given that the historically used Gleason grading system was not developed using nondirected 18-gauge needle biopsy samples nor with large numbers of radical prostatectomies in mind, it became apparent that significant modifications were needed. In 2005, the International Society of Urological Pathology (ISUP) organized a conference to discuss and modify the Gleason grading system.

2005 ISUP CONSENSUS CONFERENCE AND SUBSEQUENT MODIFICATIONS

A consensus report was published by ISUP in 2005 (6), and a number of additional studies and reviews have been published since then (7–11). In terms of very low-grade lesions, many of the cases that were diagnosed in the past as Gleason score 2 (1 + 1 = 2) adenocarcinoma would likely now be considered benign adenosis, also referred to by some authors as atypical adenomatous hyperplasia. This is in large part the result of the introduction of basal cell–specific immunohistochemical (IHC) markers over the last two decades, which show lack of basal cells in adenocarcinoma but the presence of basal cells in benign mimickers or precursor lesions of adenocarcinoma. Further, tumors that are truly very low grade (e.g., <Gleason score 5) are mostly present in the transition zone of the prostate, which is often not sampled (unless specifically targeted) by standard transrectal ultrasound-guided 18-gauge needle biopsies. Thus, it was decided that Gleason scores of <5 should almost never be rendered on these biopsies, although it is still diagnosed to some degree on incidental tumors found by transurethral resection of the prostate (TURP). The definitions of Gleason grades 3, 4, and 5 were also revised in this consensus. In brief, grade 3 lesions were narrowed to remove most (ISUP 2005) and subsequently all (ISUP 2010) cribriform patterns including glomeruloid glands (7). Grade 3 was redefined as a tumor with discrete and individual glands, often infiltrating between benign glands, and lesions with "poorly formed" glands were reclassified as Gleason grade 4. The descriptions of the patterns making up grade 5 stayed essentially unchanged.

The report also included a guide for scoring specific tumor subtypes. For example, ductal adenocarcinoma, which reflects a morphological variant of adenocarcinoma, should be scored as Gleason score 4 + 4 = 8, and small cell carcinoma should not receive a Gleason grade. Some other subtypes and morphologic variants of prostate carcinoma should be assigned based on their morphology (e.g., foamy gland carcinoma can be either grade 3 or 4 depending on the glandular architecture) although scoring some variants still stands as an unresolved issue (e.g., for colloid carcinoma, some experts suggest all should be scored as 4 + 4 = 8, whereas others indicate that underlying glandular architecture can be used to score these as low as 3 + 3 = 6).

ISSUES RELATING SPECIFICALLY TO NEEDLE BIOPSIES AND RADICAL PROSTATECTOMY SPECIMENS

The 2005 ISUP consensus meeting also examined the use of tertiary Gleason patterns in prostatectomy specimens as well as making sure that any high-grade cancer, regardless of percentage, should be included in the Gleason score of needle biopsy specimens. The suggestion of indicating tertiary pattern in radical prostatectomies came from the studies that established that the patients with Gleason score 3 + 4 = 7 with a tertiary pattern 5 often show rates of disease recurrence that is intermediate between Gleason 3 + 4 = 7 and Gleason score 8. In addition, for prostatectomy specimens, if there are clearly separable tumor nodules, then each nodule should receive a Gleason score. For prognostication, the nodule with the highest overall Gleason score should be used by clinicians, rather than an overall Gleason score based on the most common and second most common pattern in the prostatectomy specimens. On needle biopsy, if a tumor is composed of ≥95% pattern 4 and <5%Gleason pattern 3, the lower grade should be ignored and this tumor should be graded as 4 + 4 = 8. Conversely, if a tumor was >95% Gleason pattern 3 and <5% Gleason pattern 4 or 5, then the grade would be 3 + 4 = 7 and 3 + 5 = 8, respectively, since one always includes the highest grade tumor in the Gleason score on needle biopsies. On biopsy specimens, if there is a third pattern with lower grade than the two others, the lower grade should be ignored and the score should be given as the sum of the most frequent tumor grade and the highest grade.

IMPLICATIONS AND RESULTS OF THE ISUP-MODIFIED GLEASON GRADING SYSTEM

The primary purpose of a pathology grading system is to aid clinicians in stratifying patients into risk groups to help with treatment option selections. Although it is still too early to fully evaluate whether the modified Gleason grading system is superior in predicting prostate cancer–specific death, studies that have examined correlation with radical prostatectomy findings and biochemical recurrence as outcomes have generally shown the new system to perform well and when compared directly to the traditional system, as well or better (7, 9–11).

Although there are a number of implications to changes implemented by the ISUP regarding Gleason grading, the most important may be that Gleason score 6 tumors, especially if the tumor is organ confined, are now believed to be nearly universally cured by radical retropubic prostatectomy (12, 13). In fact, 10- to 15-year survival for Gleason score 6 tumors on needle biopsy are so high, even without treatment, that some investigators have raised the issue of whether to even call it carcinoma (14, 15). Although an in-depth discussion of this issue is beyond the scope of this chapter, and arguments can be made both against and for keeping the cancer label (16), it should be pointed out that studies indicating that Gleason score 6 tumors nearly never progress to metastatic disease or death were carried out on patients who were treated with surgery (12, 13, 17). Thus, it is formally possible that Gleason score 6 can "progress" or evolve into a higher grade tumor, yet there is very little definitive longitudinal data to indicate this one way or the other. For example, even when there are longitudinal data consisting of serial biopsies over time, unless the entire prostate is carefully sampled (which it cannot be unless it is removed), it is impossible to know whether a higher grade lesion identified later in time by longitudinal sampling was actually not already present in the original biopsy and simply not sampled.

Molecular evidence is being used to shed some light on this. Interestingly, individual tumor nodules that are composed of both Gleason patterns 3 and 4 often show definitive evidence of clonality between the two morphologies, both by *TMPRSS2-ERG* breakpoint analysis (18) and whole-genome sequencing that shows other breakpoints in common (18, 19). Also, at least in a few cases, it appeared that loss of one PTEN allele occurred in both the pattern 3 and 4 components, but that the pattern 4 component showed loss of the second allele, providing support for the concept that Gleason score may progress, at least at times (18). Of course, if the prostate is not removed, the clinical relevance of whether Gleason 6 tumors can progress is muted somewhat by the fact that de novo higher grade lesions could always arise over time.

■ LINGERING PROBLEMS OF THE GLEASON GRADING SYSTEM

A number of problems still remain in which there is room for improvement in the Gleason grading system. The first problem deals with interobserver reproducibility of Gleason grading, as in any system in medicine that relies somewhat on subjective assessments (e.g., radiology assessments). The problem stems from the difficulty in attempting to take a complex biological process in which the pathologist is "forced" to ascribe whole numbers to it in all cases (e.g., pathologists simply have not availed themselves of the choice to say that they are not certain of the grade), when indeed some cases simply defy clear separations in this regard. Although a significant fraction of prostate cancers contain morphological features that are relatively straightforward to classify by pathologists, there are still a number of cases that are more difficult to grade and these cases clearly lead to problems of increased interobserver variability, especially in small tumor foci. Also, it is quite clear that learning this system requires that a pathologist diagnose a large number of cases in the training setting or in a setting where they can obtain expert feedback. This issue of interobserver variation has been a problem for a long time, and there is emerging evidence that the adoption of the modified ISUP 2005 system has improved the situation (8, 9).

Another problem, which is as much a problem in tissue sampling as it is in pathologist error or lack of reproducibility, is the number of cases in which the biopsy Gleason score is different than the score rendered at radical prostatectomy. A clinical scenario in which this can be problematic is in apparent undergrading of the biopsy, where a man is found to have Gleason 3 + 3 = 6 tumor on biopsy but is found to have a higher grade tumor on radical prostatectomy, which occurs in approximately 25% to 35% of cases (20–22). This is a major problem in potential undertreatment because many programs in which men are offered active surveillance only encourage patients to enroll if they have Gleason 6 cancers or less, with the concern that lesions consisting of Gleason score 7 or higher could be life threatening (23). Although some active surveillance programs are now suggesting that select men with apparent low-volume Gleason 3 + 4 = 7 cancer should also be considered candidates for active surveillance (15), and this will render this question of limited Gleason 3 + 3 = 6 versus 3 + 4 = 7 on biopsy less of an issue. Some patients with 3 + 3 = 6 tumors on biopsy are upgraded to Gleason 4 + 3 = 7 at or higher radical prostatectomy. Although relatively rare, it is hoped that these relatively extreme types of cases could become even more rare if magnetic resonance imaging/ultrasound-fusion-guided needle biopsy is further validated and made widely available (24). In most, albeit not all, studies that have compared the concordance between needle biopsy Gleason score and radical prostatectomy Gleason score, there does seem to be improvement when using the new modified system (7, 8, 10).

Another problematic area, that was inevitably created by developing and implementing the modified ISUP grading system, is that it has now become difficult to directly compare older studies using the traditional system with newer studies using the modified system (16). For example, a number of studies have shown that by regrading cases, the percentage of tumors that contain pattern 4 has increased and the percentage that contains pattern 3 decreased (8). Thus, in comparing newer studies with older studies, these changes in grading may artificially indicate that patients with both Gleason 6 and 7 tumors have improved outcomes (the Will Rogers effect). Nevertheless, this was inevitable and should not deter pathologists from adopting the newer system as there was broad consensus on most of the proposed changes by a large international group of prostate pathology experts.

IS IT TIME FOR A MODIFIED GROUPING OF GLEASON SCORES FOR PROGNOSTIC STUDIES?

Recently, Pierorazio et al. (25) examined a large number of consecutive prostatectomy specimens and found that using the modified Gleason grading system in a modern series of patients, that grouping patients into the following prognostic categories provided excellent patient stratification when biochemical recurrence was used as the outcome measure: Gleason score ≤6 (prognostic grade group I); Gleason score 3 + 4 = 7 (prognostic grade group II); Gleason score 4 + 3 = 7 (prognostic grade group III); Gleason score 4 + 4 = 8 (prognostic grade group IV); and Gleason score 9 to 10 (prognostic grade group V). The authors indicated that the major reasons for this approach were the following: (1) although Gleason score 6 is now the lowest score rendered by most pathologists, it appears to patients that they have a 6 of 10, which instills undue fear since these tumors have an excellent prognosis overall; (2) a number of studies have shown the clear difference in outcome between Gleason score 3 + 4 = 7 and 4 + 3 = 7 tumors, justifying their separation into the new categories; and (3) Gleason score 8 tumors tend to behave significantly better than those of score 9 to 10. Of course, additional time will tell whether the combination of the modified Gleason scoring system and these newly proposed prognostic groupings will provide powerful prediction for prostate cancer–specific death.

CONCLUSIONS

The Gleason scoring system has been used to varying extents since the mid to late 1970s and it has been shown by hundreds (if not thousands) of studies that the Gleason score is a robust biomarker for predicting prostate cancer outcomes and thus guiding therapeutic choices. Although there are still some controversial issues regarding various aspects of its implementation, the 2005 (and updated 2010) modified Gleason grading system adopted by ISUP is a widely used and valuable tool. The revised system continues to employ the basic concepts introduced by Gleason—that is, that prostate cancers are heterogeneous and that different architectural patterns of glandular growth, identified at low microscopic power, are associated with varying degrees of malignant potential. Further, capturing these patterns in a Gleason score provides extremely useful information to clinicians. Future studies will certainly provide additional information to support or refute its continued use, and it is clear that emerging molecular discoveries will certainly add value as they lead to new prognostic and predictive biomarkers. The question will be whether these advances in understanding the underlying biological mechanisms and/or biomarker development and implementation will supplant or supplement this powerful, inexpensive, and simple morphology-based tool.

REFERENCES

1. Gleason DF. Classification of prostatic carcinomas. *Cancer Chemother Rep.* 1966;50(3):125–128.
2. Mellinger GT, Gleason D, Bailar J III. The histology and prognosis of prostatic cancer. *J Urol.* 1967;97(2):331-337.
3. Gleason DF. Histologic grading of prostate cancer: a perspective. *Hum Pathol.* 1992;23(3):273–279.
4. Gleason DF, Mellinger GT. Prediction of prognosis for prostatic adenocarcinoma by combined histological grading and clinical staging. *J Urol.* 1974;111(1):58–64.
5. Stamey TA, Yang N, Hay AR, McNeal JE, Freiha FS, Redwine E. Prostate-specific antigen as a serum marker for adenocarcinoma of the prostate. *N Engl J Med.* 1987;317(15):909–916.
6. Epstein JI, Allsbrook WC Jr, Amin MB, Egevad LL, Committee IG. The 2005 International Society of Urological Pathology (ISUP) Consensus Conference on Gleason Grading of Prostatic Carcinoma. *Am J Surg Pathol.* 2005;29(9):1228–1242.
7. Epstein JI. An update of the Gleason grading system. *J Urol.* 2010;183(2):433–440.
8. Delahunt B, Miller RJ, Srigley JR, Evans AJ, Samaratunga H. Gleason grading: past, present and future. *Histopathology.* 2012;60(1):75–86.
9. Brimo F, Montironi R, Egevad L, et al. Contemporary grading for prostate cancer: implications for patient care. *Eur Urol.* 2013;63(5):892–901.
10. Egevad L, Mazzucchelli R, Montironi R. Implications of the International Society of Urological Pathology modified Gleason grading system. *Arch Pathol Lab Med.* 2012;136(4):426–434.
11. Montironi R, Mazzucchelli R, Lopez-Beltran A, Scarpelli M, Cheng L. The Gleason grading system: where are we now? *Diagn Histopath.* 2011;17(10):10.
12. Miyamoto H, Hernandez DJ, Epstein JI. A pathological reassessment of organ-confined, Gleason score 6 prostatic adenocarcinomas that progress after radical prostatectomy. *Hum Pathol.* 2009;40(12):1693–1698.
13. Ross HM, Kryvenko ON, Cowan JE, Simko JP, Wheeler TM, Epstein JI. Do adenocarcinomas of the prostate with Gleason score (GS) </=6 have the potential to metastasize to lymph nodes? *Am J Surg Pathol.* 2012;36(9):1346–1352.
14. Nickel JC, Speakman M. Should we really consider Gleason 6 prostate cancer? *BJU Int.* 2012;109(5):645–646.
15. Klotz L. Active surveillance: patient selection. *Curr Opin Urol.* 2013;23(3):239–244.
16. Carter HB, Partin AW, Walsh PC, et al. Gleason score 6 adenocarcinoma: should it be labeled as cancer? *J Clin Oncol.* 2012;30(35):4294–4296.
17. Eggener SE, Scardino PT, Walsh PC, et al. Predicting 15-year prostate cancer specific mortality after radical prostatectomy. *J Urol.* 2011;185(3):869–875.
18. Sowalsky AG, Ye H, Bubley GJ, Balk SP. Clonal progression of prostate cancers from Gleason grade 3 to grade 4. *Cancer Res.* 2013;73(3):1050–1055.
19. Kovtun IV, Cheville JC, Murphy SJ, et al. Lineage relationship of Gleason patterns in Gleason score 7 prostate cancer. *Cancer Res.* 2013;73(11):3275–3284.
20. Epstein JI, Feng Z, Trock BJ, Pierorazio PM. Upgrading and downgrading of prostate cancer from biopsy to radical prostatectomy: incidence and predictive factors using the modified Gleason

grading system and factoring in tertiary grades. *Eur Urol.* 2012;61:1019–1024.

21. Bulbul MA, El-Hout Y, Haddad M, et al. Pathological correlation between needle biopsy and radical prostatectomy specimen in patients with localized prostate cancer. *Can Urol Assoc J.* 2007;1(3):264–266.
22. Fine SW, Epstein JI. A contemporary study correlating prostate needle biopsy and radical prostatectomy Gleason score. *J Urol.* 2008;179(4):1335–1338; discussion 1338–1339.
23. Ganz PA, Barry JM, Burke W, et al. National Institutes of Health State-of-the-Science Conference: role of active surveillance in the management of men with localized prostate cancer. *Ann Intern Med.* 2012;156(8):591–595.
24. Siddiqui MM, Rais-Bahrami S, Truong H, et al. Magnetic resonance imaging/ultrasound-fusion biopsy significantly upgrades prostate cancer versus systematic 12-core transrectal ultrasound biopsy. *Eur Urol.* 2013;64:713–719.
25. Pierorazio PM, Walsh PC, Partin AW, Epstein JI. Prognostic Gleason grade grouping: data based on the modified Gleason scoring system. *BJU Int.* 2013;111(5):753–760.

3.3 Evaluation of Distant Disease: The Utility of Nuclear Imaging

DIMA RASKOLNIKOV
BARIS TURKBEY
LIZA LINDENBERG
PETER L. CHOYKE
PETER A. PINTO

■ INTRODUCTION

Prostate cancer (PCa) remains the most common solid organ cancer detected in American men, as well as the second most common cause of cancer-related deaths (1). However, PCa represents a broad spectrum of diseases ranging from indolent to highly aggressive. In the era of screening with prostate-specific antigen (PSA), many men now present with disease that previously may not have been detected. This presents a diagnostic and therapeutic dilemma for clinicians. Lethal disease must now be distinguished from nonlethal disease, yet little consensus exists as to precisely how this should be done (2). Although a variety of biomarkers have been proposed, advances in imaging play an increasingly important role in this discussion. This is especially true for the evaluation of distant disease, where nuclear imaging has the potential to have the greatest impact. The role of these modalities is set to increase as we move into the post-PSA era. The purpose of this chapter is to review the current status of nuclear imaging in the evaluation of distant PCa disease.

Nuclear imaging involves the injection of a small amount of radioactive material, known as a "radiopharmaceutical," into the patient. The distribution of this material within the body is then detected by specialized imaging cameras, thus allowing for noninvasive quantitative and qualitative assessment of the extent of disease. Radiopharmaceuticals labeled with positron-emitting radionuclides are specifically detected by positron emission tomography (PET) cameras that are often combined with x-ray computed tomography (PET/CT). The relatively better resolution and quantitative capabilities make PET a desirable molecular imaging modality. PET should be distinguished from the other major category of radionuclide imaging, single-photon emission computed tomography (SPECT), in which gamma-ray-emitting radionuclides are coupled to targeting agents. SPECT cameras, which can also be combined with CT, however, have inferior resolution and sensitivity compared to PET. The clinical relevance of either approach lies in the ability to conjugate positron or single-photon radionuclides to biologically significant molecules with high affinities for their targets, thereby enabling the noninvasive detection of specific markers associated with cancers. Because neoplastic growth typically relies on abnormal upregulation of many cellular processes, PET and SPECT tracers specific to these molecular signatures have emerged as important tools in the evaluation of both localized and metastatic cancer.

From the perspective of PCa diagnosis, extensive research has recently focused on the development of novel PET tracers, each with its own set of strengths and weaknesses. This work has been motivated in large part by the limitations of previous techniques that have been used for imaging distant disease. These include CT, magnetic resonance imaging (MRI), and technetium-99m (^{99m}Tc)-labeled bone scintigraphy, the last of which is the current standard of care for detecting bone metastases in PCa. In 2000, Bubendorf et al. conducted an autopsy study of 1,589 patients with PCa (3). The authors showed that as many as 90% of patients with metastatic PCa had bone involvement. Other common sites included the lung, liver, pleura, and adrenals, in descending order of frequency. However, none of the three modalities currently used for PCa imaging is both sensitive and specific for PCa metastases in all of these sites. MRI offers the best three-dimensional anatomic imaging of localized PCa and also has excellent soft-tissue resolution. The utility of MRI has further increased with the use of higher field strength magnets, endorectal coils, and multiparametric MRI (MP-MRI). However, these advances pertain largely to localized PCa (4,5). For metastatic PCa, MRI continues to provide superior soft-tissue resolution, but suffers from low sensitivity for nodal metastases because it relies strictly on size criteria (e.g., only nodes >1 cm in diameter are considered positive) (6). Moreover, although promising improvements have been made, whole-body MRI scans are still mostly performed in research centers, and thus, coverage with MRI remains problematic. CT effectively detects bone and visceral metastases, but it is relatively insensitive for early disease in these sites and has a similarly low sensitivity for early intranodal disease. ^{99m}Tc-labelled bone scintigraphy, which is typically performed as a planar projection scan but can be obtained with a SPECT camera, has become the standard for detecting bone metastases due to its high sensitivity for osteoblastic lesions characteristic of metastatic PCa (7). However, bone scans have poor specificity in distinguishing metastases from traumatic or degenerative disease, and false positives are commonly encountered with benign conditions that have a high prevalence in patients with PCa, such as degenerative joint disease.

For all of these reasons, research has continued to focus on novel PET-based nuclear imaging modalities for distant PCa. These include PET tracers such as ^{18}F-fluorodeoxyglucose (^{18}F-FDG), ^{18}F-sodium fluoride, ^{18}F-choline and ^{11}C-choline, ^{11}C-acetate, the amino acid targets L-*methyl*-^{11}C-methionine (^{11}C-methionine) and anti-1-amino-3-(18)F-fluorocyclobutane-1-carboxylic acid (^{18}F-FACBC), 16β-18F-fluoro-5α-dihydrotestosterone (^{18}F-FDHT), as well as molecules targeting prostate-specific membrane antigen (PSMA) such as ^{8}F-DCFBC and those targeting the human epidermal growth factor receptor-2 (Her2).

^{18}F-FDG

To fuel their rapid growth, neoplastic cells typically overexpress proteins that are essential for glycolysis. This includes GLUT-1, a cell membrane glucose transporter, and hexokinase, an intracellular enzyme. ^{18}F-FDG is a fluorine-labeled glucose analog that is taken up in cells utilizing aerobic glycolysis for their energy needs. After uptake into the cell via GLUT-1, FDG is phosphorylated by hexokinase to yield FDG-6-phosphate. This molecule, however, does not undergo further metabolism and instead accumulates intracellularly. Those sites with an unusually high accumulation of ^{18}F-FDG—and thus unusually high rates of glycolysis—are suspicious for cancer. Although ^{18}F-FDG has been widely employed in the imaging of numerous cancers, it suffers from three important limitations in the imaging of PCa. First, unlike other cancers, many PCa lesions have been found to have low rates of glucose metabolism, expressing few GLUT-1 binding sites (8, 9). This is particularly problematic for low-grade, slow-growing PCa, which may be even more difficult to detect. Second, common conditions such as benign prostatic hyperplasia (BPH) and prostatitis are also characterized by increased rates of glycolysis, thereby lowering the specificity of ^{18}F-FDG for neoplastic growth (10, 11). Third, ^{18}F-FDG undergoes urinary excretion, causing significant interference with imaging of tissue adjacent to the bladder, including the prostate and surrounding tissues (12). Collectively, these obstacles limit the utility of ^{18}F-FDG in the setting of PCa (13). However, recent research has suggested possible new roles for this tracer in advanced disease. In 2013, Jadvar et al. demonstrated that ^{18}F-FDG PET/CT provides important additional prognostic information in overall survival for men with advanced castrate-resistant metastatic PCa (14). Further research is necessary to determine whether these or other findings will change the role of ^{18}F-FDG in the imaging of metastatic PCa.

^{18}F-SODIUM FLUORIDE

Despite its wide adoption, ^{99m}Tc-bone scintigraphy suffers nonspecificity and difficulties in quantitation. For this reason, there is renewed interest in ^{18}F-sodium fluoride (^{18}F-NaF), an alternative PET-based technique that can detect bone metastases with higher sensitivity than conventional bones scans (Figure 3.3.1). In one study, ^{18}F-NaF PET/CT was compared with ^{18}F-fluorocholine PET/CT (15). The two tracers were found to have similar sensitivities for bone metastases, although the authors noted that ^{18}F-NaF may be negative in sclerotic lesions that are especially dense. More compelling evidence in favor of widespread use of ^{18}F-NaF was offered in a recent prospective clinical study by Damle et al. (16). In that study, ^{18}F-NaF PET/CT was directly compared to ^{18}F-FDG PET/CT and ^{99m}Tc-bone scintigraphy for the detection of metastatic lesions in 72 patients with infiltrating ductal breast cancer, 49 patients with PCa, and 30 patients with lung carcinoma. Not only was the sensitivity and negative predictive value of ^{18}F-NaF PET/CT 100% for lesions associated with all three malignancies, but in patients with PCa, ^{18}F-NaF outperformed ^{99m}Tc-bone scintigraphy in specificity and positive predictive value as well (16). In another prospective study, Jadvar et al. compared ^{18}F-NaF with ^{18}F-FDG PET/CT in detecting occult metastatic disease after biochemical recurrence (17). In this study as well, ^{18}F-NaF proved to be the more useful tracer.

CHOLINE: ^{18}F-CHOLINE AND ^{11}C-CHOLINE

Choline kinase is an intracellular enzyme that is involved in lipid metabolism and transport, a process that is upregulated in PCa and other cancers to facilitate the rapid synthesis of cell membranes. This process can be targeted in a manner similar to that used with ^{18}F- FDG. Choline is taken up by PCa cells and converted to phosphorylcholine, which

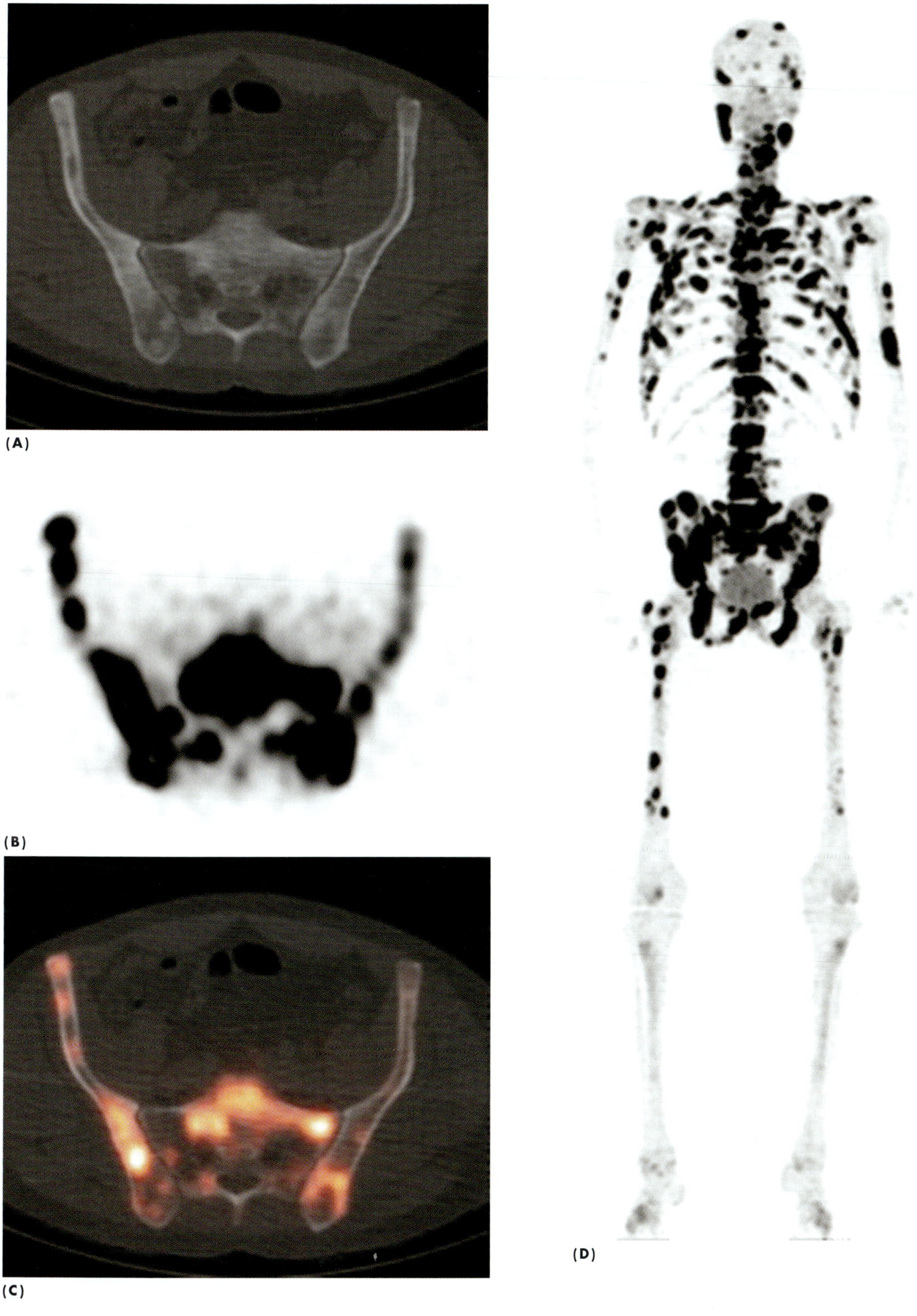

(A) (B) (C) (D)

FIGURE 3.3.1 A 54-year-old man with prostate cancer. The axial CT image (A) demonstrates diffuse osteoblastic lesions in the pelvic bone, and the axial PET (B), axial fused PET/CT (C), and coronal (D) maximum intensity projection PET images (obtained at 1 hour after injection of 18F-NaF) show increased tracer uptake in osteoblastic lesions, which is consistent with metastatic disease.

accumulates intracellularly. Theoretically, even those PCa cells that have low rates of glycolysis must still synthesize cell membranes, allowing for visualization with choline-labeled tracers. The two most common PET radiolabels are ^{11}C and ^{18}F, generating ^{11}C-choline and ^{18}F-choline, respectively. The advantage of using ^{11}C-choline is that it is chemically identical to natural choline. ^{11}C-choline PET demonstrates a sensitivity for primary and metastatic PCa ranging from 66% to 100%, with the highest sensitivity in those patients with elevated PSA (18–20). However, significant problems exist as well. First, the half-life of ^{11}C is only 20 minutes, thereby presenting the need for an on-site cyclotron. Second, choline is also taken up in benign prostatic tissue, especially in the setting of BPH (21, 22). Third, ^{11}C-choline is not sensitive to early recurrent disease (PSA < 1.0 ng/mL following prostatectomy), but progressively increases in sensitivity as PSA rises. Although Mamede et al. demonstrated that ^{11}C-choline was able to detect some instances of recurrent PCa, even in those patients with PSA values below 0.5 ng/mL, the PSA must usually be higher for reliable PCa detection (23). Nonetheless, choline uptake has not been found to correlate with tumor grade, PSA, Gleason score, tumor volume, or certain markers of cellular proliferation (24, 25). Notwithstanding these limitations, recent research has pointed to new potential uses for choline tracers in PCa. In one study, ^{11}C-choline PET/MR—as opposed to the more common ^{11}C-choline PET/CT—produced superior image quality, particularly in the pelvis (26). This suggests that future, prospective studies utilizing PET/MR may combine the sensitivity of MRI with the specificity of ^{11}C-choline PET to make an ideal PCa imaging method.

To address the short half-life of ^{11}C, ^{18}F-choline has also been investigated. Since ^{18}F has a half-life of 110 minutes, it can be produced off site and transported to medical facilities for imaging. This opens up more opportunity for its use. ^{18}F-choline has been extensively investigated outside of the United States and has shown comparable efficacy to ^{11}C-choline. Unlike ^{11}C-choline, which is excreted largely via the pancreas, there is more renal excretion with ^{18}F-choline and hence, more interfering bladder activity. However, ^{18}F-choline has proven useful for the identification of recurrent disease in patients with rising PSA after definitive treatment as well as for identifying soft-tissue and bony metastases. ^{18}F-choline is in routine use in some hospitals in Europe and Australia but, to date, it has not been used extensively in the United States.

■ ACETATE: ^{11}C-ACETATE

After uptake into the cell, acetate is converted to acetyl CoA, a substrate for the tricarboxylic acid cycle. This eventually leads to the incorporation of acetate into the cell membrane, thus making it mechanistically similar to choline as a potential PCa tracer. The tracer, ^{11}C-acetate, is chemically identical to the natural compound. Like ^{11}C-choline, ^{11}C-acetate is able to detect recurrent disease with rising PSA with similar sensitivity and specificity, and thus, there is no distinct advantage to either of the two labeled substrates. Existing studies are limited in size and have produced a broad range of sensitivities (27, 28). In addition, ^{11}C-acetate is excreted by the pancreas, so that there is little to no activity in the bladder to interfere with imaging in the pelvis (27). However, ^{11}C-acetate is not without its own limitations. First, as with ^{11}C-choline, the short half-life of ^{11}C raises the same barriers to its practical implementation. Second, normal and age-related changes in the prostate, such as BPH, cause ^{11}C-acetate uptake that is similar to that seen in PCa (29). This means that ^{11}C-acetate PET images must be interpreted with particular caution. Finally, as with ^{11}C-choline, studies have shown no correlation between ^{11}C-acetate uptake and Gleason score, PSA, or markers of tumor aggressiveness (30, 31). Despite this, the most recent studies of ^{11}C-actetate have shown promise in the setting of recurrent or metastatic disease. A 2013 meta-analysis of 23 studies by Mohsen et al. demonstrated a pooled sensitivity of 75.1% and specificity of 75.8% for primary and recurrent PCa using ^{11}C-acetate PET (32). Although the sensitivity dropped to 64% for recurrent cases, the specificity rose to 93%. The authors concluded that ^{11}C-acetate may provide important utility in this specific subset of patients. In another recent study, Yoshii et al. showed that ^{11}C-acetate may play a central role in predicting outcomes after PCa therapy with novel inhibitors of fatty acid synthase (33). Additional studies are necessary to explore all these directions.

■ AMINO ACIDS: ^{11}C-METHIONINE AND ^{18}F-FACBC

The majority of research into PET tracers for PCa has focused on glucose and fatty acid metabolism. However, a similar line of work has recently begun with molecules that target amino acid and protein metabolism. One example of this is ^{11}C-methionine, a tracer that is believed to accumulate in a variety of tumors in proportion to amino acid utilization (34). In an initial study of 348 lesions in 12 patients, Nuñez et al. found that ^{11}C-methionine PET had a sensitivity of 72.1%, compared with just 48% for ^{18}F-FDG PET (35). Further prospective studies are necessary to corroborate these findings. All the limitations of the short-lived ^{11}C radionuclide apply to this compound. More recently, a second tracer has been described, which also targets the amino acid metabolic pathway. ^{18}F-FACBC is a radiolabeled synthetic leucine analog that is taken up by PCa cells through a mechanism that remains poorly understood, but likely involves uptake by the amino acid transport mechanism. An initial report showed a sensitivity of 81.3% and specificity of 50%, although there was insufficient resolution to localize tumors to specific prostatic sextants (36). Subsequent work has reported both higher sensitivity and specificity for ^{18}F-FACBC in detecting recurrent PCa (37). A separate group also recently found ^{18}F-FACBC to be superior to ^{11}C-choline in identifying recurrent PCa, although this study was small and larger studies will be needed to establish this tracer as a part of the standard of care (38).

■ ^{18}F-FDHT

Androgen deprivation (AD) is an important tool in the treatment of patients with metastatic disease. However, this treatment is palliative, with all patients eventually progressing to a stage of androgen-independent PCa that is refractory to continued AD therapy (39). For this reason, there is an especially great need to develop and validate a noninvasive method for monitoring treatment response. To a certain extent, this has been accomplished with ^{18}F-FDHT, an androgen analog tracer. Dihydrotestosterone (DHT) binds with high affinity to the androgen receptor (AR) located in the cytoplasm, which then moves to the nucleus where it acts as a transcription factor that upregulates a number of pro-growth genes. ^{18}F-FDHT PET scans provide insight into those lesions that have active uptake for FDHT. Interestingly, not all lesions are FDHT positive, as some have already become independent of AR or have a mutated AR, and these lesions would not be expected to respond to AR treatments. An early report demonstrated a sensitivity of 57 of 59 lesions (97%) in 7 patients with progressive, metastatic PCa (40). A subsequent study of 20 patients showed similarly promising results, although there remains a paucity of research in support of this tracer since its development has so far been confined to a single institution (41). ^{18}F-FDHT has proven its use in the development of alternative inhibitors of the AR axis and is likely going to be important in the development of next-generation treatment that inhibit the AR. Significantly more work must be done, however, before ^{18}F-FDHT is adopted on a wide scale.

■ PROSTATE-SPECIFIC MEMBRANE ANTIGEN-TARGETED PET AGENTS

PSMA is a transmembrane protein expressed in prostatic epithelial cells. Not only is it highly expressed by virtually all PCa but studies have also shown its expression to correlate with tumor aggressiveness, androgen independence, metastatic disease, and disease recurrence (42). Despite these correlations, the actual role of PSMA in tumor growth is not known and inhibition of PSMA does not seem to affect survival. Nevertheless, because of its ubiquitous presence in PCa, it is an appealing target for imaging with PET. A number of PSMA-targeted tracers have been developed. Since PSMA is a transmembrane protein, it is possible to target either the internal or the external domain. The first PSMA-based imaging agent, ^{111}In capromab pendetide (tradename Prostascint), inadvertently targeted the antibody to the internal domain, limiting its utility, even though it was clinically approved and remains available today. Next-generation anti-PSMA targeting agents focused on the external domain of the receptor. Both monoclonal antibodies and low-molecular-weight radiopharmaceutical-based agents have been developed and demonstrate high uptake in PSMA-positive tumors (43, 44). A urea-based small molecule PET probe for PSMA, ^{18}F-DCFBC, has shown particular promise in identifying recurrent PCa. Unlike monoclonal antibody–based imaging, which must be performed over several days, scanning with ^{18}F-DCFBC can be performed within hours of injection. Unlike choline and acetate-based scans that are inherently nonspecific, PSMA is also a target for directing therapeutics to PCa. This not only includes targeted drugs and toxins but also includes therapeutic radioisotopes. Thus, PSMA-based imaging agents are useful not only for diagnostic purposes but also for directing future targeted therapy. In addition, PSMA-based imaging may provide unique biologic information about the tumor. In one study, Liu et al. demonstrated that prolonged AD in an in vitro model downregulated PSMA expression and, therefore, might be an indicator of successful androgen ablation and resistance (45). In addition to ^{18}F-labeled PSMA imaging agents, PSMA targeting ligands have been labeled with ^{68}Ga (46) and ^{123}I (47). Large prospective studies in humans are necessary, although PSMA is quickly emerging as a promising new target for nuclear imaging with PET.

■ HER2

Her2 is a member of the epidermal growth factor receptor family of receptor tyrosine kinases. It has been studied extensively in a wide array of cancers—particularly breast cancer—where it plays a large role in cell growth, differentiation, and migration. It is not expressed in significant quantities by normal cells but can be overexpressed in cancer. This overexpression portends a bad prognosis but also opens the opportunity for targeted inhibition by blocking the receptor, thus making Her2 a desirable target for PET imaging in PCa (48). Early preclinical work has confirmed the feasibility of this approach in other cancers with a Her2-binding Affibody labeled with ^{18}F, both before and after therapy (49, 50). Recent attention has turned to replicating these findings in PCa. In one study, Wang et al. radiolabeled Herceptin, a humanized anti-Her2 monoclonal antibody, with ^{188}Re. Treatment with Herceptin inhibited PCa growth, suggesting that Her2-based PET tracers may play an important future role in the imaging and treatment of PCa (51). In a small clinical study, Carlsson et al. demonstrated that Her2 was overexpressed in the lymph nodes that had become sites of metastatic PCa (52). As with the other recent developments in PET imaging of PCa, further research is necessary to elucidate the significance of Her2-labeled tracers.

■ CONCLUSION

As our understanding of cancer biology has grown, so too has the need for imaging modalities that can be applied to a variety of clinical situations. One especially challenging area has been the evaluation of distant disease. We have reviewed a series of promising new PET-based imaging agents that are designed to detect and characterize PCa lesions throughout the body. This field is still young, and in nearly all cases, more data are needed to clarify exactly how these modalities should be used and how they compare with each other. This will be a daunting task, but a worthwhile one. As both the technology behind nuclear imaging and our own understanding of PCa continue to improve, we will become even better positioned to treat the millions of patients diagnosed with this deadly disease.

■ REFERENCES

1. Siegel R, Naishadham D, Jemal A. Cancer statistics, 2013. *CA Cancer J Clin.* 2013;63(1):11–30.
2. Kelloff GJ, Choyke P, Coffey DS; Prostate Cancer Imaging Working Group. Challenges in clinical prostate cancer: role of imaging. *AJR Am J Roentgenol.* 2009;192(6):1455–1470.
3. Bubendorf L, Schopfer A, Wagner U, et al. Metastatic patterns of prostate cancer: an autopsy study of 1,589 patients. *Hum Pathol.* 2000;31(5):578–583.
4. Pinto PA, Chung PH, Rastinehad AR, et al. Magnetic resonance imaging/ultrasound fusion guided prostate biopsy improves cancer detection following transrectal ultrasound biopsy and correlates with multiparametric magnetic resonance imaging. *J Urol.* 2011;186(4):1281–1285.
5. Turkbey B, Mena E, Aras O, Garvey B, Grant K, Choyke PL. Functional and molecular imaging: applications for diagnosis and staging of localised prostate cancer. *Clin Oncol.* 2013;25(8):451–460.
6. Akin O, Hricak H. Imaging of prostate cancer. *Radiol Clin North Am.* 2007;45(1):207–222.
7. Bouchelouche K, Tagawa ST, Goldsmith SJ, Turkbey B, Capala J, Choyke P. PET/CT Imaging and radioimmunotherapy of prostate cancer. *Semin Nucl Med.* 2011;41(1):29–44.
8. Effert PJ, Bares R, Handt S, Wolff JM, Bull U, Jakse G. Metabolic imaging of untreated prostate cancer by positron emission tomography with 18fluorine-labeled deoxyglucose. *J Urol.* 1996;155(3):994–998.
9. Takahashi N, Inoue T, Lee J, Yamaguchi T, Shizukuishi K. The roles of PET and PET/CT in the diagnosis and management of prostate cancer. *Oncology.* 2007;72(3-4):226–233.
10. Jadvar H, Ye W, Groshen S, Conti PS. [F-18]-fluorodeoxyglucose PET-CT of the normal prostate gland. *Ann Nucl Med.* 2008;22(9):787–793.
11. Kao PF, Chou YH, Lai CW. Diffuse FDG uptake in acute prostatitis. *Clin Nucl Med.* 2008;33(4):308–310.
12. Bouchelouche K, Oehr P. Positron emission tomography and positron emission tomography/computerized tomography of urological malignancies: an update review. *J Urol.* 2008;179(1):34–45.
13. Turkbey B, Pinto PA, Choyke PL. Imaging techniques for prostate cancer: implications for focal therapy. *Nat Rev Urol.* 2009;6(4):191–203.
14. Jadvar H, Desai B, Ji L, et al. Baseline 18F-FDG PET/CT parameters as imaging biomarkers of overall survival in castrate-resistant metastatic prostate cancer. *J Nucl Med.* 2013;54(8):1195–1201.
15. Beheshti M, Vali R, Waldenberger P, et al. Detection of bone metastases in patients with prostate cancer by 18F fluorocholine and 18F fluoride PET-CT: a comparative study. *Eur J Nucl Med Mol Imaging.* 2008;35(10):1766–1774.
16. Damle NA, Bal C, Bandopadhyaya GP, et al. The role of 18F-fluoride PET-CT in the detection of bone metastases in patients with breast, lung and prostate carcinoma: a comparison with FDG PET/CT and 99mTc-MDP bone scan. *Jpn J Radiol.* 2013;31(4):262–269.
17. Jadvar H, Desai B, Ji L, et al. Prospective evaluation of 18F-NaF and 18F-FDG PET/CT in detection of occult metastatic disease in biochemical recurrence of prostate cancer. *Clin Nucl Med.* 2012;37(7):637–643.
18. Yamaguchi T, Lee J, Uemura H, et al. Prostate cancer: a comparative study of 11C-choline PET and MR imaging combined with proton MR spectroscopy. *Eur J Nucl Med Mol Imaging.* 2005;32(7):742–748.
19. Farsad M, Schiavina R, Castellucci P, et al. Detection and localization of prostate cancer: correlation of (11)C-choline PET/CT with histopathologic step-section analysis. *J Nucl Med.* 2005;46(10):1642–1649.
20. Rinnab L, Simon J, Hautmann RE, et al. [(11)C]choline PET/CT in prostate cancer patients with biochemical recurrence after radical prostatectomy. *World J Urol.* 2009;27(5):619–625.
21. Sutinen E, Nurmi M, Roivainen A, et al. Kinetics of [(11)C]choline uptake in prostate cancer: a PET study. *Eur J Nucl Med Mol Imaging.* 2004;31(3):317–324.
22. Igerc I, Kohlfurst S, Gallowitsch HJ, et al. The value of 18F-choline PET/CT in patients with elevated PSA-level and negative prostate needle biopsy for localisation of prostate cancer. *Eur J Nucl Med Mol Imaging.* 2008;35(5):976–983.
23. Mamede M, Ceci F, Castellucci P, et al. The role of 11C-choline PET imaging in the early detection of recurrence in surgically treated prostate cancer patients with very low PSA level <0.5 ng/mL. *Clin Nucl Med.* 2013;38(9):e342–e345.
24. Giovacchini G, Picchio M, Coradeschi E, et al. [(11)C]choline uptake with PET/CT for the initial diagnosis of prostate cancer: relation to PSA levels, tumour stage and anti-androgenic therapy. *Eur J Nucl Med Mol Imaging.* 2008;35(6):1065–1073.
25. Breeuwsma AJ, Pruim J, Jongen MM, et al. In vivo uptake of [11C] choline does not correlate with cell proliferation in human prostate cancer. *Eur J Nucl Med Mol Imaging.* 2005;32(6):668–673.
26. Souvatzoglou M, Eiber M, Takei T, et al. Comparison of integrated whole-body [11C]choline PET/MR with PET/CT in patients with prostate cancer. *Eur J Nucl Med Mol Imaging.* 2013;40(10):1486–1499.

27. Oyama N, Miller TR, Dehdashti F, et al. 11C-acetate PET imaging of prostate cancer: detection of recurrent disease at PSA relapse. *J Nucl Med.* 2003;44(4):549–555.
28. Albrecht S, Buchegger F, Soloviev D, et al. (11)C-acetate PET in the early evaluation of prostate cancer recurrence. *Eur J Nucl Med Mol Imaging.* 2007;34(2):185–196.
29. Kato T, Tsukamoto E, Kuge Y, et al. Accumulation of [11C] acetate in normal prostate and benign prostatic hyperplasia: comparison with prostate cancer. *Eur J Nucl Med Mol Imaging.* 2002;29(11):1492–1495.
30. Mena E, Turkbey B, Mani H, et al. 11C-Acetate PET/CT in localized prostate cancer: a study with MRI and histopathologic correlation. *J Nucl Med.* 2012;53(4):538–545.
31. Jambor I, Borra R, Kemppainen J, et al. Functional imaging of localized prostate cancer aggressiveness using 11C-acetate PET/CT and 1H-MR spectroscopy. *J Nucl Med.* 2010;51(11):1676–1683.
32. Mohsen B, Giorgio T, Rasoul ZS, et al. Application of C-acetate positron-emission tomography (PET) imaging in prostate cancer: systematic review and meta-analysis of the literature. *BJU Int.* 2013;112(8):1062–1072.
33. Yoshii Y, Furukawa T, Oyama N, et al. Fatty acid synthase is a key target in multiple essential tumor functions of prostate cancer: uptake of radiolabeled acetate as a predictor of the targeted therapy outcome. *PloS One.* 2013;8(5):e64570.
34. Miyazawa H, Arai T, Iio M, Hara T. PET imaging of non-small-cell lung carcinoma with carbon-11-methionine: relationship between radioactivity uptake and flow-cytometric parameters. *J Nucl Med.* 1993;34(11):1886–1891.
35. Nuñez R, Macapinlac HA, Yeung HW, et al. Combined 18F-FDG and 11C-methionine PET scans in patients with newly progressive metastatic prostate cancer. *J Nucl Med.* 2002;43(1):46–55.
36. Schuster DM, Taleghani PA, Nieh PT, et al. Characterization of primary prostate carcinoma by anti-1-amino-2-[(18) F]-fluorocyclobutane-1-carboxylic acid (anti-3-[(18)F] FACBC) uptake. *Am J Nucl Med Mol Imaging.* 2013;3(1):85–96.
37. Schuster DM, Savir-Baruch B, Nieh PT, et al. Detection of recurrent prostate carcinoma with anti-1-amino-3-18F-fluorocyclobutane -1-carboxylic acid PET/CT and 111In-capromab pendetide SPECT/CT. *Radiology.* 2011;259(3):852–861.
38. Nanni C, Schiavina R, Boschi S, et al. Comparison of 18F-FACBC and 11C-choline PET/CT in patients with radically treated prostate cancer and biochemical relapse: preliminary results. *Eur J Nucl Med Mol Imaging.* 2013;40(suppl 1):S11–S17.
39. Chang SS, Benson MC, Campbell SC, et al. Society of Urologic Oncology position statement: redefining the management of hormone-refractory prostate carcinoma. *Cancer.* 2005;103(1):11–21.
40. Larson SM, Morris M, Gunther I, et al. Tumor localization of 16beta-18F-fluoro-5alpha-dihydrotestosterone versus 18F-FDG in patients with progressive, metastatic prostate cancer. *J Nucl Med.* 2004;45(3):366–373.
41. Dehdashti F, Picus J, Michalski JM, et al. Positron tomographic assessment of androgen receptors in prostatic carcinoma. *Eur J Nucl Med Mol Imaging.* 2005;32(3):344–350.
42. Ross JS, Sheehan CE, Fisher HA, et al. Correlation of primary tumor prostate-specific membrane antigen expression with disease recurrence in prostate cancer. *Clin Cancer Res.* 2003;9(17):6357–6362.
43. Elsasser-Beile U, Reischl G, Wiehr S, et al. PET imaging of prostate cancer xenografts with a highly specific antibody against the prostate-specific membrane antigen. *J Nucl Med.* 2009;50(4):606–611.
44. Hillier SM, Maresca KP, Femia FJ, et al. Preclinical evaluation of novel glutamate-urea-lysine analogues that target prostate-specific membrane antigen as molecular imaging pharmaceuticals for prostate cancer. *Cancer Res.* 2009;69(17):6932–6940.
45. Liu T, Wu LY, Fulton MD, Johnson JM, Berkman CE. Prolonged androgen deprivation leads to downregulation of androgen receptor and prostate-specific membrane antigen in prostate cancer cells. *Int J Oncol.* 2012;41(6):2087–2092.
46. Roethke MC, Kuru TH, Afshar-Oromieh A, Schlemmer HP, Hadaschik BA, Fenchel M. Hybrid positron emission tomography-magnetic resonance imaging with Gallium 68 prostate-specific membrane antigen tracer: a next step for imaging of recurrent prostate cancer-preliminary results. *Eur Urol.* 2013;64(5):862–864.
47. Barrett JA, Coleman RE, Goldsmith SJ, et al. First-in-man evaluation of 2 high-affinity PSMA-avid small molecules for imaging prostate cancer. *J Nucl Med.* 2013;54(3):380–387.
48. Dowsett M, Cooke T, Ellis I, et al. Assessment of HER2 status in breast cancer: why, when and how? *Eur J Cancer.* 2000;36(2):170–176.
49. Kramer-Marek G, Kiesewetter DO, Martiniova L, Jagoda E, Lee SB, Capala J. [18F]FBEM-Z(HER2:342)-Affibody molecule—a new molecular tracer for in vivo monitoring of HER2 expression by positron emission tomography. *Eur J Nucl Med Mol Imaging.* 2008;35(5):1008–1018.
50. Kramer-Marek G, Kiesewetter DO, Capala J. Changes in HER2 expression in breast cancer xenografts after therapy can be quantified using PET and (18)F-labeled affibody molecules. *J Nucl Med.* 2009;50(7):1131–1139.
51. Wang HY, Lin WY, Chen MC, et al. Inhibitory effects of Rhenium-188-labeled Herceptin on prostate cancer cell growth: a possible radioimmunotherapy to prostate carcinoma. *Int J Radiat Biol.* 2013;89(5):346–355.
52. Carlsson J, Shen L, Xiang J, Xu J, Wei Q. Tendencies for higher co-expression of EGFR and HER2 and downregulation of HER3 in prostate cancer lymph node metastases compared with corresponding primary tumors. *Oncol Lett.* 2013;5(1):208–214.

4 Current Approaches to Prostate Cancer Staging and Risk Stratification: In the Midst of a Paradigm Shift

CHAD A. REICHARD

ERIC A. KLEIN

■ INTRODUCTION

A few key diagnostic modalities are employed in current practice to stage and risk stratify patients with prostate cancer prior to treatment. The information obtained from digital rectal examination, prostate-specific antigen (PSA), Gleason score, and imaging studies (computerized tomography [CT] scan and radionuclide bone scan), when indicated, forms the groundwork upon which clinical staging systems and more complex prognostic nomograms and/or treatment algorithms are built. The clinician's ability to estimate disease severity, communicate prognosis to the patient, and recommend a specific treatment course rests in the accuracy of the staging methodology. Over the course of the last 25 years of PSA screening, the goals of staging have changed. Early on in the PSA era, when the incidence of organ confined disease was low, the goal was to accurately detect men with nonmetastatic disease at diagnosis who would benefit from local therapy such as radical prostatectomy or external beam radiation. The current clinical staging methodologies have substantially realized this goal. Because of the marked stage migration that has occurred with widespread screening, which has led to overdetection of nonlethal tumors, the present challenge is to more accurately identify patients with indolent disease who can safely avoid initial treatment without compromising ultimate curability. This has catalyzed a shift to a staging paradigm based on tools that evaluate individual tumor biology. Therefore, to comprehensively assess prostate cancer patients, the clinician must wield an understanding of the elements that comprise clinical staging methodology, in addition to the evolving state of the biologically based criteria for staging and risk stratification. For reference, the anatomy of the prostate in relation to nearby vessels and lymph node regions is illustrated in Figure 4.1

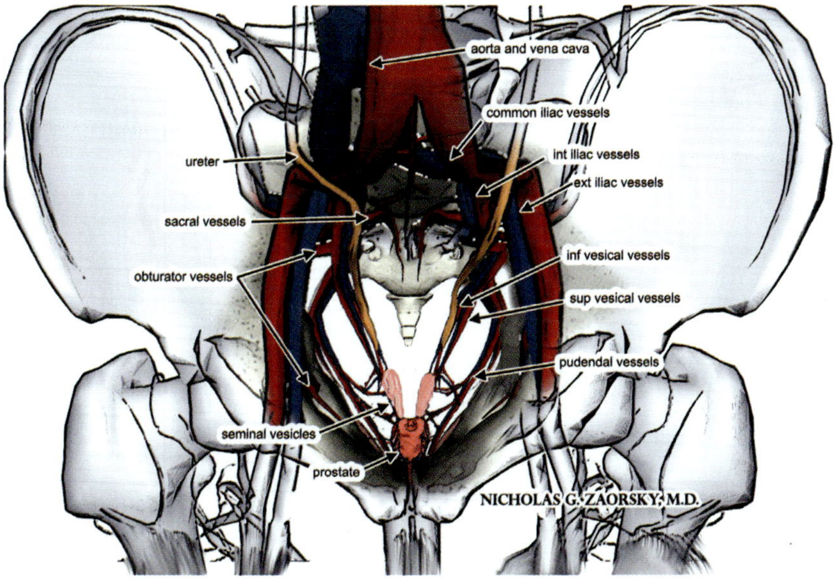

FIGURE 4.1 This figure demonstrates the anatomy of blood vessels (and their neighboring lymph node regions) relative to the prostate. The viewpoint is oriented in the antero-posterior axis, in a line from the umbilicus to the rectum.

■ CLINICAL STAGING FOR INITIAL DIAGNOSIS AND TREATMENT

AJCC–TNM

One of the most widely recognized clinicopathologic staging systems is based on the tumor-node-metastases (TNM) classification (Figure 4.2) of the American Joint Committee on Cancer (AJCC). The foundation for this system has historically been, and still remains, anatomic extent of disease. The seventh edition (2010) was updated to include Gleason score and preoperative PSA in the definition of prognostic groups. These changes referenced studies where Gleason score was the single most important predictor of prostate cancer–specific mortality and a pre-treatment PSA > 20 ng/mL was associated with a greater risk of death from prostate cancer (1, 2). In the current system, there are four prognostic subgroups (I–IV) that allow prediction of statistically significant different rates of disease-specific survival at 5, 10, and 15 years. It should be noted that surgical margin status at prostatectomy, while an important prognostic factor, is not technically included in this staging system (3–5).

National Comprehensive Cancer Network Guidelines

The current National Comprehensive Cancer Network (NCCN) prostate cancer guidelines combine prognostic groups based on the original D'Amico analysis with the addition of a very low-risk group that incorporates the Epstein criteria and a very high-risk group classified as stage T3b or T4 disease (Figure 4.3). Specific treatment

Risk Group	Criteria
Very low	T1c, PSA < 10, Gl 6, < 3 cores and no core ≥50%, PSAD < 0.15
Low	T1–T2a, PSA < 10, Gl 6
Intermediate	T2b–T2c or Gl 7 or PSA 10–20
High	T3a or Gl 8–10 or PSA > 20
Very high	T3b–T4

FIGURE 4.3 NCCN risk groups.

Primary Tumor Clinical Stages Only (T)			
Tx	Primary tumor cannot be assessed	T1a	Tumor incidental histologic finding in 5% or less of tissue resected
T0	No evidence of primary tumor	T1b	Tumor incidental histologic finding
T1	Clinically inapparent tumor neither palpable nor visible by imaging	T1c	Tumor identified by needle biopsy (for example, because of elevated)
Primary Tumor Clinical Stages (T)		**Primary Tumor Pathologic Stages (T)**	
T2	Tumor confined within prostate	pT2	Organ confined disease
T2a	Tumor involves one-half of one lobe or less	pT2a	Unilateral, one-half of one side or less
T2b	Tumor involves more than one-half of one lobe but not both lobes	pT2b	Unilateral, involving more than one-half of side, but not bilateral
T2c	Tumor involves both lobes	pT2c	Bilateral disease
T3	Tumor extends through the prostate capsule	pT3	Extraprostatic extension
T3a	Extracapsular extension (unilateral or bilateral)	pT3a	Extraprostatic extension or microscopic invasion of bladder neck
T3b	Tumor invades seminal vesicle(s)	pT3b	Seminal vesicle invasion
T4	Tumor is fixed or invades adjacent structures other than seminal vesicles	pt4	Invasion or rectum, levators, and/or pelvic wall
Clinical Lymph Nodes (N)		**Pathologic Lymph Nodes (N)**	
Nx	Regional lymph nodes not assessed	pNx	Regional nodes not sampled
N0	No regional lymph node metastasis	pN0	No positive regional nodes
N1	Regional lymph node metastasis	pN1	Regional lymph node metastasis
Distant Metastasis (M)			
M0	No distant metastasis		
M1	Distant metastasis		
M1a	Nonregional lymph node(s)		
M1b	Bone metastasis		
M1c	Other site(s) with or without bone disease		

FIGURE 4.2 AJCC–TNM prostate cancer.

algorithms accompany each of the risk-stratified subgroups. Of particular contemporary interest are the recommendations for active surveillance. According to the guidelines, patients eligible for active surveillance are those in the very low-risk group with a life expectancy less than 20 years or those in the low-risk group with a life expectancy less than 10 years as calculated using the Social Security Administration tables. This difference in recommendation based on life expectancy is in part due to data that show patients with low-risk disease versus very low-risk disease have a relative risk of 1.89 (95% confidence interval [CI] 1.21–2.95) for Gleason score upgrade and 2.06 (95% CI 1.19–3.57) for nonorgan-confined cancer (6, 7). These guidelines generically suggest treatment for patients on active surveillance that develop progressive disease, noting that specific criteria for progression have not been definitively outlined, but that a change in risk group is a reasonable surrogate marker of progression.

Kattan Nomograms

The initial Kattan nomogram added evidence-based objectivity to the clinician's ability to predict probability of organ-confined disease based on the input of pretreatment PSA, biopsy tumor grade, and clinical stage (8). This allowed more accurate risk stratification of patients in the PSA era. This prognostic tool was further elaborated with development of nomograms for pretreatment prediction of the probability of remaining free from biochemical recurrence following prostatectomy, external beam radiotherapy, or brachytherapy for localized prostate cancer defined as clinical stage T1 to T3a (9–11). This nomogram has been updated and validated to be useful in predicting indolent disease in patients with clinically localized, stage T1c or T2a and biopsy Gleason score 6 prostate cancer (12). Iremashvili et al. demonstrated that the Kattan nomogram was well calibrated to estimate probability of clinically insignificant cancer in a contemporary prostatectomy cohort of 370 patients with biopsy Gleason 6 prostate cancer, outperforming many other available nomograms (Figure 4.4) (13). In addition to the nomograms included in this study, there are a variety of other contemporary nomograms that take into account similar variables in both pre- and posttreatment scenarios that have been validated in different patient cohorts (10, 14–18).

D'Amico Risk Stratification

To further refine the prognostic precision of disease staging prior to treatment, D'Amico stratified patients with prostate cancer into three separate risk groups: low-risk (clinical stage T1 to 2a, PSA ≤ 10 ng/mL, and Gleason score ≤6), intermediate-risk (stage T2b, PSA > 10 but <20 ng/mL or Gleason score 7), or high-risk disease (stage T2c, PSA > 20 ng/mL or Gleason score 8–10). A significant association with

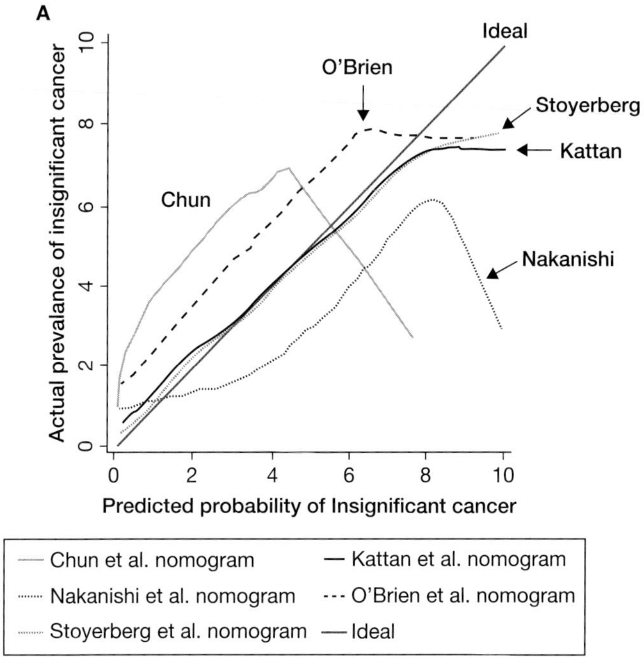

FIGURE 4.4 Comparative performance of nomograms.
Source: From Ref. (13). Iremashvili V, Soloway MS, Pelaez L, Rosenberg DL, Manoharan M. Comparative validation of nomograms predicting clinically insignificant prostate cancer. *Urology.* 2013;81(6):1202–1208. Reprinted with permission from Elsevier.

absence of disease at 10 years after radical prostatectomy was demonstrated: 83% for low-risk, 46% for intermediate-risk, and 29% for high-risk disease (19). The American Urological Association uses a similar schema to define low-, intermediate-, and high-risk groups.

Epstein Criteria

The aim of the Epstein criteria is to predict pathologically insignificant prostate cancer based mainly on needle biopsy, although it does take PSA into account. According to the criteria, insignificant prostate cancer is identified by clinical stage T1c, biopsy Gleason score less than or equal to 6, fewer than 3 positive biopsy cores, less than or equal to 50% prostate cancer involvement in any core, and PSA density less than 0.15 ng/mL/g (20). Although these criteria form the basis for the low-risk groups that some algorithms recommend for active surveillance, they neither have been specifically studied directly in the context of an active surveillance cohort nor have the Epstein criteria been validated with long-term follow-up as a good surrogate for low risk of prostate cancer–related death. In addition, studies have shown that as many as 8% of cancers that qualified as being insignificant using the Epstein criteria were not organ confined based on postsurgical pathology (21, 22). In another study, radical prostatectomy cases that met Epstein criteria preoperatively were more likely to have insignificant disease by either the classical (organ-confined, Gleason score ≤6, and tumor volume ≤0.5 cm^3) or more liberal definition (organ confined, Gleason ≤6, tumor of any volume) of insignificant disease and more likely to have organ-confined tumors. The sensitivity, specificity, positive predictive value (PPV), and negative predictive value (NPV) varied widely among the end points, with sensitivity (74%) and NPV (86%) best for the classical definition of insignificant disease and specificity (74%) and PPV (92%) best for organ-confined disease. The authors concluded that the Epstein criteria predict for a high likelihood of organ-confined disease and the absence of biochemical failure up to 5 years after radical prostatectomy, but that the criteria are insufficiently robust to predict the presence of biologically insignificant disease (23).

Cancer of the Prostate Risk Assessment Score

Recognizing that there can be a range of prognoses and outcomes even within the specific risk subgroups of staging tools/guidelines already described, the Cancer of the Prostate Risk Assessment (CAPRA) score represents an attempt to provide a more discriminatory assessment of disease risk and prognosis. It was developed using data from the Cancer of the Prostate Strategic Urologic Research Endeavor registry. The score ranges from 0 to 10 and includes input from five clinical variables (PSA, Gleason score, clinical stage, % of positive biopsy cores, and age), which are similar to the variables included in the Kattan nomograms (Figure 4.5). It has been independently validated in a large German cohort as accurate in predicting recurrence-free survival after radical prostatectomy as well as specific pathologic outcomes (24, 25).

The CAPRA Scoring System*

Variable	Level	Points
PSA (ng/ml.)	2.0–6.0	0
	6.1–10.0	1
	10.1–20	2
	20.1–30	3
	>30	4
Biopsy Gleason score	1–3/1–3	0
(primary/secondary grade)	1–3/4–5	1
	4–5/1–5	3
Clinical T-stage	T1/T2	0
	T3a	1
Positive biopsy cores	<34%	0
	≥34%	1
Age, y	<50	0
	≥50	1

CAPRA indicates cancer of the prostate risk assessment; PSA, prostate-specific antigen.
***CAPRA score (0 to 10) is the total of points in each category.**

FIGURE 4.5 The CAPRA scoring system.
Source: Reprinted with permission from the American Cancer Society.

Imaging Modalities

A variety of imaging modalities have also been employed in an attempt to add sensitivity to clinical staging and risk prognostication in patients with prostate cancer. CT scan is not sensitive enough to provide meaningful clinical information regarding patients with localized prostate cancer. CT scan along with radionuclide bone scan are only recommended for patients with high-risk disease based on studies that have shown the risk of radiographically detectable metastases in intermediate- and low-risk disease to be very low. On the contrary, magnetic resonance imaging (MRI) and magnetic resonance spectroscopy have been widely studied in a variety of clinical scenarios and have a more controversial role in the staging and risk stratification aspects of prostate cancer management. According to the NCCN guidelines, multiparametric MRI (mpMRI) may be considered to exclude the presence of an anterior cancer if the PSA level continues to rise despite repeatedly negative systematic prostate biopsy; however, it is not recommended for routine use (26).

MRI in Patients on Active Surveillance

The role of MRI as an additional criterion for inclusion in clinical nomograms used to predict insignificant prostate cancer has been evaluated (27). These nomograms have been applied to active surveillance situations (28, 29). However, it has been suggested that two implementations of mpMRI could, if proven, make active surveillance unnecessary: (1) If mpMRI was used prior to biopsy so that based on imaging characteristics, patients could be excluded from undergoing biopsy based on PSA alone, thus avoiding unnecessary diagnosis of clinically insignificant prostate cancer; and 2) if low-grade, low-volume lesions found with mpMRI-guided or template-mapped prostate biopsies could be reclassified as a noncancerous entity (30, 31). However, these goals, if feasible, are unlikely to be realized in the near future given the massive paradigm shift in prostate cancer management they represent. Thus, it is likely prudent to continue to evaluate MRI as one data point in a collection of multiple inputs necessary to increase the accuracy of prostate cancer staging.

One clinical question that MRI has been used to address is the likelihood of upstaging on repeat biopsy in men on active surveillance, and thus whether repeat biopsy could be avoided given certain imaging characteristics. Vargas et al. used MRI in 388 men with low-risk prostate cancer on initial assessment (Gleason 6, PSA < 10 ng/mL, and clinical stage T2a or less). Three radiologists independently scored each MRI on a 1 to 5 scale, where 1 and 2 were deemed low risk for significant cancer. Although upgrading was seen in 79 of 388 (20%) of men overall, an MRI score of 1 or 2 had an NPV of 0.96 to 1 for upgrading, suggesting that men with a low-risk MRI could avoid repeat biopsy. The PPV of an MRI score of 5 was 0.87 to 0.98, with greater agreement between MRI scores for the two more experienced readers (32). Similarly, Margel et al. report the use of mpMRI in 60 men suitable for active surveillance. Twenty-three of 60 (38%) had a negative MRI, with 24 of 60 (40%) having an MRI that showed concordance with the biopsy results (defined as a tumor of <1 cm) and the remaining 13 of 60 (22%) suggesting unexpectedly large tumor volumes on MRI that led to reclassification with confirmatory biopsy in 10 of 13 (77%). The proportion of men who were reclassified in the negative MRI was low (2.5%) and slightly higher in the concordant group (10.7%) (33).

Mullins et al. examined 50 men in an active surveillance program with a mean follow-up of 47.5 months and found that mpMRI demonstrated 97% specificity and 90% NPV for the detection of a pathological-index lesion (cancer present in the same prostate sextant in two separate surveillance biopsies). The prevalence of MRI-detected lesions was low at 20%, as is expected in an active surveillance population. Biopsy reclassification occurred in 40% of men with an MRI lesion compared to 12.5% of men without; however, when only men who met all active surveillance criteria were examined, there was no significant difference in biopsy reclassification due to MRI findings. These studies were also read by a single radiologist with 10 years of experience in prostate imaging. Thus, this study lacks the ability to demonstrate interobserver reliability, but does underscore the importance of clinical expertise as a contributing factor to the utility of prostate MRI (34). Given these figures, some patients might choose to forgo a repeat biopsy if their MRI was negative or concordant.

^{11}C-choline Positron Emission Tomography/Computerized Tomography Scan

CT alone is not sensitive enough to be clinically useful in patients with high pretest probability of localized prostate cancer. However, ^{11}C-choline positron emission tomography (PET)/CT has been shown to have equal sensitivity and greater specificity for the presence of lymph node metastasis when compared with two other pretreatment nomograms (Briganti and Kattan) in a cohort of 57 patients with intermediate- or high-risk prostate cancer. The baseline sensitivity for all three methods is, however, a relatively low, 60%. PET/CT had an overall specificity of 97.6% compared to the nomograms at 73.8% and 64.3%; however, this difference did not reach statistical significance in area-under-the-curve analysis. The diameter of the metastatic deposit directly correlated with rate of detection (0/6 metastatic deposits <2 mm were detected, compared with 7/9 deposits >10 mm in diameter). Lymph node metastases outside of the standard boundaries of pelvic lymph node dissection were detected in 4 of 57 patients. ^{11}C-choline PET/CT, however, is not useful for the determination of local extent of disease (35, 36).

Summary

These clinical staging systems, nomograms, and use of adjunctive imaging have proved invaluable in aiding the clinician to determine a patient's likelihood of clinically localized disease and to counsel them effectively regarding their potential benefit from immediate local therapy in regard to cure. However, they are unable to distinguish between indolent and aggressive disease. This in turn has led to a high rate of overtreatment of nonlethal tumors in patients who could otherwise delay treatment-associated morbidity or perhaps avoid it altogether. This highlights the need for the development of biologically based predictors of individual disease aggressiveness that can accurately predict the presence of worrisome disease on needle biopsy and other pretreatment criteria.

■ MOLECULAR AND GENOMIC MODALITIES: IMPROVING PROGNOSTIC PRECISION

The previously reviewed clinical and imaging metrics as applied to localized prostate cancer are based solely on clinical and pathologic features (e.g., biopsy Gleason grade, PSA, clinical stage). Recent large studies have demonstrated the shortcomings of the current state of prostate cancer risk stratification. The Prostate Intervention Versus Observation Trial suggested that radical prostatectomy does not reduce mortality compared to observation (37). The Scandinavian Prostate Cancer Group 4 trial showed only a modest benefit of surgery over conservative management (a projected prostate cancer–specific mortality rate after 15 years of 14.6% vs. 20.7%, respectively). Although prostatectomy prevented cancer deaths in this study, a large number of patients had tumors that were not life threatening within the follow-up range of 15 years. In contrast, one in seven of the patients who underwent prostatectomy recurred and died of prostate cancer (38).

The 2011 National Institutes of Health consensus statement on the role of active surveillance in the management of patients with clinically localized prostate cancer estimates that only 10% of men who are eligible for active surveillance choose this approach. This low number has been attributed to a wide variety of factors such as patient and clinician anxiety, the need for repeated biopsy, and the imprecision of available clinical prognosticators of disease aggressiveness or progression. Thus, several molecular and genetic tests have been recently developed and studied in hopes of refining the clinician's ability to more accurately determine an individual's risk by analyzing specific prostate tumor genes. These tests have been studied as stand-alone risk stratification metrics as well as in conjunction with existing clinical tools (39).

Prostate Cancer Antigen-3

This biomarker is a single gene product noncoding mRNA expressed only in the prostate, which is measured clinically via urine assays (40, 41). It is highly overexpressed in prostate cancer compared with benign tissue. This test has been employed in a wide variety of clinical scenarios. It has been associated with the likelihood of a positive initial or repeat prostate biopsy (42–44). However, studies are conflicted as to whether prostate cancer antigen-3 (PCA3) correlates with prostate cancer aggressiveness (45–49). A study of urinary TMPRSS2:ERG and PCA3 in an active surveillance cohort seemed to stratify the risk of having aggressive cancer as defined by tumor volume or Gleason score (50). A comparative effectiveness review demonstrated that PCA3 had a higher diagnostic accuracy than total PSA increases, but strength of evidence was low (limited confidence in effect estimates). In addition, strength of evidence was insufficient to conclude that PCA3 testing leads to improved health outcomes (51). However, a study combining PCA3 with other expressed prostatic secretion biomarkers such as TXNRD1-mRNA, PSA-mRNA, and TMPRSS2:ERG fusion mRNA was found to improve stratification of NCCN active surveillance candidates by reducing the risk of upstaging in patients with a negative test by almost eight times and reducing the risk of being both upstaged and upgraded by about five times while increasing the prevalence of upstaging in the positive test group by a factor of two (52). When PCA3 was combined with best clinical judgment in regard to the decision for repeat biopsy after a previous negative prostate biopsy, it was found that 64% of repeat biopsies could have been avoided when compared with 26% for best clinical judgment alone. Combining best clinical judgment with the PCA3 test resulted in an NPV of 99% for cancers with Gleason score greater than or equal to 7 (53). Ongoing re-evaluation of the data on the ability of PCA3 to aid in risk stratification is necessary, especially as experience with active surveillance continues to grow.

Prolaris (Myriad Genetic Laboratories)

This is a genetic test based on analysis of cell cycle progression (CCP) genes. The assay quantitatively measures the RNA expression levels of 46 genes involved in tumor cell division. These specific genes were chosen for the assay based on the strength of correlation with prostate tumor cell proliferation. The levels of gene expression were found to directly correlate with risk of prostate cancer–specific disease progression. This correlation is reported as the CCP score, which is calculated as the average expression of 31 CCP genes, normalized to 15 housekeeper genes. The initial study examining the prognostic value of the CCP score after prostatectomy demonstrated that it accurately predicted biochemical recurrence. This study also included a transurethral resection of the prostate (TURP) cohort for which the CCP score was the most important variable for prediction of time to death from prostate cancer in both univariate analysis (hazard ratio 2.92; 95% CI 2.38–3.57, $P = 6.1 \times 10^{-22}$) and the final multivariate analysis (hazard ratio 2.57; 95% CI 1.93–3.43, $P = 8.2 \times 10^{-11}$), and was stronger than all other prognostic factors. The CCP score was subsequently applied to a group of patients obtained from six British cancer registries from 1990 to 1996. Inclusion criteria were patients with clinically localized prostate cancer diagnosed by needle biopsy managed conservatively (i.e., patients treated by surgery or radiation within 6 months of diagnosis were excluded). In this study, the score was found to have the most robust independent predictive value of all variables examined for prostate cancer death outcome (54, 55). Thus, the clinical implication is to use the test to better distinguish which low- or intermediate-risk patients are suitable candidates for active surveillance, from those who are potentially at higher risk and may have a greater benefit from more rigorous monitoring or progression immediately to therapy. In a validation study of a contemporary prostatectomy cohort of 413 patients in which 19.9% of patients had disease recurrence, the CCP score was demonstrated to significantly improve the precision of the prediction of disease recurrence over CAPRA-S score alone. In addition, a score that combined CAPRA-S and CCP was validated. This combined score demonstrated consistent outcome prediction through a wide range of clinical risk (56).

Oncotype DX Prostate Cancer Assay (Genomic Health)

This is a gene expression test based on analysis of genes from multiple different cellular pathways involved in prostate cancer cells such as stromal response, cellular organization, androgen, and stress response. The test is a 17-gene assay that was shown to predict for clinical recurrence (local, metastatic, or prostate cancer–related death) in long-term follow-up after radical prostatectomy and then validated in a prospective clinical study of 395 needle biopsy specimens of patients with low- to low-intermediate-risk prostate cancer with the primary endpoints defined as clinical recurrence, prostate cancer death, and adverse pathology at radical prostatectomy (57). The results of the test are reported as a genomic prostate score (GPS) ranging from 0 to 100 (a score of zero, correlating to the lowest percent chance of adverse pathology). In binary analyses adjusting for biopsy Gleason score, the GPS was found to be predictive of high grade (dominant pattern Gleason score ≥4) (odds ratio [OR] per 20 GPS units: 2.3; CI 1.5–3.7, $P < 0.001$) and/or nonorgan-confined disease (OR per 20 GPS units: 1.9; CI 1.3–3.0, $P = 0.003$) at radical prostatectomy. Similar to the Prolaris assay, it was found to have a wide distribution of score values when applied to patients at each level of clinical risk (both according to NCCN guidelines and CAPRA score) such that a patient in the NCCN very low-risk group with a low GPS score would have a more favorable prognosis than a NCCN very low-risk patient with a high GPS score. Similarly, for example, a patient with a CAPRA score of 2 has a 66% average probability of adverse pathology, but with addition of GPS to risk assessment, patients with a CAPRA score of 2 have anywhere from 35% to 82% probability of adverse pathology (Figure 4.6). (58, 59) In multivariable analysis of the clinical validation study referenced earlier, adjusting for significant clinical covariates did not diminish the GPS score's ability to predict high-grade and/or nonorgan-confined pathology. The ORs for each 20-point increase in GPS adjusted for continuous CAPRA score was 2.1 (95% CI 1.4–3.2), adjusted for NCCN risk group; the OR was 1.9 (95% CI 1.3–2.8), and adjusted for age, PSA, clinical stage, and biopsy Gleason score; the OR was 1.9 (95% CI 1.2–28) as well. This demonstrated that the GPS adds additional clinically meaningful prognostic precision above and beyond the previously existing and validated multivariable clinical risk stratification tools (57).

In contrast to the Prolaris assay, which bases the risk score solely on the biology of the tumor sampled by biopsy, the Oncotype DX assay was developed to predict the biology of the entire prostate (Figure 4.7). From an initial gene discovery study, 288 genes were identified that were similarly predictive of clinical recurrence (as assessed by standardized hazard ratios) in both primary and highest Gleason pattern of specimens that were microdissected from radical prostatectomy specimens. This result demonstrated that certain genes could predict tumor aggressiveness regardless of the Gleason pattern tumor in which they were assessed. Eighty-one of the most predictive of the 288 genes used in the radical prostatectomy study were then analyzed in tumor from prostate needle biopsies, 58 of which were found to be predictive of high-grade and/or nonorgan-confined with a false discovery rate of less than 10%. Thus, even if only low-grade tumor is sampled by biopsy, the GPS score will still be high if

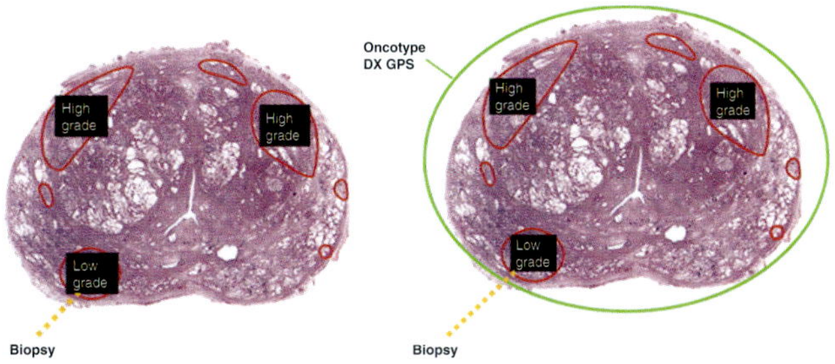

FIGURE 4.7 Conceptual demonstration of the ability of Oncotype DX to capture the entire biology of the prostate even though only one tumor was sampled and assayed.

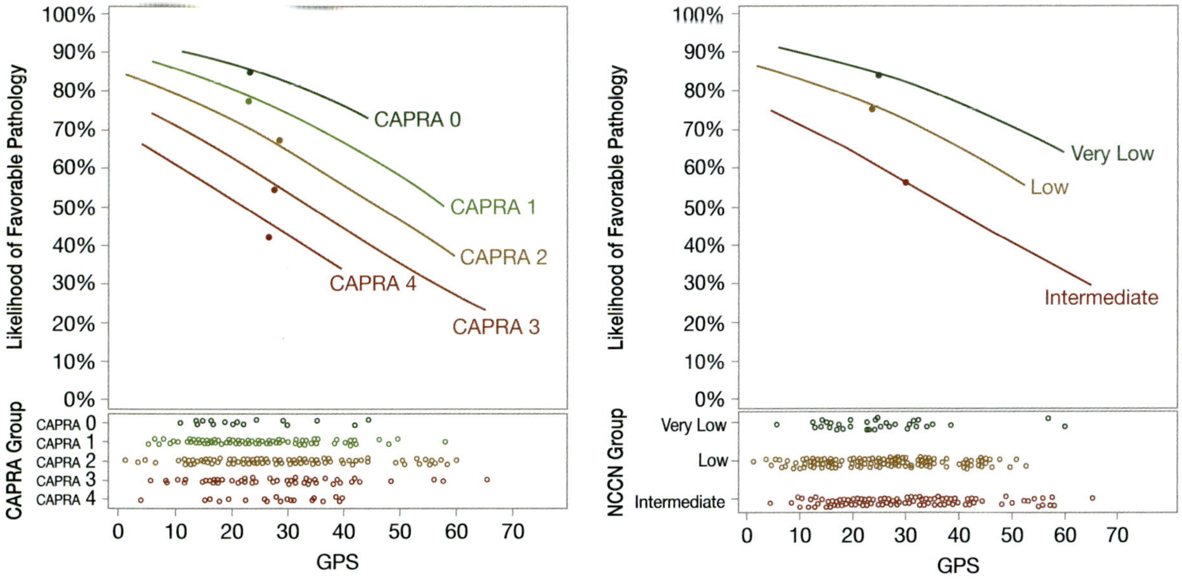

FIGURE 4.6 Distribution of GPS scores within CAPRA and NCCN risk groups (open circles) and probability of favorable pathology at each level of clinical risk, incorporating GPS (curves).

Source: From Ref. (57). Klein EA, Cooperberg MR, Magi-Galluzzi C, et al. A 17-gene assay to predict prostate cancer aggressiveness in the context of gleason grade heterogeneity, tumor multifocality, and biopsy undersampling. *Eur Urol.* 2014;pii: S0302-2838(14)00414-X. Reprinted with permission from Elsevier.

there is high-grade disease present elsewhere in the prostate. Conversely, a low-risk Prolaris score does not entirely eliminate the possibility of a more aggressive lesion that was simply missed on prostate biopsy. This advantage addresses important concerns of understaging and biopsy undersampling that have inhibited the more widespread adoption of active surveillance in clinical practice.

Clinical Application of Genomic Tools

Further study will be necessary to compare the various genetic tests previously described and determine whether there are any particular clinical scenarios in which one test outperforms the other. In addition, these tests represent outcomes from first generation assays from which subsequent study and new technical platforms, such as whole-exome sequencing, could provide further prognostic precision. These changes will need to be re-validated in light of the simultaneous development of current and future therapeutic modalities that active surveillance is compared to as well. Given the continued rapid evolution that will likely characterize the field of prostate cancer genomics, a simplified clinical metric is helpful to keep in perspective the end result that the clinician is trying to achieve by implementing any of the genetic tests in combination with previously described clinical nomograms. Patients with a "good" gene signature on genomic analysis can be counseled for active surveillance. In addition, patients on active surveillance can be counseled if and when their cancer progresses to needing treatment based on a change in gene signature (Figure 4.8).

Active surveillance even in the setting of current clinical staging and risk prognostication methods has rendered very positive results with a variety of studies demonstrating cancer-specific survival rates at or near 100%. However, as previously stated, these studies represent a fraction of the number of men who are eligible for active surveillance. To safely increase the number of patients who are managed with active surveillance, the NPV of the nomograms that are developed with the addition of the aforementioned genetic tools needs to be as high as possible so that the cancer-specific survival rates of patients who are managed with active surveillance do not fall below those who are immediately treated. This is especially true as the average age of the patient under active surveillance decreases (60). One model that represents an implementation of a simple clinical risk stratification system without addition of genomic testing demonstrated encouraging outcomes for active surveillance compared to immediate prostatectomy. The model, based on a hypothetical cohort of one million simulated patients aged 40 to 90 years with low-risk prostate cancer defined as (T-stage ≤ T2a, Gleason score ≤ 6, and PSA level ≤ 10 ng/mL), projected that 2.8% of men on active surveillance versus 1.6% of men with immediate radical prostatectomy would die of their disease in 20 years. It predicted that the average increase in life expectancy associated with immediate radical prostatectomy was 1.8 months (61). If results such as these can be improved upon with addition of genomic analysis, this will, in addition, hopefully provide more assurance for men who would be eligible for active surveillance, but choose against it due to the ongoing anxiety of living with a cancer diagnosis or the need for frequent testing.

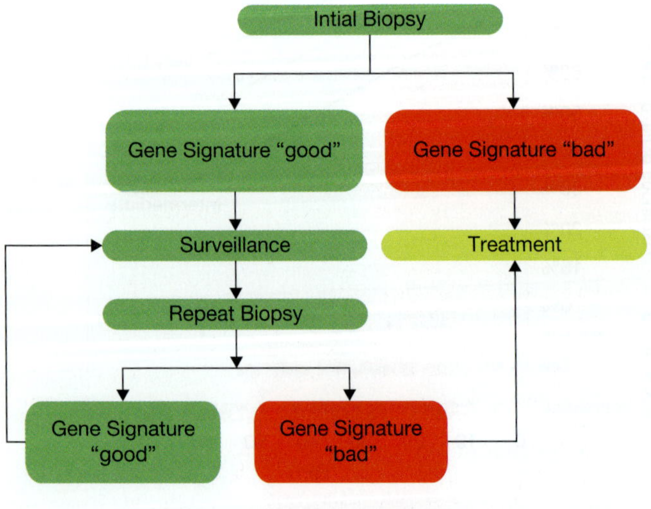

FIGURE 4.8 Clinical algorithm of a biopsy-based gene expression signature for choosing and managing active surveillance patients. *Source:* Reprinted with permission from Ref. (59). Klein EA. A genomic approach to active surveillance: a step toward precision medicine. *Asian J. Androl.* 2013;15(3):340–341. doi:10.1038/aja.2012.140.

■ CONCLUSION

The staging and risk stratification of prostate cancer is in the midst of a transition from solely a clinicopathologic-based system to one that includes molecular and genomic tools as well as various radiographic modalities. Further refinements to currently available clinical decision-making tools (i.e., Gleason grade, palpable extent of tumor, PSA, and nomograms based on these variables) are unlikely to yield the additional predictive power needed to confidently distinguish between patients with aggressive versus indolent disease. Improved decision-making tools developed by integrating new imaging techniques along with future refinements in genomic and molecular analyses will hopefully provide more adequate assurance of a patient's indolent disease status such that clinicians and patients alike can more comfortably choose active surveillance.

■ REFERENCES

1. Roach M III, Weinberg V, Sandler H, Thompson I. Staging for prostate cancer: time to incorporate pretreatment prostate-specific antigen and Gleason score? *Cancer.* 2007;109(2):213–220.
2. van der Kwast TH, Collette L, Van Poppel H, et al. Impact of pathology review of stage and margin status of radical prostatectomy specimens (EORTC trial 22911). *Virchows Arch.* 2006;449(4):428–434.

3. Chuang AY, Nielsen ME, Hernandez DJ, Walsh PC, Epstein JI. The significance of positive surgical margin in areas of capsular incision in otherwise organ confined disease at radical prostatectomy. *J Urol.* 2007;178(4 pt 1):1306–1310.
4. Freedland SJ, Aronson W, Presti JC Jr, et al. Should a positive surgical margin following radical prostatectomy be pathological stage T2 or T3? Results from the SEARCH database. *J Urol.* 2003;169(6):2142–2146.
5. Edge S, Byrd DR, Compton CC, Fritz AG, Greene FL, Trotti A. *AJCC Cancer Staging Manual.* 7th ed. New York, NY: Springer; 2010.
6. Klotz L. Active surveillance: patient selection. *Curr Opin Urol.* 2013;23(3):239–244.
7. Tosoian JJ, JohnBull E, Trock BJ, et al. Pathologic outcomes in men with low-risk and very low-risk prostate cancer: implications on the practice of active surveillance. *J Urol.* 2013;190:1218–1222.
8. Kattan MW, Stapleton AM, Wheeler TM, Scardino PT. Evaluation of a nomogram used to predict the pathologic stage of clinically localized prostate carcinoma. *Cancer.* 1997;79(3):528–537.
9. Kattan MW, Eastham JA, Stapleton AM, Wheeler TM, Scardino PT. A preoperative nomogram for disease recurrence following radical prostatectomy for prostate cancer. *J Natl Cancer Inst.* 1998;90(10):766–771.
10. Kattan MW, Potters L, Blasko JC, et al. Pretreatment nomogram for predicting freedom from recurrence after permanent prostate brachytherapy in prostate cancer. *Urology.* 2001;58(3): 393–399.
11. Kattan MW, Zelefsky MJ, Kupelian PA, Scardino PT, Fuks Z, Leibel SA. Pretreatment nomogram for predicting the outcome of three-dimensional conformal radiotherapy in prostate cancer. *J Clin Oncol.* 2000;18(19):3352–3359.
12. Dong F, Kattan MW, Steyerberg EW, et al. Validation of pretreatment nomograms for predicting indolent prostate cancer: efficacy in contemporary urological practice. *J Urol.* 2008;180(1): 150–154; discussion 154.
13. Iremashvili V, Soloway MS, Pelaez L, Rosenberg DL, Manoharan M. Comparative validation of nomograms predicting clinically insignificant prostate cancer. *Urology.* 2013;81(6):1202–1208.
14. Stephenson AJ, Kattan MW, Eastham JA, et al. Prostate cancer-specific mortality after radical prostatectomy for patients treated in the prostate-specific antigen era. *J Clin Oncol.* 2009;27(26):4300–4305.
15. Stephenson AJ, Scardino PT, Eastham JA, et al. Preoperative nomogram predicting the 10-year probability of prostate cancer recurrence after radical prostatectomy. *J Natl Cancer Inst.* 2006;98(10):715–717.
16. Makarov DV, Trock BJ, Humphreys EB, et al. Updated nomogram to predict pathologic stage of prostate cancer given prostate-specific antigen level, clinical stage, and biopsy Gleason score (Partin tables) based on cases from 2000 to 2005. *Urology.* 2007;69(6):1095–1101.
17. Kattan MW, Eastham JA, Wheeler TM, et al. Counseling men with prostate cancer: a nomogram for predicting the presence of small, moderately differentiated, confined tumors. *J Urol.* 2003;170(5):1792–1797.
18. Zelefsky MJ, Kattan MW, Fearn P, et al. Pretreatment nomogram predicting ten-year biochemical outcome of three-dimensional conformal radiotherapy and intensity-modulated radiotherapy for prostate cancer. *Urology.* 2007;70(2):283–287.
19. D'Amico AV, Whittington R, Malkowicz SB, et al. Biochemical outcome after radical prostatectomy, external beam radiation therapy, or interstitial radiation therapy for clinically localized prostate cancer. *JAMA.* 1998;280(11):969–974.
20. Epstein JI, Walsh PC, Carmichael M, Brendler CB. Pathologic and clinical findings to predict tumor extent of nonpalpable (stage t1 c) prostate cancer. *JAMA.* 1994;271(5):368–374.
21. Bastian PJ, Mangold LA, Epstein JI, Partin AW. Characteristics of insignificant clinical T1c prostate tumors. A contemporary analysis. *Cancer.* 2004;101(9):2001–2005.
22. Jeldres C, Suardi N, Walz J, et al. Validation of the contemporary epstein criteria for insignificant prostate cancer in European men. *Eur Urol.* 2008;54(6):1306–1313.
23. Lee MC, Dong F, Stephenson AJ, Jones JS, Magi-Galluzzi C, Klein EA. The Epstein criteria predict for organ-confined but not insignificant disease and a high likelihood of cure at radical prostatectomy. *Eur Urol.* 2010;58(1):90–95.
24. May M, Knoll N, Siegsmund M, et al. Validity of the CAPRA score to predict biochemical recurrence-free survival after radical prostatectomy. Results from a European multicenter survey of 1,296 patients. *J Urol.* 2007;178(5):1957–1962; discussion 1962.
25. Cooperberg MR, Freedland SJ, Pasta DJ, et al. Multiinstitutional validation of the UCSF cancer of the prostate risk assessment for prediction of recurrence after radical prostatectomy. *Cancer.* 2006;107(10):2384–2391.
26. Dickinson L, Ahmed HU, Allen C, et al. Magnetic resonance imaging for the detection, localisation, and characterisation of prostate cancer: recommendations from a European consensus meeting. *Eur Urol.* 2011;59(4):477–494.
27. Shukla-Dave A, Hricak H, Akin O, et al. Preoperative nomograms incorporating magnetic resonance imaging and spectroscopy for prediction of insignificant prostate cancer. *BJU Int.* 2012;109(9):1315–1322.
28. Lagemaat MW, Scheenen TW. Role of high-field MR in studies of localized prostate cancer. *NMR Biomed.* 2014;27:67–79.
29. Moore CM, Ridout A, Emberton M. The role of MRI in active surveillance of prostate cancer. *Curr Opin Urol.* 2013;23(3):261–267.
30. Ahmed HU. Multiparametric magnetic resonance imaging findings in men with low-risk prostate cancer followed using active surveillance. *BJU Int.* 2013;111(7):1011–1013.
31. Ahmed HU, Arya M, Freeman A, Emberton M. Do low-grade and low-volume prostate cancers bear the hallmarks of malignancy? *Lancet Oncol.* 2012;13(11):e509–e517.
32. Vargas HA, Akin O, Afaq A, et al. Magnetic resonance imaging for predicting prostate biopsy findings in patients considered for active surveillance of clinically low risk prostate cancer. *J Urol.* 2012;188(5):1732–1738.
33. Margel D, Yap SA, Lawrentschuk N, et al. Impact of multiparametric endorectal coil prostate magnetic resonance imaging on disease reclassification among active surveillance candidates: a prospective cohort study. *J Urol.* 2012;187(4):1247–1252.
34. Mullins JK, Bonekamp D, Landis P, et al. Multiparametric magnetic resonance imaging findings in men with low-risk prostate cancer followed using active surveillance. *BJU Int.* 2013;111(7):1037–1045.
35. Schiavina R, Scattoni V, Castellucci P, et al. 11C-choline positron emission tomography/computerized tomography for preoperative lymph-node staging in intermediate-risk and high-risk prostate cancer: comparison with clinical staging nomograms. *Eur Urol.* 2008;54(2):392–401.
36. Martorana G, Schiavina R, Corti B, et al. 11C-Choline positron emission tomography/computerized tomography for tumor localization of primary prostate cancer in comparison with 12-Core biopsy. *J Urol.* 2006;176(3):954–960.
37. Wilt TJ, Brawer MK, Jones KM, et al. Radical prostatectomy versus observation for localized prostate cancer. *N Engl J Med.* 2012;367(3):203–213.
38. Holmberg L, Bill-Axelson A, Steineck G, et al. Results from the Scandinavian Prostate Cancer Group Trial Number 4: a randomized controlled trial of radical prostatectomy versus watchful waiting. *J Natl Cancer Inst Monogr.* 2012; 2012(45):230–233.
39. Ganz PA, Barry JM, Burke W, et al. National Institutes of Health State-of-the-Science Conference: role of active surveillance in the management of men with localized prostate cancer. *Ann Intern Med.* 2012;156(8):591–595.
40. Bussemakers MJ, van Bokhoven A, Verhaegh GW, et al. DD3: a new prostate-specific gene, highly overexpressed in prostate cancer. *Cancer Res.* 1999;59(23):5975–5979.

41. Sokoll LJ, Ellis W, Lange P, et al. A multicenter evaluation of the PCA3 molecular urine test: pre-analytical effects, analytical performance, and diagnostic accuracy. *Clin Chim Acta.* 2008;389(1–2):1–6.
42. Deras IL, Aubin SM, Blase A, et al. PCA3: a molecular urine assay for predicting prostate biopsy outcome. *J Urol.* 2008;179(4):1587–1592.
43. Marks LS, Fradet Y, Deras IL, et al. PCA3 molecular urine assay for prostate cancer in men undergoing repeat biopsy. *Urology.* 2007;69(3):532–535.
44. Haese A, de la Taille A, van Poppel H, et al. Clinical utility of the PCA3 urine assay in European men scheduled for repeat biopsy. *Eur Urol.* 2008;54(5):1081–1088.
45. Nakanishi H, Groskopf J, Fritsche HA, et al. PCA3 Molecular urine assay correlates with prostate cancer tumor volume: implication in selecting candidates for active surveillance. *J Urol.* 2008;179(5):1804–1810.
46. van Gils MP, Hessels D, Hulsbergen-van de Kaa CA, et al. Detailed analysis of histopathological parameters in radical prostatectomy specimens and PCA3 urine test results. *Prostate.* 2008;68(11):1215–1222.
47. Hessels D, van Gils MP, van Hooij O, et al. Predictive value of PCA3 in urinary sediments in determining clinico-pathological characteristics of prostate cancer. *Prostate.* 2010;70(1):10–16.
48. Miller K. Words of wisdom. Re: PCA3 score before radical prostatectomy predicts extracapsular extension and tumor volume. Whitman EJ, Groskopf J, Ali A, et al. J Urol 2008;180:1975–8; discussion 1978-9. *Eur Urol.* 2009;56(1):218–219.
49. Whitman EJ, Groskopf J, Ali A, et al. PCA3 score before radical prostatectomy predicts extracapsular extension and tumor volume. *J Urol.* 2008;180(5):1975–1978; discussion 1978–1979.
50. Lin DW, Newcomb LF, Brown EC, et al. Urinary TMPRSS2:ERG and PCA3 in an active surveillance cohort: results from a baseline analysis in the Canary Prostate Active Surveillance Study. *Clin Cancer Res.* 2013;19(9):2442–2450.
51. Bradley LA, Palomaki GE, Gutman S, Samson D, Aronson N. Comparative effectiveness review: prostate cancer antigen 3 testing for the diagnosis and management of prostate cancer. *J Urol.* 2013;190:389–398.
52. Whelan C, Kawachi M, Smith DD, et al. EPS biomarkers improve stratification of NCCN active surveillance candidates: performance of secretion capacity and TMPRSS2:ERG models. *J Urol.* 2014;191:220–226.
53. Tombal B, Andriole GL, de la Taille A, et al. Clinical judg ment versus biomarker prostate cancer gene 3: which is best when determining the need for repeat prostate biopsy? *Urology.* 2013;81(5):998–1004.
54. Cuzick J, Swanson GP, Fisher G, et al. Prognostic value of an RNA expression signature derived from cell cycle proliferation genes in patients with prostate cancer: a retrospective study. *Lancet Oncol.* 2011;12(3):245–255.
55. Cuzick J, Berney DM, Fisher G, et al. Prognostic value of a cell cycle progression signature for prostate cancer death in a conservatively managed needle biopsy cohort. *Br J Cancer.* 2012;106(6):1095–1099.
56. Cooperberg MR, Simko JP, Cowan JE, et al. Validation of a cell-cycle progression gene panel to improve risk stratification in a contemporary prostatectomy cohort. *J Clin Oncol.* 2013;31(11):1428–1434.
57. Klein EA, Cooperberg MR, Magi-Galluzzi C, et al. A 17-gene assay to predict prostate cancer aggressiveness in the context of gleason grade heterogeneity, tumor multifocality, and biopsy undersampling. *Eur Urol.* 2014;pii: S0302-2838(14)00414-X.
58. Klein EA, Michael Crager MK, Magi-Galluzzi C, et al.; Glickman Urological and Kidney Institute, Cleveland Clinic, Cleveland, OH; Genomic Health, Redwood City, CA; Pathology and Laboratory Medicine Institute, Cleveland Clinic, Cleveland, OH. Identification of prostate cancer-expressed microRNAs associated with clinical recurrence (cR) and prostate cancer-specific survival (PCSS) following radical prostatectomy (RP). *J Clin Oncol.* 2012;30 (suppl 5):Abstr 21.
59. Klein EA. A genomic approach to active surveillance: a step toward precision medicine. *Asian J Androl.* 2013;15(3):340-341.
60. Liu D, Lehmann HP, Frick KD, Carter HB. Active surveillance versus surgery for low risk prostate cancer: a clinical decision analysis. *J Urol.* 2012;187(4):1241–1246.
61. Xia J, Trock BJ, Cooperberg MR, et al. Prostate cancer mortality following active surveillance versus immediate radical prostatectomy. *Clin Cancer Res.* 2012;18(19):5471–5478.

5.1 Novel Molecular and Genotype Profiling in Prostate Cancer: The Future of Screening, Diagnosis, and Staging

HEESUN SHIN
ISMAEL A. VERGARA
ANIRBAN P. MITRA
TIMOTHY J. TRICHE
ELAI DAVICIONI

INTRODUCTION

Recent advances in genomic technologies have expanded our knowledge of complex biological processes that are believed to drive prostate carcinogenesis. These advances are beginning to be leveraged by emerging laboratory tests that may be useful for improved prostate cancer screening, diagnosis, and risk stratification. In this chapter, we will outline the limitations of current clinical tools and highlight several examples of emerging tests that use the wealth of information encoded in the genome toward improving prostate cancer disease and patient management.

A ROLE FOR GENOMIC-BASED BIOMARKERS IN SCREENING, DISEASE DIAGNOSIS AND CLASSIFICATION, AND CLINICAL TREATMENT DECISION MAKING

Emerging molecular genetic tests capitalize on one or more "layers" of genomic information primarily through assays that measure chromosomal aberrations, DNA sequence mutations, epigenetic modifications, RNA or protein expression/modification, and changes in the concentration of metabolites. This is especially important in prostate cancer where capturing a variety of biological variables in addition to clinical and pathological features can ultimately improve characterization of an individual patient's disease. It is hoped that armed with more detailed information regarding the genomic profile of a tumor, physicians will be able to make better treatment and management decisions in a disease whose clinical course is highly heterogeneous. Genomic-based biomarkers encompass a variety of molecular and genetic mutational markers that are suitable for use in cancer detection and diagnostic strategies (Table 5.1.1). Among the most common molecular events in prostate cancer progression are androgen receptor (AR) splicing or amplification (1, 2), gene fusion or rearrangement of ETS transcription factors (i.e., TMPRSS2:ERG gene fusion) (3), loss of PTEN function (PI3K activation) (4), and germline mutations in HOXB13 (5, 6). However, in contrast to many other solid tumors such as lung and colon cancer, which often have mutations (e.g., p53 and k-Ras mutations) on diagnosis that define 30%–40% of tumors of the affected population, prostate cancer genomes are not dominated by any such "driver" mutations (7). In prostate cancer, it appears that the more prevalent genetic alterations occur during progression to advanced stage disease (8) and perhaps greater utility can be detected through measurement of specific expression signatures that represent multiple biological pathways important to prostate carcinogenesis early on (9, 10). Numerous new molecular and genetic tests for prostate cancer are under development and in early commercialization that target specific clinical decision points for prostate cancer disease. In this chapter, we will provide an overview of some of these emerging tests that are representative of current strategies for leveraging more genomic information for prostate cancer screening, disease diagnosis, risk stratification, and prediction of treatment response (Figure 5.1.1).

Table 5.1.1 Examples of different types of genomic biomarkers

Category	Biomarker Type	Biomarker Candidates	Commonly Used Specimens	Commonly Used Profiling Technology/ Platform	Prostate Cancer Examples	References/Reviews
Genotype	Genomic	Germline/ Somatic SNPs	Tissue, blood, urine	NGS (whole genome/exome sequencing), SNP arrays	SNPs in LEPR, RNASEL, IL4, CYR1, ARVCF, HOXB13	Lin et al. (55) *Cancer Epidemiol Biomarkers Prev* (2011). Xu et al. (6) *Human Genetics* (2013)
		Copy number variations	Tissue, blood, urine	aCGH, NGS	The duplication at 14q32.33 encompasses IGHG3 gene	Ledet et al. (51) *The Prostate* (2013)
		Gene fusions	Tissue, blood, urine	NGS (whole genome/ exome and transcriptome sequencing [RNA-seq]), microarrays	TMPRSS2-ERG,CTAGE5-KHDRBS3, USP9Y-TTTY15	Shancheng Ren et al. (56) *Cell Research* (2012)
	Epigenomic	Methylations, histone modifications	Tissue, blood, urine	ChIP-Chip, NGS (ChIP-seq, MeDIP-Seq, MethylC-seq)	hypermethylation of GSTP1, MGMT, AR, ER, CDKN2A genes	Majumdar et al. (57) *Curr Genomics* (2011)
Molecular Phenotype	Transcriptomic	mRNAs and ncRNAs	Tissue	NGS (RNA-seq), microarrays	STEAP4, multi-gene/transcript signatures*	Karnes et al. (36) *Journal of Urology* (2013)
		Splice variants (SVs)	Tissue	NGS (RNA-seq)	Androgen receptor splice variants	Guo et al. (58) *Cancer Res.* (2009)
	Proteomic	Proteins	Tissue, serum, plasma, urine	iTraq, MRM, SRM, MS	PEBP-1, PIN1, cIAP2, MIF, Caveolin-1	Wood et al. (59) *Nature Reviews Urology* (2013)
	Metabolomic	Metabolites	Tissue, serum, plasma, urine	Nuclear magnetic resonance (NMR), Mass spectrometry (MS)	sarcosine	Sreekumar et al. (60) *Nature* (2009)
Cellular components	Other	CTC	Blood, urine	CellSearch, CTC-chip	CTCs coexpressing epithelial, mesenchymal, and stem cell markers in progressive metastases	Danila et al. (61) *Clin Cancer Res* (2011). Cann et al. (46) *PloS one* (2012). Armstrong et al. (62) *Mol Cancer* Res (2011)
		Cell-free RNA/ DNA	Serum, plasma, urine	RT-qPCR, NGS	PCADM-1, PCA3	Sita-Lumsden et al. (49) *British Journal of Cancer* (2013). Wroclawski et al. (48) *Tumor Biol* (2013)
		Exosomes	Serum, plasma, urine	Flow cytometry, MS	PCA-3 and TMPRSS2:ERG in exosomes isolated from urine of prostate cancer patients	Zhang et al. (63) *Clin Cancer Res* (2011). Jansen et al. (64) *Mol Cell Proteomics* (2009). Nilsson et al. (65) *Br J Cancer* (2009)

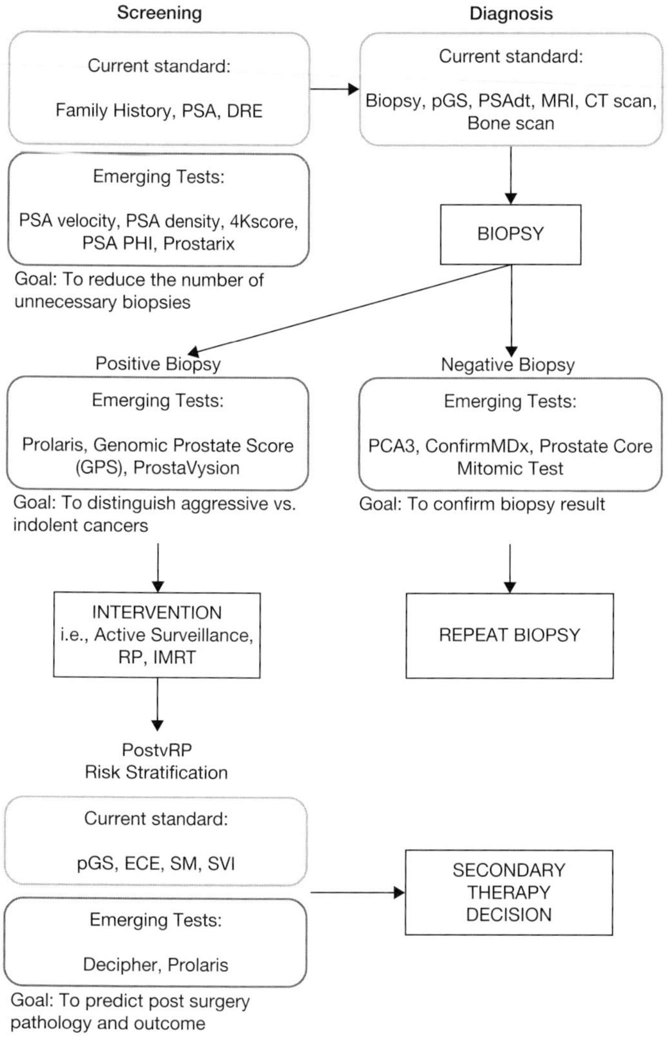

FIGURE 5.1.1 Summary of emerging molecular tests at different clinical decision-making points for prostate cancer screening, diagnosis, and risk-stratification.

■ CURRENT CHALLENGES AND OPPORTUNITIES IN PROSTATE CANCER SCREENING

A family history of prostate cancer as well as prostate-specific antigen (PSA) measurement and digital rectal examination (DRE) are the key variables used for screening and early detection of prostate cancer. Though highly sensitive, PSA measurement provides poor specificity for clinically significant disease detection and if used inappropriately results in too many patients getting unnecessary biopsies, leading to overdiagnosis and overtreatment of many indolent tumors that can be managed more conservatively (11, 12). PSA concentrations above 4.0 ng/mL have about 30% positive predictive value, meaning that only one in three men biopsied for elevated PSA will have prostate cancer detected on subsequent biopsy (13). While in May of 2012 the U.S. Preventive Services Task Force made a recommendation against the use of PSA-based screening for healthy men, citing that the harms associated with biopsy or treatment initiated by PSA screening outweighed the potential benefits (14–16), others are calling for more refined approaches to use PSA for earlier, "smarter" screening of true at-risk populations.

In an effort to improve the accuracy and reduce the number of unnecessary biopsies, various derivatives or modifications of measurement of PSA have been developed, including PSA velocity, PSA density, 4Kscore™ (Opko Health, Inc.), and PSA Prostate Health Index (PHI) (Beckman Coulter, Inc.). A recent study by Catalona et al., for example, has demonstrated that the use of PHI improves prostate cancer detection accuracy in comparison with PSA, particularly in the 2 to 10 ng/mL PSA range, reporting that at 95% sensitivity, the specificity of PHI was 16.0% compared with 6.5% for PSA. The AUC of prostate cancer detection was also significantly greater for PHI (AUC 0.70) than for PSA (AUC 0.53) (17). Though new PSA derived approaches have been somewhat successful, there appears to be an upper limit for PSA-based test specificity. Non-PSA-based molecular tests currently under development include Prostarix™ (Metabolon, Inc.), which is based on the measurement of various metabolites that are reported to be specific to prostate cancer.

Since a family history of prostate cancer is one of the most significant risk factors for developing the disease (18–20), identifying inherited genetic susceptibility through genotyping is another promising complement that can be used to refine more generalized screening strategies. Several studies have demonstrated the utility of detecting germline single nucleotide polymorphisms (SNPs) as a means for identifying men at a high risk for developing prostate cancer (21–23). Furthermore, advances in genetic screening are being enabled by rapidly developing genomic technologies facilitating the identification and validation of new prostate cancer susceptibility loci. For example, using a custom Illumina genotyping array, the Collaborative Oncological Gene-Environment Study (COGS) recently identified 23 novel loci that are susceptible to variation in prostate cancer. To date, 77 prostate cancer susceptibility loci have been identified, which are thought to account for approximately 30% of the prostate cancer familial risk. When these SNPs were combined in a risk model, the top 1% of men in the highest risk stratum had a 4.7-fold higher risk than the population average (24). Coupling PSA screening only for at-risk individuals based on the measurement of prostate cancer susceptibility loci may emerge as an approach to increase specificity for disease detection and reduce PSA testing that triggers unnecessary interventions.

■ CURRENT CHALLENGES AND OPPORTUNITIES IN PROSTATE CANCER DIAGNOSIS

Each year an estimated 1,000,000 men in the United States alone undergo a diagnostic core-needle biopsy to sample the prostate and to confirm a diagnosis of prostate cancer—mostly triggered by elevated PSA findings. However, prostate biopsies, particularly multiple repeat re-biopsies, have associated risks that include developing serious infection/sepsis, cases of which are rising as many strains of hospital bacteria have developed antibiotic resistance (25). Measurement of prostate cancer antigen 3 (PCA3), a noncoding RNA detectable in post-DRE urine using the FDA-approved Progensa assay was developed to rule out the need for subsequent biopsy in men with previous negative biopsy findings but persistently high PSA. Tissue-based tests, such as ConfirmMDx™ (MDxHealth, Inc.) and Mitomics Prostate Core Test™ (Mitomics, Inc.), are genomic-based biopsy tests that try to predict occult prostate cancer missed by standard 10 to 12 core biopsy, which samples approximately 1% to 3% of the prostate gland by measuring a "field effect" of the cancerous tissue on the surrounding nonneoplastic cells. ConfirmMDx™ identifies epigenetic events associated with cancer progression, that is, hypermethylation of genes, glutathione-S-transferase P1 (GSTP1) and adenomatous polyposis coli (APC) in prostate tumor tissue compared with the benign prostate (26). Recently, Trock et al. evaluated these DNA methylation biomarkers prospectively in the setting of repeat biopsy after an initial negative biopsy, and showed that while GSTP1 showed modest performance measures (negative predictive value [NPV] = 0.80, sensitivity = 0.43), APC methylation yielded an NPV of 0.96 and a sensitivity of 0.95. This result shows that analysis of epigenetic biomarkers in biopsy tissue may provide for increased specificity over urine- or blood-based PSA and PCA3 testing although validation in larger prospective cohorts is needed (27). Similarly, Prostate Core Mitomic Test™, which measures a mitochondrial genomic alteration (i.e., deletion), has also been assessed for its performance in predicting the absence of cancer on repeat biopsy. This test showed sensitivity and specificity of 84% and 54%, respectively, with the area under the ROC curve (AUC) of 0.75 and NPV of 91% in a validation study of 101 patients (28). Therefore, genomic assessment of the "field effect" in prostate cancer may ultimately overcome the under-sampling issue inherent in the standard biopsy procedure.

Once a diagnosis of prostate cancer is confirmed histologically, determining the clinical significance of the disease and how it should be optimally managed is a major area of focus for emerging diagnostic tests. ProstaVysion™ (Bostwick Laboratories, Inc.) measures two of the most common genetic events in prostate carcinogenesis, ERG gene fusion and PTEN tumor suppressor gene loss. Although these markers have been extensively studied in the literature, little clinical validation data on this assay have been produced to show how the information from this test should be used to guide patient management. More data is available on the Prolaris® test (Myriad Genetics, Inc.) that was developed to predict prostate cancer–specific mortality from analysis of gene expression on prostate biopsy. Prolaris® defines a prognostic score from the expression of 31 cell cycle progression (CCP) genes and 15 housekeeper genes that were selected based upon the most informative prognostic genes from similar tests developed for diagnosing breast cancer (9, 29). CCP genes are more highly expressed in actively proliferating cells, and therefore represent an indirect measure of the growth rate and inherent aggressiveness of the tumor. More recently, the Genomic Prostate Score (Genomic Health, Inc.) is being marketed as a test that can be used to better select patients that can safely defer definitive treatment in favor of active surveillance. Again, no data has been presented that this test may improve decision making for men considering active surveillance for very low–risk or low-risk prostate cancer over currently available guidelines. Instead, the data that has been presented are based on radical prostatectomy series that by today's guidelines could be candidates for active surveillance. While these emerging genomic-based tests are certainly promising, additional clinical studies in patients actually being managed with active surveillance are warranted.

■ CURRENT CHALLENGES AND OPPORTUNITIES IN PROSTATE CANCER RISK STRATIFICATION

The role of multimodal therapy in high-risk prostate cancer has been established through several randomized clinical trials. Intensification of therapy on men at risk for developing potentially lethal prostate cancer aims primarily at preventing or at least delaying the onset of metastatic disease. For example, current clinical guidelines recommend adjuvant radiotherapy for patients who present with postoperative pT3 disease or positive surgical margins. However, this may lead to overtreatment of many of these men who would not have had a recurrence after surgery alone (30). An emerging genomic-based risk stratification test, the Decipher® (GenomeDx Biosciences, Inc.) prostate cancer classifier was developed for intermediate to high-risk prostate cancer patients who are candidates for multimodal therapy postradical prostatectomy (10, 31, 32). Decipher® is the first test in prostate cancer that is the result of a genome-wide search for markers that predict early clinical metastasis postradical prostatectomy. The test was developed by profiling over 1.4 million expressed RNA markers including all of the known approximately 22,000 protein-coding genes and many noncoding RNAs in over 500 formalin-fixed paraffin-embedded (FFPE) primary tumor specimens from patients treated with radical prostatectomy at the Mayo Clinic. The Decipher® test results are based on a set of 22 expressed RNA biomarkers that represent multiple biological pathways involved in the development of metastatic disease, such as cell adhesion and migration, cell cycle control, immune system modulation, and tumor motility (10).

A novel aspect of this analysis was the inclusion of ncRNAs, which have been highlighted recently for their involvement in carcinogenesis (33–35) in addition to the typical RNA features from protein coding genes. Also notable, the endpoint used for development of this test was early clinical metastasis after initial postradical prostatectomy PSA recurrence. Using this measure for aggressive prostate cancer may avoid reflexive treatment intensification

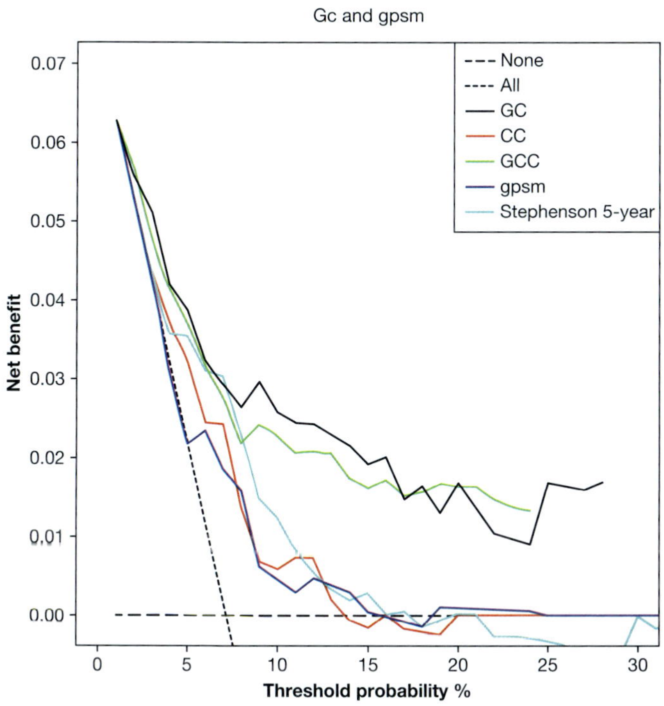

FIGURE 5.1.2 Survival decision curve analysis comparing the net benefit of Decipher® (GC) and Decipher® combined with clinical variables (GCC) against clinical-only models (CC) (clinical variables, GPSM, and Stephenson nomogram). Performance of models is compared with extremes of classifying all patients as at risk for clinical metastasis (thus warranting treatment of all patients; sloping gray dotted line), versus classifying no patients at risk (thus treating none; horizontal black-dashed line). The "decision-to-treat" threshold, the probability of metastasis used to trigger the decision to treat, is varied from 0 to 1, with sensitivity and specificity of each prediction model calculated at each threshold to determine net benefit. An optimal classifier has high net benefit above the gray dotted "treat all" line. At a wide range of "decision-to-treat" thresholds, the net benefit of the Decipher® is superior. GPSM (Gleason score, preoperative PSA, SVI, and margins prediction model developed at Mayo Clinic); Stephenson 5 year (Stephenson nomogram derived 5-year probability of survival). Individual clinicopathologic factors: Path GS, pathological Gleason score; Preop PSA, preoperative prostate specific antigen; SVI, seminal vesicle invasion; ECE, extracapsular extension; SM+; positive surgical margins; N+, lymph node involvement.

solely based on rising PSA, which is often a relatively nonspecific predictor of death due to prostate cancer. In a prospectively designed study of a high-risk population of 1,010 men treated with radical prostatectomy, Decipher® was shown to provide independent prediction of metastasis over clinical variables in multivariable analysis with an AUC of 0.79 (36). Furthermore, decision curve analysis revealed that the increased predictive power of Decipher® translated into a greater "net benefit" (e.g., reducing unnecessary overtreatment after RP in comparison to clinical prediction models and commonly used nomograms) (Figure 5.1.2). It is noteworthy that in conjunction with analytical and clinical validity (31,36), Decipher® has been also evaluated for clinical utility, and more specifically, for its influence on urologist treatment recommendations for patients at risk of metastasis (37,38). These studies showed that adjuvant treatment recommendations changed in 37% of cases on average following review of Decipher® test results in comparison to pre-Decipher® decision making based on pathology alone (Figure 5.1.3).

THE FUTURE OF MOLECULAR SCREENING AND STAGING METHODS

The discovery and development of novel molecular and genetic biomarkers for prostate cancer diagnosis and prognosis have been empowered by high-throughput genomic technologies such as microarrays and genome sequencing. The so-called Next Generation Sequencing (NGS), a massively parallel DNA sequencing technology (39,40), has been used to evaluate the spectrum of DNA alterations seen in advanced prostate cancer using FFPE biopsy tissue, which is an important step toward identifying novel therapeutic targets for individual patients with castrate-resistant prostate cancer (41). Clinical application of this technology, such as the MI-ONCOSEQ effort at the Michigan Oncology Sequencing Center, has begun to give hope of using clinical genomics to better sequence the delivery of current and novel systemic agents.

As NGS whole genome or exome sequencing (8,42) becomes more established and cost-effective, the ability to comprehensively identify genetic mutations will eventually lead to in-depth and informed disease predisposition determination in addition to treatment decision making for affected individuals. In addition, the application of these technologies to more accessible, noninvasive sources of biosamples such as the blood (39) and urine to enable examination of circulating tumor cells (43–46), exosomes (47), and cell free DNAs and RNAs (48), including miRNAs (49), would significantly expand the utility across the spectrum of disease management, especially in situations where tumor tissue is not easily available in many cases (e.g., bone metastases).

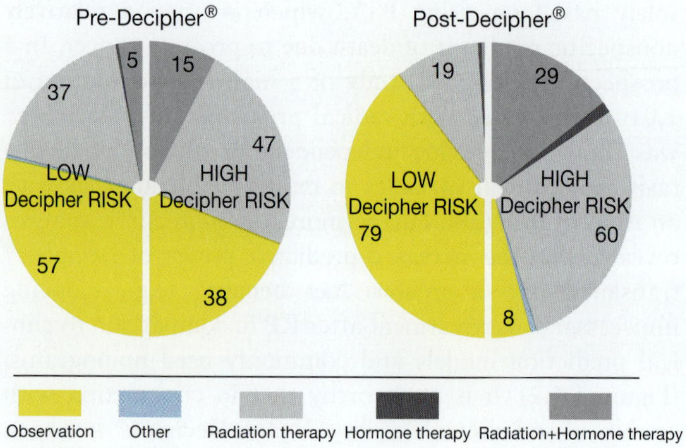

FIGURE 5.1.3 Breakdown of treatment recommendations pre-Decipher® and post-Decipher® for low and high-risk groups determined by Decipher® in the adjuvant setting. Pre-Decipher® treatment recommendations are shown on left, post-Decipher® treatment recommendation are shown on right. Numbers indicate the % of patient cases for which a specific treatment recommendation was made in the respective group (100% for each risk group).

While we continue to explore the genomic heterogeneity of prostate carcinogenesis and its relationship to the diverse clinical outcomes observed in prostate cancer disease (50), undoubtedly the plethora of genomic data, such as whole genome sequences, structural genomic rearrangements (7), DNA copy number variations (51), epigenomes (52,53) (i.e., DNA methylation and chromatin modification), transcriptomes (RNAs including ncRNAs and splice variants), proteomes (proteins), and metabolomes (metabolites), that are becoming available will continue to provide a wellspring for emerging genomic tests. The real bottleneck for innovation, however, remains the extensive clinical validation and demonstration of clinical utility for each treatment decision point in large numbers of patients demanded by clinicians. As analytical methodologies to measure the layers of the genome become more cost-effective and as the data itself becomes more ubiquitous, ultimately this may lead to integrative "omics" approaches using network-based systems biology methods (54) to understand the underlying biology of the patient and his tumor.

REFERENCES

1. Newmark JR, Hardy DO, Tonb DC, et al. Androgen receptor gene mutations in human prostate cancer. *Proc Natl Acad Sci U S A*. 1992;89(14):6319–6323.
2. Visakorpi T, Hyytinen E, Koivisto P, et al. In vivo amplification of the androgen receptor gene and progression of human prostate cancer. *Nat Genet*. 1995;9(4):401–406.
3. Bastus NC, Boyd LK, Mao X, et al. Androgen-induced TMPRSS2:ERG fusion in nonmalignant prostate epithelial cells. *Cancer Res*. 2010;70(23):9544–9548.
4. Krohn A, Diedler T, Burkhardt L, et al. Genomic deletion of PTEN is associated with tumor progression and early PSA recurrence in ERG fusion-positive and fusion-negative prostate cancer. *Am J Pathol*. 2012;181(2):401–412.
5. Ewing CM, Ray AM, Lange EM, et al. Germline mutations in HOXB13 and prostate-cancer risk. *N Engl J Med*. 2012;366(2):141–149.
6. Xu J, Lange EM, Lu L, et al. HOXB13 is a susceptibility gene for prostate cancer: results from the International Consortium for Prostate Cancer Genetics (ICPCG). *Hum Genet*. 2013;132(1):5–14.
7. Baca SC, Prandi D, Lawrence MS, et al. Punctuated evolution of prostate cancer genomes. *Cell*. 2013;153(3):666–677.
8. Kumar A, White TA, MacKenzie AP, et al. Exome sequencing identifies a spectrum of mutation frequencies in advanced and lethal prostate cancers. *Proc Natl Acad Sci U S A*. 2011;108(41):17087–17092.
9. Cuzick J, Swanson GP, Fisher G, et al. Prognostic value of an RNA expression signature derived from cell cycle proliferation genes in patients with prostate cancer: a retrospective study. *Lancet Oncol*. 2011;12(3):245–255.
10. Erho N, Crisan A, Vergara IA, et al. Discovery and validation of a prostate cancer genomic classifier that predicts early metastasis following radical prostatectomy. *PloS One*. 2013;8(6):e66855.
11. Andriole GL, Crawford ED, Grubb RL 3rd, et al. Prostate cancer screening in the randomized Prostate, Lung, Colorectal, and Ovarian Cancer Screening Trial: mortality results after 13 years of follow-up. *J Natl Cancer Inst*. 2012;104(2):125–132.
12. Schroder FH, Hugosson J, Roobol MJ, et al. Prostate-cancer mortality at 11 years of follow-up. *N Engl J Med*. 2012;366(11):981–990.
13. Catalona WJ, Richie JP, Ahmann FR, et al. Comparison of digital rectal examination and serum prostate specific antigen in the early detection of prostate cancer: results of a multicenter clinical trial of 6,630 men. *J Urol*. 1994;151(5):1283–1290.
14. Andriole GL, Crawford ED, Grubb RL 3rd, et al. Mortality results from a randomized prostate-cancer screening trial. *N Engl J Med*. 2009;360(13):1310–1319.
15. Schroder FH, Hugosson J, Roobol MJ, et al. Screening and prostate-cancer mortality in a randomized European study. *N Engl J Med*. 2009;360(13):1320–1328.
16. Etzioni R, Gulati R, Cooperberg MR, Penson DM, Weiss NS, Thompson IM. Limitations of basing screening policies on screening trials: the US Preventive Services Task Force and Prostate Cancer Screening. *Med Care*. 2013;51(4):295–300.
17. Catalona WJ, Partin AW, Sanda MG, et al. A multicenter study of [-2]pro-prostate specific antigen combined with prostate specific antigen and free prostate specific antigen for prostate cancer detection in the 2.0 to 10.0 ng/ml prostate specific antigen range. *J Urol*. 2011;185(5):1650–1655.
18. Bruner DW, Moore D, Parlanti A, Dorgan J, Engstrom P. Relative risk of prostate cancer for men with affected relatives: systematic review and meta-analysis. *Int J Cancer*. 2003;107(5):797–803.
19. Johns LE, Houlston RS. A systematic review and meta-analysis of familial prostate cancer risk. *BJU Int*. 2003;91(9):789–794.
20. Kicinski M, Vangronsveld J, Nawrot TS. An epidemiological reappraisal of the familial aggregation of prostate cancer: a meta-analysis. *PloS One*. 2011;6(10):e27130.
21. Kader AK, Sun J, Reck BH, et al. Potential impact of adding genetic markers to clinical parameters in predicting prostate biopsy outcomes in men following an initial negative biopsy: findings from the REDUCE trial. *Eur Urol*. 2012;62(6):953–961.
22. Sun J, Kader AK, Hsu FC, et al. Inherited genetic markers discovered to date are able to identify a significant number of men at considerably elevated risk for prostate cancer. *Prostate*. 2011;71(4):421–430.
23. Eeles RA, Kote-Jarai Z, Al Olama AA, et al. Identification of seven new prostate cancer susceptibility loci through a genome-wide association study. *Nat Genet*. 2009;41(10):1116–1121.
24. Eeles RA, Olama AA, Benlloch S, et al. Identification of 23 new prostate cancer susceptibility loci using the iCOGS custom genotyping array. *Nat Genet*. 2013;45(4):385–391, 391.e1-2.
25. Loeb S, Vellekoop A, Ahmed HU, et al. Systematic review of complications of prostate biopsy. *Eur Urol*. 2013;64:876–892.
26. Henrique R, Jeronimo C, Teixeira MR, et al. Epigenetic heterogeneity of high-grade prostatic intraepithelial neoplasia: clues for clonal progression in prostate carcinogenesis. *Mol Cancer Res*. 2006;4(1):1–8.

27. Trock BJ, Brotzman MJ, Mangold LA, et al. Evaluation of GSTP1 and APC methylation as indicators for repeat biopsy in a high-risk cohort of men with negative initial prostate biopsies. *BJU Int.* 2012;110(1):56–62.
28. Robinson K, Creed J, Reguly B, et al. Accurate prediction of repeat prostate biopsy outcomes by a mitochondrial DNA deletion assay. *Prostate Cancer Prostatic Dis.* 2010;13(2):126–131.
29. Cuzick J, Berney DM, Fisher G, et al. Prognostic value of a cell cycle progression signature for prostate cancer death in a conservatively managed needle biopsy cohort. *Br J Cancer.* 2012;106(6):1095–1099.
30. Swanson GP, Basler JW. Prognostic factors for failure after prostatectomy. *J Cancer.* 2010;2:1–19.
31. Ross AE, Feng FY, Ghadessi M, et al. A genomic classifier predicting metastatic disease progression in men with biochemical recurrence after prostatectomy. *Prostate cancer and prostatic diseases.* 2014;17(1):64–69.
32. Den RB, Feng FY, Showalter TN, et al. A genomic prostate cancer classifier predicts biochemical failure and metastasis in patients following post operative radiation therapy. *Int J Radiat Oncol Biol Phys.* 2014;89(5):1038–1046.
33. Du Z, Fei T, Verhaak RG, et al. Integrative genomic analyses reveal clinically relevant long noncoding RNAs in human cancer. *Nat Struct Mol Biol.* 2013;20:908–913.
34. Vergara IA, Erho N, Triche TJ, et al. Genomic "Dark Matter" in prostate cancer: exploring the clinical utility of ncRNA as biomarkers. *Front Genet.* 2012;3:23.
35. Prensner JR, Iyer MK, Balbin OA, et al. Transcriptome sequencing across a prostate cancer cohort identifies PCAT-1, an unannotated lincRNA implicated in disease progression. *Nat Biotechnol.* 2011;29(8):742–749.
36. Karnes RJ, Bergstralh EJ, Davicioni E, et al. Validation of a genomic classifier that predicts metastasis following radical prostatectomy in an at risk patient population. *J Urol.* 2013;190:2047–2053.
37. Badani K, Thompson DJ, Buerki C, et al. Impact of a genomic classifier of metastatic risk on postoperative treatment recommendations for prostate cancer patients: a report from the DECIDE study group. *Oncotarget.* 2013;4(4):600–609.
38. Badani K, Thompson DJ, Brown G, et al. Effect of a genomic classifier test on clinical practice decisions for patients with high-risk prostate cancer after surgery. *BJU international.* 2014; doi: 10.1111/bju.12789.
39. Heitzer E, Ulz P, Belic J, et al. Tumor associated copy number changes in the circulation of patients with prostate cancer identified through whole-genomc sequencing. *Genome Med.* 2013;5(4):30.
40. Roychowdhury S, Iyer MK, Robinson DR, et al. Personalized oncology through integrative high-throughput sequencing: a pilot study. *Sci Translat Med.* 2011;3(111):111ra21.
41. Beltran H, Yelensky R, Frampton GM, et al. Targeted next-generation sequencing of advanced prostate cancer identifies potential therapeutic targets and disease heterogeneity. *Eur Urol.* 2013;63(5):920–926.
42. Barbieri CE, Baca SC, Lawrence MS, et al. Exome sequencing identifies recurrent SPOP, FOXA1 and MED12 mutations in prostate cancer. *Nat Genet.* 2012;44(6):685–689.
43. Attard G, Swennenhuis JF, Olmos D, et al. Characterization of ERG, AR and PTEN gene status in circulating tumor cells from patients with castration-resistant prostate cancer. *Cancer Res.* 2009;69(7):2912–2918.
44. de Bono JS, Scher HI, Montgomery RB, et al. Circulating tumor cells predict survival benefit from treatment in metastatic castration-resistant prostate cancer. *Clin Cancer Res.* 2008;14(19):6302–6309.
45. Danila DC, Anand A, Sung CC, et al. TMPRSS2-ERG status in circulating tumor cells as a predictive biomarker of sensitivity in castration-resistant prostate cancer patients treated with abiraterone acetate. *Eur Urol.* 2011;60(5):897–904.
46. Cann GM, Gulzar ZG, Cooper S, et al. mRNA-Seq of single prostate cancer circulating tumor cells reveals recapitulation of gene expression and pathways found in prostate cancer. *PloS One.* 2012;7(11):e49144.
47. Duijvesz D, Luider T, Bangma CH, Jenster G. Exosomes as biomarker treasure chests for prostate cancer. *Eur Urol.* 2011;59(5):823–831.
48. Wroclawski ML, Serpa-Neto A, Fonseca FL, et al. Cell-free plasma DNA as biochemical biomarker for the diagnosis and follow-up of prostate cancer patients. *Tumour Biol.* 2013;34:2921–2927.
49. Sita-Lumsden A, Dart DA, Waxman J, Bevan CL. Circulating microRNAs as potential new biomarkers for prostate cancer. *Br J Cancer.* 2013;108(10):1925–1930.
50. Berger MF, Lawrence MS, Demichelis F, et al. The genomic complexity of primary human prostate cancer. *Nature.* 2011;470(7333):214–220.
51. Ledet EM, Hu X, Sartor O, Rayford W, Li M, Mandal D. Characterization of germline copy number variation in high-risk African American families with prostate cancer. *Prostate.* 2013;73(6):614–623.
52. Lister R, Pelizzola M, Dowen RH, et al. Human DNA methylomes at base resolution show widespread epigenomic differences. *Nature.* 2009;462(7271):315–322.
53. Lin PC, Giannopoulou EG, Park K, et al. Epigenomic alterations in localized and advanced prostate cancer. *Neoplasia.* 2013;15(4):373–383.
54. Weischenfeldt J, Simon R, Feuerbach L, et al. Integrative genomic analyses reveal an androgen-driven somatic alteration landscape in early-onset prostate cancer. *Cancer Cell.* 2013;23(2):159–170.
55. Lin DW, Fitzgerald LM, Fu R, et al. Genetic variants in the LEPR, CRY1, RNASEL, IL4, and ARVCF genes are prognostic markers of prostate cancer-specific mortality. *Cancer epidemiology, biomarkers & prevention: a publication of the American Association for Cancer Research, cosponsored by the American Society of Preventive Oncology.* 2011;20(9):1928–1936.
56. Ren S, Peng Z, Mao JH, et al. RNA-seq analysis of prostate cancer in the Chinese population identifies recurrent gene fusions, cancer-associated long noncoding RNAs and aberrant alternative splicings. *Cell research.* 2012;22(5):806–821.
57. Majumdar S, Buckles E, Estrada J, Koochekpour S. Aberrant DNA methylation and prostate cancer. *Current genomics.* 2011; 12(7):486–505.
58. Guo Z, Yang X, Sun F, et al. A novel androgen receptor splice variant is up-regulated during prostate cancer progression and promotes androgen depletion-resistant growth. *Cancer research.* 2009;69(6):2305–2313.
59. Wood SL, Knowles MA, Thompson D, Selby PJ, Banks RE. Proteomic studies of urinary biomarkers for prostate, bladder and kidney cancers. *Nature reviews Urology.* 2013; 10(4):206–218.
60. Sreekumar A, Poisson LM, Rajendiran TM, et al. Metabolomic profiles delineate potential role for sarcosine in prostate cancer progression. *Nature.* 2009;457(7231):910–914.
61. Danila DC, Fleisher M, Scher HI. Circulating tumor cells as biomarkers in prostate cancer. *Clinical cancer research: an official journal of the American Association for Cancer Research.* 2011; 17(12):3903–3912.
62. Armstrong AJ, Marengo MS, Oltean S, et al. Circulating tumor cells from patients with advanced prostate and breast cancer display both epithelial and mesenchymal markers. *Molecular cancer research: MCR.* 2011;9(8):997–1007.
63. Zhang HG, Grizzle WE. Exosomes and cancer: a newly described pathway of immune suppression. *Clinical cancer research: an official journal of the American Association for Cancer Research.* 2011;17(5):959–964.
64. Jansen FH, Krijgsveld J, van Rijswijk A, et al. Exosomal secretion of cytoplasmic prostate cancer xenograft-derived proteins. *Molecular & cellular proteomics: MCP.* 2009;8(6):1192–1205.
65. Nilsson J, Skog J, Nordstrand A, et al. Prostate cancer-derived urine exosomes: a novel approach to biomarkers for prostate cancer. *British journal of cancer.* 2009;100(10):1603–1607.

5.2 Genomics and Risk Assessment

HAO G. NGUYEN
MATTHEW R. COOPERBERG
PETER R. CARROLL

■ INTRODUCTION

For the last 20 years, risk assessment in prostate cancer has heavily relied on prostate-specific antigen (PSA), clinical staging, the extent of biopsy tissue involvement, and Gleason score. The currently available biomarkers and clinical features that clinicians use to differentiate indolent, low-risk cancer from the clinically significant, high-risk cancer that could progress to incurable, metastatic cancer could be improved. The problem of overdiagnosis and overtreatment of low-risk cancer has stemmed, in part, from routine PSA screening, lack of a biomarker to precisely identify clinically significant disease, and also from the failure to implement the current risk stratification in a consistent way.

Recent advances in genome analysis technology have allowed researchers to accelerate the genomic characterization of prostate cancer. Genomic data from a personalized analysis will very likely position clinicians to better stratify risks of progression and offer patients a more precise treatment option thereby avoiding both over- and undertreatment. RNA assessment through RT-PCR and/or microarray gene chips can now be accomplished using small samples from a needle biopsy to provide gene expression data on early to late stage prostate cancer. This chapter will highlight the current and future integration of genomic data into the current system to aid clinicians in risk stratification of prostate cancer.

■ CURRENT SYSTEM OF RISK ASSESSMENT AND THE NEED FOR INTEGRATING GENOMIC DATA

The goal of an optimal risk assessment system is to provide precise information on the biological aggressiveness of the cancer and to accurately differentiate which patients are at risk of disease progression, and therefore which will require treatment. Such precise genomic information may decrease the uncertainty for the clinicians and the patients when deciding the best treatment modalities. Urologists use pretreatment information including age, race/ethnicity, family history, PSA value, digital rectal examination (DRE), PSA density, prostate volume, previous biopsy status, urinary symptoms, and transrectal ultrasound findings to predict risk of a positive biopsy. D'Amico risk stratification is now widely used to counsel patients on treatment modality. Cooperberg et al. developed the Cancer of the Prostate Risk Assessment (CAPRA) score based on the above criteria but also added several important risk factors such as the percentage of positive cores, primary and secondary Gleason pattern on biopsy, and age at diagnosis (1). Once a patient has been diagnosed with prostate cancer, urologists generally use a variety of risk assessment tools including the D'Amico risk stratification, Kattan nomogram, Partin table, or CAPRA score to decide on treatment modality. However, treatment decision varies considerably across practices, often driven by age, comorbidities, socioeconomic factors, and so forth, as well as by both physician and patient preferences/bias (2, 3).

D'Amico and colleagues used PSA level, Gleason score, and clinical staging to stratify patients into the three risk groups to predict biochemical recurrence after local therapy (4). In addition, the Stephenson model or Cancer of the Prostate Risk Assessment score (CAPRA-S) were also used to predict biochemical recurrence after prostatectomy with C-index of 0.72 and 0.73 respectively (5). These risk stratification systems exhibited reasonably predictive accuracy (4, 6, 7).

In patients with pathologic features that carry a higher risk of recurrence after radical prostatectomy, contemporary practices rely on pathologic staging, Gleason score, volume of disease, surgical margin status, months until PSA recurrence, and PSA kinetics following surgery to predict risk of biochemical recurrence (8). However, the decision whether to proceed with adjuvant or salvage therapy is not always a clear-cut decision.

One limitation of the current risk stratification systems is the lack of genomic data, which could provide a more personalized assessment. There are several scenarios in which genomic data can further refine the current system. Approximately 30% of patients with low Gleason, aggressive disease on active surveillance do receive treatment due to disease progression (9). Patients with low-to-intermediate risk cancer in which biopsy showed high-volume Gleason 3+3 (>1/3 cores or >50% in one core) or in patients with small amount of secondary Gleason 4 pattern (1 core positive or less than 10% of core) are generally thought not to be ideal candidates for active surveillance in most community practices and are recommended to proceed with local treatment. However, most patients in this category could harbor low-risk indolent disease and would be reasonable candidates for active surveillance. Genomic data are not generally used to determine if these patients will progress over a period of time or harbor more aggressive disease during treatment counseling of patients in most community practices.

Genomic analysis of the biopsy core can yield crucial information on the biology of the cancer and therefore allow for better counseling of men in this group on whether to proceed with treatment or continue active surveillance. For example, Prolaris (46-gene expression signature) and Decipher genomic tests are currently available to evaluate prostate cancer aggressiveness and predict outcomes for disease progression following prostatectomy (10–12). The Prolaris and the Oncotype DX Prostate Cancer assay (17-gene expression signature) can be performed on RNA extracted from just 1 to 2 mm of cancer core tissue (13). Such individualized information will allow more precision in identifying men who harbor less aggressive cancer and with low risk of cancer progression, and hence could be managed by active surveillance. These tests are discussed below.

■ DIFFERENT TECHNOLOGIES TO OBTAIN GENOMIC DATA

Gene Expression Microarray

cDNA expression arrays or "gene chips" allow objective assessment of thousands of genes involved in tumorigenesis. The advancements in robotic technology have paved the way for development of commercially available gene chips that contain collections of microscopic DNA spots on a solid for researchers using biomarker discovery or for validation studies (14–16). Maturation of microarray platforms leads to the identification and development several multigene signatures that are currently integrated into clinical practice (i.e., Prolaris, Decipher, and Oncotype DX). These subsets of gene signatures help clinicians predict tumor aggressiveness or relapse after local therapy.

Whole Genome Sequencing

Whole genome sequencing (WGS) provides the DNA sequence of the entire 3 billion base pairs of the human genome. It allows detailed detection of point mutations, amplifications, deletions, and rearrangements, but also provides extensive information about the sequences in the intergenic regions that may not be relevant. This approach is powerful, providing a detailed map of a specific cancer tissue genome, and may uncover novel driver mutations and rearrangements in prostate cancer pathogenesis (17). For instance, a complete whole genome, sequencing of localized prostate cancer revealed a new PTEN-interacting protein MAGI2 that was not previously identified in prostate cancer development (18).

Whole Exome Sequencing

Whole exome sequencing (WES) only sequences the coding regions of the genome (2%) and is less costly. However, it is limited to sequencing only the area of previously described genes and cannot identify new driver mutations, complex rearrangements, or regulatory regions that may be important in driving the expression of oncogenes or suppressing the expression of tumor suppressor genes (19). Using exome sequencing of advanced prostate cancer, studies by Grasso et al. and Barbieri et al. identified novel recurrent mutations of FOXA1, an AR collaborating factor, MED12, SPOP, and multiple chromatin and histone-modifying genes. There recurrent mutations are implicated in altering the gene expression profile that drives cancer progression (20, 21).

Transcriptome Sequencing

Transcriptome sequencing (RNA-seq) is a powerful and cost-effective method to measure the expression of mRNAs and miRNAs, allowing assessment of genome-wide gene expression patterns. It is not only able to identify known genes but can also provide information about novel coding and noncoding RNA levels, gene fusions, and alternative splice variants of genes. One limitation to this approach, however, is the high error rate and the requirement for independent validation using other methods such as RT-PCR (19).

Gene Copy Number Analysis

High-resolution array comparative genomic hybridization is a method to accurately provide genome-wide information on specific whole, or partial, chromosomal gains or losses and genomic rearrangement. Compared with WGS or WES, aCGH in general requires less bioinformatics supports, has a slightly lower cost, and requires as little as 0.5 μg of DNA to provide accurate data on gene copy number. Hence, specific gene copy number information is attainable from a small needle biopsy (22). Using this technology, Paris et al. showed that a set of gene copy number alteration (Genomic Evaluators of Metastatic Prostate Cancer [GEMCaP]) can predict risk of recurrence with 80% accuracy (23).

Ribosome Profiling

Ribosome profiling refers to the sequencing of mRNAs that are in the process of actively being translated. It can identify translationally regulated genes or gene signatures that are involved in tissue invasion, cell proliferation, and cancer progression. Using ribosomal profiling, one can compare actively translated genes from a primary tumor to a metastatic lesion to pinpoint a group of translationally regulated genes associated with advanced disease and progression (24).

■ EXISTING GENOMIC DATA THAT CAN BE INTEGRATED INTO RISK ASSESSMENT

Recently, transcriptome, exome resequencing, and DNA copy number alteration analysis of 218 prostate cancer samples confirmed three major pathways that had previously been implicated in the pathogenesis of prostate cancer (RB signaling, PIK/AKT signaling, and RAS/RAF signaling) (25). The most common genetic alterations found in prostate cancer were deletion of PTEN on 10q23.31, RB1 on 13q14.2, TP53 on 17p31.1, and NKX3.1 on 8p21. Fusion of ERG and TMPRSS2 were found in early stage prostate cancer. The most common amplified regions included MYC on 8q24.21 and NCOA2 on 8q13.3 found in early disease while AR gene amplification is found mostly in metastatic prostate cancer. The pattern of copy number alterations was also identified as a key prognostic indicator of disease progression, independent of Gleason score (23, 26). Although these genomic alterations have been strongly associated with clinically significant cancer, their usage in risk assessment has not been translated in the clinic setting, but will prove to be an exciting advancement in the future. Some of the genomic alterations that could be used as prognostic or predictive markers are summarized in Table 5.2.1.

Genomic Risk Assessment for Prostate Cancer Detection

Abnormal DRE and/or abnormal PSA value lack the required sensitivity to detect prostate cancer; the predictive value of DRE with PSA in detecting clinically significant cancer ranges from 25% to 40%. A PSA range between 4 and 10 most often resulted in a 60% to 70% negative biopsy rate. At the same time, prostate cancer is detected in 17% to 27% of patients with PSA from 1 to 4 (27). Furthermore, a repeat saturation biopsy also detected cancer in about 18% to 43% of cases that had been missed after the first biopsy in men with elevated PSA (28, 29). Hence PSA alone is not an ideal tool to reliably predict cancer. PSA can also be measured in unbounded form, termed free PSA. A lower percentage of free PSA is correlated with a higher probability of detecting prostate cancer. Catalona et al. demonstrated that a cutoff value of <25% has a sensitivity of 95% in detecting prostate cancer, while avoiding 25% of unnecessary biopsies (30).

Currently, the Prostate Health Index ([PHI] Beckman Coulter) and four-kallikrein panel ([4K panel] OPKO Diagnostics) are available molecular biomarkers to improve sensitivity and specificity of predicting cancer for men with PSA > 2 ng/mL who are considering biopsy. The PHI is a panel of total PSA, free PSA, and pro-PSA that has been validated in multicenter studies, which showed a significant increase in prostate cancer detection when compared to PSA and free PSA (31, 32). Similarly, the 4K panel, consisting of total PSA, free PSA, intact PSA, and kallikrein-related peptidase 2, significantly improved predictive accuracy in detecting cancer in a large validation study by Vickers et al. (33).

The PCA3 (Progensa) urinary marker is currently approved by the FDA to help risk stratify men after a negative biopsy. This test measures the mRNA level of prostate cancer antigen 3 (higher level in cancer tissue than adjacent noncancerous tissue in 95% of the 56 tumors studied). A score of less than 35 is associated with lower likelihood of prostate cancer with the AUC of 0.693 compared with the AUC of 0.612 for serum PSA (34). The TMPRSS2-ERG fusion (transmembrane protease serine 2 implicated in tumor metastasis) has been reported to be one of the earliest genetic events in prostate cancer tumorigenesis and is detected in approximately 50% of prostate cancers (35, 36). A few studies have demonstrated improvements in sensitivity and predictive value of detecting prostate cancer using the TMPRSS2-ERG fusion transcript and PCA-3 (prostate cancer antigen-3 is overexpressed in 95% prostate cancer) urine assay with up to 90% specificity and 80% sensitivity (37–39).

Several studies reported that assessing DNA methylation pattern of specific genes (GSTP1 and APC) from initially negative biopsy tissue can provide a high negative predictive value (NPV) and improve both sensitivity and specificity for detecting cancer in subsequent biopsy in men with high index of suspicion for cancer (40, 41). These studies had led to the development of the ConfirmMDx test, commercially available to clinicians for risk assessment after the initial negative biopsy. These tools can be used concurrently to increase the probability of a positive prostate biopsy.

■ Table 5.2.1 Potential genomic alterations that can be translated into prognostic and predictive biomarkers

Tissue- and Serum-Based Biomarker of Cell Cycle Progression and Signaling Pathways	Functions	References
Cyclin D1	overexpression is linked to poor prognosis after prostatectomy	(57)
c-myc	overexpression is linked to poor prognosis after prostatectomy	(58, 59)
p16	overexpression is linked to poor prognosis after prostatectomy	(60)
Retinoblastoma (Rb), p53	loss of function involved in tumor initiation and progression	(61)
Loss of hMSH2 expression	lower recurrence rates after prostatectomy	(62)
PTEN and p27	loss or decreased expression involved in tumor initiation and progress	(63–66)
PI3kinase/AKT/mTOR signaling cascade	activation leads to tumor progression	(67)
PAR-2	overexpression is linked to PCa metastasis	(68)
EZH2	overexpression is linked to PCa metastasis	(69)
H3K27Me3	overexpression is associated with biochemical recurrence	(70)
AMACR	expression is associated with risk of prostate cancer	(71)
TGF-β1 and IL-6	overexpression is linked to disease progression and biochemical recurrence	(72)
TMPRSS2-ERG,PCA3	diagnosing prostate cancer	(73)
Ras/Raf signaling	activation leads to tumor progression	(74, 75)
AR	overexpression and mutation is associated with CRPC progression	(76)
NKX3.1	loss or decreased expression involved in tumor initiation and progress	(77)
NCOA2	overexpression is linked to PCa metastasis	(78)

Genomic Risk Assessment Prior to Local Therapy

Uncertainty still exists among physicians and patients about the best course of treatment after their cancer diagnosis, mainly due to under-sampling from biopsy. Recent advances in genomic biomarkers have been geared toward improving accuracy of risk stratification beyond Gleason score, PSA, tumor volume, and clinical staging. Cuzick et al. reported that by assessing the expression of cell cycle progression (CCP) genes in prostatectomy specimens and in biopsy samples of men with localized disease, this expression profile added a substantial amount of prognostic information regarding disease progression. Subsequently, these studies lead to the development of the Prolaris test (42, 43). The CCP was further validated in a large contemporary cohort (12). Klein et al. introduced the 17-gene signature assay (Oncotype DX) to evaluate disease aggressiveness from paraffin-embedded biopsy tissue with significant improvement in predicting clinical progression (44–45). Cooperberg et al. validated this multigene signature assay in a large cohort of men with low to low-intermediate risk prostate cancer who were candidates for active surveillance (46). Currently, both the Prolaris and Onxotype Dx are available to offer patients with low-to-intermediate–risk cancer more information on their prostate cancer diagnosis, hence giving them more certainty on deciding treatment options.

Genomic Risk Assessment for Prostate Cancer Recurrence After Local Therapy

The main tools urologists use to predict cancer outcome after local therapy are a combination pre- and posttreatment PSA, PSA velocity and doubling time, PSA density, pathological staging, Gleason grade, surgical margin status, and the Kattan nomogram or Partin table (47, 48). However, there are limitations with these tools since they do not give insight into the biology of the cancer. These tools could overestimate or underestimate risk of recurrence after radical prostatectomy and may not give physicians and patients the best information, especially when deciding whether to proceed to adjuvant therapy or elect to undergo careful follow–up with salvage therapy (49). The Prolaris, Decipher, and Oncotype DX prostate assays are commercially available genomic tests to offer patients more precise information about their risk of recurrence after prostatectomy, independent of pathological staging and Gleason score (10, 12, 46, 50). In addition, validation studies are underway to bring other genomic tests such as gene copy number alteration into this space (23, 51).

Genomic Risk Assessment for Developing Castration-Resistant Prostate Cancer (CRPC)

Using genomic data as biomarkers in assessing progression to CRPC or responses to chemotherapy is still in the early stages of development. Translation of basic science results into clinically valuable biomarkers for diagnosis, prognosis, and selective therapy is critical in addressing the challenges of treating metastatic castration-resistant prostate cancer (mCRPC). However, characterization of such biomarkers on a genomic level is expected to greatly impact the way we detect and treat metastatic PCa. Currently, there are several potential biomarkers that are in development for clinical utility in CRPC. The number of circulating tumor cells and distinct patterns of chromosome copy number alterations have been reported to be useful in predicting the risk of progression to CRPC and overall survival in CRPC (52, 53). Genomic analysis of these CTC showed 70% of the mutations were present in matched lymph node and primary core tissue, hence CTC genomics could hold potential in guiding treatment of mCRPC in the clinic.

Furthermore, genomic data could be used to predict antiandrogen resistance in CRPC patients undergoing second generation antiandrogen therapy, allowing clinicians to choose a more appropriate therapy. Studies by Joseph et al. showed that 3 out of 29 patients receiving the second generation antiandrogen ARN-509 in the phase 1 dose escalation trial developed de novo AR F876L mutation. This is a missense mutation in the AR ligand-biding domain that confers agonistic activity to both Enzalutamide and ARN-509 (54). Patients with AR F876L mutation will generally fail the second generation antiandrogen therapies, but may have other mutations such as RAS/RAF mutations or PTEN loss, which may steer therapy toward using RAS pathway inhibitors (e.g., sorafenib, vemurafenib) or PI3 kinase pathway inhibitors (e.g., BKM120, BAY 80-6946) instead of Enzalutamide (54).

■ FUTURE PERSPECTIVE

As we move into the era of personalized medicine, there is a high demand for biomarkers that can: (a) reduce overtreatment of low-risk prostate cancer and (b) reduce under treatment. To increase utility in the clinic, besides confirming validity, the biomarkers assay should be easy to use and interpret, have a rapid turnaround for results, and be reproducible. Next, the issue of diffusing the knowledge and clinical uses of the genomic biomarkers to both specialists and primary care providers plus the general public is of crucial importance to overcome in order to bring genomic biomarkers into clinical practice. This could be addressed with clinical guidelines and in training of physicians. An example of such integration is seen in the NCCN guideline for HER2 assays used in targeted therapy for Stage IV breast cancer (55). Finally, validation studies should follow REMARK guidelines to ensure the standardization of methods and predictive validity of the biomarkers. The REMARK guidelines recommend to researchers a list of criteria on study design, patient selection, methods of specimen retrieval and preservation, statistical analysis, data reporting, and the relation of the marker to standard prognostic variables (56).

■ CONCLUSION

The variability of clinical progression and the molecular heterogeneity of prostate cancer continue to pose a challenge for clinicians in selecting the more personalized management strategies (effective, efficient, and necessary) for contemporary patients. Genomic risk assessment will complement and augment standard risk assessment tools of the cancer (and very likely the host with time).

■ REFERENCES

1. Cooperberg MR, Freedland SJ, Pasta DJ, et al. Multiinstitutional validation of the UCSF cancer of the prostate risk assessment for prediction of recurrence after radical prostatectomy. *Cancer.* 2006;107(10):2384–2391.
2. Bechis SK, Carroll PR, Cooperberg MR. Impact of age at diagnosis on prostate cancer treatment and survival. *J Clin Oncol.* 2011;29(2):235–241.
3. Cooperberg MR, Broering JM, Carroll PR. Time trends and local variation in primary treatment of localized prostate cancer. *J Clin Oncol.* 2010;28(7):1117–1123.
4. D'Amico AV, Whittington R, Malkowicz SB, et al. Biochemical outcome after radical prostatectomy, external beam radiation therapy, or interstitial radiation therapy for clinically localized prostate cancer. *JAMA.* 1998;280(11):969–974.
5. Punnen S, Freedland SJ, Presti JC Jr, et al. Multi-institutional validation of the CAPRA-S score to predict disease recurrence and mortality after radical prostatectomy. *Eur Urol.* 2014;65(6):1171–1177.
6. Cooperberg MR, Pasta DJ, Elkin EP, et al. The University of California, San Francisco Cancer of the Prostate Risk Assessment score: a straightforward and reliable preoperative predictor of disease recurrence after radical prostatectomy. *J Urol.* 2005;173(6):1938–1942.
7. Stephenson AJ, Scardino PT, Eastham JA, et al. Preoperative nomogram predicting the 10-year probability of prostate cancer recurrence after radical prostatectomy. *J Natl Cancer Inst.* 2006;98(10):715–717.
8. Freedland SJ, Humphreys EB, Mangold LA, et al. Risk of prostate cancer-specific mortality following biochemical recurrence after radical prostatectomy. *JAMA.* 2005;294(4):433–439.
9. Dall'Era MA, Albertsen PC, Bangma C, et al. Active surveillance for prostate cancer: a systematic review of the literature. *Eur Urol.* 2012;62(6):976–983.
10. Karnes RJ, Bergstralh EJ, Davicioni E, et al. Validation of a genomic classifier that predicts metastasis following radical prostatectomy in an at risk patient population. *J Urol.* 2013;190(6):2047–2053.
11. Freedland SJ, Gerber L, Reid J, et al. Prognostic utility of cell cycle progression score in men with prostate cancer after primary external beam radiation therapy. *Int J Radiat Oncol Biol Phys.* 2013;86(5):848–853.
12. Cooperberg MR, Simko JP, Cowan JE, et al. Validation of a cell-cycle progression gene panel to improve risk stratification in a contemporary prostatectomy cohort. *J Clin Oncol.* 2013;31(11):1428–1434.
13. Knezevic D, Goddard AD, Natraj N, et al. Analytical validation of the Oncotype DX prostate cancer assay–a clinical RT-PCR assay optimized for prostate needle biopsies. *BMC Genomics.* 2013;14(1):690.
14. Chee M, Yang R, Hubbell E, et al. Accessing genetic information with high-density DNA arrays. *Science.* 1996;274(5287):610–614.
15. Schena M, Shalon D, Davis RW, Brown PO. Quantitative monitoring of gene expression patterns with a complementary DNA microarray. *Science.* 1995;270(5235):467–470.
16. Grouse LH, Munson PJ, Nelson PS. Sequence databases and microarrays as tools for identifying prostate cancer biomarkers. *Urology.* 2001;57(4, suppl 1):154–159.
17. Stadler ZK, Schrader KA, Vijai J, Robson ME, Offit K. Cancer genomics and inherited risk. *J Clin Oncol.* 2014;32(7):687–698.

18. Berger MF, Lawrence MS, Demichelis F, et al. The genomic complexity of primary human prostate cancer. *Nature.* 2011;470(7333):214–220.
19. Rizzo JM, Buck MJ. Key principles and clinical applications of "next-generation" DNA sequencing. *Cancer Prev Res (Phila).* 2012;5(7):887–900.
20. Barbieri CE, Baca SC, Lawrence MS, et al. Exome sequencing identifies recurrent SPOP, FOXA1 and MED12 mutations in prostate cancer. *Nat Genet.* 2012;44(6):685–689.
21. Grasso CS, Wu YM, Robinson DR, et al. The mutational landscape of lethal castration-resistant prostate cancer. *Nature.* 2012;487(7406):239–243.
22. Przybytkowski E, Aguilar-Mahecha A, Nabavi S, Tonellato PJ, Basik M. Ultradense array CGH and discovery of micro-copy number alterations and gene fusions in the cancer genome. *Methods Mol Biol.* 2013;973:15–38.
23. Paris PL, Weinberg V, Albo G, et al. A group of genome-based biomarkers that add to a Kattan nomogram for predicting progression in men with high-risk prostate cancer. *Clin Cancer Res.* 2010;16(1):195–202.
24. Hsieh AC, Liu Y, Edlind MP, et al. The translational landscape of mTOR signalling steers cancer initiation and metastasis. *Nature.* 2012;485(7396):55–61.
25. Taylor BS, Schultz N, Hieronymus H, et al. Integrative genomic profiling of human prostate cancer. *Cancer Cell.* 2010;18(1):11–22.
26. Cher ML, Bova GS, Moore DH, et al. Genetic alterations in untreated metastases and androgen-independent prostate cancer detected by comparative genomic hybridization and allelotyping. *Cancer Res.* 1996;56(13):3091–3102.
27. Thompson IM, Pauler DK, Goodman PJ, et al. Prevalence of prostate cancer among men with a prostate-specific antigen level < or =4.0 ng per milliliter. *N Engl J Med.* 2004;350(22):2239–2246.
28. Campos-Fernandes JL, Bastien L, Nicolaiew N, et al. Prostate cancer detection rate in patients with repeated extended 21-sample needle biopsy. *Eur Urol.* 2009;55(3):600–606.
29. Walz J, Graefen M, Chun FK, et al. High incidence of prostate cancer detected by saturation biopsy after previous negative biopsy series. *Eur Urol.* 2006;50(3):498–505.
30. Catalona WJ, Partin AW, Slawin KM, et al. Use of the percentage of free prostate-specific antigen to enhance differentiation of prostate cancer from benign prostatic disease: a prospective multicenter clinical trial. *JAMA.* 1998;279(19):1542–1547.
31. Catalona WJ, Partin AW, Sanda MG, et al. A multicenter study of [-2]pro-prostate specific antigen combined with prostate specific antigen and free prostate specific antigen for prostate cancer detection in the 2.0 to 10.0 ng/ml prostate specific antigen range. *J Urol.* 2011;185(5):1650–1655.
32. Stephan C, Vincendeau S, Houlgatte A, Cammann H, Jung K, Semjonow A. Multicenter evaluation of [-2]proprostate-specific antigen and the prostate health index for detecting prostate cancer. *Clin Chem.* 2013;59(1):306–314.
33. Vickers AJ, Gupta A, Savage CJ, et al. A panel of kallikrein marker predicts prostate cancer in a large, population-based cohort followed for 15 years without screening. *Cancer Epidemiol Biomarkers Prev.* 2011;20(2):255–261.
34. Day JR, Jost M, Reynolds MA, Groskopf J, Rittenhouse H. PCA3: from basic molecular science to the clinical lab. *Cancer Lett.* 2011;301(1):1–6.
35. Tomlins SA, Rhodes DR, Perner S, et al. Recurrent fusion of TMPRSS2 and ETS transcription factor genes in prostate cancer. *Science.* 2005;310(5748):644–648.
36. Mosquera JM, Mehra R, Regan MM, et al. Prevalence of TMPRSS2-ERG fusion prostate cancer among men undergoing prostate biopsy in the United States. *Clin Cancer Res.* 2009;15(14):4706–4711.
37. Hessels D, Smit FP, Verhaegh GW, Witjes JA, Cornel EB, Schalken JA. Detection of TMPRSS2-ERG fusion transcripts and prostate cancer antigen 3 in urinary sediments may improve diagnosis of prostate cancer. *Clin Cancer Res.* 2007;13(17):5103–5108.
38. Salami SS, Schmidt F, Laxman B, et al. Combining urinary detection of TMPRSS2:ERG and PCA3 with serum PSA to predict diagnosis of prostate cancer. *Urol Oncol.* 2013;31(5):566–571.
39. Bussemakers MJ, van Bokhoven A, Verhaegh GW, et al. DD3: a new prostate-specific gene, highly overexpressed in prostate cancer. *Cancer Res.* 1999;59(23):5975–5979.
40. Trock BJ, Brotzman MJ, Mangold LA, et al. Evaluation of GSTP1 and APC methylation as indicators for repeat biopsy in a high-risk cohort of men with negative initial prostate biopsies. *BJU Int.* 2012;110(1):56–62.
41. Troyer DA, Lucia MS, de Bruïne AP, et al. Prostate cancer detected by methylated gene markers in histopathologically cancer-negative tissues from men with subsequent positive biopsies. *Cancer Epidemiol Biomarkers Prev.* 2009;18(10):2717–2722.
42. Cuzick J, Berney DM, Fisher G, et al. Prognostic value of a cell cycle progression signature for prostate cancer death in a conservatively managed needle biopsy cohort. *Br J Cancer.* 2012;106(6):1095–1099.
43. Cuzick J, Swanson GP, Fisher G, et al. Prognostic value of an RNA expression signature derived from cell cycle proliferation genes in patients with prostate cancer: a retrospective study. *Lancet Oncol.* 2011;12(3):245–255.
44. Knezevic D, Goddard AD, Natraj N, et al. Analytical validation of the Oncotype DX prostate cancer assay - a clinical RT-PCR assay optimized for prostate needle biopsies. *BMC Genomics.* 2013;14:690.
45. Klein EA, Maddala T, Millward C, et al. Development of a needle biopsy-based genomic test to improve discrimination of clinically aggressive from indolent prostate cancer. *J Clin Oncol.* 2012;30 (suppl; abst 4560).
46. Klein EA, Cooperberg MR, Magi-Galluzzi C, et al. A 17-gene assay to predict prostate cancer aggressiveness in the context of Gleason grade heterogeneity, tumor multifocality, and biopsy undersampling. *Eur Urol.* 2014;66(3):550–560.
47. Graefen M, Karakiewicz PI, Cagiannos I, et al. International validation of a preoperative nomogram for prostate cancer recurrence after radical prostatectomy. *J Clin Oncol.* 2002;20(15): 3206–3212.
48. Pound CR, Partin AW, Epstein JI, Walsh PC. Prostate-specific antigen after anatomic radical retropubic prostatectomy. Patterns of recurrence and cancer control. *Urol Clin North Am.* 1997;24(2):395–406.
49. Greene KL, Meng MV, Elkin EP, et al. Validation of the Kattan preoperative nomogram for prostate cancer recurrence using a community based cohort: results from cancer of the prostate strategic urological research endeavor (capsure). *J Urol.* 2004;171 (6 pt 1):2255–2259.
50. Erho N, Crisan A, Vergara IA, et al. Discovery and validation of a prostate cancer genomic classifier that predicts early metastasis following radical prostatectomy. *PLoS One.* 2013;8(6):e66855.
51. Kattan MW. Evaluating a marker's contribution to a nomogram: the GEMCaP example. *Clin Cancer Res.* 2010;16(1):1–3.
52. de Bono JS, Scher HI, Montgomery RB, et al., Circulating tumor cells predict survival benefit from treatment in metastatic castration-resistant prostate cancer. *Clin Cancer Res.* 2008;14(19):6302–6309.
53. Friedlander TW, Roy R, Tomlins SA, et al. Common structural and epigenetic changes in the genome of castration-resistant prostate cancer. *Cancer Res.* 2012;72(3):616–625.
54. Joseph JD, Lu N, Qian J, et al. A clinically relevant androgen receptor mutation confers resistance to second-generation antiandrogens enzalutamide and ARN-509. *Cancer Discov.* 2013;3(9):1020–1029.
55. Theriault RL, Carlson RW, Allred C, et al. Breast cancer, version 3.2013: featured updates to the NCCN guidelines. *J Natl Compr Canc Netw.* 2013;11(7):753–760; quiz 761.
56. McShane LM, Altman DG, Sauerbrei W, et al. Reporting recommendations for tumor marker prognostic studies. *J Clin Oncol.* 2005;23(36):9067–9072.

57. Aaltomaa S, Eskelinen M, Lipponen P. Expression of cyclin A and D proteins in prostate cancer and their relation to clinopathological variables and patient survival. *Prostate.* 1999;38(3):175–182.
58. Bernard D, Pourtier-Manzanedo A, Gil J, Beach DH. Myc confers androgen-independent prostate cancer cell growth. *J Clin Invest.* 2003;112(11):1724–1731.
59. Bubendorf L, Kononen J, Koivisto P, et al. Survey of gene amplifications during prostate cancer progression by high-throughout fluorescence in situ hybridization on tissue microarrays. *Cancer Res.* 1999;59(4):803–806.
60. Jarrard DF, Modder J, Fadden P, et al. Alterations in the p16/pRb cell cycle checkpoint occur commonly in primary and metastatic human prostate cancer. *Cancer Lett.* 2002;185(2):191–199.
61. Osman I, Drobnjak M, Fazzari M, Ferrara J, Scher HI, Cordon-Cardo C. Inactivation of the p53 pathway in prostate cancer: impact on tumor progression. *Clin Cancer Res.* 1999;5(8):2082–2088.
62. Prtilo A, Leach FS, Markwalder R, et al. Tissue microarray analysis of hMSH2 expression predicts outcome in men with prostate cancer. *J Urol.* 2005;174(5):1814–1818; discussion 1818.
63. Warde N. Prostate cancer: loss of PTEN promotes progression of prostate cancer in an androgen-independent manner. *Nat Rev Urol.* 2011;8(8):412.
64. Sircar K, Yoshimoto M, Monzon FA, et al. PTEN genomic deletion is associated with p-Akt and AR signalling in poorer outcome, hormone refractory prostate cancer. *J Pathol.* 2009;218(4):505–513.
65. Dreher T, Zentgraf H, Abel U, et al. Reduction of PTEN and p27kip1 expression correlates with tumor grade in prostate cancer. Analysis in radical prostatectomy specimens and needle biopsies. *Virchows Arch.* 2004;444(6):509–517.
66. Facher EA, Law JC. PTEN and prostate cancer. *J Med Genet.* 1998;35(9):790.
67. De Velasco MA, Uemura H. Preclinical remodeling of human prostate cancer through the PTEN/AKT pathway. *Adv Urol.* 2012;2012:419348.
68. Wilson S, Greer B, Hooper J, et al. The membrane-anchored serine protease, TMPRSS2, activates PAR-2 in prostate cancer cells. *Biochem J.* 2005;388(pt 3):967–972.
69. Varambally S, Dhanasekaran SM, Zhou M, et al. The polycomb group protein EZH2 is involved in progression of prostate cancer. *Nature.* 2002;419(6907):624–629.
70. Pellakuru LG, Iwata T, Gurel B, et al. Global levels of H3K27me3 track with differentiation in vivo and are deregulated by MYC in prostate cancer. *Am J Pathol.* 2012;181(2):560–569.
71. Jiang N, Zhu S, Chen J, Niu Y, Zhou L. A-methylacyl-CoA racemase (AMACR) and prostate-cancer risk: a meta-analysis of 4,385 participants. *PLoS One.* 2013;8(10):e74386.
72. Reis ST, Pontes-Júnior J, Antunes AA, et al. Tgf-beta1 expression as a biomarker of poor prognosis in prostate cancer. *Clinics (Sao Paulo).* 2011;66(7):1143–1147.
73. Salagierski M, Schalken JA. PCA3 and TMPRSS2-ERG: promising biomarkers in prostate cancer diagnosis. *Cancers (Basel).* 2010;2(3):1432–1440.
74. Wang XS, Shankar S, Dhanasekaran SM, et al. Characterization of KRAS rearrangements in metastatic prostate cancer. *Cancer Discov.* 2011;1(1):35–43.
75. Bakin RE, Gioeli D, Sikes RA, Bissonette EA, Weber MJ. Constitutive activation of the Ras/mitogen-activated protein kinase signaling pathway promotes androgen hypersensitivity in LNCaP prostate cancer cells. *Cancer Res.* 2003;63(8):1981–1989.
76. Mitsiades N. A road map to comprehensive androgen receptor axis targeting for castration-resistant prostate cancer. *Cancer Res.* 2013;73(15):4599–4605.
77. Bhatia-Gaur R, Donjacour AA, Sciavolino PJ, et al. Roles for Nkx3.1 in prostate development and cancer. *Genes Dev.* 1999;13(8):966–977.
78. Taylor BS, Schultz N, Hieronymus H, et al. Integrative genomic profiling of human prostate cancer. *Cancer Cell.* 2010;18(1):11–22.

5.3 Future Direction: Novel Urine and Serum Markers

WALEED A. HASSEN

Prostate cancer remains a significant source of morbidity and mortality in the Western world (1). The introduction of prostate-specific antigen (PSA) in the 1980s has certainly led to a significant increase in prostate cancer diagnosis and many would argue an improvement in prostate cancer mortality. PSA, however, has low specificity and results in many needless diagnostic interventions (2). PSA screening also leads to an increase in the diagnosis of indolent cancers with its inherent burdens on the individual as well as society (3). This chapter reviews promising blood- and urine-based markers beyond PSA for the detection of prostate cancer. For reference, the markers described in this chapter are illustrated in Figure 5.3.1.

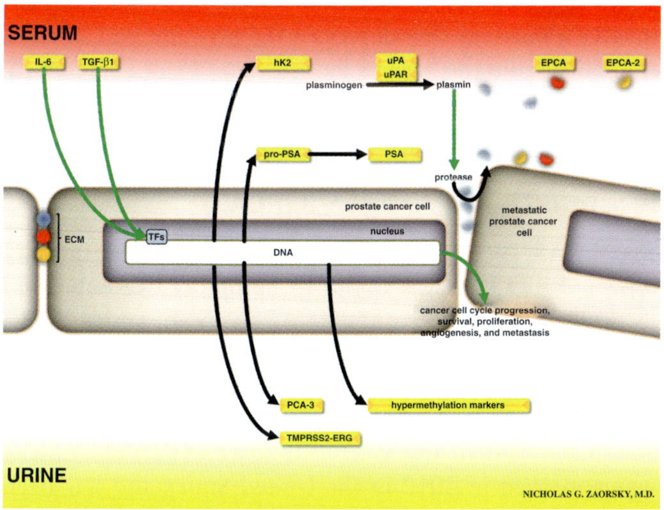

FIGURE 5.3.1 Novel serum and urine markers for the detection of prostate cancer.
Abbreviations: ECM = extracellular matrix; EPCA = early prostate cancer antigen; hK2 = human Kallikrein 2; IL-6 = interleukin 6; PCA3 = prostate cancer antigen 3; pro-PSA = pro-prostate specific antigen; TMPRSS2-ERG = (transmembrane protease, serine 2)-(ETS-related genes) promoter; TF = transcription factor; TGF-β1/R = transforming growth factor-beta 1 and receptor; uPA/R = urokinase plasminogen activator and receptor.
Note: black arrow = produces / converted to; green arrow = stimulates; orange boxes with black text represent novel markers.

BLOOD-BASED MARKERS

PSA Isoforms

Free PSA (fPSA) has three different isoforms in serum: pro-PSA (pPSA), BPH-associated PSA (BPSA), and intact or inactive PSA (iPSA) (4). pPSA is cleaved by various serum proteases into PSA (4). Elevated levels of pPSA were shown to improve prostate cancer detection as well as reduce unnecessary biopsies when compared with PSA or fPSA alone (5, 6). In a prospective study of 268 men, Guazzoni et al. recently reported that pPSA improved the detection of prostate cancer on biopsy over total PSA (tPSA), fPSA, or PSA density (PSAD) by 10% (7). Jansen et al. also showed that pPSA increased the prostate cancer predictive value and specificity over total and fPSA (8). There was also the suggestion that pPSA may increase the detection of more aggressive forms of cancer (Gleason score ≥ 7). The ability of pPSA to detect more aggressive forms of cancer was also demonstrated by Makarov et al. (9). pPSA measurements in serum and tissue were associated with an increased probability of treatment necessity among 71 men enrolled in an active surveillance protocol for prostate cancer.

The Beckman Coulter Prostate Health Index (PHI) is a proprietary equation that incorporates pPSA. It is calculated as [(pPSA/fPSA) × tPSA]. The PHI has also been shown to increase both prostate cancer detection and perhaps predict more aggressive disease when compared with PSA or standard pathologic features alone (7, 8).

Human Kallikrein 2

Human kallikrein-related peptidase 2 (hK2) is a secreted serine protease from the same gene family as PSA with very similar sequence homology (10). Studies have shown that serum hK2 improves the prediction of prostate cancer when combined with PSA and fPSA (11, 12). There is also the suggestion that hk2 may be able to predict more aggressive disease. Elevated serum levels of hK2 have been shown to predict extracapsular extension in radical prostatectomy specimens (13). Serum hK2 levels also correlated with adverse pathologic features and biochemical recurrence in a cohort of over 800 men undergoing radical prostatectomy (14). Others have not confirmed this data however, and its use therefore remains controversial (15).

Urokinase Plasminogen Activator (uPA)

uPA is a serum protease that binds to the uPA receptor (uPAR) and converts plasminogen to plasmin. This subsequently leads to protease activation and the degradation of extracellular matrix proteins. This degradation has been implicated in cancer growth and progression (16). This link to progression is highlighted by the fact that increased levels of both uPA and uPAR have been linked to metastatic disease in numerous malignancies (17, 18). Elevated levels of uPA and uPAR have been shown to have potential in both diagnostic and prognostic applications. The addition of uPAR to PSA and fPSA isoforms significantly improved the prediction model for prostate cancer diagnosis from an area under the curve (AUC) of 0.61 to 0.75 (19). Given its role in disease progression, uPA(R) appears to be associated with aggressive disease. In a large retrospective cohort of patients who underwent radical prostatectomy, elevated preoperative uPA and uPAR levels were correlated with both aggressive disease and recurrent disease (20). Elevated levels have also been correlated with metastatic disease to the bone (21).

Transforming Growth Factor-Beta 1 (TGF-β1)

TGF-β1 is a protein that is involved in numerous biological processes including regulating cellular proliferation, differentiation, angiogenesis, and apoptosis. TGF-β1 appears to play a role in prostate cancer progression. Preoperative levels of TGF-β1 predicted for adverse pathological features (extra-capsular extension, seminal vesicle invasion, and lymph node involvement) as well as biochemical recurrence after prostatectomy (22). Its value remains controversial, however, as others have not been able to replicate this data (23, 24).

Interleukin-6 (IL-6) Ligand and Receptor

IL-6 is a cytokine that is expressed by a variety of cell types and is involved in hematopoesis as well as immune response modulation. IL-6 appears to be a growth factor that drives prostate cancer growth by activation of the androgen receptor (25, 26). IL-6 also appears to promote the growth of androgen-independent cell lines in vitro (27). A few studies have shown that IL-6 may be a useful prognostic marker as elevated levels are correlated with advanced disease and survival (28, 29). Recently, in a small study of 51 patients Terracciano et al. were able to demonstrate that an elevated ratio of IL-6 to its receptor predicted higher-grade disease on radical prostatectomy, potentially making it useful as a marker for active surveillance (30). When incorporated into a nomogram, IL-6, along with TGF-β1, was shown to improve the ability to predict biochemical progression over standard criteria (31).

Early Prostate Cancer Antigen (EPCA)

EPCA is a nuclear matrix protein that may be of utility in both a diagnostic and prognostic capacity. Nuclear matrix proteins assist with maintaining the structure of the nuclear membrane. EPCA was initially found to be preferentially expressed in histologically negative prostate tissue in patients who eventually developed prostate cancer (32). Subsequently, a blood-based assay for EPCA was shown to have a diagnostic specificity and sensitivity of 94 and 92% respectively in a small cohort of patients (33). Larger retrospective studies also demonstrated similar diagnostic specificity and sensitivity as well as the ability of EPCA and EPCA-2 to discriminate between localized and advanced disease (AUC 0.89) (34, 35). While there was a lot of enthusiasm and public interest for EPCA-2 when first presented, subsequent studies could not validate the performance of EPCA-2, and methodologic deficiencies were alleged. EPCA-2 was included here because of the significant popular press that was generated, but it is no longer in clinical use and several studies regarding EPCA-2 were subsequently retracted (36).

■ URINE-BASED MARKERS

The noninvasive nature of urine, as well as its proximity to the prostate, makes it a potentially ideal source of biomarkers for prostate cancer. Prostate cancer cells pass directly into the urethra via prostatic ducts (37). It has been suggested that the accurate collection of urine should involve a massage that depresses the prostate by 1 cm and is applied from the base to the apex and from the laterally to the median sulcus for each lobe. This should then be repeated three times (38).

Prostate Cancer Antigen 3 (PCA3)

The PCA3 gene (initially referred to as DD3), initially reported in 1999, was found to be highly overexpressed in prostate cancer (39). The PCA3 assay measures PCA3 mRNA as well as PSA mRNA. The PSA mRNA is not upregulated in prostate cancer and is used to normalize for the amount of prostate-specific mRNA in the sample. This ratio is then reported as a score. The PCA3 assay was approved in 2012 in the United States and has been approved in Europe since 2006 to assist in deciding on the need for a repeat biopsy. PCA3 has been found to improve the AUC for the detection of prostate cancer in numerous studies by 5% to 10%. PCA3, however, is plagued with the same issues of balancing sensitivity and specificity that PSA is. Using a PCA3 cutoff score of 35 for example yields a specificity of 72% and a sensitivity of 58%. PCA3, however, is not influenced by inflammation, age, 5-alpha reductase use, or prostate volume (40–44).

Although some studies have suggested that PCA3 may be useful in predicting more aggressive disease, larger studies have contradicted this. Taken together it does not appear that PCA3 is useful in predicting tumor aggressiveness (45–50). PCA3 has also not been shown to predict progression in prostate patients who are on an active surveillance program (44).

TMPRSS2-ERG Fusion

Gene rearrangements have been described in malignancies particularly hematologic cancers. The most common rearrangement in prostate cancer is the fusion of the TMPRSS2 (a gene transcriptional promoter) and the oncogene ERG. This rearrangement has been shown to occur in 80% of prostate cancer specimens (51). Transcripts of these fusion products have been reported in the urine of up to 40% of prostate cancer patients (52–54). In an attempt to improve the diagnostic accuracy, studies have evaluated combining PCA3 with TMPRSS2-ERG. In a study of 48 patients undergoing a prostate biopsy, combining TMPRSS2-ERG with PCA3 increased the diagnostic accuracy over PSA alone from an AUC of 0.72 to 0.88 (55). Other studies have shown improved diagnostic accuracy using both TMPRSS2-ERG and PCA3 as well although with more modest gains (56).

DNA Hypermethylation

Aberrant methylation of DNA has been associated with many malignancies including prostate cancer. The most studied marker is Glutathione S-transferase pi 1 (GSTP1). Hypermethylation of GSTP1 has been shown in a series of small studies to theoretically be able to improve the detection of prostate cancer with specificities ranging from 93% to 100% and sensitivities of approximately 50% to 75% (57–60). A larger multi-institutional study, involving 337 prebiopsy urine samples, used a panel of hypermethylation markers (GSTP1, RARbeta2, and APC). The negative predictive value in this cohort was 87% for patients who had a PSA between 4 and 10 ng/mL suggesting its possible utility in biopsy decision making (61).

■ CONCLUSIONS

Numerous biomarkers in both serum and urine have shown promise in improving the detection of prostate cancer; however, their utility in curbing overdiagnosis and more accurately predicting prognosis has remained a challenge. In all likelihood, panels of markers and other decision-making tools such as nomograms will better characterize the heterogeneity of prostate cancer phenotypes and require further validation.

■ REFERENCES

1. Siegel R, Naishadham D, Jemal A. Cancer statistics, 2012. *CA Cancer J Clin*. 2012;62(1):10–29.
2. Heijnsdijk EA, der Kinderen A, Wever EM, Draisma G, Roobol MJ, de Koning HJ. Overdetection, overtreatment and costs in prostate-specific antigen screening for prostate cancer. *Br J Cancer*. 2009;101(11):1833–1838.
3. Etzioni R, Penson DF, Legler JM, et al. Overdiagnosis due to prostate-specific antigen screening: lessons from U.S. prostate cancer incidence trends. *J Natl Cancer Inst*. 2002;94(13):981–990.
4. Mikolajczyk SD, Marks LS, Partin AW, Rittenhouse HG. Free prostate-specific antigen in serum is becoming more complex. *Urology*. 2002;59(6):797–802.
5. Mikolajczyk SD, Marker KM, Millar LS, et al. A truncated precursor form of prostate-specific antigen is a more specific serum marker of prostate cancer. *Cancer Res*. 2001;61(18): 6958–6963.
6. Sokoll LJ, Wang Y, Feng Z, et al. [-2]proenzyme prostate specific antigen for prostate cancer detection: a national cancer institute early detection research network validation study. *J Urol*. 2008;180(2):539–543; discussion 543.
7. Guazzoni G, Nava L, Lazzeri M, et al. Prostate-specific antigen (PSA) isoform p2PSA significantly improves the prediction of prostate cancer at initial extended prostate biopsies in patients with total PSA between 2.0 and 10 ng/ml: results of a prospective study in a clinical setting. *Eur Urol*. 2011;60(2):214–222.
8. Jansen FH, van Schaik RH, Kurstjens J, et al. Prostate-specific antigen (PSA) isoform p2PSA in combination with total PSA and free PSA improves diagnostic accuracy in prostate cancer detection. *Eur Urol*. 2010;57(6):921–927.
9. Makarov DV, Isharwal S, Sokoll LJ, et al. Pro-prostate-specific antigen measurements in serum and tissue are associated with treatment necessity among men enrolled in expectant management for prostate cancer. *Clin Cancer Res*. 2009;15(23):7316–7321.
10. Yousef GM, Diamandis EP. The new human tissue kallikrein gene family: structure, function, and association to disease. *Endocr Rev*. 2001;22(2):184–204.
11. Becker C, Piironen T, Pettersson K, Hugosson J, Lilja H. Clinical value of human glandular kallikrein 2 and free and total prostate-specific antigen in serum from a population of men with prostate-specific antigen levels 3.0 ng/mL or greater. *Urology*. 2000;55(5):694–699.
12. Nam RK, Diamandis EP, Toi A, et al. Serum human glandular kallikrein-2 protease levels predict the presence of prostate cancer among men with elevated prostate-specific antigen. *J Clin Oncol*. 2000;18(5):1036–1042.
13. Haese A, Graefen M, Becker C, et al. The role of human glandular kallikrein 2 for prediction of pathologically organ confined prostate cancer. *Prostate*. 2003;54(3):181–186.
14. Steuber T, Vickers AJ, Serio AM, et al. Comparison of free and total forms of serum human kallikrein 2 and prostate-specific antigen for prediction of locally advanced and recurrent prostate cancer. *Clin Chem*. 2007;53(2):233–240.
15. Kurek R, Nunez G, Tselis N, et al. Prognostic value of combined "triple"-reverse transcription-PCR analysis for prostate-specific antigen, human kallikrein 2, and prostate-specific membrane antigen mRNA in peripheral blood and lymph nodes of prostate cancer patients. *Clin Cancer Res*. 2004;10(17): 5808–5814.
16. Andreasen PA, Kjøller L, Christensen L, Duffy MJ. The urokinase-type plasminogen activator system in cancer metastasis: a review. *Int J Cancer*. 1997;72(1):1–22.
17. Andreasen PA, Egelund R, Petersen HH. The plasminogen activation system in tumor growth, invasion, and metastasis. *Cell Mol Life Sci*. 2000;57(1):25–40.
18. Mazar AP, Henkin J, Goldfarb RH. The urokinase plasminogen activator system in cancer: implications for tumor angiogenesis and metastasis. *Angiogenesis*. 1999;3(1):15–32.
19. Steuber T, Vickers A, Haese A, et al. Free PSA isoforms and intact and cleaved forms of urokinase plasminogen activator receptor in serum improve selection of patients for prostate cancer biopsy. *Int J Cancer*. 2007;120(7):1499–1504.
20. Shariat SF, Roehrborn CG, McConnell JD, et al. Association of the circulating levels of the urokinase system of plasminogen activation with the presence of prostate cancer and invasion, progression, and metastasis. *J Clin Oncol*. 2007;25(4):349–355.

21. Miyake H, Hara I, Yamanaka K, Gohji K, Arakawa S, Kamidono S. Elevation of serum levels of urokinase-type plasminogen activator and its receptor is associated with disease progression and prognosis in patients with prostate cancer. *Prostate.* 1999;39(2):123–129.
22. Shariat SF, Walz J, Roehrborn CG, et al. Early postoperative plasma transforming growth factor-beta1 is a strong predictor of biochemical progression after radical prostatectomy. *J Urol.* 2008;179(4):1593–1597.
23. Lange I, Hammerer P, Knabbe C, Graefen M, Schmahl M, Huland H. [Plasma TGF-beta1 concentrations in patients with prostate carcinoma or benign prostatic hyperplasia]. *Urologe A.* 1998;37(2):199–202.
24. Wolff JM, Fandel TH, Borchers H, Jakse G. Serum concentrations of transforming growth factor-beta 1 in patients with benign and malignant prostatic diseases. *Anticancer Res.* 1999;19(4A):2657–2659.
25. Giri D, Ozen M, Ittmann M. Interleukin-6 is an autocrine growth factor in human prostate cancer. *Am J Pathol.* 2001;159(6):2159–2165.
26. Hobisch A, Eder IE, Putz T, et al. Interleukin-6 regulates prostate-specific protein expression in prostate carcinoma cells by activation of the androgen receptor. *Cancer Res.* 1998;58(20): 4640–4645.
27. Lee SO, Lou W, Hou M, de Miguel F, Gerber L, Gao AC. Interleukin-6 promotes androgen-independent growth in LNCaP human prostate cancer cells. *Clin Cancer Res.* 2003;9(1):370–376.
28. Nakashima J, Tachibana M, Horiguchi Y, et al. Serum interleukin 6 as a prognostic factor in patients with prostate cancer. *Clin Cancer Res.* 2000;6(7):2702–2706.
29. Michalaki V, Syrigos K, Charles P, Waxman J. Serum levels of IL-6 and TNF-alpha correlate with clinicopathological features and patient survival in patients with prostate cancer. *Br J Cancer.* 2004;90(12):2312–2316.
30. Terracciano D, Bruzzese D, Ferro M, et al. Soluble interleukin-6 receptor to interleukin-6 (sIL6R/IL-6) ratio in serum as a predictor of high Gleason sum at radical prostatectomy. *Oncol Lett.* 2011;2(5):861–864.
31. Kattan MW, Shariat SF, Andrews B, et al. The addition of interleukin-6 soluble receptor and transforming growth factor beta1 improves a preoperative nomogram for predicting biochemical progression in patients with clinically localized prostate cancer. *J Clin Oncol.* 2003;21(19):3573–3579.
32. Dhir R, Vietmeier B, Arlotti J, et al. Early identification of individuals with prostate cancer in negative biopsies. *J Urol.* 2004;171(4):1419–1423.
33. Paul B, Dhir R, Landsittel D, Hitchens MR, Getzenberg RH. Detection of prostate cancer with a blood-based assay for early prostate cancer antigen. *Cancer Res.* 2005;65(10):4097–4100.
34. Leman ES, Cannon GW, Trock BJ, et al. EPCA-2: a highly specific serum marker for prostate cancer. *Urology.* 2007;69(4):714–720.
35. Zhao Z, Ma W, Zeng G, Qi D, Ou L, Liang Y. Preoperative serum levels of early prostate cancer antigen (EPCA) predict prostate cancer progression in patients undergoing radical prostatectomy. *Prostate.* 2012;72(3):270–279.
36. Diamandis EP. Cancer biomarkers: can we turn recent failures into success? *J Natl Cancer Inst.* 2010;102(19):1462–1467.
37. Fujita K, Pavlovich CP, Netto GJ, et al. Specific detection of prostate cancer cells in urine by multiplex immunofluorescence cytology. *Hum Pathol.* 2009;40(7):924–933.
38. Vlaeminck-Guillem V, Ruffion A, André J, Devonec M, Paparel P. Urinary prostate cancer 3 test: toward the age of reason? *Urology.* 2010;75(2):447–453.
39. Bussemakers MJ, van Bokhoven A, Verhaegh GW, et al. DD3: a new prostate-specific gene, highly overexpressed in prostate cancer. *Cancer Res.* 1999;59(23):5975–5979.
40. Marks LS, Fradet Y, Deras IL, et al. PCA3 molecular urine assay for prostate cancer in men undergoing repeat biopsy. *Urology.* 2007;69(3):532–535.
41. Deras IL, Aubin SM, Blase A, et al. PCA3: a molecular urine assay for predicting prostate biopsy outcome. *J Urol.* 2008;179(4):1587–1592.
42. Chun FK, de la Taille A, van Poppel H, et al. Prostate cancer gene 3 (PCA3): development and internal validation of a novel biopsy nomogram. *Eur Urol.* 2009;56(4):659–667.
43. Roobol MJ, Schröder FH, van Leeuwen P, et al. Performance of the prostate cancer antigen 3 (PCA3) gene and prostate-specific antigen in prescreened men: exploring the value of PCA3 for a first-line diagnostic test. *Eur Urol.* 2010;58(4):475–481.
44. Tosoian JJ, Loeb S, Kettermann A, et al. Accuracy of PCA3 measurement in predicting short-term biopsy progression in an active surveillance program. *J Urol.* 2010;183(2):534–538.
45. Nakanishi H, Groskopf J, Fritsche HA, et al. PCA3 molecular urine assay correlates with prostate cancer tumor volume: implication in selecting candidates for active surveillance. *J Urol.* 2008;179(5):1804–1809; discussion 1809-1810.
46. Bostwick DG, Gould VE, Qian J, Susani M, Marberger M. Prostate cancer detected by uPM3: radical prostatectomy findings. *Mod Pathol.* 2006;19(5):630–633.
47. Whitman EJ, Groskopf J, Ali A, et al. PCA3 score before radical prostatectomy predicts extracapsular extension and tumor volume. *J Urol.* 2008;180(5):1975–1978; discussion 1978–1979.
48. Hessels D, van Gils MP, van Hooij O, et al. Predictive value of PCA3 in urinary sediments in determining clinico-pathological characteristics of prostate cancer. *Prostate.* 2010;70(1):10–16.
49. van Gils MP, Hessels D, Hulsbergen-van de Kaa CA, et al. Detailed analysis of histopathological parameters in radical prostatectomy specimens and PCA3 urine test results. *Prostate.* 2008;68(11):1215–1222.
50. Auprich M, Chun FK, Ward JF, et al. Critical assessment of preoperative urinary prostate cancer antigen 3 on the accuracy of prostate cancer staging. *Eur Urol.* 2011;59(1):96–105.
51. Tomlins SA, Rhodes DR, Perner S, et al. Recurrent fusion of TMPRSS2 and ETS transcription factor genes in prostate cancer. *Science.* 2005;310(5748):644–648.
52. Laxman B, Tomlins SA, Mehra R, et al. Noninvasive detection of TMPRSS2:ERG fusion transcripts in the urine of men with prostate cancer. *Neoplasia.* 2006;8(10):885–888.
53. Hessels D, Smit FP, Verhaegh GW, Witjes JA, Cornel EB, Schalken JA. Detection of TMPRSS2-ERG fusion transcripts and prostate cancer antigen 3 in urinary sediments may improve diagnosis of prostate cancer. *Clin Cancer Res.* 2007;13(17):5103–5108.
54. Rice KR, Chen Y, Ali A, et al. Evaluation of the ETS-related gene mRNA in urine for the detection of prostate cancer. *Clin Cancer Res.* 2010;16(5):1572–1576.
55. Salami SS, Schmidt F, Laxman B, et al. Combining urinary detection of TMPRSS2:ERG and PCA3 with serum PSA to predict diagnosis of prostate cancer. *Urol Oncol.* 2013;31(5):566–571.
56. Tomlins SA, Aubin SM, Siddiqui J, et al. Urine TMPRSS2:ERG fusion transcript stratifies prostate cancer risk in men with elevated serum PSA. *Sci Transl Med.* 2011;3(94):94ra72.
57. Gonzalgo ML, Nakayama M, Lee SM, De Marzo AM, Nelson WG. Detection of GSTP1 methylation in prostatic secretions using combinatorial MSP analysis. *Urology.* 2004;63(2):414–418.
58. Harden SV, Sanderson H, Goodman SN, et al. Quantitative GSTP1 methylation and the detection of prostate adenocarcinoma in sextant biopsies. *J Natl Cancer Inst.* 2003;95(21): 1634–1637.
59. Crocitto LE, Korns D, Kretzner L, et al. Prostate cancer molecular markers GSTP1 and hTERT in expressed prostatic secretions as predictors of biopsy results. *Urology.* 2004;64(4):821–825.
60. Hoque MO, Topaloglu O, Begum S, et al., Quantitative methylation-specific polymerase chain reaction gene patterns in urine sediment distinguish prostate cancer patients from control subjects. *J Clin Oncol.* 2005;23(27):6569–6575.
61. Baden J, Green G, Painter J, et al. Multicenter evaluation of an investigational prostate cancer methylation assay. *J Urol.* 2009;182(3):1186–1193.

5.4 Morphometric and Systems Pathology: The Future of Screening, Diagnosis, and Staging

MICHAEL J. DONOVAN
FAISAL M. KHAN
RICHARD SCOTT
GERARDO FERNANDEZ
CARLOS CORDON-CARDO

INTRODUCTION

Over the past 15 years, there has been a gradual transition in the focus of translational oncologic medicine to a patient-centric, systems platform that incorporates host/tumor molecular profiling, medical genetics-genomics, liquid biopsies (e.g., exosomes), and peptide screening as part of a "whole patient" treatment paradigm (1–7). Such transformative and integrative approaches require advancements in multiple clinical and scientific subspecialties including basic disease biology, translational medicine, biophysics, image analysis, and theoretical modeling. One of the key challenges is how best to effectively manage this voluminous and complex data stream starting with acquisition, storage, quality control, in silico modeling, and finally creating access for the clinician/care-giver to a user-friendly, accurate tool that is able to guide decisions surrounding early diagnosis, management, and treatment.

This chapter focuses on how these comprehensive, information-driven approaches will be applied in the early detection and management of men diagnosed with prostate cancer. Findings such as age-based prostate-specific antigen (PSA) thresholds, suspicious digital rectal exam, family history, and ethnic background have resulted in men being subjected to unnecessary biopsies with subsequent overdiagnosis and overtreatment of mostly indolent disease. Furthermore, approximately 75% of the 1.3 million men in the United States who undergo a prostate biopsy receive a negative result and it is believed that around 25% of these men actually do have cancer somewhere in the gland but it was missed due to sampling (8, 9). These facts combined with the observed increased morbidity associated with the prostate needle biopsy illustrate the need for improved detection techniques, not only to find cancer but to ultimately identify the clinically significant disease (10, 11).

FUTURE OF SCREENING AND DIAGNOSIS

Given that the current clinical variables are decidedly limited, advancements in imaging and fluid-based detection assays will aid not only in the identification of prostate cancer but also in finding aggressive disease, ultimately guiding appropriate patients to specific treatment options (12–14). Although MRI has emerged as a promising noninvasive diagnostic imaging modality, the lack of end user reproducibility and consistency for finding high-risk disease and the associated imaging cost have created challenges for routine clinical adoption (15). Noteworthy is that future innovative methods that couple multiparametric MRI with computer-assisted image analytics based on tissue registration and decision support methods should improve the detection of prostate cancer including indolent vs. aggressive disease (16, 17).

Another significant area of development is fluid analytics and the use of urine and blood samples to aid in the diagnostic process. The more novel approaches utilize highly accurate exosome-RNA signatures from nondigital rectal exam urine specimens (18). By employing a multigene signature derived from stable microvesicles/exosome RNA in the urine, both the patient and treating physician (i.e., urologist or primary care doctor in the future) will be able to dynamically monitor the disease process without the need for biopsy or even immediate intervention. It is hypothesized that screening in the future will include an initial PSA combined with other serum markers and an exosome-urine test linked, at an appropriate time, to advanced imaging techniques for the identification and early treatment of high-risk disease.

TREATMENT, STAGING, AND THE APPLICATION OF RISK STRATIFICATION THROUGH SYSTEMS "PRECISE" PATHOLOGY

Once diagnosed with prostate cancer, the patient must make a decision on a treatment plan with relatively limited information as to what is the optimal choice for their disease. Unfortunately, for patients with prostate cancer a comprehensive or systems view is currently limited to the integration of patient-specific clinical-only attributes such as age, ethnicity, serum PSA, imaging (to determine clinical stage), and subjective features from the diagnostic prostate needle biopsy or prostatectomy specimen including tumor differentiation (i.e., Gleason grade and score) and volume (% and length). There are no routine ancillary tests performed.

Although the development of various clinical statistical instruments such as nomograms has provided a mechanism to interrogate such variables, most urologists rely on basic prognostic features of stage, grade, and PSA along with clinical judgment to define and understand individual risk, predict health outcomes, and provide recommendations for treatment. The existing predictive tools do provide some benefit; however, the majority of contemporary patients are considered midrange, where nomograms are neither accurate nor particularly helpful for decision making. There have been several recent attempts to augment the current clinical nomograms by introducing gene expression data and serum markers; however, the lack of sufficient clinical efficacy/utility based on limited patient numbers and price has hampered their broad clinical adoption (19).

SYSTEMS "PRECISE" PATHOLOGY PLATFORM

Specifically in prostate cancer, there are many variables that are not amenable to the gene expression "grind and find" approach, notably issues surrounding sampling, subjectivity on histologic grading/volume of disease, and molecular tumor heterogeneity. These limitations are inherently linked as there is no a priori method or technology to identify and biopsy an index or high-risk lesion. Furthermore, current practice with a 10- to 12-core transrectal ultrasound (TRUS) biopsy approach only samples approximately 1% of the entire prostate gland. In addition, with the use of PSA screening, the majority of men diagnosed with prostate cancer today have low-volume disease, so even with improvements in MRI-guided biopsy, sampling and molecular variability will continue to be limiting factors. Precise pathology preserves the intact specimen from which the original diagnosis was made and provides a quantitative (morphometric) assessment of the overall architecture and composition of the tumor while incorporating biological attributes through advanced multiplex immunofluorescent (IF) biomarker techniques (20–22).

Unlike other solid tumors which incorporate additional criteria to define a risk state (e.g., estrogen receptor [ER] and Her2 status in breast cancer), prostate cancer, particularly in the biopsy, relies on the subjective assignment of a Gleason grade to drive a treatment decision. Over the years, a number of investigators have sought to quantitatively identify and classify additional histologic features as a way to further refine the interpretive limitations of the Gleason grading system. This has included nuclear morphometric approaches that incorporate nuclear size, shape, and chromatin organization (e.g., DNA content) and the development of computer-assisted decision support tools to quantify subtle morphologic changes to allow for a more reproducible discrimination between Gleason grades (23, 24). Unfortunately, the majority of these approaches have either not been able to associate features with specific outcome data or have been hampered by the inability to produce reliable stable metrics across large cohorts for validation and broad clinical application.

The precise pathology method extracts high-content morphologic characteristics from the histologic digital image using both preprocessed H&E and IF-stained prostate tissue specimens. By applying various sophisticated techniques that deconstruct the overall tumor histology, quantitative nuclear and cytoplasmic (morphometric and biologic) features become components of multivariate outcome models for de novo patients. Figure 5.4.1A–C illustrates the H&E and IF segmented and feature-classified images from a prostate needle biopsy. The discrete histologic and biomarker attributes (e.g., Androgen Receptor and Ki67) are easily identified through color annotation (22). Further advancements have propelled this field toward more IF morphometric analytics which removes the H&E staining variability while preserving the organizational properties of tumor. Through de-convolution and various threshold algorithms, challenges of nuclear segmentation, overlapping and irregularly stained nuclei, as well as biomarker distribution in various compartments (e.g., nuclear vs. epithelial cytoplasm vs. stroma) have been addressed. Further enhancements will include the application of Voronoi region—seed diagrams (Figure 5.4.2)—and the resultant combination of these algorithms with biomarker distribution patterns to ultimately add further

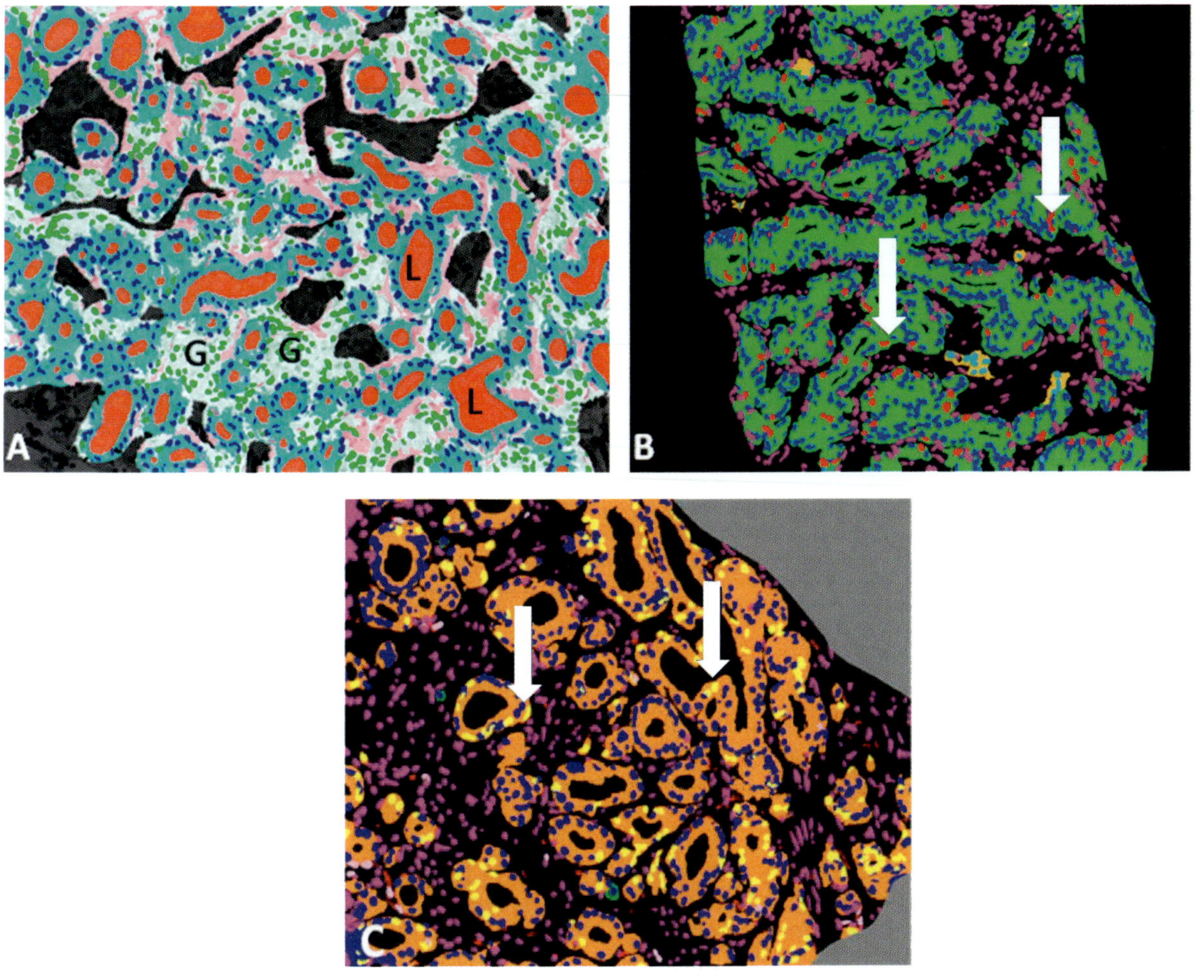

FIGURE 5.4.1 A–C. Representative H&E and Multiplex Immunofluorescent (MIF) images of three different prostate needle biopsy cases. (A) postsegmented H&E image of a well-differentiated Gleason score 6 prostate needle biopsy with a relatively small number of tumor cells that are a distance from gland lumens reflecting less transition to a Gleason grade 4 (A, gland lumens (L, red); tumor cells a distance from gland lumens, green, G). Two MIF postsegmented images of well-differentiated Gleason Score 6 prostate cancer: (B) with a range of nuclear AR intensity levels (lowest blue – highest red, white arrow) in CK18+ (green) tumor epithelial nuclei; and (C) with abundant levels of Ki67 (yellow) in AMACR (brown) + tumor epithelial nuclei. 200X.

content to the field of functional-histologic-biometric morphometry.

The derived systems-based (precise) pathology models utilize the patient's clinical data and intact formalin-fixed, paraffin-embedded (FFPE) tissue specimen to construct a baseline phenotype for defining a clinical risk stage. These biologic-quantitative models also provide a biomarker profile that is linked to treatment and outcome end points. The systems precise pathology platform represents a major advance in the practice of tissue-based pathology through its integration of molecular and imaging data with the patient's clinical record. Over the years, these modeling efforts have proved successful in accurately stratifying patients either at the time of diagnosis using features in the biopsy to guide appropriate treatment (i.e., surgery, radiation, active surveillance) or the prostatectomy specimen for incorporating additional monitoring or even the use of adjuvant therapy postintervention.

The employment of multivariate modeling in prostate cancer staging and treatment serves two broad categories, which include prognostic, time-dependent risk outcome models, that is, probability of disease progression over a specific time period based on a series of variables (e.g., clinical, genetic), and predictive models, which are more closely aligned with response to treatment (targeted therapy, radiation) and the presence of a tumor-specific phenotype. For decades, the primary methodology for linking variables with outcome was the Cox Proportional Hazards Model (25); however, when hundreds of features are generated, as in a systems disease analysis, the Cox method is neither reliable nor accurate. As a result, a variety of novel mathematical methods representing the latest advances in artificial intelligence and statistical analytics have been adapted including Random Forrests, neural networks, and support vector machines (26). Recent advances in this field have employed semi-supervised learning techniques to help address limitations when dealing with censored data (27). Indeed, these

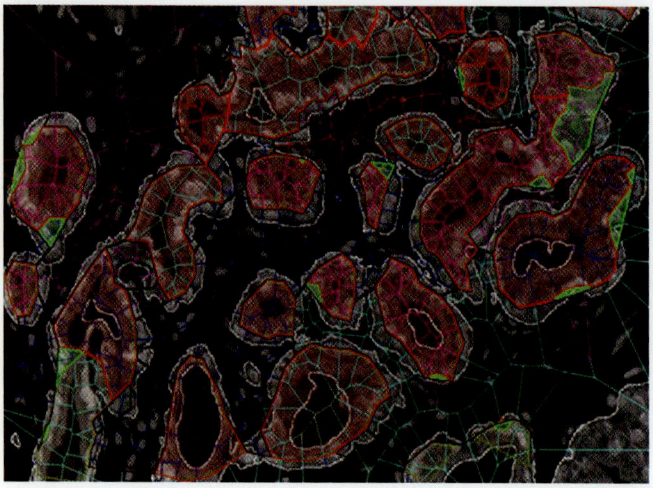

FIGURE 5.4.2 Immunofluorescent "Voronoi" derived image of prostate cancer stained with the epithelial marker Cytokeratin 18 and the nuclear stain DAPI (4′6-diamidino-2-phenylindole) from a formalin-fixed, paraffin-embedded prostate needle biopsy.

tools will become even more important for the effective integration and assessment of patient-specific content-rich protein and genomic/genetic profiles when defining a treatment course or determining a response to therapy.

■ CONCLUSIONS

Systems precise pathology represents a methodological shift in translational–diagnostic/prognostic pathology. The technical advances outlined above for prostate cancer exemplify some of the ways in which phenotypic characteristics contained within the diagnostic specimen (tissue or fluid) can be routinely extracted and employed, in a clinical setting, for routine patient management. This suggests that the incorporation of a systems-based approach using functional histology, quantitative biomarker expression, and advanced mathematics should provide a useful framework for further advancing personalized medicine and selective therapy design. By incorporating the patient's own specimen, the treating physician (together with the "primary care pathologist") is able to construct a disease blueprint beneficial for optimizing health outcomes, reducing adverse events from drugs that are otherwise likely to fail and thereby providing a rational framework for a more dynamic, long-term personalized treatment regimen.

■ REFERENCES

1. Auffray C, Chen Z, Hood L. Systems medicine: the future of medical genomics and healthcare. *Genome Med.* 2009;1:1–11.
2. Vidal M. A unifying view of 21st century systems biology. *FEBS Lett.* 2009;583:3891–3894.
3. Ginsburg GS, Willard HF. Genomic and personalized medicine: foundations and applications. *Trans Res.* 2009;154:277–287.
4. Mornzova D, Mara MA. Genomics applications of next-generation sequencing technologies in functional genomics. *Genomics.* 2008;2:255–264.
5. Bauca JM, Martinex-Morillo E, Diamandis EP. Peptidomics of urine and other biofluids for cancer diagnostics. *Clin Chem.* 2013;60:1–9.
6. Proteomic profiling of exosomes leads to the identification of novel biomarkers for prostate cancer. *PLoS One.* 2013;8:e82589.
7. Duijvesz D, Luider T, Bangma CH, Jenster G. Exosomes as biomarker treasure chests for prostate cancer. *Eur Urol.* 2011;59:823–831.
8. Babaian RJ, Toi A, Kamoi K, et al. A comparative analysis of sextant and an extended 11-core multisite directed biopsy strategy. *J Urol.* 2000;163:152–157.
9. Shariat S, Roehrborn C. Using biopsy to detect prostate cancer. *Rev Urol.* 2008;10:262–280.
10. Rosario D, Lane JA, Metcalfe C, et al. Short term outcomes of prostate biopsy in men tested for cancer by prostate specific antigen: prospective evaluation within ProtecT study. *BMJ.* 2012;344:d7894.
11. Gonzalez CM, Averch T, Boyd lA, et al. AUA/SUNA White Paper on the Incidence, Prevention and Treatment of Complications Related to Prostate Needle Biopsy. *Linthicum, MD: AUA Education and Research, Inc*; 2012.
12. Leake JL, Hardman R, Ojili V, et al. Prostate MRI: access to and current practice of prostate MRI in the United States. *J Am Coll Radiol.* 2014;11:156–160.
13. Sapre N, Selth LA. Circulating microRNAs as biomarkers of prostate cancer: the state of play. *Prostate Cancer.* 2013;2013:539680.
14. Hessvik NP, Sandvig K, Llorente A. Exosomal miRNAs as biomarkers for prostate cancer. *Front Genet.* 2013;4:1–9.
15. Murphy G, Haider M, Ghai S, et al. The expanding role of MRI in prostate cancer. *AJR Am J Roentgenol.* 2013;201:1229–1238.
16. Rastinhad AR, Turkbey B, Salami SS, et al. Improving detection of clinically significant prostate cancer: MRI/TRUS fusion-guided prostate biopsy. *J Urol.* 2013. [Epub ahead of print].
17. Bonekamp D, Bonekamp S, Mullins JK, et al. Multiparametric magnetic resonance imaging characterization of prostate lesions in the active surveillance population: incremental value of magnetic resonance imaging for prediction of disease reclassification. *J Comput Assit Tomogr.* 2013;37:948–956.
18. Nilsson J, Skog J, Nordstrand A, et al. Prostate cancer-derived urine exosomes: a novel approach to biomarkers for prostate cancer. *Br J Cancer.* 2009;100:1603–1607.
19. Miyake H, Fujisawa M. Prognostic prediction following radical prostatectomy for prostate cancer using conventional as well as molecular biological approaches. *Int J Urol.* 2013;20:301–311.
20. Cordon-Cardo C, Kotsianti A, Verbel DA, et al. Improved prediction of prostate cancer recurrence through systems pathology. *J Clin Invest.* 2007;117:1876–1883.
21. Donovan MJ, Hamann S, Clayton M, et al. A systems pathology approach for the prediction of prostate cancer progression after radical prostatectomy. *J Clin Oncol.* 2008;26:3923–3929.
22. Donovan MJ, Khan FM, Fernandez G, et al. Personalized prediction of tumor response and cancer progression on prostate needle biopsy. *J Urol.* 2009;182:123–130.
23. Veltri RW, Christudass CS, Isharwal S. Nuclear morphometry, nucleomics and prostate cancer progression. *Asian J Androl.* 2012;14:375–384.
24. Sparks R, Madabhushi A. Statistical shape model for manifold regularization: Gleason grading of prostate histology. *Comput Vis Image Underst.* 2013;117:1138–1146.
25. Cox DR. Regression models and life-tables (with Discussion). *J Roy Stat Soc.* 1972;34:187–220.
26. Boyce S, Fan Y, Watson RW, et al. Evaluation of prediction models for the staging of prostate cancer. *BMC Med Inform Decis Mak.* 2013;136:1–10.
27. Khan, F, Liu, Q.Transduction of semi-supervised regression targets in survival analysis for medical prognosis. *Biological Data Mining Workshop (BioDM), IEEE 11th International Conference on Data Mining ICDM*; 2011:1018–1025.

5.5.1 PET: The Future of Screening, Diagnosis, and Staging for Prostate Cancer

MATHEW L. THAKUR

EDOUARD J. TRABULSI

SUNG M. KIM

CHARLES M. INTENZO

LEONARD G. GOMELLA

INTRODUCTION

Over the past two decades, Positron Emission Tomography (PET) has become one of the most indispensible tools in the management of oncologic diseases. It has continued to play a vital role in diagnosis, prognosis, and screening. PET is a three-dimensional imaging technique that can provide unique molecular and metabolic information on the disease, leading the way to identify and monitor genomic modulation that forms the basis of oncogenesis on a cellular level. Today, PET is primarily driven by a glucose analogue labeled with a radionuclide, fluorine-18, injected systemically that provides molecular characterization essential for the management of many diseases. Glucose is taken up by cells, indicating their metabolic activity by the virtue of their regional glucose consumption. The F-18 then is trapped within the cells due to phosphorylation of glucose.

The positrons emitted by these radionuclides travel a short distance (up to 2 mm) and encounter an electron, resulting in emission of two 511 keV gamma rays in the opposite direction. The PET gantry then detects the annihilation electrons in coincidence, and computers reconstruct sectional images of the tissue into which the positron-emitting radionuclide was deposited. This oversimplified PET process forms the basis of its worldwide expanding role in medical practice. The global interest in this technology has led to the study and use of many other positron-emitting radionuclides. This enlarging the library of compounds has contributed to the assessment of biological processes and transduction pathways that govern neurologic, cardiovascular, and oncologic diseases and their treatment.

This chapter focuses only on the role of PET in the management of prostate cancer. It gives an overview of this enormously large, highly successful, yet often challenging imaging modality. It must be stressed that PET is complemented by computerized tomography (CT) in a hybrid imaging modality approach. This merger of imaging techniques has allowed PET to take a pivotal role in the screening, diagnosis, and staging of the majority of neoplasms.

Prostate cancer is a common, yet heterogeneous and biologically complex disease. As the leading solid tumor in men in the United States, prostate cancer is associated with significant controversy, high morbidity, and considerable emotional and financial cost. As a result of the heterogeneity and the biological complexity of prostate cancer, it creates challenges in screening, diagnosing, differentiating indolent from aggressive disease, determining the effectiveness of therapeutic interventions, and detecting its recurrence. Accurate staging of the high-risk patient is vital for the multidisciplinary management of prostate cancer. In order to address many of these needs, molecules have been developed and evaluated specifically for PET imaging of prostate cancer (1,2). A few promising agents are reviewed below that outline the current status of PET imaging in the management of prostate cancer. The mechanisms of the radionuclides used in the detection of prostate cancer and described in this chapter are illustrated in Figure 5.5.1.1.

F-18-FDG

Primary Imaging

This radiopharmaceutical, which has contributed so extensively to the management of oncologic diseases in general, has played a limited role in the diagnosis and staging of prostate cancer (3). This weakness of F-18-FDG is attributed to many parameters which include the poor uptake of the tracer in slow growing prostate cancer, its nonspecific uptake in normal and benign masses, and its extensive accumulation in the urinary bladder in proximity to the prostate gland. Similarly, F-18-FDG uptake in benign prostate hyperplasia (3) and in prostatitis (4) can lead to false-positive imaging results that may result in overtreatment. Despite these limitations, in one study in men with Gleason score of 7 or greater, sensitivity of 80% and positive predictive value of 87% were reported (5).

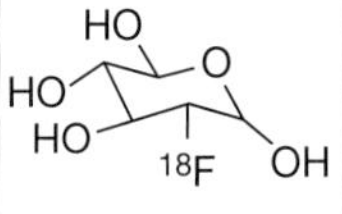

^{18}F-FDG

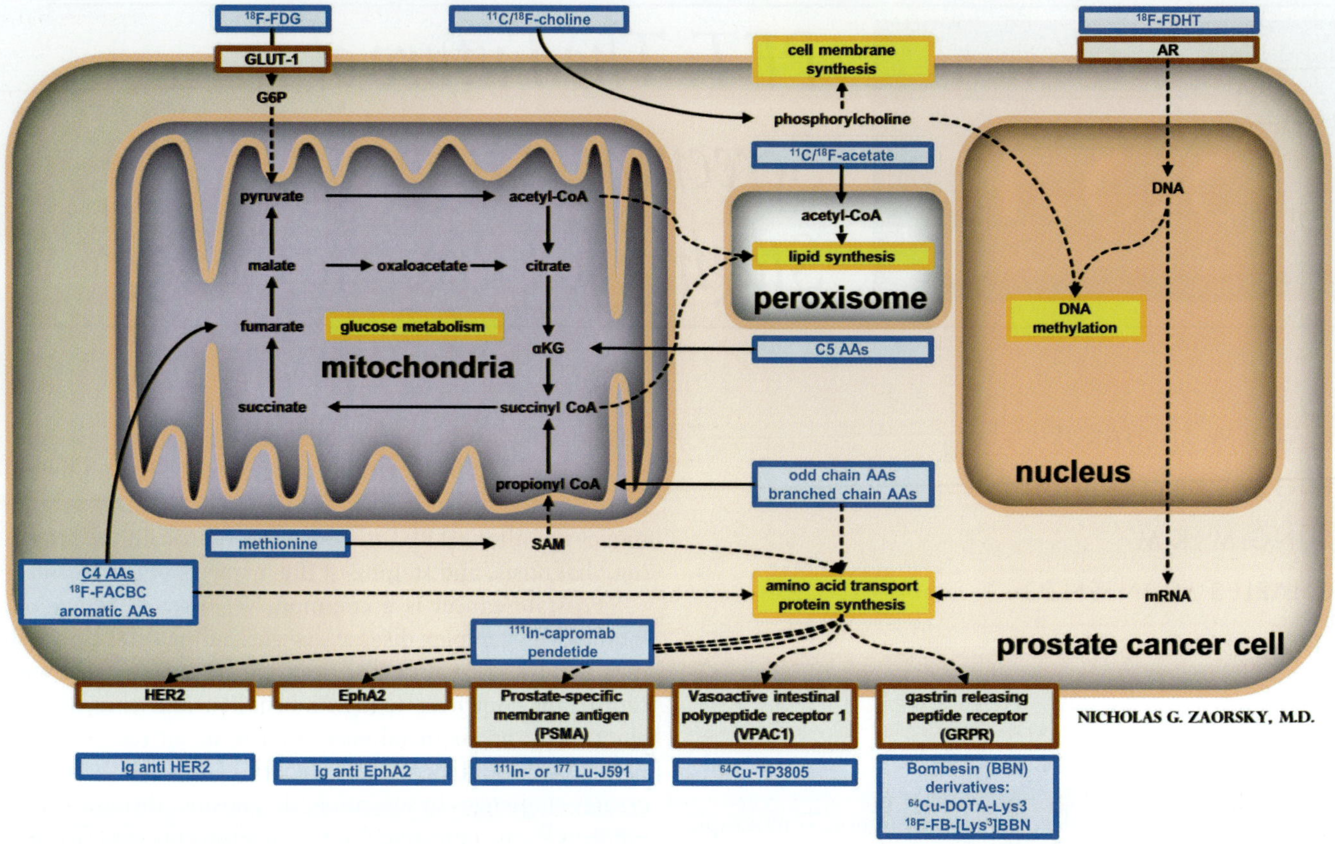

FIGURE 5.5.1.1 Radionuclides in the detection of prostate cancer. The mechanisms of the radionuclides (blue boxes) used in the detection of prostate cancer are displayed. Currently, ^{18}F-FDG is the most frequently used radionuclide for detecting metastatic disease; followed by ^{11}C/^{18}F-choline and ^{11}C/^{18}F-acetate. These biomarkers help detect intracellular processes (yellow boxes), including glucose metabolism, lipid synthesis, and cell membrane synthesis. Novel radionuclides include androgen receptor (AR) ligands, amino acid (AA) derivatives (e.g. anti-1-amino-3-1-^{18}F-fluorocyclobutane-1-carboxylic acid [anti-^{18}F-FACBC]), and ligands to protein biomarkers (brown boxes) specific to prostate cancer cells.
Note: solid arrows = "converted to"; dashed arrows = "involved in" / "leads to"; Figure adapted from Zaorsky et al. A paradigm shift from anatomic to functional and molecular imaging in the detection of recurrent prostate cancer. *Future Oncol.* 2014;10(3):457–474.

However, much greater sensitivity (85%), specificity (100%), positive predictive value (100%), and negative predictive value (68%) were reported for detection of pelvic nodes with metastatic disease (6). Furthermore, F-18-FDG has been found to be useful in staging of advanced prostate cancer in patients with rising PSA and to have significant advantages over In-111–Capromab Pendetide scintigraphy in the detecting of metastatic disease (7).

Staging

A large portion of prostate cancer patients suffer from rising PSA following definitive local therapy. Additional treatment decisions rely on determining if the disease recurrence is in the prostatic bed or has metastasized elsewhere. Results of several studies indicate with high sensitivity and specificity that F-18-FDG PET imaging can be useful in staging the disease in such a group of patients (8,9). Another study in a limited number of patients also showed decreased quantitative regimens of chemotherapy (10). Despite the occasional encouraging reports, the use of F-18-FDG in the routine management of prostate cancer patients has remained limited and the search has continued in the development of improved agents that may address these issues with greater utility.

C-11/F-18-Acetate

Acetate is a common anion in biology and is primarily utilized in the form of acetyl coenzyme-A (CoA) in the synthesis of fatty acids. In prostate cancer cells, extensive involvement of fatty acid synthesis pathways has been suggested (11) and the importance of CoA synthetase in C-11-acetate cell uptake has been demonstrated (12). The lack of urinary excretion of C-11-acetate contrasts with the extensive bladder uptake of F-18-FDG and adds to the potential utility of C-11 acetate in PET imaging of prostate cancer.

A comparative study of C-11-acetate with F-18-FDG in a small group of patients with prostate cancer concluded that the C-11-acetate was a more sensitive tracer than F-18-FDG (13). Similarly, a recent study in which 107 men were imaged with C-11-acetate before radical prostatectomy demonstrated that C-11-acetate was more sensitive for

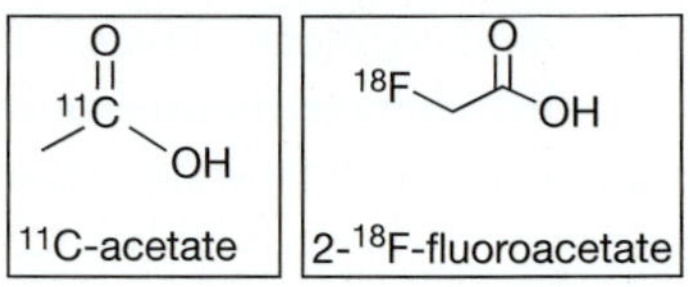

diagnosis of nodal metastatic disease than current imaging methods (14). C-11-acetate may also be useful in prostate cancer recurrence in patients who had been treated with radiation or had prostatectomy; however, false positive rates of approximately 15% were reported (15). C-11-acetate therefore remains a promising radiopharmaceutical in the management of prostate cancer patients.

The physical half-life of 20 minutes for C-11, however, prevents it from use in most institutions that do not have their own cyclotron required for the production of C-11. Due to its longer half-life (110 min), F-18 has been chosen as a tracer for acetate (16). Just as for F-18-FDG, the longer half-life of F-18-acetate permits its regional commercial availability. One study in cynomolgus monkeys reported that F-18 acetate is not a physiologically comparable analogue of C-11-acetate (17). In rodents, however, several fold greater tumor uptake with F-18-acetate than C-11-acetate was observed (16). The true potential of F-18-acetate in prostate cancer patients largely remains unexplored.

C-11 and F-18-Choline

Choline plays an important role in cell membrane synthesis and phospholipid metabolism and functions as a methyl donor for DNA methylation. Choline supports cell proliferation through its role in cell membrane synthesis. Prostate cancer cells show elevated levels of choline and certain choline metabolites (17, 18).

Under aerobic conditions, prostate tumors exhibit higher H3-choline uptake than that of C-14-acetate and F-18-FDG (19). In hypoxia, however, tumor uptake of choline is lower than that of acetate and F-18-FDG (19). Choline has been radiolabeled both with C-11 and F-18 and studied in patients (20–25).

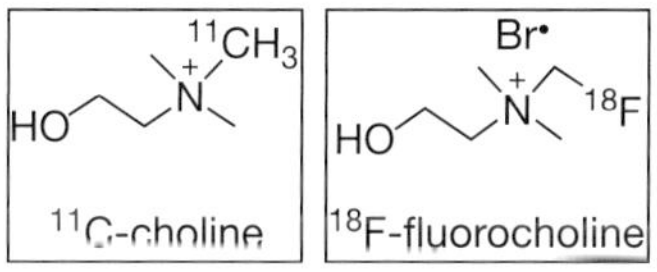

Overall, both tracers have shown significant promise for detecting primary, recurrent, and metastatic prostate cancer. In staging prostate cancer, some uncertainty remains as to its diagnostic sensitivity in patients with low levels of PSA following radical prostatectomy, external-beam therapy, and brachytherapy (22). The low sensitivity at low PSA values may limit the use of F-18-choline in prostate cancer salvage therapy. A similar conclusion has been drawn by another group in imaging recurrent prostate cancer in which they noted that the imaging results were dependent on the PSA level. Abnormal tumor activity was noted in 88% of the patients with PSA levels > 1.1 ng/mL (23). A Zurich group reported that F-18-choline PET imaging promises to play an important role to determine therapeutic treatment in patients with recurrent prostate cancer (24).

With C-11-choline, false positives were reported in patients with benign prostatic hyperplasia (25). The technique, however, has been found to be useful in detecting lymph nodes and distant metastatic lesions (25). For detecting primary tumors, these tracers have shown conflicting results with the sensitivity ranging from 55% to 87% for C-11-choline (26). The uptake of both C-11-choline and F-18-choline overlaps among cancerous, benign prostatic hyperplasia, and prostate cancer and did not correlate with tumor grade, PSA, Gleason score, tumor volume, or with cellular proliferation (26). Although C-11-choline promises to be useful in imaging nodal metastases, detecting local recurrence, and visualizing distant metastases, with high sensitivity, the use of C-11-choline has remained limited only to a few centers, primarily because of the short half-life of C-11. As noted previously, F-18 has a longer half-life, facilitating commercial use. This form of choline has renal excretion which may lead to bladder activity artifacts (26).

F-18-Sodium Fluoride (F-18-NaF)

For prostatic cancer, bone is the most common site for metastatic lesions. Technetium-99m–based tracers underestimate the burden of bone metastases and cannot provide quantitative measure for determination of therapeutic responses (27). The uptake of fluoride ions in hydroxyapatite is long known. Therefore, F-18-NaF, a long-standing agent, has resurfaced as a viable imaging agent due to the wide availability of PET/CT scanners. In addition, the recent shortage of Tc-99m and the recent reimbursement approval by the Centers for Medicare and Medicaid Services have contributed to its resurgence.

In a study of the efficacy of Tc-99m methylene bisphosphonate planar bone scintigraphy, SPECT, F-18-NaF PET, and F-18-NaF PET/CT were performed and compared in 25 patients with newly diagnosed prostate cancer with a Gleason score of > 8 and PSA levels of > 20 ng/mL. Sensitivity and specificity were 70% and 57%, respectively, for planar bone scintigraphy, 92% and 82% for SPECT, 100% and 62% for F-18-NaF PET, and 100% and 100% for F-18-NaF PET/CT. This efficacy of F-18-NaF PET/CT in the detection of occult bone metastases enhances patient management (27). The very high sensitivity and specificity is preferable and may impact the clinical management of patients with high-risk prostate cancer (Figure 5.5.1.2) (28). It can be debated if detecting 10 bone metastatic lesions by one technique versus 20 by the other in the same patient truly impacts the therapeutic management of the patient. The high false-positive rate, however, is a concern since it may lead to overtreatment. A true utility of F-18-NaF in daily routine application will be determined by the cost and by its availability as compared with the current standard techniques.

■ FUTURE DIRECTIONS

During the past two decades, great strides have been made by PET imaging with F-18-FDG and many other novel compounds discussed here. With the limitations of some of these agents noted in the management of prostate

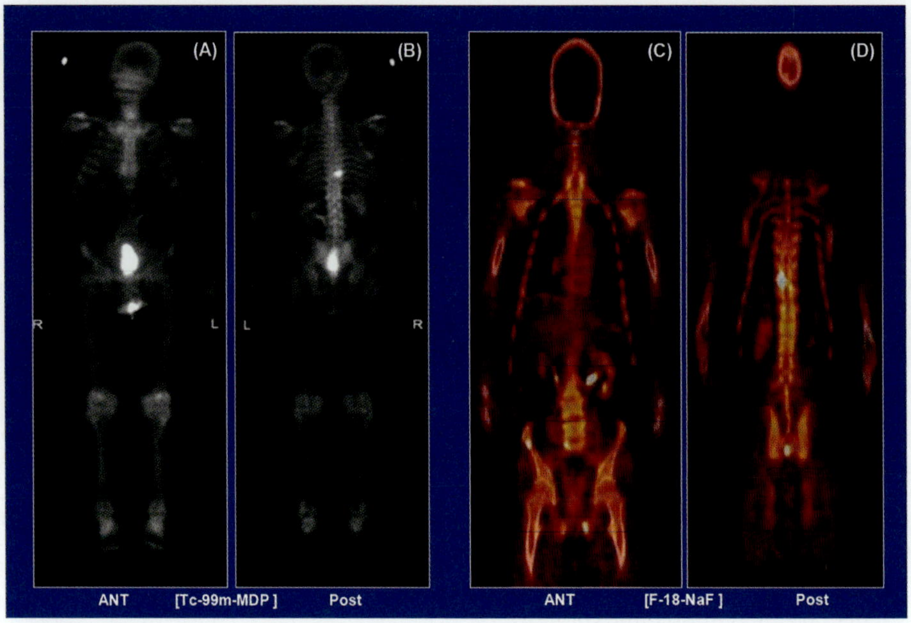

FIGURE 5.5.1.2 Seventy-one-year-old man with prostate cancer. Tc-99m-MDP bone scan (A and B) shows suspicious single metastatic lesion in T9. The F-18-NaF scan (C and D) shows multiple metastatic bone lesions in T9, sacrum, and right-iliac crest S1 and S3.

cancer, numerous disease-specific radiopharmaceuticals are being explored for this common disease. Many other agents are currently under study for the radiopharmaceutical imaging of prostate cancer and are beyond the scope of this chapter.

There is a compelling need to develop more effective imaging to accurately screen for and stage prostate cancer. Newer approaches to drug discovery are generally based on the improved understanding of the biochemical pathways that govern the pathogenesis of the diseases at a molecular level.

Androgens promote prostate growth and help maintain its biological functions. Several androgen receptor (AR) specific agents have been investigated (28–30) including 16-beta-(F-18)-fluoro-5-alpha, dihydrotestosterone (F-18-FDHT). Similarly, anti-1-amino-3-1-F-18-fluorocyclobutane-1-carboxylic acid (anti-F-18-FACBC) has been shown to accumulate in prostate cancer with relatively little renal excretion (31). These agents have paved the way to innovative approaches to address several issues that remain challenging in the management of prostate cancer patients.

Targeting mutated gene mRNAs or genomic products expressed on prostate cancer cell surface can provide an excellent imaging approach. Incorporated with these novel biomolecules, specific for given genomic biomarkers, is an array of positron emitting radionuclides other than F-18. These include agents such as Cu-64 (t ½ = 12.7 hr), Cu-62 (t ½ = 9.8 min), I-124 (t ½ = 4.2 d), Zr-89 (t ½ = 3.26 d), Ga-68 (t ½ = 68 min), and C-11 (t ½ = 20 min) (32–34). Our own preliminary data in humans with breast cancer that targets a genomic biomarker, VPAC1 with a Cu-64-labeled specific biomolecule, promises to selectively identify malignant lesions from benign masses by PET or positron emission mammography (PEM). This imaging may spare millions of patients from anxiety and trauma associated with unnecessary biopsies and conserve billions of health care dollars in the United States (33). VPAC1 receptors are also expressed on the cells of prostate cancer of all types. This provides us with an opportunity to diagnose and stage prostate cancer in patients with the same Cu-64 biomarker. With the lack of urinary excretion, this biomarker adds to its virtues in prostate cancer imaging (34). Such genomic-based imaging agents and others in development will enhance PET utilization in diagnosis, staging, and perhaps in the future may find a role in screening. The recent addition of PET/MRI hybrid imaging will further invigorate PET utility in the management of patients with prostate cancer (35). Lastly, radionuclide targeting of prostate cancer–specific miRNAs 19 to 25 nucleotides long may have utility in the diagnosis and treatment of prostate cancer (36).

■ REFERENCES

1. Hong H, Zhang Y, Sun J, Cai W. Positron emission tomography imaging of prostate cancer. *Amino Acids*. 2010;39:11–27.
2. Kelloff GJ, Choyke P, Coffey DS; Prostate Cancer Imaging Working Group. Challenges in clinical prostate cancer: role of imaging. *AJR Am J Roentgenol*. 2009;192(6):1455–1470.
3. Salminen E, Hogg A, Binns D, Frydenberg M, Hicks R. Investigations with FDG-PET scanning in prostate cancer show limited value for clinical practice. *Acta Oncol.* 2002;41(5):425–429.

4. Kao PF, Chou YH, Lai CW. Diffuse FDG uptake in acute prostatitis. *Clin Nucl Med.* 2008;33(4):308–310.
5. Minamimoto R, Uemura H, Sano F, et al. The potential of FDG-PET/CT for detecting prostate cancer in patients with an elevated serum PSA level. *Ann Nucl Med.* 2011;25(1):21–27.
6. Chang CH, Wu HC, Tsai JJ, Shen YY, Changlai SP, Kao A. Detecting metastatic pelvic lymph nodes by 18F-2-deoxyglucose positron emission tomography in patients with prostate-specific antigen relapse after treatment for localized prostate cancer. *Urol Int.* 2003;70(4):311–315.
7. Jadvar H. Prostate cancer: PET with 18F-FDG, 18F- or 11C-Acetate, and 18F- or 11C-Choline. *J Nucl Med.* 2011;52(1):81–89.
8. Chang CH, Wu HC, Tsai JJ, Shen YY, Changlai SP, Kao A. Detecting metastatic pelvic lymph nodes by 18F-2-deoxyglucose positron emission tomography in patients with prostate-specific antigen relapse after treatment for localized prostate cancer. *Urol Int.* 2003;70(4):311–315.
9. Schöder H, Herrmann K, Gönen M, et al. 2-[18F]fluoro-2-deoxyglucose positron emission tomography for the detection of disease in patients with prostate-specific antigen relapse after radical prostatectomy. *Clin Cancer Res.* 2005;11(13):4761–4769.
10. Jadvar H. Molecular imaging of prostate cancer with 18F-fluorodeoxyglucose PET. *Nat Rev Urol.* 2009;6(6):317–323.
11. Vāvere AL, Kridel SJ, Wheeler FB, Lewis JS. 1-11C-acetate as a PET radiopharmaceutical for imaging fatty acid synthase expression in prostate cancer. *J Nucl Med.* 2008;49(2):327–334.
12. Yun M, Bang SH, Kim JW, Park JY, Kim KS, Lee JD. The importance of acetyl coenzyme A synthetase for 11C-acetate uptake and cell survival in hepatocellular carcinoma. *J Nucl Med.* 2009;50(8):1222–1228.
13. Oyama N, Akino H, Kanamaru H, et al. 11C-acetate PET imaging of prostate cancer. *J Nucl Med.* 2002;43(2):181–186.
14. Haseebuddin M, Dehdashti F, Siegel BA, et al. 11-C-acetate PET/CT before radical prostatectomy: nodal staging and treatment failure prediction. *J Nucl Med.* 2013;54(5):699–706.
15. Sandblom G, Sörensen J, Lundin N, Häggman M, Malmström PU. Positron emission tomography with C11-acetate for tumor detection and localization in patients with prostate-specific antigen relapse after radical prostatectomy. *Urology.* 2006;67(5):996–1000.
16. Ponde DE, Dence CS, Oyama N, et al. F-18 fluoroacetate: a potential acetate analog for prostate tumor imaging--in vivo evaluation of F-18 fluoroacetate versus 11C-acetate. *J Nucl Med.* 2007;48(3):420–428.
17. Lindhe O, Sun A, Ulin J, Rahman O, Långström B, Sörensen J. F-18 fluoroacetate is not a functional analogue of C-11-acetate in normal physiology. *Eur J Nucl Med Mol Imaging.* 2009;36(9):1453–1459.
18. Brogsitter C, Zöphel K, Kotzerke J. F-18 Choline, C-11 choline and C-11 acetate PET/CT: comparative analysis for imaging prostate cancer patients. *Eur J Nucl Med Mol Imaging.* 2013;40 (suppl 1):18–27.
19. Hara T, Bansal A, DeGrado TR. Effect of hypoxia on the uptake of [methyl-3H] choline, [1-14C] acetate and [18F]FDG in cultured prostate cancer cells. *Nucl Med Biol.* 2006;33(8):977–984.
20. Reischl G, Bieg C, Schmiedl O, Solbach C, Machulla HJ. Highly efficient automated synthesis of [(11)C]choline for multi dose utilization. *Appl Radiat Isot.* 2004;60(6):835–838.
21. DeGrado TR, Coleman RE, Wang S, et al. Synthesis and evaluation of 18F-labeled choline as an oncologic tracer for positron emission tomography: initial findings in prostate cancer. *Cancer Res.* 2001;61(1):110–117.
22. Picchio M, Castellucci P. Clinical indications of C-choline PET/CT in prostate cancer patients with biochemical relapse. *Theranostics.* 2012;2(3):313–317.
23. Kwee SA, Coel MN, Lim J. Detection of recurrent prostate cancer with 18F-fluorocholine PET/CT in relation to PSA level at the time of imaging. *Ann Nucl Med.* 2012;26(6):501–507.
24. Soyka JD, Muster MA, Schmid DT, et al. Clinical impact of 18F-choline PET/CT in patients with recurrent prostate cancer. *Eur J Nucl Med Mol Imaging.* 2012;39(6):936–943.
25. Chen J, Zhao Y, Li X, et al. Imaging primary prostate cancer with 11C-Choline PET/CT: relation to tumour stage, Gleason score and biomarkers of biologic aggressiveness. *Radiol Oncol.* 2012;46(3):179–188.
26. Turkbey B, Mena E, Aras O, Garvey B, Grant K, Choyke PL. Functional and molecular imaging: applications for diagnosis and staging of localised prostate cancer. *Clin Oncol (R Coll Radiol).* 2013;25:451–460.
27. Jadvar H. Molecular imaging of prostate cancer: PET radiotracers. *AJR Am J Roentgenol.* 2012;199(2):278–291.
28. Parent EE, Dence CS, Sharp TL, Welch MJ, Katzenellenbogen JA. Synthesis and biological evaluation of a fluorine-18-labeled nonsteroidal androgen receptor antagonist, N-(3-[^{18}F]fluoro-4-nitronaphthyl)-cis-5-norobornene-endo-2,3-dicarboxylic imide. *Nucl Med Biol.* 2006;33:615–624.
29. Larson SM, Morris M, Gunther I, et al. Tumor localization of 16beta-^{18}F-fluoro-5alpha-dihydrotestosterone versus ^{18}F-FDG in patients with progressive, metastatic prostate cancer. *J Nuclear Med.* 2004;45:366–373.
30. Dehdashti F, Picus J, Michalski JM, et al. Positron tomographic assessment of androgen receptors in prostatic carcinoma. *Eur J Nucl Med Mol Imaging.* 2005;32:344–350.
31. Oka S, Hattori R, Kurosaki F, et al. A preliminary study of anti-1-amino-3-^{18}F-fluorocyclobutyl-1-carboxylic acid for the detection of prostate cancer. *J Nucl Med.* 2007;48:46–55.
32. Fonge H, Leyton JV. Positron emission tomographic imaging of iodine 124 anti-prostate stem cell antigen-engineered antibody fragments in LAPC-9 tumor-bearing severe combined immunodeficiency mice. *Mol Imaging.* 2013;12(3):191–202.
33. Thakur ML, Zhang K, Berger A, et al. VPAC1 receptors for imaging breast cancer: a feasibility study. *J Nucl Med.* 2013;54(7):1019–1025.
34. Zhang K, Aruva MR, Shanthly N, et al. PET imaging of VPAC1 expression in experimental and spontaneous prostate cancer. *J Nucl Med.* 2008;49(1):112–121.
35. Boss A, Bisdas S, Kolb A, et al. Hybrid PET/MRI of intracranial masses: initial experiences and comparison to PET/CT. *J Nucl Med.* 2010;51(8):1198–1205.
36. Deng JH, Deng Q, Kuo CH, Delaney SW, Ying SY. MiRNA targets of prostate cancer. *Methods Mol Biol.* 2013;936:357–369.

DCE MRI and MR Spectroscopy: The Future of Screening, Diagnosis, and Staging

5.5.2

VICTOR SAI
ANTONIO C. WESTPHALEN

Although T1- and T2-weighted MR sequences are the workhorse for assessing prostate morphology and identifying potential areas of pathology, their accuracy is limited in T2 isointense prostate tumors and a variety of nonneoplastic etiologies of T2 hypointensity including inflammation, hemorrhage, scarring, and treatment changes. Recent advances in physiologic and functional sequences including diffusion-weighted imaging, dynamic contrast-enhanced (DCE) MRI, and MR spectroscopy have improved overall detection accuracy and have supplemented traditional T1- and T2-weighted imaging (1–5). In this chapter, we will address DCE and MR spectroscopy methods.

■ DCE MRI

DCE MRI is a physiologic imaging method based on the fact that most prostate cancers demonstrate increased angiogenesis, which like many other cancers leads to earlier and more intense enhancement and faster wash-out compared with normal tissue. After gadolinium injection, the signal intensity of prostate tissue is measured as a function of time, and by comparison to the signal curve from a nearby artery, the underlying tissue permeability and microvascular flow can be calculated. Increased tissue permeability and increased microvascular volume and flow correlate with higher likelihood of underlying cancer (1,4).

In addition to tissue permeability, the DCE series can assess tissue wash-in and wash-out characteristics. Both rapid wash-in and rapid wash-out are also associated with increased likelihood of underlying cancer (2,6). Using the wash-in rate, Kim et al. noted that the sensitivity/specificity for prostate cancer was 96%/97% using DCE MRI compared with 75%/53% using T2-weighted sequence alone (2). The use of DCE also improves staging through better detection of extracapsular extension with Bloch et al. reporting greater than 25% improvement in sensitivity with DCE compared with T2-weighted MRI alone (7, 8). This is valuable in preoperative planning since extracapsular extension and seminal vesicle invasion may necessitate more extensive surgical resection. Figure 5.5.2.1 is an example of a patient with biopsy-proven prostate cancer in the left lateral apex; the T2-weighted sequence does not demonstrate any appreciable abnormality, but DCE MRI demonstrates both rapid wash-in and rapid wash-out suggesting underlying malignancy.

■ MR SPECTROSCOPY

MR spectroscopy assesses underlying tissue metabolism by identifying metabolites through their different chemical shifts in response to the magnetic field. Normal prostate tissue demonstrates high citrate concentration and relatively low choline. Prostate cancer tissue spectra demonstrate increased choline and decreased citrate, and therefore an increased choline-to-citrate ratio is the most reliable marker of malignancy, particularly in the peripheral zone. Depending on the number of standard deviations above the mean of the ratio of (choline+creatine)/citrate, a score from 1 to 5 can be assessed for each voxel, with a score of 1 representing a ratio less than 1 SD above the mean and 5 representing ≥ 4 SDs above the mean. A score of 4 or 5 is generally used to identify cancer (9). Figure 5.5.2.1 demonstrates significantly increased choline and decreased citrate in the region of biopsy-proven prostate cancer.

MR spectroscopy has been shown to improve prostate cancer detection and localization (1, 3) and cancer volume measurement in the peripheral zone (10). The combined sensitivity/specificity for combined MRI and MR

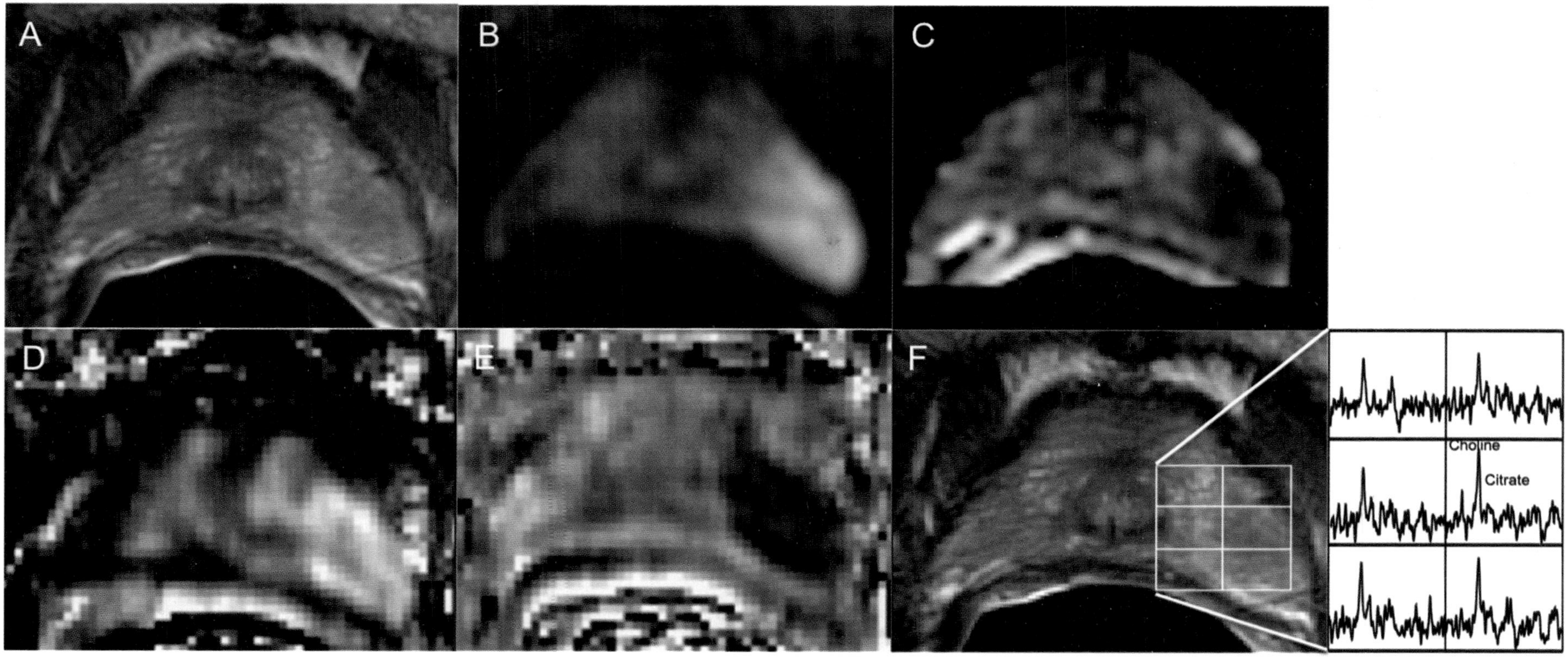

FIGURE 5.5.2.1 (A) T2 weighted, (B) DWI, (C) ADC, (D) wash-in DCE MRI, (E) wash-out DCE MRI, and (F) MR spectroscopy sequences in this patient with biopsy-proven prostate cancer in the left lateral apex who demonstrates no significant T2 signal abnormality (A). Diffusion-weighted imaging with corresponding ADC demonstrates restricted diffusion in the left lateral apex (B, C), and both wash-in and wash-out DCE show rapid wash-in and wash-out (D, E). MR spectroscopy demonstrates increased choline peaks and decreased citrate peaks suggestive of cancer.

spectroscopy is 91%/95% (11). In addition to improving detection accuracy, the use of MR spectroscopy has also demonstrated improvement in prostate cancer staging, particularly in the detection of extracapsular extension (12–14). However, some studies have demonstrated similar accuracy with or without spectroscopy (15) and others have suggested an unacceptably high number of false positives (16), which can occur from stromal benign prostatic hyperplasia, prostatitis, or inclusion of signal from the seminal vesicles. MR spectroscopy can also be limited by low sensitivity due to partial volume averaging in smaller cancers.

■ CONCLUSION

DCE MRI and MR spectroscopy are valuable complementary tools to T1/T2 and diffusion weighted images for accurate diagnosis and staging of prostate cancers, and they should be part of any comprehensive prostate MRI. Many recent studies have demonstrated significant added value of DCE and spectroscopy when used together, including a combined DCE and spectroscopy accuracy of 85% (16), improvement in prostate cancer localization and characterization (1, 5), and nearly double the detection of cancer in a patient cohort with previous negative transrectal ultrasound-guided biopsy compared with those undergoing repeat ultrasound-guided biopsy (17). Staging accuracy is also improved with the use of both DCE and spectroscopy as a result of greater accuracy in detection of extracapsular extension (3, 7, 8, 13, 14). Increasing use of 3T field strength, improvements in sequence design and postprocessing software, and greater understanding of the correlation between pathophysiology observed on functional imaging and actual pathology will result in even greater utility of these newer sequences.

■ REFERENCES

1. Fütterer JJ, Heijmink SWTPJ, Scheenen TWJ, et al. Prostate cancer localization with dynamic contrast-enhanced MR imaging and proton MR spectroscopic imaging. *Radiology.* 2006;241(2):449–458.
2. Kim JK, Hong SS, Choi YJ, et al. Wash-in rate on the basis of dynamic contrast-enhanced MRI: usefulness for prostate cancer detection and localization. *J Magn Reson Imaging.* 2005;22(5):639–646.
3. Kurhanewicz J, Vigneron DB, Hricak H, Narayan P, Carroll P, Nelson SJ. Three-dimensional H-1 MR spectroscopic imaging of the in situ human prostate with high (0.24-0.7-cm3) spatial resolution. *Radiology.* 1996;198(3):795–805.
4. Ocak I, Bernardo M, Metzger G, et al. Dynamic contrast-enhanced MRI of prostate cancer at 3 T: a study of pharmacokinetic parameters. *Am J Roentgenol.* 2007;189(4):849.
5. van Dorsten FA, van der Graaf M, Engelbrecht MR, et al. Combined quantitative dynamic contrast-enhanced MR imaging and (1)H MR spectroscopic imaging of human prostate cancer. *J Magn Reson Imaging.* 2004;20(2):279–287.
6. Engelbrecht MR, Huisman HJ, Laheij RJ, et al. Discrimination of prostate cancer from normal peripheral zone and central gland tissue by using dynamic contrast-enhanced MR imaging. *Radiology.* 2003;229(1):248–254.
7. Bloch BN, Furman-Haran E, Helbich TH, et al. Prostate cancer: accurate determination of extracapsular extension with high-spatial-resolution dynamic contrast-enhanced and T2-weighted MR imaging–initial results. *Radiology.* 2007;245(1):176–185.
8. Bloch BN, Genega EM, Costa DN, et al. Prediction of prostate cancer extracapsular extension with high spatial resolution dynamic contrast-enhanced 3-T MRI. *Eur Radiol.* 2012;22(10): 2201–2210.
9. Jung JA, Coakley FV, Vigneron DB, et al. Prostate depiction at endorectal MR spectroscopic imaging: investigation of a standardized evaluation system. *Radiology.* 2004;233(3):701–708.
10. Coakley FV, Kurhanewicz J, Lu Y, et al: Prostate cancer tumor volume: measurement with endorectal MR and MR spectroscopic imaging. *Radiology.* 2002;223(1):91–97.
11. Scheidler J, Hricak H, Vigneron DB, et al. Prostate cancer: localization with three-dimensional proton MR spectroscopic imaging–clinicopathologic study. *Radiology.* 1999;213(2):473–480.
12. Hricak H. MR imaging and MR spectroscopic imaging in the pre-treatment evaluation of prostate cancer. *Br J Radiol.* 2005;78 Spec No 2:S103–S111.
13. Wang L, Hricak H, Kattan MW, Chen HN, Scardino PT, Kuroiwa K. Prediction of organ-confined prostate cancer: incremental value of MR imaging and MR spectroscopic imaging to staging nomograms. *Radiology.* 2006;238(2):597–603.
14. Zakian KL, Sircar K, Hricak H, et al. Correlation of proton MR spectroscopic imaging with gleason score based on step-section pathologic analysis after radical prostatectomy. *Radiology.* 2005;234(3):804–814.
15. Weinreb JC, Blume JD, Coakley FV, et al. Prostate cancer: sextant localization at MR imaging and MR spectroscopic imaging before prostatectomy–results of ACRIN prospective multi-institutional clinicopathologic study. *Radiology.* 2009;251 (1):122–133.
16. Perdona S, Di Lorenzo G, Autorino R, et al. Combined magnetic resonance spectroscopy and dynamic contrast-enhanced imaging for prostate cancer detection. *Urol Oncol.* 2013;31:761–765.
17. Sciarra A, Panebianco V, Ciccariello M, et al. Value of magnetic resonance spectroscopy imaging and dynamic contrast-enhanced imaging for detecting prostate cancer foci in men with prior negative biopsy. *Clin Cancer Res.* 2010;16(6):1875–1883.

5.5.3 Future Direction: Contrast Ultrasound

SANJAY KASTURI

EDOUARD J. TRABULSI

ETHAN J. HALPERN

■ INTRODUCTION

Prostate cancer is the most commonly diagnosed cancer in American males, with over 238,000 new cases and over 29,000 deaths expected in 2013, accounting for 28% of newly diagnosed cancer in American men (1). Since its inception in 1968 transrectal ultrasound (TRUS) imaging of the prostate occupies a central role in the diagnosis of prostate cancer. However, conventional TRUS imaging of the prostate is not without pitfalls. Though prostate cancer is traditionally described as hypoechoic lesions on ultrasound (US), it may manifest as isoechoic lesions (40%) or even hyperechoic ones (1%) (2). Our own data suggest that imaging findings on grayscale US are a poor predictor of prostate cancer (3). Furthermore, in one autopsy series, grayscale TRUS demonstrated only a 30% sensitivity for detection of prostatic malignancy (4). This chapter reviews the current literature on US adjuncts for prostate biopsies including color Doppler US, power Doppler US, three-dimensional US (3D US), and elastography, but largely focuses on contrast-enhanced ultrasound (CEUS).

■ COLOR AND POWER DOPPLER US

The tumor biology of prostate cancer and the associated neoplastic angiogenesis result in hypervascular lesions, which may be evaluated with Doppler imaging. Previously, our group analyzed preoperative color Doppler imaging and correlated Doppler findings with final pathologic grade and stage, as well as with biochemical recurrence in men with biopsy-proven prostate cancer. We reported that pathologic outcomes (tumor grade and seminal vesicle invasion) and relapse rates were worse in those men who demonstrated increased flow on preoperative color Doppler compared with those with normal flow patterns (5). Based on this observation, the clinical value of color Doppler US seems evident. To date, several investigators have studied the utility in color Doppler US to improve cancer detection. However, the data are conflicting. Initial reports had wide variations in sensitivities and specificities (6, 7). More recent data from our group also confirms that color Doppler US by itself does not have the sensitivity to replace random biopsy templates (8). However, color Doppler is a useful adjunct, as targeted cores had a higher cancer detection rate than random cores and abnormal color flow was strongly associated with higher Gleason scores 8–10 (9).

Power Doppler US differs from traditional color Doppler US in that power Doppler displays the amplitude of the Doppler signal, while color Doppler displays the frequency of the Doppler shift. Power Doppler has two main advantages over color Doppler. First, power Doppler is more sensitive to slow flow and better for depicting smaller vessels. Second, power Doppler is less angle dependent than conventional color Doppler. This allows one to better track blood vessel continuity when a vessel changes its course. Despite these theoretical advantages, our own studies have failed to demonstrate added benefits of power Doppler over color Doppler (3, 8).

Finally, though prostatic adenocarcinoma is hypervascular and will have large supplying vessels, the neoplastic microvessels themselves are below the resolution of convention color and power Doppler. However, CEUS represents an evolving technological modality that can address this aforementioned problem to image neovascularity, as will be discussed later in this chapter.

■ 3D US

Hamper et al. first examined the utility of 3D US in 16 men undergoing TRUS-guided prostate biopsy. Investigators performed a sextant biopsy and targeted biopsies in any hypoechoic lesion on conventional 2D or 3D. They found subjective improvement in lesion visualization but offered no statistical advantage of 3D imaging (10). In a later study of 180 patients, Mitterberger and colleagues performed 3D

TRUS staging imaging prior to radical prostatectomy and compared these preoperative findings to final pathologic staging. Overall, 3D TRUS had an 84% sensitivity and 96% specificity in identifying macroscopic extracapsular extension (11). To date, the role of 3D TRUS–guided prostate biopsy has yet to be determined.

■ CEUS

CEUS utilizes intravenous microbubble agents that are 1 to 10 microns in diameter. These microbubbles are either air- or gas-filled bubbles, coated with albumin or phospholipid polymers, and are sufficiently small to traverse the rich microvasculature of prostatic adenocarcinoma. Acoustic energy applied to the microbubbles may cause them to rupture or resonate, thereby enhancing the vascular signal and providing improved signal to noise for visualization of vascular anatomy. CEUS affords the opportunity to visualize neovessels that would be missed by conventional Doppler and to identify potentially neoplastic areas.

CEUS is typically performed through Doppler imaging or grayscale harmonic imaging. Both color and power Doppler CEUS employ high mechanical index (MI) US waves. While high MI waves produce an intense Doppler signal by rupturing a large portion of available microbubbles, they do so in larger vessels before microbubbles can enter neoplastic microcirculation. This in turn limits imaging of neovascularity within suspicious areas. Conversely, grayscale harmonic imaging can be performed with lower MI in order to visualize harmonic signals that return from microbubbles that resonate without rupturing as they course into smaller malignant microvessels. Microbubble persistence into the neovasculature may be further enhanced with intermittent imaging modes that reduce the rate of microbubble rupture and destruction.

Finally, flash replenishment is a grayscale imaging technique that utilizes an initial high-energy pulse that destroys microbubbles followed by a series of lower energy pulses that visualize microbubble reentry into the microvasculature. The low-energy pulses result in a harmonic signal from resonating microbubbles as these bubbles enter the microvasculature. This harmonic signal is imaged over multiple frames that are combined in a maximum intensity projection image, thereby highlighting the ultrastructure of malignant microvessels. For simplicity, our discussion will generalize CEUS into Doppler and grayscale harmonic imaging, both of which may be used to visualize vascularity associated with prostate cancer and to guide targeted biopsy of the prostate.

Initial results from our institution utilizing CEUS with color and power Doppler and harmonic grayscale imaging in 301 patients yielded an overall cancer detection rate of 35%, with carcinoma found in 15.5% of targeted cores compared with 10.4% of sextant cores ($P < 0.01$). In addition, individual targeted CEUS cores were twice as likely to return cancer ($OR = 2.0$, $P < 0.001$) as compared with traditional sextant cores (12). However, even though targeted biopsies alone detected 11% of cancers, this modality also missed cancer 20% of the time. In a similar study by Frauscher et al. in 230 subjects, the authors noted an overall cancer detection rate of 30%, including 24.4% rate by targeted cores compared with 22.6% rate by systematic cores (10-core template). In contrast to our findings, the difference in overall cancer detection between targeted and systematic cores was not statistically significant ($P = 0.58$). Despite this, targeted cores were 2.6 times more likely to yield cancer than systematic cores (10.4% versus 5.3%, $P < 0.001$) (13). In this report, CEUS alone missed cancer in only 5.6% of cases. In another large study of 380 patients, Pelzer et al. reported similar findings. These investigators noted that CEUS missed cancer detection in 10.2% of cases (14). Though this missed detection rate is inferior to that reported by Frauscher, it underscores the overall added value of CEUS. Furthermore, in a small study of 35 patients, Seitz and colleagues reported that contrast-enhanced TRUS performed significantly better than traditional TRUS in detecting cancer. The authors noted that on a per-patient basis, contrast-enhanced TRUS was superior to conventional TRUS with sensitivity, specificity, positive predictive value, and negative predictive values of 71%, 50%, 91.7%, and 18.2% versus 45.2%, 75%, 93.3%, and 18% respectively ($P = 0.004$, McNemar test) (15). Interestingly, Colleselli and colleagues reported superior cancer detection rates by CEUS than conventional US with 10-core biopsies in glands <20 cc (88.1% vs. 69%) and 20 to 30 cc (80.8% vs. 70.4%, $P < 0.5$), but failed to show appreciable difference in detection for higher prostate volumes (16).

Several studies have shown that CEUS may also detect more aggressive and clinically significant cancers than conventional methods. In a large study of 690 men with PSA > 1.25 ng/mL or free-to-total PSA < 18%, Mitterberger et al. demonstrated a higher mean Gleason score in cores obtained utilizing CEUS than traditional grayscale imaging (6.8 vs. 5.4, $P < 0.003$). The range of Gleason scores was also higher for CEUS than for traditional grayscale US (6 or greater vs. 4–6) (17). In our most recent experience, CEUS is also more accurate at finding higher grade cancer, as Gleason 7 cancer was found in 55% of targeted cores versus in 17% of systematic cores ($P < 0.001$). In addition, targeted cores had higher volume disease (≥50% core involvement) (18). It should be noted that men in this study were randomized to pretreatment with 2 weeks of dutasteride (see below) and had an abnormal DRE, elevated PSA, or PSA velocity of greater than 0.75ng/mL/y.

Despite these promising results, the acceptance of CEUS should be tempered by its shortcomings, as others have demonstrated no benefit of CEUS in the detection of prostate cancer. Taverna and associates examined prostate cancer detection in a screening population of men (PSA 2.5 ng/mL–9.9 ng/mL) using traditional US (n = 100), color Doppler US (n = 100), and CEUS (n = 100). Patients undergoing traditional US had systematic biopsies, while patients undergoing color Doppler US or CEUS had both targeted and systematic biopsies. Overall, investigators found a 29.3% prostate cancer detection rate; however, they did not find a significant difference among the three groups ($P = 0.329$). Furthermore, color Doppler US and CEUS had poor sensitivities, specificities, and accuracy of 23%, 68%, 53% and 54%, 42%, 47%, respectively (19).

To better differentiate neoplastic and benign areas of the prostate several investigators have examined blood flow patterns with CEUS. Zhao and colleagues assigned a 5-point subjective blood flow scale (previously described by our group) during CEUS in 106 men undergoing prostate biopsy. They noted that increased blood flow during CEUS correlated not only with the presence of cancer, but also with higher Gleason sums ($r = 0.66$, $r = 0.61$, $P < 0.001$) (20). Using micro-flow imaging (MFI), a type of flash replenishment technique, Xie et al. performed both grayscale systematic biopsies and targeted MFI CEUS biopsies. The authors described 4 types of MFI patterns. They found that the sensitivity, specificity, accuracy, and positive and negative predictive values for MFI were 81.1%, 84.3%, 83.3%, 68.6%, and 91.3%, respectively. The authors also noted Gleason scores of cancers with MFI patterns 3 (7.09) or 4 (7.51) were significantly higher than those with patterns 1 (6.17) or 2 (6.59) ($P = 0.001$, $P = 0.005$, $P < 0.001$, $P < 0.001$) (21). These studies highlight the importance of grading schemes to improve the diagnostic capability of CEUS.

In order to increase the efficacy of CEUS, several investigators have utilized pharmacologic augmentation of prostatic microcirculation. Morrelli et al. evaluated the use of vardenafil 20 mg given 1 hour prior to CEUS in 150 men with a PSA of 4 ng/mL or greater. All subjects had a standard 12-core biopsy with grayscale US, and then they had targeted biopsies under CEUS and vardenafil-enhanced CEUS. The authors reported higher cancer detection rates with vardenafil-enhanced CEUS compared with normal CEUS and standard US (41.2% vs. 22.7% vs. 8.1%, $P < 0.005$ and < 0.001, respectively) (22). Conversely, 5α-reductase inhibitors (5ARIs) should decrease blood flow to areas of "high noise" such as those harboring benign prostatic hyperplasia or chronic prostatitis. Initial reports showed promise. In small cohort of 36 patients, Mitterberger et al. demonstrated that a 2 week course of dutasteride decreased blood flow to benign prostatic tissue but not to cancerous areas (23). However, in a large randomized, double-blind trial, our group pretreated 272 patients with dutasteride for 2 weeks and found no difference in cancer detection in the dutasteride group compared with placebo in both targeted (15.3% vs. 17.3%, $P = 0.35$) and sextant core biopsies (7.8% vs. 9.1%, $P = 0.21$) (18). These mixed results underscore the need to refine CEUS technology.

■ ELASTOGRAPHY

Elastography or sonoelastography has been introduced more recently as an adjunct for TRUS to improve detection of prostate cancer. Elastography takes advantage of the fact that cancerous prostate tissue is more dense and, therefore, less elastic than normal gland tissue. Several techniques have been devised to measure tissue elasticity in vivo, including manual compression, vibro-acoustography, Acoustic Radiation Force Impulsion (ARFI), and shear wave imaging (24). In the simplest model of manual compression, an elastogram is generated when the operator compresses and decompresses a target area, and the resulting changes in the reflected radiofrequency pattern are translated into a color-coded map of tissue strain. ARFI and shear wave imaging provide newer methods for elastography that do not require manual tissue compression and may therefore be less subject to differences in operator technique.

Koenig and colleagues noted that in targeted sextant biopsies in 404 patients, cancerous tissues cores demonstrated abnormalities 84.1% of the time on elastograms (25). In the largest elastography study to date in 492 men, Pallwein et al. performed elastography with prospective scoring of lesions prior to systematic 10-core biopsy. The authors reported an overall cancer detection rate of 25.4%. Elastography demonstrated sensitivity and specificity of 86% and 72%, respectively, with a negative predictive value of 91.4% (26). Our group reported in 137 subjects that targeted cores are almost twice as likely to yield a cancer diagnosis than random cores (OR = 1.84, $P = 0.004$) (9). However, elastography detected no abnormality in 53.8% of areas ultimately found to have neoplasia. Though more research is needed, these studies demonstrate the promise of elastography.

■ FUTURE DIRECTIONS

In order to increase the affinity of microbubbles to target neoplastic areas, several investigators have investigated targeted contrast agents. A major limitation in this endeavor is that US microbubble contrast agents remain within the vasculature and cannot be targeted directly to antigens on prostate cancer tissue. Nonetheless, it is possible to target these microbubbles to antigens within neovessels, such as VEGFR2. Tardy et al. examined the utility of BR55, a VEGFR2-specific contrast agent against SonoVue™ (Bracco Diagnostic, Italy). Though both contrast agents showed early phase enhancement, the SonoVue™ was rapidly eliminated. However, BR55 showed late phase enhancement due to VEGFR2 binding. Theoretically, in humans, this late stage binding will allow improvement in target to background discrimination and will result in improved yield of CEUS-targeted biopsies (27). A similar study by Fischer et al. also demonstrated superiority of a VEGFR2-targeted agent over a nonspecific agent in both early inflow analysis and specific accumulation in prostate cancer after 20 minutes (28). Both reports demonstrate promising advances in antigen-specific targeting for the future of CEUS.

■ CONCLUSION

Given the recent controversy over PSA screening and the detection of clinically insignificant prostate cancer, the onus of diagnosing clinically relevant prostate cancer with minimal morbidity is more important now than ever. CEUS and elastography are two emerging adjuncts to conventional TRUS that may allow selective detection of higher grade prostate cancer, and are therefore likely to play an important future role in prostate cancer care. The United States Preventative Service Task Force cited the morbidity of prostate biopsies including biopsy-related infections (29). Both CEUS and elastography may be able to mitigate these risks, as CEUS-targeted biopsies require fewer than half the number of cores as compared with systematic biopsy for diagnosis of cancer (30). Taken together, all these data support the continued investigation of CEUS and elastography as important adjuncts to conventional TRUS.

■ REFERENCES

1. Siegel R, Naishadham D, Jemal A. Cancer Statistics, 2013. *CA Cancer J Clin.* 2013;63(11):11–30.
2. Shinohara K, Wheeler T, Scardino P. The appearance of prostate cancer on transrectal ultrasonography: correlation of imaging and pathological examinations. *J Urol.* 1989;142(1):76–82.
3. Halpern E, Strup S. Using gray scale, color and power Doppler sonography to detect prostatic cancer. *AJR Am J Roentgenol.* 2000;174(3):623–627.
4. Delongchamps N, de la Roza G, Jones R, Jumbelic M, Haas GP. Saturation biopsies on autopsied prostates for detecting and characterizing prostate cancer. *BJU Int.* 2009;103(1):49–54.
5. Ismail M, Petersen R, Alexander A, Newschaffer C, Gomella LG. Color Doppler imaging in predicting the biologic behavior of prostate cancer: correlation with disease-free survival. *Urology.* 1997;50(6):906–912.
6. Rifkin M, Sudakoff G, Alexander A. Prostate: techniques, results, and potential applications of color Doppler US scanning. *Radiology.* 1993;186(2):509–513.
7. Newman J, Bree R, Rubin JM. Prostate cancer: diagnosis with color Doppler sonography with histologic correlation of each biopsy site. *Radiology.* 1995;195(1):86–90.
8. Halpern E, Frauscher F, Strup S, Nazarian LN, O'Kane P, Gomella LG. Prostate: high-frequency Doppler US imaging for cancer detection. *Radiology.* 2002;225(1):71–77.
9. Nelson E, Slotoroff C, Gomella G, Halpern EJ. Targeted biopsy of the prostate: the impact of color Doppler imaging and elastography on prostate cancer detection and Gleason score. *Urology.* 2007;70(6):1136–1140.
10. Hamper U, Trapanotto V, DeJong M, Sheth S, Caskey CI. Three-dimensional US of the prostate: early experience. *Radiology.* 1999;212(3):719–723.
11. Mitterberger M, Pinggera G, Pallwein L, et al. The value of three-dimensional transrectal ultrasonography in staging prostate cancer. *BJU Int.* 2007;100(1):47–50.
12. Halpern E, Ramey J, Strup S, Frauscher F, McCue P, Gomella LG. Detection of prostate carcinoma with contrast-enhanced sonography using intermittent harmonic imaging. *Cancer.* 2005;104(11):2373–2383.
13. Frauscher F, Klauser A, Volgger H, et al. Comparison of contrast enhanced color Doppler targeted biopsy with conventional systematic biopsy: impact on prostate cancer detection. *J Urol.* 2002;167(4):1648–1652.
14. Pelzer A, Bektic J, Berger A, et al. Prostate cancer detection in men with prostate specific antigen 4 to 10 ng/ml using a combined approach of contrast enhanced color Doppler targeted and systematic biopsy. *J Urol.* 2005;173(6):1926–1929.
15. Seitz M, Gratzke C, Schlenker B, et al. Contrast-enhanced transrectal ultrasound (CE-TRUS) with cadence-contrast pulse sequence (CPS) technology for the identification of prostate cancer. *Urol Oncol.* 2011;29(3):295–301.
16. Colleselli D, Bektic J, Schaefer G, et al. The influence of prostate volume on prostate cancer detection using combined approach of contrast-enhanced ultrasonography-targeted and systematic grey-scale biopsy. *BJU Int.* 2007;100(6):1264–1267.
17. Mitterberger M, Pinggera G, Horninger W, et al. Comparison of contrast enhanced color Doppler targeted biopsy to conventional systematic biopsy: impact on Gleason score. *J Urol.* 2007;178(2):464–468.
18. Halpern E, Gomella G, Forsberg F, McCue PA, Trabulsi EJ. Contrast enhanced transrectal ultrasound for the detection of prostate cancer: a randomized, double-blind trial of dutasteride pretreatment. *J Urol.* 2012;188(5):1739–1745.
19. Taverna G, Morandi G, Seveso M, et al. Colour Doppler and microbubble contrast agent ultrasonography do not improve cancer detection rate in transrectal systematic prostate biopsy sampling. *BJU Int.* 2011;108(11):1723–1727.
20. Zhao H, Luo J, Xu H, et al. The value of contrast-enhanced transrectal ultrasound in predicting the nature of prostate disease and the Gleason score of prostate cancer by a subjective blood flow grading scale. *Urol Int.* 2011;87(2):165–170.
21. Xie S, Li F, Li H, et al. Value of contrast-enhanced sonography with micro flow imaging in the diagnosis of prostate cancer. *J Clin Ultrasound.* 2011;39(7):371–377.
22. Morelli G, Pagni R, Mariani C, et al. Results of vardenafil mediated power Doppler ultrasound, contrast enhanced ultrasound and systematic random biopsies to detect prostate cancer. *J Urol.* 2011;185(6):2126–2131.
23. Mitterberger, Pinggera G, Horninger W, et al. Dutasteride prior to contrast enhanced colour Doppler ultrasound prostate biopsy increases prostate cancer detection. *Eur Urol.* 2008;53(1):112–117.
24. Gennisson J, Deffieux T, Fink M, Tanter M. Ultrasound elastography: principles and techniques. *Diagn Interv Imaging.* 2013;94(5):487–495.

25. Konig, Scheipers U, Pesavento A, Lorenz A, Ermert H, Senge T. Initial experiences with real-time elastography guided biopsies of the prostate. *J Urol.* 2005;174(1):115–117.
26. Pallwein L, Mitterberger M, Pinggera G, et al. Sonoelastography of the prostate: comparison with systematic biopsy findings in 492 patients. *Eur J Radiol.* 2008;65(2):304–310.
27. Tardy I, Ponchon S, Theraulaz M, et al. Ultrasound molecular imaging of VEGFR2 in a rate prostate tumor model using BR55. *Invest Radiol.* 2010;45(10):573–578.
28. Fischer T, Thomas A, Tardy I, et al. Vascular endothelial growth factor receptor 2-specific molecular ultrasound detection of prostate cancer in a rat model. *Invest Radiol.* 2010;45(10):675–684.
29. Moyer V. U.S. Preventive Services Task Force. Screening for prostate cancer: U.S. Preventive Service Task Force recommendation statement. *Ann Intern Med.* 2012;157(2):120–134.
30. Wink M, Frauscher F, Cosgrove D, et al. Contrast-enhanced ultrasound and prostate cancer; a multicenter European research coordination project. *Eur Urol.* 2008;54(5):982–992.

6 Counseling Patients With Clinically Localized, High-Risk Prostate Cancer

JONATHAN L. SILBERSTEIN
JAMES A. EASTHAM

Serum prostate-specific antigen (PSA) screening has resulted in a dramatic shift toward detection of prostate cancer at earlier stages of disease, with a decrease in the number of men with metastatic disease at the time of their diagnosis (1). Despite this trend toward the diagnosis of lower risk prostate cancer in the PSA era, 20% to 35% of newly diagnosed patients are classified as high risk, based on PSA level, prostate biopsy Gleason score, and/or clinical examination (2). Those diagnosed with clinically localized, high-risk prostate cancer are at greater risk of failing local therapy after radical prostatectomy (RP) or radiation therapy (RT), with subsequent higher rates of disease progression and prostate cancer–specific mortality (PCSM) than lower risk prostate cancer patients. Because anticipated outcomes for local treatment options are significantly worse, men with high-risk cancer require different counseling than their lower risk counterparts, including discussion of anticipated oncologic outcomes, recovery of functional outcomes, and the potential need for secondary therapies.

While controversy exists regarding the need to treat men with low-risk prostate cancer, men with clinically localized, high-risk cancer unequivocally benefit from treatment as long as the man is of reasonable age and health. In the U.S. Prostate Cancer Intervention Versus Observation Trial (PIVOT), men with intermediate- and high-risk prostate cancer demonstrated an improved PCSM with RP compared with observation (3). Similar findings were reported in the Scandinavian Prostate Cancer Group (SPCG) Study 4 randomizing men with prostate cancer to RP or observation (4). Finally, the randomized trial SPCG-7 demonstrated improvement in both PCSM and overall survival with RT plus androgen deprivation therapy (ADT) compared with ADT alone (5). Thus, while the preferred treatment paradigm has yet to be defined, local therapy in men with clinically localized, high-risk prostate cancer is certainly preferable to observation or ADT alone. Unfortunately, no appropriately powered randomized trials have compared outcomes following the various active forms of local treatment. Nevertheless, physicians can counsel patients based on the guidance from several population-based and institutionally based retrospective studies that have reported oncologic and quality-of-life (QoL) outcomes following treatment. In offering guidance, it is important that the physician take into account the patient's overall clinical health and baseline urinary and erectile function, as well as the patient's individualized preferences. In this chapter, we are reviewing important considerations for men with clinically localized, high-risk prostate cancer, including treatment options and strategies for counseling these men.

■ ESTABLISHING REALISTIC EXPECTATIONS

Patients with newly diagnosed, clinically localized, high-risk prostate cancer must be counseled regarding the risk their cancer poses to them. These men should be informed that much of the current attention in the media and the scientific literature suggesting that prostate cancer screening should be discouraged and that this disease is overtreated in the majority of men is not applicable to their situation (6). In PIVOT, 731 men were randomized to RP or observation. While the study showed no overall benefit for surgery compared with observation (7), the subgroup of men meeting the National Comprehensive Cancer Network (NCCN) definition of high-risk disease who were treated with RP had significant reductions in PCSM at 12 years compared with the observation arm (9.1% vs. 17.5%, $P = .04$). Although many prostate cancers may not need immediate treatment, cancers with high-risk features carry a significant risk for progression to metastasis and cancer-specific death; therefore, men with high-risk features are poor candidates for observation.

Approximately 30,000 men die of prostate cancer every year in the United States. Although the majority have high-risk features at the time of their diagnosis, not all men with clinically localized, high-risk prostate cancer will die of their disease (8). Depending on the definition of high-risk disease, local treatment with either RP or RT results in progression-free probability of 49% to 80% (9). Furthermore, in the event that the patient is not "cured" with local treatment, death from prostate cancer is not likely to be imminent; there is frequently a long interval from diagnosis to death, on the order of years to decades, rather than weeks to months (10). Results from a recent multi-institutional study demonstrated that men with clinically localized, high-risk prostate cancer treated with RP had a 15-year PCSM of 19%, which was significantly less than the 31% (95% confidence interval [CI], 26%–57%) mortality rate from competing causes (11). Finally, for patients who do not respond to local treatment, tremendous advances have been made in the treatment of metastatic prostate cancer. Since 2004, six new therapies, all providing survival benefit for patients with metastatic disease, have been approved by the U.S. Food and Drug Administration (12).

Conveying information about risk and potential recurrence after local therapy may be challenging, but it is critical for the patient to have an adequate perspective about his cancer. Once the patient has a better understanding of the risk his cancer poses, a more in-depth conversation regarding treatment options and goals can commence.

■ DEFINING CLINICALLY LOCALIZED, HIGH-RISK PROSTATE CANCER

Prostate cancer is not a uniform disease, meaning every cancer does not carry the same risk and thus the same prognosis. As such, no one treatment strategy is appropriate for every newly diagnosed patient. Even within the subsets of patients characterized as high risk there is significant heterogeneity with a wide diversity of clinical features influencing oncologic outcomes.

It is unclear how to best define high-risk disease. Yossepowitch and colleagues reviewed eight common definitions of high-risk prostate cancer (Table 6.1) (9). These definitions ranged from single clinical features such as clinical stage T3 (cT3) to multivariable models relying on several clinical factors. Depending on the definition of high risk, outcomes after treatment varied tremendously (Figure 6.1). This study highlights the importance of considering the definition of high risk when comparing outcomes between studies.

The American Urological Association, the European Association of Urology, and the NCCN all define high risk in a similar fashion, with patients presenting one or more of the following three characteristics: PSA > 20 ng/mL or Gleason grade ≥ 4+4 or clinical examination ≥ T3 (the American Urological Association uses clinical examination of ≥T2c). While risk-based groupings allow simple categorization of patients, they fail to distinguish the diversity of outcomes within any one group. For example, these groupings fail to distinguish a patient with multiple high-risk features from a patient with a single high-risk feature such that although both men are considered at high risk, they may have very different prognoses (13, 14). An alternative, although more complex, strategy for cate gorizing men into risk groups is to determine individualized risk through the use of multivariable models or nomograms. Nomograms incorporate multiple risk factors that are proportionately weighted to their relative contribution, allowing more accurate assessment of the probability of treatment failure or, more important, the likelihood of metastatic progression or prostate cancer–specific survival.

■ Table 6.1 Eight high-risk prostate cancer definitions based on preoperative variables

Definition No.	High-Risk Definition	Description	No. Pts (% Cohort)
1	Biopsy 8–10	Poorly differentiated Ca (4)	274 (6)
2	Preop PSA 20 ng/mL or greater		275 (6)
3	1992 TNM cT3	Locally advanced Ca (3)	144 (3)
4	PSA 20 ng/mL or greater, 1992 TNM cT2C or greater, or biopsy GS 8–10	D'Amico high risk definition (1)	957 (20)
5	Nomogram 5-y PFP 50% or less	Preop nomogram, 60% or less PFP is entry criterion for Ca + Leukemia Group B Trial 90203	391 (8)
6	PSA 20 ng/mL or greater, 1992 TNM cT3 or greater, or biopsy GS 8–10	National Comprehensive Ca Network guidelines for clinically localized high risk Ca (6)	605 (13)
7	PSA 15 ng/mL or greater, 1992 TNM cT2B or greater, or biopsy GS 8–10	Entry criteria into neoadjuvant chemotherapy trials for high risk pts (21, 22)	1,752 (37)
8	Preop PSA velocity greater than 2 ng/mL/y	Increased risk of prostate Ca specific mortality after RP or radiotherapy (12)	952 (38)[a]

[a]Percentage of 2,521 patients with calculable preoperative PSA velocity.

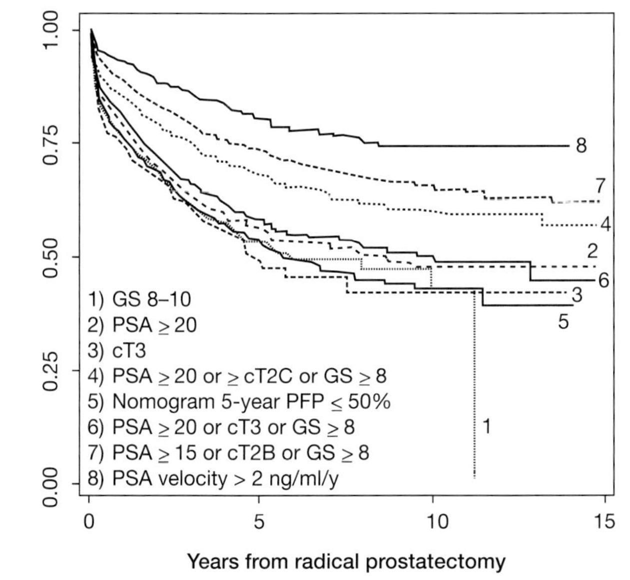

Numbers at risk:

1)	274	110	51	28	11	2	1
2)	275	146	106	66	30	14	4
3)	144	63	34	13	6	2	1
4)	957	557	375	213	112	36	10
5)	391	198	124	75	35	11	3
6)	605	295	179	100	42	16	4
7)	1752	1094	727	429	230	76	20
8)	952	564	308	163	65	10	1

FIGURE 6.1 PFP for patients with high-risk prostate cancer by various definitions treated with RP alone.

No one model for predicting risk is perfect; all are subject to the limitations of clinical assessment based on PSA, digital rectal examination, and prostate biopsy Gleason score. Clinical staging with digital rectal examination is subjective and lacks clinical precision; approximately 25% of patients classified with cT3 disease are down-staged to organ-confined disease at the time of RP (15). PSA levels reflect not only the burden of cancer, but also the volume of benign prostatic hyperplasia and the presence of inflammation. Gleason score is subjective, and thus dependent on the interpretation of the individual pathologist. In addition, a prostate biopsy does not sample the entire gland. Changes in Gleason grading between the biopsy specimen and the RP specimen have been demonstrated to occur in 36% of cases at tertiary care centers with expert dedicated genitourinary pathologists (16). The potential for error in each of these clinical features underscores the importance of using multivariable models that use all available data rather than any single parameter.

Workup to Better Define the Extent of the Patient's Disease

Patients with high-risk prostate cancer may have regional or distant metastasis at diagnosis. Before counseling the patient on treatment options, the extent of the disease must be defined. The NCCN recommends technetium 99m (Tc99m) bone scintigraphy in any patient with NCCN-defined high-risk cancer (PSA > 20 ng/mL or clinical stage ≥ T3 or Gleason score ≥ 8) or any patient with cT2 disease and PSA > 10 ng/mL. Pelvic computed tomography (CT) or magnetic resonance imaging (MRI) is recommended only in patients with ≥ cT3 disease or nomogram probability >10% for lymph node involvement (17). At Memorial Sloan-Kettering Cancer Center, prostate MRI is routinely performed prior to treatment since it may assist with treatment planning (either RP or RT). This is of particular importance for patients with high-risk disease, as they are at risk for extraprostatic extension. Knowing the location and extent of extraprostatic extension may better allow the clinician to plan the appropriate treatment for the individual patient.

Because of the lack of specificity and sensitivity of bone scintigraphy, newer imaging modalities are being explored, such as fluorodeoxyglucose ^{18}F positron emission tomography (PET), ^{11}C-choline–acetate PET, ^{18}F-fluorodihydrotestosterone PET, or single-photon emission CT scanning. Although various metabolic tracers combined with PET or PET/CT are encouraging and may have increased ability to detect bone lesions when compared with traditional Tc99m bone scintigraphy (18), one of the more promising new imaging modalities is whole-body MRI, which has the ability to detect both bony and soft tissue lesions and has the potential to replace other modalities used to evaluate for metastatic disease. Recent investigators have demonstrated that whole-body MRI may be more sensitive than bone scintigraphy in detecting metastatic lesions without any loss of specificity and equally effective as CT scanning for detecting adenopathy (19). Emerging imaging modalities to better assess the presence of micrometastatic lesions are likely to become an increasingly integral step in the evaluation of the high-risk patient.

■ TREATMENT OPTIONS

Multiple treatment options are available for patients with clinically localized, high-risk prostate cancer. For patients with life expectancy > 5.5 years, RP or RT plus ADT are both preferred options according to NCCN guidelines (20). However, the CaPSURE database, a provider-based registry from a number of community-based urology practices, has demonstrated that 41% of high-risk patients receive ADT alone, compared with 24% and 28% who undergo RP or RT, respectively (21). Monotherapy with ADT is not curative, has the potential for significant harm, reduces QoL, and is not indicated for patients with asymptomatic localized disease. The reasons for the continued use of ADT as the primary treatment option in this population are unclear, but this practice is strongly discouraged.

Surgery

Historically, RP has not been a widely used treatment option for men with clinically localized, high-risk prostate cancer due to high rates of biochemical failure, coupled with the perception that surgical morbidity was higher in these men than in those with low- or intermediate-risk cancer. Improvements in surgical technique and the associated outcomes have led some to question the view that surgery not be performed in the high-risk setting. The precise description of pelvic anatomy by Walsh and Donker led to a refinement in surgical approach, making for a safer and more reproducible procedure (22). This dramatically reduced convalescence and morbidity, with an associated improvement in functional recovery following RP. Results from recent surgical series suggest that continence can be preserved in most cases and is not influenced by disease risk. Furthermore, in selected cases, potency may be preserved as well (23). Although biochemical recurrence (BCR) rates remain greater for patients with high-risk than lower risk disease, it has become increasingly clear that oncologic outcomes following RP rival or may surpass those of RT plus ADT. Additionally, surgery provides excellent local control (24) and can readily be combined with either adjuvant or salvage RT, which is well tolerated with minimal impact on functional outcomes. Although RP remains underused in men with clinically localized, high-risk disease, recent Surveillance, Epidemiology and End Results (SEER) data suggest that the use of RP alone in this setting has increased from 2% in 1998 to 10% in 2005 (25). Provided that the patient is an adequate surgical candidate and that the tumor has not invaded adjacent organs (cT4), RP is a reasonable treatment option.

Progression-free probability after RP for patients with clinically localized, high-risk prostate cancer has been examined in multiple series and ranges from 49% to 80% at 5 years depending on the definition of high-risk disease (9,26,27). More recent publications have placed a greater emphasis on PCSM because this is a more meaningful outcome. Stephenson and colleagues examined a multi-institutional cohort of more than 12,000 prostate cancer patients treated with RP and noted the 15-year PCSM was 19% for patients classified as high risk (11). This result compares favorably with the 50% to 70% PCSM reported for similar-risk patients from unscreened populations who received no curative treatment (28).

RP is one of the most complex operations performed by urologists. Outcomes are sensitive to the surgeon's experience and to the technique and approach used by the individual surgeon (29–31). It should be noted that, because of the high risk of extraprostatic extension, surgical considerations for this population are different from men with lower risk disease. As in every RP, the most important goal is removing all local disease and achieving a negative surgical margin. Even after adjusting for other prognostic factors, a positive surgical margin has been associated with as much as a fourfold increased risk for BCR (32). Importantly, unlike other prognostic factors such as PSA or Gleason score, a positive surgical margin is modifiable and dependent on surgical technique. While controversy exists regarding the role (staging vs. therapeutic) and extent of pelvic lymphadenectomy at the time of RP, our bias is to perform a complete pelvic lymph node dissection including the external iliac, obturator, and hypogastric nodes. RP may be curative for patients with limited regional nodal metastasis, and knowing the histologic status of the nodes may guide future treatment (33). In one series, progression-free probability following RP was reported to be as high as 79% 2 years after RP alone for patients with one positive node and a Gleason score < 7 in the RP specimen (34). Even in men experiencing BCR in the setting of positive lymph nodes, clinical progression is not necessarily imminent, with many men experiencing a prolonged survival (35,36).

Despite encouraging long-term results after RP in men with clinically localized, high-risk prostate cancer, many men still experience BCR. As such, strong consideration should be given to enrollment in a clinical trial. Of particular interest are trials with neoadjuvant chemo-hormonal therapy followed by RP, such as the currently accruing Cancer and Leukemia Group B randomized phase III study of RP alone versus neoadjuvant docetaxel plus ADT before RP (NCT00430183) (37). The goals of such trials are to obtain optimal local control while also addressing the potential metastatic component of the disease, as is the paradigm in multiple other malignancies (38–40).

Radiation Therapy

For high-risk patients who elect curative treatment with RT, level 1 evidence demonstrated a significant survival advantage with RT plus ADT rather than RT alone. The European Organisation for Research and Treatment of Cancer (EORTC) 22863 study recruited 415 men diagnosed with cT1-2 World Health Organization (WHO) grade 3 prostate cancer, or cT3-4 N0-1 M0 prostate cancer of any histologic grade, and compared RT plus adjuvant ADT (for 3 years) with RT alone (41). With a median follow-up period of 66 months, combination therapy yielded significantly better overall survival than RT alone (78% vs. 62%, $P = .001$). Updated results from this study were recently published, confirming the initial findings and demonstrating 10-year overall survival rates of 40% in patients receiving RT alone and 58% in those allocated to combined treatment (hazard ratio [HR] 0.60, 95% CI 0.45–0.80, $P = .0004$) (42). This landmark study clearly demonstrated that RT plus ADT is the standard of care for high-risk patients. Subsequent studies have focused on the length of time ADT needs to be administered. While short-term ADT before and during RT has been shown to improve cancer control and overall survival compared with no ADT (43), it may not be as effective as longer durations of ADT.

With a 5.2-year median follow-up, the 5-year overall survival rate was 85.3% with 3 years of adjuvant ADT and 80.6% with 6 months of adjuvant ADT (HR 1.43; 96.4% CI 1.04–1.98) (44). Current NCCN guidelines recommend 2 to 3 years of neoadjuvant/concomitant/adjuvant ADT for patients with high-risk cancers, whereas European Association of Urology guidelines recommend 3 years of adjuvant ADT for these patients. Thus, the patient at high risk should receive a minimum of 2 years of ADT and should be informed of the potential harms that may negatively impact QoL, such as decreased libido, erectile dysfunction, vasomotor symptoms, impaired cognitive function, and metabolic abnormalities.

Modern RT techniques allow the administration of higher doses of radiation to the prostate without increasing adverse effects by using CT images and computer software to specifically conform the RT to the prostate. Higher radiation doses (often referred to as dose escalation) have been demonstrated to result in improved BCR-free survival (45–48) and in one study improved metastases-free survival (47). A recent retrospective study found that for patients with high-risk prostate cancer, RT doses greater than 81 Gy were associated with reduced rates of BCR (49). The NCCN guidelines currently recommend that high-risk patients should receive doses up to 81 Gy (17).

Surgery Versus Radiation Therapy

Although no adequately powered randomized controlled trials have compared RT (with or without ADT) with RP, recent publications may provide some insight and be used for counseling patients. The majority of these studies focus on oncologic outcomes from single centers or population-based data sets (50, 51). Zelefsky and colleagues compared progression to metastasis and PCSM in a matched cohort of 2,380 prostate cancer patients treated with RP or RT (51). To account for potential differences in outcome related to practitioner experience, the study included only patients treated by two experienced surgeons or by four radiation oncologists focused on patients with prostate cancer. All patients treated surgically underwent an open RP with pelvic lymph node dissection, and patients who underwent RT received a prescription dose ≥81 Gy. After adjustment for case mix, RP in the whole cohort was associated with a reduced risk for metastasis (HR 0.35, 95% CI 0.19–0.65, $p < .001$) and PCSM (HR 0.32, 95% CI 0.13–0.80, $p < .015$). Note that the magnitude of the difference in outcome between treatment types was greatest for patients with higher-risk cancers (Figure 6.2). When the analysis was restricted to patients with NCCN-defined high-risk prostate cancer, the likelihood of dying of prostate cancer was more than double if RT was used (9.5%; 95% CI 4.9%– 17.9%) rather than RP (3.8%; 95% CI 1.2%–11.5%).

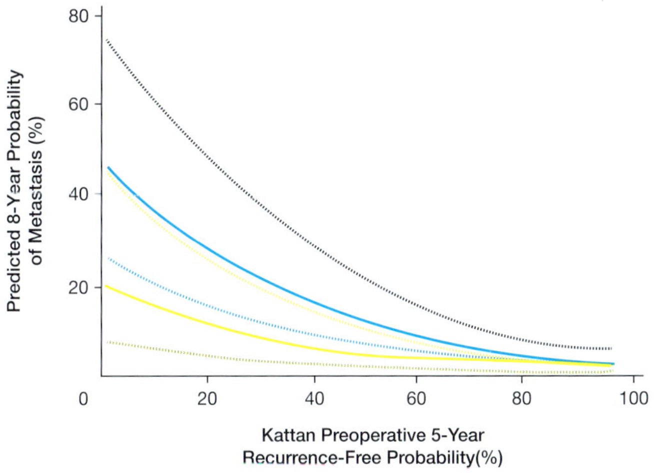

FIGURE 6.2 Predicted 8-year probability of metastases by preoperative nomogram risk, separately by treatment. Blue: radiation; gold: surgery. Dotted lines are 95% CIs. Probabilities are adjusted for a patient at the mean age for the cohort (64 years) treated at the end of the study (2002).

Similar conclusions have been reached using population-based datasets (50, 52, 53). Abdollah et al., using SEER data, noted significantly lower mortality rates (both PCSM and non-PCSM) after RP than RT at 10 years for men younger than 70 years of age (52). For patients 70 to 79 years of age, there was no significant difference in PCSM between RP and RT groups, although both modalities demonstrated significantly better outcomes than observation. For patients older than 80 years, RT was associated with lower rates of PCSM and non-PCSM than RP. In a separate study, Cooperberg et al. compared the outcomes of patients who received RP, RT, or primary ADT in the CaPSURE database (53). After adjusting for age and cancer risk, the HR for PCSM relative to RP was 2.21 (95% CI 1.50–3.24) for RT and 3.22 (95% CI 2.16–4.81) for ADT. The authors noted that the benefit of RP over other treatments increased with increasing baseline cancer risk. For example, patients in the highest-risk group had a 10-year rate of PCSM dramatically lower with RP (HR 36, 95% CI 21–57) than with RT (HR 46, 95% CI 29–68). Ongoing randomized controlled trials comparing RP with RT do exist but will take many years before they reach maturity (54). In the interim, retrospective studies provide increasing evidence that RP should be considered a standard treatment option for men with clinically localized, high-risk prostate cancer.

Functional Outcomes of Surgery Versus Radiation Therapy

Oncologic outcomes are not the only consideration for patients with clinically localized, high-risk prostate cancer. QoL outcomes are also an important consideration for many patients. Understanding an individual's specific concerns with respect to QoL, as well as his baseline erectile function, urinary continence, and lower urinary tract symptoms, is paramount to helping him in his decision-making process (55). Similar to cancer outcomes, little data exist in terms of randomized trials evaluating QoL measures following RP relative to RT. As such, data must be extrapolated from reported results of tertiary referral centers and population-based cohorts, although the best of these studies include few men with high-risk disease (56–58). Despite these limitations, some clear patterns emerge and may be informative to patients. All treatment is associated with at least temporary diminution of QoL with adverse effects on urinary and sexual function (58–60). Collectively, comparative studies indicate that RP is associated with an increased rate of urinary incontinence, RT is associated with greater urinary irritation and tends to have an adverse impact on bowel function, all treatments have a long-term negative impact on sexual QoL, and the differences between these treatments tend to equilibrate over time (61). These negative treatment effects are likely to be exacerbated in high-risk patients because of the need for adjuvant or salvage therapies. For patients who elect RT, adjuvant ADT has an added negative impact on QoL (58). Similarly, patients who receive adjuvant or salvage interventions after RP are likely to experience further adverse effects on health-related QoL (62–64).

■ MULTIDISCIPLINARY APPROACH

Once the practitioner has ruled out radiographic evidence of metastatic disease, discussed the natural history of clinically localized, high-risk prostate cancer, and reviewed the oncologic and functional outcome data for various treatment options, almost invariably the patient will then turn to the physician and ask, "What should I do?" The answer to this question should not come from a single physician or from several physicians in one specialty area. It is imperative that patients receive counseling from physicians in multiple fields who specialize in the management of prostate cancer. Ideally, these physicians will work together as part of a multidisciplinary team to most reliably present the patient with all of his treatment options and revealing all of the biases of the physicians involved (65). Relying on a single physician or a single type of specialist may not present a full picture. In addition, patients with high-risk prostate cancer have a fair probability of receiving treatment from urologic surgeons, medical oncologists, and radiation therapists over the course of their disease management. Starting these relationships early will likely enhance patient satisfaction with their care.

■ SUMMARY

Advising the high-risk prostate cancer patient is difficult, in large part due to the paucity of high-quality data comparing outcomes of different treatment modalities. Furthermore, ambiguity with clinical staging and lack of sensitive imaging modalities limit a clear definition of high-risk disease without pathologic staging. There is strong evidence that intervention with curative intent results in improvements in metastasis-free survival, prostate cancer–specific survival, and overall survival compared with observation. Unfortunately, although cure is possible for many patients, for others, initial local treatment may fail and require local adjuvant, salvage, or systemic therapy.

Counseling patients with high-risk disease is fraught with a number of pitfalls, and much of the initial management involves (re)educating the patient on how and why his disease may be different from a friend or relative with prostate cancer, and how that may impact his treatment options or recommendations. Ultimately, the physician must convey the same information content to all patients with newly diagnosed prostate cancer, review the natural history of the disease, rule out metastases (in selected patients), discuss available treatment options including risks, try to tailor those treatments to what is best for the individual needs and desire of the patient, and encourage the patient to seek other opinions. Although the same pieces of information are being conveyed, the data and recommendations are different for men with high-risk disease and should be presented as such. In the future, genetic tests and improved imaging modalities may help us to better characterize an individual's disease and guide the best therapy. Until that time, emphasizing to the patient the limitations of available data is critical in any complete discussion.

■ REFERENCES

1. Etzioni R, Gulati R, Falcon S, Penson DF. Impact of PSA screening on the incidence of advanced stage prostate cancer in the United States: a surveillance modeling approach. *Med Decis Making.* 2008;28:323–331.
2. Shao YH, Demissie K, Shih W, et al. Contemporary risk profile of prostate cancer in the United States. *J Natl Cancer Inst.* 2009;101:1280–1283.
3. Wilt TJ, Brawer MK, Jones KM, et al. Radical prostatectomy versus observation for localized prostate cancer. *N Engl J Med.* 2012;367:203–213.
4. Bill-Axelson A, Holmberg L, Ruutu M, et al. Radical prostatectomy versus watchful waiting in early prostate cancer. *N Engl J Med.* 2011;364:1708–1717.
5. Widmark A, Klepp O, Solberg A, et al. Endocrine treatment, with or without radiotherapy, in locally advanced prostate cancer (SPCG-7/SFUO-3): an open randomised phase III trial. *Lancet.* 2009;373:301–308.

6. U.S. Preventive Services Task Force. *Screening For Prostate Cancer: Current Recommendation.* http://www. uspreventiv eservicestaskforce.org/prostatecancerscreening.htm. Updated May 2012. Accessed May 15, 2013.
7. Vickers AJ, Eastham JA, Scardino PT. Radical prostatectomy versus observation for prostate cancer. *N Engl J Med.* 2012;367:1467–1468; author reply 8-9.
8. Siegel R, Naishadham D, Jemal A. Cancer statistics, 2012. *CA Cancer J Clin.* 2012;62:10–29.
9. Yossepowitch O, Eggener SE, Bianco FJ Jr, et al. Radical prostatectomy for clinically localized, high risk prostate cancer: critical analysis of risk assessment methods. *J Urol.* 2007;178:493–499; discussion 9.
10. Pound CR, Partin AW, Eisenberger MA, Chan DW, Pearson JD, Walsh PC. Natural history of progression after PSA elevation following radical prostatectomy. *JAMA.* 1999;281:1591–1597.
11. Stephenson AJ, Kattan MW, Eastham JA, et al. Prostate cancer-specific mortality after radical prostatectomy for patients treated in the prostate-specific antigen era. *J Clin Oncol.* 2009;27:4300–4305.
12. Shore N, Mason M, de Reijke TM. New developments in castrate-resistant prostate cancer. *BJU Int.* 2012;109(suppl 6):22-32.
13. Gontero P, Spahn M, Tombal B, et al. Is there a prostate-specific antigen upper limit for radical prostatectomy? *BJU Int.* 2011;108:1093–1100.
14. Spahn M, Joniau S, Gontero P, et al. Outcome predictors of radical prostatectomy in patients with prostate-specific antigen greater than 20 ng/mL: a European multi-institutional study of 712 patients. *Eur Urol.* 2010;58:1–7; discussion 10-11.
15. Carver BS, Bianco FJ Jr, Scardino PT, Eastham JA. Long-term outcome following radical prostatectomy in men with clinical stage T3 prostate cancer. *J Urol.* 2006;176:564–568.
16. Epstein JI, Feng Z, Trock BJ, Pierorazio PM. Upgrading and downgrading of prostate cancer from biopsy to radical prostatectomy: incidence and predictive factors using the modified Gleason grading system and factoring in tertiary grades. *Eur Urol.* 2012;61:1019–1024.
17. National Comprehensive Cancer Network. *NCCN Clinical Practice Guidelines in Oncology: Prostate Cancer; Version 2.2013.* Page PROS-1. http://www.nccn.org/professionals/physician_gls/pdf/prostate.pdf. Updated March 11, 2013. Accessed May 17, 2013.
18. Tombal B, Lecouvet F. Modern detection of prostate cancer's bone metastasis: is the bone scan era over? *Adv Urol.* 2012;2012:893193.
19. Lecouvet FE, El Mouedden J, Collette L, et al. Can whole-body magnetic resonance imaging with diffusion-weighted imaging replace Tc 99m bone scanning and computed tomography for single-step detection of metastases in patients with high-risk prostate cancer? *Eur Urol.* 2012;62:68–75.
20. Mohler JL, Armstrong AJ, Bahnson RR, et al. Prostate cancer, Version 3.2012: featured updates to the NCCN guidelines. *J Natl Compr Canc Netw.* 2012;10:1081–1087.
21. Cooperberg MR, Broering JM, Carroll PR. Time trends and local variation in primary treatment of localized prostate cancer. *J Clin Oncol.* 2010;28:1117–1123.
22. Walsh PC, Donker PJ. Impotence following radical prostatectomy: insight into etiology and prevention. *J Urol.* 1982;128:492–497.
23. Loeb S, Smith ND, Roehl KA, Catalona WJ. Intermediate-term potency, continence, and survival outcomes of radical prostatectomy for clinically high-risk or locally advanced prostate cancer. *Urology.* 2007;69:1170–1175.
24. Paparel P, Cronin AM, Savage C, Scardino PT, Eastham JA. Oncologic outcome and patterns of recurrence after salvage radical prostatectomy. *Eur Urol.* 2009;55:404–410.
25. Lowrance WT, Elkin EB, Yee DS, et al. Locally advanced prostate cancer: a population-based study of treatment patterns. *BJU Int.* 2012;109:1309–1314.
26. D'Amico AV, Whittington R, Malkowicz SB, et al. Pretreatment nomogram for prostate-specific antigen recurrence after radical prostatectomy or external-beam radiation therapy for clinically localized prostate cancer. *J Clin Oncol.* 1999;17:168–172.
27. Ward JF, Slezak JM, Blute ML, Bergstralh EJ, Zincke H. Radical prostatectomy for clinically advanced (cT3) prostate cancer since the advent of prostate-specific antigen testing: 15-year outcome. *BJU Int.* 2005;95:751–756.
28. Cuzick J, Fisher G, Kattan MW, et al. Long-term outcome among men with conservatively treated localised prostate cancer. *Br J Cancer.* 2006;95:1186–1194.
29. Bianco FJ Jr, Vickers AJ, Cronin AM, et al. Variations among experienced surgeons in cancer control after open radical prostatectomy. *J Urol.* 2010;183:977–982.
30. Saranchuk JW, Kattan MW, Elkin E, Touijer AK, Scardino PT, Eastham JA. Achieving optimal outcomes after radical prostatectomy. *J Clin Oncol.* 2005;23:4146–4151.
31. Silberstein JL, Su D, Glickman L, et al. A case-mix-adjusted comparison of early oncological outcomes of open and robotic prostatectomy performed by experienced high volume surgeons. *BJU Int.* 2013;111:206–212.
32. Yossepowitch O, Eastham JA. Radical prostatectomy for high-risk prostate cancer. *World J Urol.* 2008;26:219–224.
33. Bader P, Burkhard FC, Markwalder R, Studer UE. Disease progression and survival of patients with positive lymph nodes after radical prostatectomy. Is there a chance of cure? *J Urol.* 2003;169:849–854.
34. von Bodman C, Godoy G, Chade DC, et al. Predicting biochemical recurrence-free survival for patients with positive pelvic lymph nodes at radical prostatectomy. *J Urol.* 2010;184:143–148.
35. Briganti A, Blute ML, Eastham JH, et al. Pelvic lymph node dissection in prostate cancer. *Eur Urol.* 2009;55:1251–1265.
36. Messing EM, Manola J, Yao J, et al. Immediate versus deferred androgen deprivation treatment in patients with node-positive prostate cancer after radical prostatectomy and pelvic lymphadenectomy. *Lancet Oncol.* 2006;7:472–479.
37. Eastham JA, Kelly WK, Grossfeld GD, Small EJ. Cancer and Leukemia Group B (CALGB) 90203: a randomized phase 3 study of radical prostatectomy alone versus estramustine and docetaxel before radical prostatectomy for patients with high-risk localized disease. *Urology.* 2003;62(suppl 1):55–62.
38. Carlson RW, Allred DC, Anderson BO, et al. Metastatic breast cancer, version 1.2012: featured updates to the NCCN guidelines. *J Natl Compr Canc Netw.* 2012;10:821–829.
39. Montie JE, Clark PE, Eisenberger MA, et al. Bladder cancer. *J Natl Compr Canc Netw.* 2009;7:8–39.
40. Walsh TN, Noonan N, Hollywood D, Kelly A, Keeling N, Hennessy TP. A comparison of multimodal therapy and surgery for esophageal adenocarcinoma. *N Engl J Med.* 1996;335:462–467.
41. Bolla M, Collette L, Blank L, et al. Long-term results with immediate androgen suppression and external irradiation in patients with locally advanced prostate cancer (an EORTC study): a phase III randomised trial. *Lancet.* 2002;360:103–106.
42. Bolla M, Van Tienhoven G, Warde P, et al. External irradiation with or without long-term androgen suppression for prostate cancer with high metastatic risk: 10-year results of an EORTC randomised study. *Lancet Oncol.* 2010;11:1066–1073.
43. Jones CU, Hunt D, McGowan DG, et al. Radiotherapy and short-term androgen deprivation for localized prostate cancer. *N Engl J Med.* 2011;365:107–118.
44. Bolla M, de Reijke TM, Van Tienhoven G, et al. Duration of androgen suppression in the treatment of prostate cancer. *N Engl J Med.* 2009;360:2516–2527.
45. Dearnaley DP, Sydes MR, Graham JD, et al. Escalated-dose versus standard-dose conformal radiotherapy in prostate cancer: first results from the MRC RT01 randomised controlled trial. *Lancet Oncol.* 2007;8:475–487.
46. Peeters ST, Heemsbergen WD, Koper PC, et al. Dose-response in radiotherapy for localized prostate cancer: results of the Dutch multicenter randomized phase III trial comparing 68 Gy of radiotherapy with 78 Gy. *J Clin Oncol.* 2006;24:1990–1996.

47. Pollack A, Zagars GK, Starkschall G, et al. Prostate cancer radiation dose response: results of the M. D. Anderson phase III randomized trial. *Int J Radiat Oncol Biol Phys.* 2002;53:1097–1105.
48. Zietman AL, Bae K, Slater JD, et al. Randomized trial comparing conventional-dose with high-dose conformal radiation therapy in early-stage adenocarcinoma of the prostate: long-term results from proton radiation oncology group/american college of radiology 95-09. *J Clin Oncol.* 2010;28:1106–1111.
49. Zelefsky MJ, Pei X, Chou JF, et al. Dose escalation for prostate cancer radiotherapy: predictors of long-term biochemical tumor control and distant metastases-free survival outcomes. *Eur Urol.* 2011;60:1133–1139.
50. Liu L, Coker AL, Du XL, Cormier JN, Ford CE, Fang S. Long-term survival after radical prostatectomy compared to other treatments in older men with local/regional prostate cancer. *J Surg Oncol.* 2008;97:583–591.
51. Zelefsky MJ, Eastham JA, Cronin AM, et al. Metastasis after radical prostatectomy or external beam radiotherapy for patients with clinically localized prostate cancer: a comparison of clinical cohorts adjusted for case mix. *J Clin Oncol.* 2010;28:1508–1513.
52. Abdollah F, Sun M, Thuret R, et al. A competing-risks analysis of survival after alternative treatment modalities for prostate cancer patients: 1988-2006. *Eur Urol.* 2011;59:88–95.
53. Cooperberg MR, Vickers AJ, Broering JM, Carroll PR. Comparative risk-adjusted mortality outcomes after primary surgery, radiotherapy, or androgen-deprivation therapy for localized prostate cancer. *Cancer.* 2010;116:5226–5234.
54. Donovan JL, Lane JA, Peters TJ, et al. Development of a complex intervention improved randomization and informed consent in a randomized controlled trial. *J Clin Epidemiol.* 2009;62:29–36.
55. Lepor H. Radical prostatectomy for long-term functional and oncologic outcomes. *Eur Urol.* 2012;61:676–678.
56. Litwin MS, Gore JL, Kwan L, et al. Quality of life after surgery, external beam irradiation, or brachytherapy for early-stage prostate cancer. *Cancer.* 2007;109:2239–2247.
57. Pardo Y, Guedea F, Aguilo F, et al. Quality-of-life impact of primary treatments for localized prostate cancer in patients without hormonal treatment. *J Clin Oncol.* 2010;28:4687–4696.
58. Sanda MG, Dunn RL, Michalski J, et al. Quality of life and satisfaction with outcome among prostate-cancer survivors. *N Engl J Med.* 2008;358:1250–1261.
59. Huang GJ, Sadetsky N, Penson DF. Health related quality of life for men treated for localized prostate cancer with long-term followup. *J Urol.* 2010;183:2206–2212.
60. Penson DF, McLerran D, Feng Z, et al. 5-year urinary and sexual outcomes after radical prostatectomy: results from the prostate cancer outcomes study. *J Urol.* 2005;173:1701–1705.
61. Boorjian SA, Eastham JA, Graefen M, et al. A critical analysis of the long-term impact of radical prostatectomy on cancer control and function outcomes. *Eur Urol.* 2012;61:664–675.
62. Chade DC, Eastham J, Graefen M, et al. Cancer control and functional outcomes of salvage radical prostatectomy for radiation-recurrent prostate cancer: a systematic review of the literature. *Eur Urol.* 2012;61:961–971.
63. Moinpour CM, Hayden KA, Unger JM, et al; Southwest Oncology Group. Health-related quality of life results in pathologic stage C prostate cancer from a Southwest Oncology Group trial comparing radical prostatectomy alone with radical prostatectomy plus radiation therapy. *J Clin Oncol.* 2008;26:112–120.
64. Thompson IM Jr, Tangen CM, Paradelo J, et al. Adjuvant radiotherapy for pathologically advanced prostate cancer: a randomized clinical trial. *JAMA.* 2006;296:2329–2335.
65. Gomella LG, Lin J, Hoffman-Censits J, et al. Enhancing prostate cancer care through the multidisciplinary clinic approach: a 15-year experience. *J Oncol Pract.* 2010;6:e5–e10.

II

Treatment for Low-Risk, Localized Disease

7 Active Surveillance for Prostate Cancer: An Overview

LAURENCE KLOTZ

Early detection of prostate cancer was introduced in North America in the late 1980s with the advent and widespread adoption of prostate-specific antigen (PSA) testing. The result was an almost immediate dramatic spike in the number of new cases of prostate cancer, as the large reservoir of "prevalent" cases was diagnosed within a few years. This spike eventually attenuated as the pool of prevalent cases diminished and eventually returned close to baseline. Mortality from prostate cancer began to fall around this time (1995) and has continued to do so. There has been a 40% reduction in prostate cancer mortality rates in North America, and much of this has to do with early detection.

The price of early detection, however, is the increased risk of overdiagnosis and overtreatment. Prostate cancer is widely prevalent; the likelihood of harboring the disease is equal to one's age as a percentage, according to the Sakr autopsy studies (1). The strategy of PSA testing and biopsy at relatively mildly increased levels results in the diagnosis of a great number of men with extremely slow-growing, "latent" disease. Most, although not all, of these men have microfoci of Gleason 6 cancer. Since the advent of PSA testing, the management of virtually all newly diagnosed patients who have greater than a 10-year life expectancy has been surgery or radiation.

In 2011, the U.S. Preventive Services Task Force (USPSTF) applied a level "D" recommendation to PSA screening (2). A level D recommendation means that there is no basis for using the test, since the risks outweigh the benefits. This recommendation was based on an extensive analysis of PSA testing, but the crux of the concern was the high risk of overdiagnosis of clinically insignificant disease and the high risk of overtreatment of that disease. The task force was also concerned about the lack of a consensus regarding indications for a biopsy and the threshold for an abnormal PSA.

Overdiagnosis is a malady of modern medicine. Physicians have embraced new diagnostic tools with enthusiasm. These offer the promise of disease diagnosis at a more treatable and more curable point in the disease trajectory. In addition, as evidence mounts on the importance of mild abnormalities in affecting long-term health, disease definitions are often redefined to include mild abnormalities. The unintended and often unanticipated consequence of this is a stage shift toward diagnosis of much earlier conditions, and the diagnosis of "disease" in many patients who would never have been diagnosed before death in the absence of the screening test.

In the prostate cancer field, we are at the forefront in grappling with the overdiagnosis problem, but many other disease sites share this with us. Overdiagnosis and overtreatment of disease occurs across the medical spectrum, including diabetes, chronic renal failure, hypertension, and breast, lung, and thyroid cancer.

Overdiagnosis, when recognized, can be reduced, and the impact minimized. Solutions include restricting screening attempts to higher risk individuals and reducing the burden of therapy by avoiding unnecessary treatment. This is the rationale for active surveillance in prostate cancer.

Many clinicians in the field believe that the USPSTF erred in making a level D recommendation. The clinicians cite the declining mortality from prostate cancer in screened populations, and the results of the ERSPC, which showed a 30% reduction in prostate cancer mortality with screening, a benefit that is likely to increase with further follow-up. However, the task force recommendation was driven not by blindness to the mortality benefit but by awareness of the risks of overdiagnosis and overtreatment, along with the well-known adverse effects of treatment.

Prostate cancer clinicians have a choice. They can object strenuously to the task force recommendation, or they can wake up and hear the music. The task force recommendation is a call for change and action. If the number needed to treat can be reduced by selective therapy, PSA screening will warrant a second and more positive look.

In this sense, active surveillance not only improves quality of life and reduces side effects of therapy but also saves lives. How can less treatment improve prostate cancer mortality? Consider the following: PSA screening saves lives by early detection. However, it can result in overtreatment. This has made it unpalatable to health policy experts and patients. Thus, PSA screening has been discouraged, prostate cancers will be diagnosed late, and prostate cancer mortality will increase. Active surveillance, by reducing overtreatment and the number needed to treat to avoid each death, will make PSA screening more attractive. This will likely increase the appeal of PSA testing to these constituencies, the number of screened patients will increase, and lives will be saved!

Historically, conservative management was termed watchful waiting, based on the concept that local therapy was of little or no benefit, since most patients had very indolent disease and those with more aggressive cancer were not likely to be cured. For these patients, it was determined at the time of diagnosis that there was no role for curative therapy, and patients were treated palliatively when distant metastatic disease became symptomatic or local progression was apparent (3). In some countries, particularly Scandinavia and the United Kingdom, this was the standard of care for newly diagnosed patients. In North America, this approach was taken for those with a limited life expectancy due to age or comorbidity.

In contrast, the concept of active surveillance is that immediate therapy for men whose disease is likely to be indolent should be deferred, in most cases indefinitely, but implemented for evidence of risk reclassification for more aggressive disease (4, 5). In contrast to watchful waiting, the intent is curative, not palliative; it involves close monitoring and disease re-assessment, rather than a hands-off approach; and it is appropriate for men of all ages and health states, not just those with limited life expectancy.

The rationale for this is based on the following assumptions. Prostate cancer has a high prevalence, and clinically significant disease is often detected. In most cases, patients with clinically insignificant disease can be differentiated from those with more aggressive cancer by clinical and pathological parameters. Definitive treatment has significant quality-of-life effects and costs. During surveillance, patients who harbor more aggressive disease can be identified and receive definitive treatment without reducing the likelihood of cure significantly. Finally, the psychological burden of living with untreated cancer has less impact on quality of life than unnecessary treatment. In fact, all of these assumptions have been demonstrated to be true in most cases, notwithstanding that there are occasional exceptions.

■ EVIDENCE TO SUPPORT THE ACTIVE SURVEILLANCE CONCEPT

Autopsy studies have demonstrated a high incidence of occult prostate cancer in men dying of other causes. This incidence is roughly equal to age as a percentage; about 30% in men younger than 40, 50% in men in their 50s, and 80% in men older than 80 (1). A recent comparative trial of autopsies in men in Japan and Russia, neither population being exposed to PSA screening, showed that although the prevalence of cancer in both groups was high, the incidence of prostate cancer in Japanese prostates was similar to that of Russian (white) men aged 20 years. Strikingly, the rate of Gleason 7 or higher cancer in the Japanese prostates was considerably greater, about 50% of all prostates (6). Unsuspected prostate cancer was diagnosed in 25% of men enrolled in the Prostate Cancer Prevention Trial (PCPT), in which routine biopsies were performed at the completion of the trial (7). In men with a normal PSA and digital rectal examination (DRE), 15% harbored prostate cancer. This is striking compared to the 3% lifetime risk of prostate cancer mortality. There is no doubt that PSA-driven biopsies identify this insignificant disease in many patients.

There are three components to the surveillance approach:

1. Patient selection
2. Monitoring during surveillance
3. Triggers for definitive intervention
   - Selection of patients who are at low risk of progression
   - Frequency and type of monitoring during active surveillance
   - Criteria for switching from surveillance to definitive therapy

■ PATIENT SELECTION

There is a range of selection criteria in the prospective active surveillance series (8–17). This reflects the risk tolerance of the investigators. At the minimum, patients with minimal volume of low-grade disease and a PSA less than 10 are considered candidates. The most widely used definition for minimal volume is the Epstein criteria, defining such patients as having no more than two positive cores, no involvement greater than 50% on any one core, and a PSA density less than 0.15 (9, 18). This is based on clinical characteristics predictive of the traditional Stamey definition of insignificant disease, namely less than 0.5 cc of Gleason 6 or less cancer. The Epstein criteria predicted the presence of organ-confined disease in 93%, although 20% harbored Gleason 7 cancer or had extra prostatic extension (19).

A re-analysis of the definition of clinically insignificant disease based on patients having a radical prostatectomy in the ERSPC study found that a more realistic definition was less than 1.4 cc of cancer. This group used a similar approach to Stamey, stratifying patients by cancer volume and identifying the 50th percentile for volume, which identified the threshold for clinically insignificant disease (20). This has led many to view the Epstein criteria as overly stringent.

Some groups have used a more inclusive definition to include all patients with favorable risk prostate cancer according to the D'Amico definition, that is, Gleason 6 or less and PSA less than 10. Finally, there is mounting evidence that a small amount of Gleason 4 cancer in a field of Gleason 3 (i.e., 3 + 4 = 7) is also very indolent. Thus, many centers offer surveillance to these patients, particularly for those older than 65 years. In patients with more than a 10-year life expectancy, the percentage of Gleason 4 should be no more than 10%.

Several groups prefer to perform a confirmatory biopsy before offering patients surveillance (12). Others defer the biopsy for up to 1 year after the diagnostic biopsy. There is no evidence that the timing of this biopsy has any effect on long-term outcome, even if higher grade disease is identified.

In a prospective experience in Toronto, led by this author, eligibility criteria consisted of clinical stage T1c or T2a prostate cancer, a Gleason score ≤6, and a serum PSA ≤10 ng/mL (21). For patients older than 70 years, less stringent criteria were applied (Gleason score ≤ 7 [3 + 4], and/or PSA ≤ 15 ng/mL).

Although there is a consensus that Gleason ≤6 cancers are the primary candidates for active surveillance, there is increasing evidence that predominant Gleason 3 with a minority component of pattern 4 also have an indolent course. Grade inflation has been a real phenomenon since 2005, with the shift in the Gleason scoring system to include any higher grade cancer in the secondary score, regardless of how small the amount. The biopsy needle tangentially cutting a Gleason 3 acinus producing the appearance of cancer cells lacking a lumen (a characteristic of Gleason 4 pattern) is partly responsible for this. In one series, the proportion of biopsies with Gleason 7 cancer increased from 26% to 68% after the introduction of the 2005 Gleason modifications, mostly at the expense of Gleason 6 cancers (22). This suggests that a grade migration has occurred and that Gleason 3 + 4 may be similar in its behavior to what used to be called Gleason 6.

Three series (23–25) have reported the results of the subset of men in this category (with Gleason 3 + 4) managed with surveillance. All studies have shown that their risk of progression requiring treatment is as low or lower than men with Gleason 3 + 3.

Other factors must also be taken into consideration. Young age is not a contraindication to surveillance. The observation that 30% of men in their 30s harbor prostate cancer is incontrovertible proof that most "latent" prostate cancer is not destined to progress, even over a very long period. However, younger patients are exposed to the risk of progression for a longer period of time. They also, of course, have a longer period of time to experience the adverse quality-of-life effects of treatment, particularly erectile dysfunction and incontinence. Although these side effects are more common in older men after treatment (26), they are more devastating in younger men. However, most experts at least agree that extensive Gleason 6 disease in a young man (younger than 50 years) should be treated.

African Americans have been known for many years to have an increased incidence and mortality from prostate cancer. A recent study of African American men with low-risk disease having a radical prostatectomy showed that they had higher rates of upgrading (33% vs. 13%), positive margins (19% vs. 6%), and PSA recurrence (27). Therefore, race should be taken into account, but like age, it is not a contraindication to surveillance.

Multiparametric magnetic resonance imaging (MRI) has an emerging role in improving patient selection. One prospective study of 60 men selected for surveillance used the finding of a tumor greater than 1 cm in diameter (approximately corresponding to a 0.5 cc sphere) as a threshold for significant disease. Among the 22% of patients who had this finding, 80% had more than Epstein criteria on repeat biopsy (28). Among those who did not, 90% were not reclassified. A recent report from MSKCC of 388 men on surveillance who had an MRI showed that the negative predictive value of a negative MRI was 96% to 100% (29).

■ STRATEGY FOR MONITORING

Patients are followed up with serial PSA, DRE, and repeat biopsy. Multiparametric MRI has been incorporated by many groups. Our approach is to perform PSA q 3 months for 2 years and then q 6 months for life. A confirmatory biopsy is performed within the first year, and then every 3 to 5 years until 80 years of age (30). More recently, MP MRI is performed for patients who have adverse PSA kinetics (a PSA doubling time [PSADT] <3 years), a substantial increase in volume of Gleason 6 disease on repeat biopsy, or progression to Gleason 3 + 4 in a patient who wishes to remain on surveillance. Other groups perform MP MRI routinely in men considering surveillance.

PSA kinetics is a sensitive marker for risk of progression, but lacks the specificity to be a reliable trigger for intervention (31). In the Sunnybrook cohort, all those patients who died of prostate cancer had a short PSADT, less than 1.6 years. In the cohort, the median PSADT was 7 years, and 20% had a doubling time less than 3 years. In the 300 stable patients in this study, none of whom progressed clinically or pathologically, 50% had a PSA trigger at some point during their follow-up (32).

The probability that higher grade disease will be detected on repeat biopsy has been reported to be between 8% and 28% (33, 34). In most cases, the upgrading represents the results of sampling, rather than true disease progression. In our series, upgrading occurred in 20% at the confirmatory biopsy. Interestingly, the likelihood of upgrading increased according to the time since the diagnostic biopsy, at the rate of 1% per year. This may approximate the likelihood of spontaneous true biological progression of Gleason 3 to higher patterns (35).

Prevention of Progression

An intervention that would reduce the likelihood of disease progression by stabilizing existing disease is of great interest to patients and clinicians. One approach has been to use a 5-alpha reductase inhibitor, dutasteride. Both this drug and finasteride, a similar drug in the same class, showed a significant reduction in the diagnosis of low-grade prostate cancer in the REDUCE and PCPT trials, respectively (31, 36). Thus, it was reasoned, perhaps they would be effective in men harboring these cancers.

In the REDEEM trial, 302 men were randomly assigned to treatment with either dutasteride or placebo for 3 years (37). All patients had low-risk disease and met Epstein criteria for active surveillance (T1c or T2a prostate cancer, PSA < 11 ng/mL, a Gleason score ≤6, ≤3 positive cores on biopsy with ≤50 positivity on any one core). Repeat biopsies were performed at 18 and 36 months. The primary endpoint was time to progression (defined by an increase in Gleason score to >6, involvement of >3 cores, >50% involvement of any one core, or treatment for prostate cancer [RT, radical prostatectomy, and hormonal ablation]).

Treatment with dutasteride significantly decreased or delayed the risk of prostate cancer reclassification to higher risk disease (an increase in volume or grade of disease) compared with placebo (54 of 144 [38%] vs. 70 of 145 [48%], hazard ratio 0.62, 95% confidence interval 0.43–0.89). There was no evidence of an increase in the number of patients with high-grade prostate cancer on the final biopsy. (The study was not powered to identify a 0.5% increase in high-grade cancer, the outcome of the PCPT and REDUCE trials.)

These results are provocative and require longer term follow-up and validation before 5-ARI is widely adopted for men on surveillance. However, in those men on surveillance who have BPH and LUTS, it is completely reasonable to manage them with 5-ARIs, with the expectation that their clinical symptoms will improve and there may be an added benefit of a reduction in the likelihood that they will require definitive intervention.

■ OUTCOMES

The available data on patient outcomes with active surveillance come from observation studies. Several randomized studies have compared radical prostatectomy to watchful waiting, without the opportunity for delayed intervention, and provide important information about natural history.

Phase 2 Studies

Several large prospective cohorts of active surveillance have been reported. These studies have all found an extremely low rate of progession to metastatic disease or prostate cancer mortality in the intermediate term. The majority of patients remained on surveillance; approximately 30% have been treated (30, 38–45).

The most mature series, from Toronto, reported on 450 patients managed with an initial approach of active surveillance (30). For the first 5 years of the study, patients, if older than 70 years, with favorable risk disease (D'Amico criteria) or intermediate-risk disease (PSA ≤ 15 or Gleason 3 + 4) were offered this approach. Definitive treatment was recommended for a PSADT of 3 years or less, histologic progression, or clinical progression. This experience was reported in 2010 and has been updated recently. The current cohort comprises 841 patients. Median age was 69 years. Median follow-up is 7 years (range 0.5–20 years). The overall survival was 82%. Thirty-two percent were treated. The 10-, 15-, and 20-year overall survival was 77%, 58%, and 50%, respectively.

Among the 841 patients, there were 14 (1.7%) deaths from prostate cancer. Of the 14 patients who died of prostate cancer, 7 patients received RT, 2 received RP, 3 received hormones, 1 had no treatment, and 1 refused treatment. Among the remaining 827 patients, none have clinical metastatic disease. The 10-, 15-, and 20-year actuarial CSS was 97.9%, 93.5%, and 86.3%, respectively.

At 5, 10, 15, and 20 years, 77%, 63%, 52.3%, and 52.3% of patients, respectively, remain untreated and on surveillance. Two hundred nine patients were treated after a period of surveillance. Of these, 44 (21%) had PSA failure. This represents 5% of the overall cohort (44/841). In the patients treated radically, the bNED survival from the time of diagnosis at 5 and 10 years was 80% and 66%, respectively. The 5- and 10-year bNED figures from the time of treatment were 94% and 75%, respectively. Forty-four patients were treated with surgery and 138 with radiation. Eleven percent of the surgery patients and 22% of the radiation patients had PSA failure. The bNED survival after surgery at 5, 10, and 15 years was 90%, 90%, and 72%, respectively. In patients treated with radiation, it was 82%, 61%, and 47%. This difference in bNED failure between surgery and radiation was significant (P = .031). The cumulative hazard ratio for dying of other causes versus prostate cancer was 9.7:1. In men older than 70 years, who are at a greater risk for other causes of death, this ratio was 12.7; in men younger than 70 years, the ratio was 5.8.

The concept of active surveillance is further supported by data from the Health Professionals Follow-Up

Study, in which 3,331 men were diagnosed with prostate cancer between 1986 and 2007. In this cohort, treatment was deferred for at least 1 year in 10% (45). The cohort included both active surveillance patients and those untreated due to age and/or comorbidity. At 7 years, 50% remained untreated. Multivariate analysis adjusting for significant predictors of progression showed no difference in the rate of metastatic disease or prostate cancer mortality between the active surveillance and radical intervention groups.

Randomized Trials

Both the Scandinavian Prostate Cancer Group 4 (SPCG4) trial (46) and the PIVOT trial (47) have compared radical prostatectomy with watchful waiting (WW). Neither trial offered delayed intervention to the watchful waiting group. The SPCG4 study showed a 50% mortality reduction in the treatment group. A mortality reduction was seen in the low-risk group. However, this likely reflected the fact that the SPCG4 cohort was a non-PSA screened group that did not have the benefit of volume migration seen in a screened population. Diagnosis was by aspiration in most cases. Further, the prostate cancer mortality in the RP group in this study was 6% at 12 years and 10% in the WW group. In our surveillance cohort, it was 3.2% at 12 years. This difference emphasizes the difference in patient selection between the cohorts. The SPCG4 results in the "low-risk" patients should not be interpreted as relevant to the outcome in screen-detected, low-risk patients (48). The PIVOT study showed a modest benefit of treatment for intermediate- and high-risk groups, but no benefit at all in favorable risk patients.

A landmark study in the United Kingdom, the ProtecT trial, is nearing completion. In that study, patients were randomized to surveillance, RP, or radiation therapy (49). All patients, including intermediate and high risk, were randomized between these three management strategies. Patients on surveillance had serial PSA, but did not have serial biopsies unless clinically indicated. This trial was initiated in 2001 and has enrolled about 2,050 patients. This trial, when completed, should provide very reliable data about the incremental mortality associated with an initial expectant approach, if any. It is possible, on the basis of what we know today, that active surveillance may be associated with a slight absolute increase in prostate cancer mortality. This difference is almost certain to be small; at the most, 1% at 15 years. If true, this should not undermine the case for active surveillance. As mentioned earlier, a selective approach to therapy is required to make PSA screening palatable and therefore provide men with high-grade disease the benefit of early detection without excessive overtreatment of the low-risk patients. Thus, in the long run, many more lives would be saved.

Quality-of-Life Benefits

Active surveillance has two benefits: the avoidance of treatment-related side effects and the legitimization of screening based on reducing overtreatment. The quality-of-life benefits are obvious to clinicians and patients. A stringent decision analysis that evaluated quality of life in a hypothetical 65-year-old healthy male with low-risk prostate cancer found a higher quality-adjusted life year with surveillance than any other treatment option (50). A sensitivity analysis showed that this finding was robust.

Another issue to consider is the patient's personal preferences. Some patients have difficulty coping with the psychological aspects of living with untreated cancer (51). These patients tend to have a history of anxiety disorders, suffer from social isolation, and lack of family support (52).

Such patients require more personal and psychological support and may indeed elect to have their disease treated definitively.

Education and reassurance are critical. Consider the zeitgeist of cancer: that it is an aggressive, frequently lethal disease that must be treated aggressively. This creates fear that drives a great deal of unnecessary intervention. However, some key facts communicated clearly to the patient can dramatically reduce this fear. Some of these statements include the following:

What you have is not a real disease.
Most men your age have this but don't know it.
It is really a "pseudo-cancer" or a "pseudo-disease."
The chance of dying of other causes is 10 times greater than the chance of dying of prostate cancer.

Improved communication undoubtedly enhances the acceptability of surveillance and reduces patient anxiety (53).

One of the concerns associated with repeated biopsy of the prostate is the risk of urosepsis with each biopsy, and the risk of erectile dysfunction in men having repeated biopsy (54). The increased risk of ED in men having three or more biopsies was based on annual biopsy. It is possible that a less frequent biopsy schedule (i.e., every 3–5 years) may not have this effect. Nonetheless, an unmet need is to develop biomarkers or imaging studies that can replace the biopsy as a means for identifying higher risk patients.

■ REFERENCES

1. Sakr WA, Grignon DJ, Crissman JD, et al. High grade prostatic intraepithelial neoplasia (HGPIN) and prostatic adenocarcinoma between the ages of 20–69: an autopsy study of 249 cases. *In Vivo*. 1994;8(3):439–443.
2. Moyer VA. U.S. Preventive Services Task Force Screening for prostate cancer: U.S. Preventive Services Task Force recommendation statement. *Ann Intern Med*. 2012;157(2):120–134.
3. Dahabreh IJ, Chung M, Balk EM, et al. Active surveillance in men with localized prostate cancer: a systematic review. *Ann Intern Med*. 2012;156:582.

4. *National Comprehensive Cancer Network (NCCN) Guidelines*. www.nccn.org. Accessed May 15, 2013.
5. Thompson I, Thrasher JB, Aus G, et al. Guideline for the management of clinically localized prostate cancer: 2007 update. *J Urol*. 2007;177:2106.
6. Zlotta AR, Egawa S, Pushkar D, et al. Prevalence of prostate carcinoma and its precursor lesions in Russian Caucasian and Japanese men in autopsy specimens: a prospective comparative international study with central pathology review. Presented at 27th Congress of European Association of Urology; February 25, 2013; Milan, Italy.
7. Thompson IM, Goodman PJ, Tangen CM, et al. The influence of finasteride on the development of prostate cancer. *N Engl J Med*. 2003;349(3):215–224.
8. Klotz L. Active surveillance for favorable-risk prostate cancer: who, how and why? *Nat Clin Pract Oncol*. 2007;4:692.
9. Dall'Era MA, Cooperberg MR, Chan JM, et al. Active surveillance for early-stage prostate cancer: review of the current literature. *Cancer*. 2008;112:1650.
10. Anast JW, Andriole GL, Bismar TA, et al. Relating biopsy and clinical variables to radical prostatectomy findings: can insignificant and advanced prostate cancer be predicted in a screening population? *Urology*. 2004;64:544.
11. Cupp MR, Bostwick DG, Myers RP, Oesterling JE. The volume of prostate cancer in the biopsy specimen cannot reliably predict the quantity of cancer in the radical prostatectomy specimen on an individual basis. *J Urol*. 1995;153:1543.
12. Eggener SE, Mueller A, Berglund RK, et al. A multi-institutional evaluation of active surveillance for low risk prostate cancer. *J Urol*. 2009;181:1635.
13. Epstein JI, Chan DW, Sokoll LJ, et al. Nonpalpable stage T1c prostate cancer: prediction of insignificant disease using free/total prostate specific antigen levels and needle biopsy findings. *J Urol*. 1998;160:2407.
14. Cupp MR, Bostwick DG, Myers RP, Oesterling JE. The volume of prostate cancer in the biopsy specimen cannot reliably predict the quantity of cancer in the radical prostatectomy specimen on an individual basis. *J Urol*. 1995;153:1543.
15. Irwin MB, Trapasso JG. Identification of insignificant prostate cancers: analysis of preoperative parameters. *Urology*. 1994;44:862.
16. Epstein JI, Walsh PC, Carmichael M, Brendler CB. Pathologic and clinical findings to predict tumor extent of nonpalpable (stage T1c) prostate cancer. *JAMA*. 1994;271:368.
17. Noguchi M, Stamey TA, McNeal JE, Yemoto CM. Relationship between systematic biopsies and histological features of 222 radical prostatectomy specimens: lack of prediction of tumor significance for men with nonpalpable prostate cancer. *J Urol*. 2001;166:104.
18. Bastian PJ, Mangold LA, Epstein JI, Partin AW. Characteristics of insignificant clinical T1c prostate tumors. A contemporary analysis. *Cancer*. 2004;101:2001.
19. Lee MC, Dong F, Stephenson AJ, et al. The Epstein criteria predict for organ-confined but not insignificant disease and a high likelihood of cure at radical prostatectomy. *Eur Urol*. 2010;58:90.
20. Wolters T, Roobol MJ, van Leeuwen PJ, et al. A critical analysis of the tumor volume threshold for clinically insignificant prostate cancer using a data set of a randomized screening trial. *J Urol*. 2011;185(1):121–125.
21. Klotz L. Active surveillance for prostate cancer: trials and tribulations. *World J Urol*. 2008;26:437.
22. Helpap B, Egevad L. The significance of modified Gleason grading of prostatic carcinoma in biopsy and radical prostatectomy specimens. *Virchows Arch*. 2006;449(6):622–627.
23. Choo R, Klotz L, Danjoux C, et al. Feasibility study: watchful waiting for localized low to intermediate grade prostate carcinoma with selective delayed intervention based on prostate specific antigen, histological and/or clinical progression. *J Urol*. 2002;167(4):1664–1669.
24. Cooperberg MR, Cowan JE, Hilton JF, et al. Outcomes of active surveillance for men with intermediate-risk prostate cancer. *J Clin Oncol*. 2011;29(2):228–234.
25. Bul M, van den Bergh RC, Zhu X, et al. Outcomes of initially expectantly managed patients with low or intermediate risk screen-detected localized prostate cancer. *BJU Int*. 2012;110(11):1672–1677.
26. Loeb S, Roehl KA, Helfand BT, Catalona WJ. Complications of open radical retropubic prostatectomy in potential candidates for active monitoring. *Urology*. 2008;72:887.
27. Sundi D, Ross AE, Humphreys EB, et al. African American men with very low-risk prostate cancer exhibit adverse oncologic outcomes after radical prostatectomy: should active surveillance still be an option for them? *J Clin Oncol*. 2013;31:2991–2997.
28. Margel D, Yap SA, Lawrentschuk N, et al. Impact of multiparametric endorectal coil prostate magnetic resonance imaging on disease reclassification among active surveillance candidates: a prospective cohort study. *J Urol*. 2012;187:1247.
29. Vargas HA, Akin O, Afaq A, et al. Magnetic resonance imaging for predicting prostate biopsy findings in patients considered for active surveillance of clinically low risk prostate cancer. *J Urol*. 2012;188(5):1732–1738.
30. Klotz L, Zhang L, Lam A, et al. Clinical results of long-term follow-up of a large, active surveillance cohort with localized prostate cancer. *J Clin Oncol*. 2010;28:126.
31. Vickers AJ, Savage C, O'Brien MF, Lilja H. Systematic review of pretreatment prostate-specific antigen velocity and doubling time as predictors for prostate cancer. *J Clin Oncol*. 2009;27(3):398–403.
32. Loblaw A, Zhang L, Lam A, et al. Comparing prostate specific antigen triggers for intervention in men with stable prostate cancer on active surveillance. *J Urol*. 2010;184(5):1942–1946.
33. Patel MI, DeConcini DT, Lopez-Corona E, et al. An analysis of men with clinically localized prostate cancer who deferred definitive therapy. *J Urol*. 2004;171:1520.
34. Choo R, Do V, Sugar L, et al. Comparison of histologic grade between initial and follow-up biopsy in untreated, low to intermediate grade, localized prostate cancer. *Can J Urol*. 2004; 11:2118.
35. Jain S, Vesprini D, Mamedov A, et al. Gleason upgrading with time in a large, active surveillance cohort with long-term follow-up. ASCO 2013 Genitourinary Cancers Symposium. February 14–16, 2013; Orlando, FL.
36. Andriole GL, Bostwick DG, Brawleyetal OW. Effect of dutasteride on the risk of prostate cancer. *N Engl J Med*. 2010;362(13):1192–1202.
37. Fleshner NE, Lucia MS, Egerdie B, et al. Dutasteride in localised prostate cancer management: the REDEEM randomised, double-blind, placebo-controlled trial. *Lancet*. 2012;379:1103.
38. Stattin P, Holmberg E, Bratt O, et al. Surveillance and deferred treatment for localized prostate cancer. Population based study in the National Prostate Cancer Register of Sweden. *J Urol*. 2008;180:2423.
39. Khatami A, Ali K, Aus G, et al. PSA doubling time predicts the outcome after active surveillance in screening-detected prostate cancer: results from the European randomized study of screening for prostate cancer, Sweden section. *Int J Cancer*. 2007;120:170.
40. Dall'Era MA, Konety BR, Cowan JE, et al. Active surveillance for the management of prostate cancer in a contemporary cohort. *Cancer*. 2008;112:2664.
41. Carter HB, Kettermann A, Warlick C, et al. Expectant management of prostate cancer with curative intent: an update of the Johns Hopkins experience. *J Urol*. 2007;178:2359.
42. van As NJ, Norman AR, Thomas K, et al. Predicting the probability of deferred radical treatment for localised prostate cancer managed by active surveillance. *Eur Urol*. 2008;54:1297.

43. van den Bergh RC, Roemeling S, Roobol MJ, et al. Gleason score 7 screen-detected prostate cancers initially managed expectantly: outcomes in 50 men. *BJU Int*. 2009;103:1472.
44. Duffield AS, Lee TK, Miyamoto H, et al. Radical prostatectomy findings in patients in whom active surveillance of prostate cancer fails. *J Urol*. 2009;182:2274.
45. Shappley WV III, Kenfield SA, Kasperzyk JL, et al. Prospective study of determinants and outcomes of deferred treatment or watchful waiting among men with prostate cancer in a nationwide cohort. *J Clin Oncol*. 2009;27:4980.
46. Bill-Axelson A, Holmberg L, Ruutu M, et al. Radical prostatectomy versus watchful waiting in early prostate cancer. *N Engl J Med*. 2011;364:1708.
47. Wilt TJ, Brawer MK, Jones KM, et al. Radical prostatectomy versus observation for localized prostate cancer. *N Engl J Med*. 2012;367:203.
48. Klotz L, Thompson I. Early prostate cancer—treat or watch? *N Engl J Med*. 2011;365(6):569.
49. http://www.clinicaltrials.gov/ Accessed June 15, 2014.
50. Hayes JH, Ollendorf DA, Pearson SD, et al. Active surveillance compared with initial treatment for men with low-risk prostate cancer: a decision analysis. *JAMA*. 2010;304:2373.
51. Latini DM, Hart SL, Knight SJ, et al. The relationship between anxiety and time to treatment for patients with prostate cancer on surveillance. *J Urol*. 2007;178:826.
52. Goh AC, Kowalkowski MA, Bailey DE Jr, Kazer MW, Knight SJ, Latini DM. Perception of cancer and inconsistency in medical information are associated with decisional conflict: a pilot study of men with prostate cancer who undergo active surveillance. *BJU Int*. 2012;110(2 pt 2):E50–E56.
53. Bailey DE, Mishel MH, Belyea M, et al. Uncertainty intervention for watchful waiting in prostate cancer. *Cancer Nurs*. 2004;27:339.
54. Fujita K, Landis P, McNeil BK, Pavlovich CP. Serial prostate biopsies are associated with an increased risk of erectile dysfunction in men with prostate cancer on active surveillance. *J Urol*. 2009;182:2664.

8 Treatment of Low-Risk, Localized Prostate Cancer: A Holistic Approach With Diet

JILLIAN SCAMBIA
ANNIE DARVES-BORNOZ
AARON KATZ

INTRODUCTION

Prostate cancer (PC) is the most common cancer among men in the United States, second to nonmelanoma skin cancer (1). It is also one of the leading causes of cancer death among men of all races. Early detection of PC, due to the introduction of the prostate-specific antigen (PSA) blood test, has been attributed to being one factor involved in lowering the PC mortality rate in the past decades. Although PSA testing is routinely used for PC screening, concerns have emerged regarding the lack of evidence that screening itself is what directly decreases mortality.

The United States Preventative Services Task Force recommended against screening for PC using PSA for healthy men in 2011. This was based on studies that concluded the harms related to subsequent evaluation and treatment outweighed the small reduction in PC-specific mortality in patients screened with a PSA test. However, it is important to note that PSA testing demonstrating a sustained trending rise or in conjunction with tests such as PSA velocity, the *PC gene 3* (PCA3), and the percentage free PSA can enhance the value of using PSA as a screening tool (2).

With a dramatic increase in the diagnosis of asymptomatic PC, drastically different treatment modalities are being explored for these patients compared with those diagnosed with aggressive disease. Before considering major surgery, radiation, or androgen deprivation therapy, which have a myriad of adverse effects, clinicians are turning to active surveillance or watchful waiting in these low-risk populations (3). One recommendation for management of low-risk patients is to make lifestyle changes including dietary modifications, incorporation of supplements, introduction of aerobic exercise, and meditation or stress reduction techniques. These simple alterations can act as both treatment and prevention of disease. Furthermore, for all grades of PC, nutritional interventions complement conventional treatments and are important in improving outcomes and quality of life.

There is increasing evidence from epidemiologic surveys and from laboratory, intervention, and case-control studies that diet and lifestyle play a crucial role in PC biology and tumorigenesis. This applies to both the development and the progression of PC. The information presented in this chapter about a holistic approach to the treatment of low-risk localized PC summarizes the key evidence for the role of different dietary components and their effect on PC prevention and progression. Most nutrients and supplements outlined in this chapter also have the added benefit of being beneficial for the cardiovascular system, bone health, and the prevention of other cancers. The dietary factors that influence the development of prostate cancer are illustrated in Figure 8.1.

EPIDEMIOLOGY OF PROSTATE CANCER

The most recent data from the Surveillance Epidemiology and End Results database estimate that 241,740 men were diagnosed with prostate cancer and over 28,000 died of the disease in the United States in 2012 (4). Autopsy studies have demonstrated that 60% to 70% of older men have some area showing cancer within the prostate (5, 6). It is estimated that a 50-year-old man has a lifetime risk of 42% of developing prostate cancer, but only a 9.5% risk of developing the disease clinically and being diagnosed and a 2.9% risk of dying from prostate cancer (7). Thus, prostate cancer is extremely prevalent; however, many cases of the disease can remain clinically insignificant due to its protracted course.

The stage of prostate cancer is a major predictor of survival rates as men with local and regional disease had 5-year survival rates nearing 100%, while patients with distant metastasis had a 5-year survival of only 28% (8). Due to the increase in screening, there has been an increase in incidence of organ-confined and regional disease and a decrease in incidence of metastatic disease (9).

The incidence of prostate cancer differs greatly geographically. The disease is most prevalent in Scandinavia and North America and lowest in Asia (4, 10).

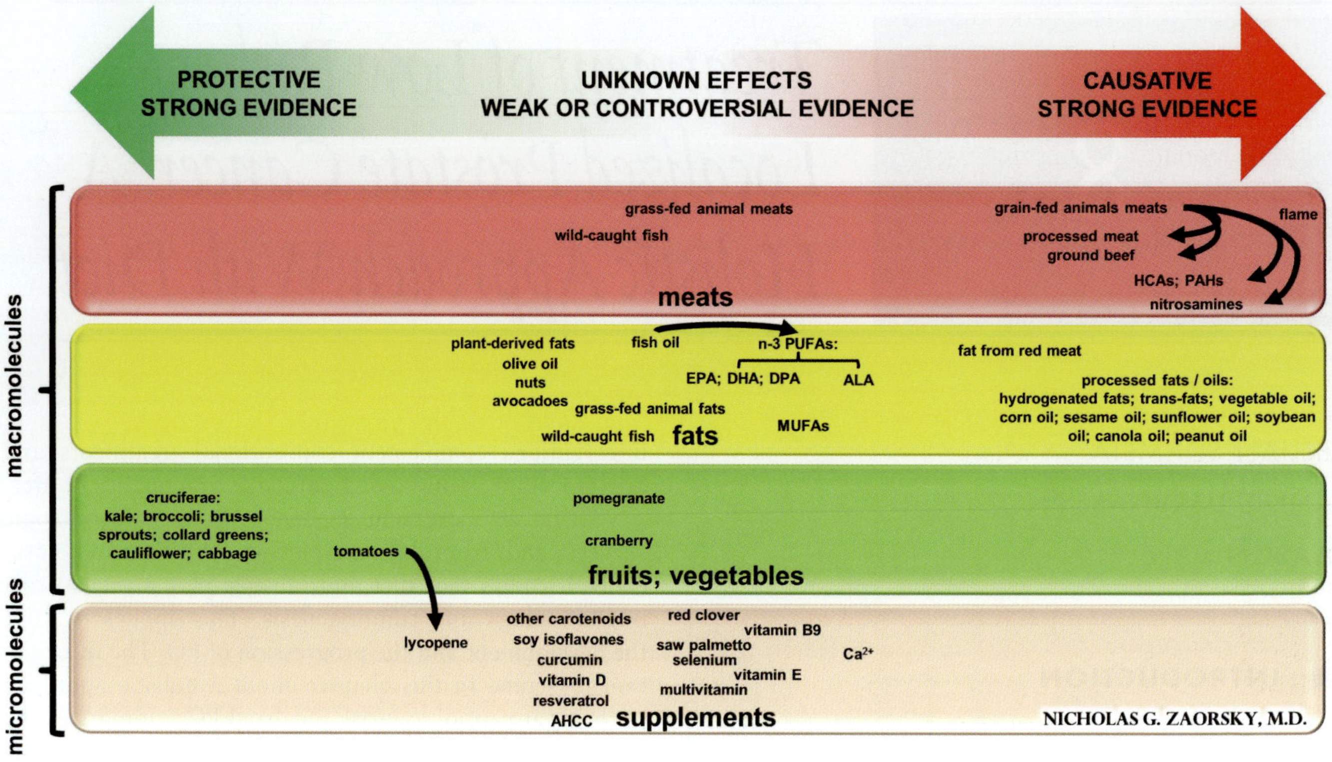

FIGURE 8.1 Dietary factors that influence the development of prostate cancer. The macro- and micromolecules that have been associated with causation or prevention of prostate cancer are illustrated. In general, the main macromolecules associated with an increased risk of prostate cancer are grain-fed, processed, and/or burned meat; and processed fats/oils. In contrast, the main macromolecules associated with protection against prostate cancer are cruciferous vegetables. Notably, there is not enough evidence to recommend for or against many macromolecules, and all micromolecules.

Abbreviations: AHCC = active hexose correlated compound; ALA = alpha-linolenic acid; DHA = docosahexaenoic acid; DPA = docosapentaenoic acid; EPA = eicosapentaenoic acid; HCA = heterocyclic amines; n-3 PUFAs = long-chain omega-3 polyunsaturated fatty acids; PAH = polycyclic aromatic hydrocarbons.

The incidence also varies with race. African Americans have the highest incidence of prostate cancer of any race or ethnicity in the United States (between 2005 and 2009, 236.0 per 100,000 men annually). This is in contrast to other groups living in the United States, including white American males (146.9 per 100,000 men annually), Asian/ Pacific Islanders (85.4 per 100,000), American Indian/Alaska Natives (78.4 per 100,000), and Hispanics (125.9 per 100,000) (4).

Other risk factors include advancing age and family history. From 2005 to 2009, the median age of diagnosis was 67 years of age, with close to 90% of diagnoses occurring at age 55 and older. In addition, older men are more likely to be diagnosed with high-risk prostate cancer leading to lower overall and cancer-specific survival (4). Risk of prostate cancer is double for a male who has one affected first-degree relative (11–15). For males with more than one affected relative, risk is further increased (13). Age of onset in affected first-degree relatives is also important, as younger age of onset correlates with increased risk as well (13, 16).

Diet and lifestyle have also been identified as risk factors for PC, which will be discussed in this chapter. The role of obesity is still unclear. Many studies show that excess body weight (defined by body mass index) does not lead to increased cases of prostate cancer (17–19), although some studies have shown a positive association (20, 21). However, it has been shown more conclusively that obesity is associated with cases of higher grade and fatal prostate cancer (22, 23).

■ PATHOPHYSIOLOGY OF PROSTATE CANCER

Prostate cancer occurs when normal semen-secreting prostate gland cells mutate into cancer cells. It is classified as an adenocarcinoma, meaning glandular in nature. The region of the prostate gland where the adenocarcinoma is most common is the peripheral zone. This area of the prostate can be assessed during a digital rectal exam (DRE), which is why the DRE is an important part of the physical exam in male patients.

Initially, small clumps of cancer cells remain confined to otherwise normal prostate glands, a condition known as prostatic intraepithelial neoplasia (PIN). PIN can present as low grade or high grade, and although there is no proof that PIN is a cancer precursor, it is well recognized to be closely associated with the development of invasive cancer. Chronic inflammation, which damages epithelial cells, results in proliferative lesions and is a likely precursor to PIN or PC; prostatisis has therefore been associated with a high risk of PC.

Over time, these cancer cells begin to multiply and spread to the surrounding prostate tissue (prostatic stroma) forming a tumor. Eventually, the tumor may grow large enough to invade nearby organs such as the seminal vesicles, the rectum, and the neighboring lymph nodes and can even spread hematogenously.

Prostate cancer is considered a malignant tumor because it has the potential to metastasize. PC most commonly metastasizes to the bones and lymph nodes and may invade rectum, bladder, urethra, and lower ureters after local progression. The route of metastasis to bone is believed to be hematogenous due to the prostatic venous plexus, which drains the prostate, connecting with the vertebral veins of the lumbar spine.

■ IMPACT OF FOOD ON PROSTATE CANCER

Meat

A recent case-control study of 982 men demonstrated that high consumption of processed meat, including ground beef, was associated with aggressive PC. Ground beef showed the strongest association followed by well-done meat. Consumption of rare- or less-cooked meat was not associated with an increased risk of PC (24). Overcooked meats and those prepared on an open flame contain heterocyclic amines (HCAs), polycyclic aromatic hydrocarbons, and carcinogenic chemicals formed from cooking muscle meat such as beef, pork, fowl, and fish (25). Researchers have identified 17 different HCAs resulting from the cooking of meats that may pose human cancer risk.

The largest prospective study to date for high-risk patient populations examined the association of meat and HCA intake on PC risk in 7,949 African American men. It demonstrated that African American men who were part of the quantile of highest consumption of red meat cooked at high temperatures had a 22% higher risk of PC over a 10-year period than men in the lowest consumption quantile (26).

It is also advisable to avoid smoked and cured meats, which contain nitrosamines. Lean protein and meat from grass-fed animals when eaten sparingly, cooked at low temperatures, are the preferred choice. Grass-fed animal meat contains high levels of vitamin E, glutathinone, conjugated linoleic acid, and lower levels of saturated fat compared to grain-fed animals (27).

Fats

A recent study followed up PC patients over 5 years, and those who consumed the most saturated fat (from meat and dairy) had more than three times the risk of dying from PC compared with patients in the trial who consumed the least amount of saturated fat. A long-term prospective study reported the findings of serum levels of *trans* fatty acids, specifically *trans* fats resulting from the hydrogenation of vegetable oils, which are associated with an increased risk of PC.

There have been inconsistent results regarding the relationship of omega-3 fatty acids and PC risks in the recent literature. A meta-analysis published in 2013 provided evidence to clarify the variable results regarding the association of long-chain omega-3 polyunsaturated fatty acids or the individual components—eicosapentaenoic acid (EPA), docosahexaenoic acid (DHA), docosapentaenoic acid (DPA)—with PC risk. It was determined that high blood level of DPA is associated with a reduced risk of PC, whereas high blood level of EPA and DHA in combination is associated with increase high-grade prostate tumor risk (28).

Alpha-linolenic acid (ALA) is the essential omega-3 fatty acid precursor of EPA and DHA, which are known to have anti-inflammatory and possibly anti-cancer properties. Yet results indicate that people with measurably high ALA are at an increased risk for PC. Dietary ALA is most commonly obtained through the consumption of meat and thus is used as a marker in many studies. Most, but not all studies, have found that there is a correlation between high dietary ALA and PC risks.

Men who include fish in their diet have been reported to have lower risk for PC due to the abundance of omega-3 fatty acids in fish.

Cruciferous Vegetables

Cruciferous vegetables belong to the Brassicaceae family and include leafy greens such as kale, cauliflower, broccoli, Brussels sprouts, cabbage, bok choy, and collard greens. They are high in vitamin C, soluble fiber, and phytochemicals sulforaphane and indole-3 carbinol (I3C) (29). Phytochemicals exhibit anti-inflammatory activity and anticarcinogenic properties including induction of cell cycle arrest, inhibition of tumor invasion and angiogenesis, inhibition of extracellular signal-regulated kinases, proteasome degradation, and alteration of phase I and phase II biotransformation enzyme expression (30). Sulforaphane has been shown to have proapoptotic properties in PC cells both in vitro and in vivo, and I3C has demonstrated antiproliferative and antimetastatic properties in animal models of PC (31).

In men with newly diagnosed PC, a preliminary study showed a 41% decreased risk of PC in men consuming greater than two servings of cruciferous vegetables per week, compared with those eating less than one serving per week. The protective effect is believed to be due to the high concentrations of the carotenoids, luteins, and zeaxanthins, as well as their stimulatory effects on the breakdown of environmental carcinogens associated with PC. Cruciferous vegetables also contain phytoestrogens. With regard to phytoestrogens, it is more appropriate that we examine isoflavones, the most researched of the phytoestrogens, which are commonly found in soy and red clover (32).

Soy Isoflavones

Soy is high in isoflavones. Isoflavones are characterized as phytoestrogens due to their estrogen activity. These compounds may reduce 5α-reductase activity, induce differentiation of prostate cells, and modulate estrogen receptors, which inhibit androgen activity (33). Genistein is one of the most abundant active isoflavones in soy. It has been shown to inhibit both androgen-dependent and androgen-independent prostate cancer cell growth in vitro (34).

Isoflavone supplementation may be beneficial in men with localized disease. In a study of men with biochemical recurrent prostate cancer, isoflavones proved to have biological activity as shown by a decline in the slope of PSA (34). A meta-analysis of six case-control and two cohort studies (35), as well as the U.S. Multiethnic Cohort Study (36), showed a reduction in the risk of prostate cancer in males with high soy consumption. The latter study also found a 30% reduction in risk of being diagnosed with advanced disease. It is postulated that Asian soy-based diets contribute to the lower rates of prostate cancer in this population.

Red Clover

Red clover contains isoflavones, which are metabolized into phytoestrogens in the body, as discussed in the previous section. A recent study showed that daily oral administration of 60 mg of red clover isoflavone extract was well tolerated, caused no side effects, and demonstrated significant decreases in total PSA levels by more than 30% (37). Patients should notify their general practitioner or urologist if they are taking these supplements without recommendation because the potential development of PC could be masked by a reduction in PSA values secondary to the intake of phytoestrogens.

Lycopene

Lycopene has been proposed to protect against PC through various properties including decreased lipid oxidation, inhibition of cancer cell proliferation, and most notably potent antioxidant properties (38). Tomatoes are the primary source of lycopene, although trace amounts can be obtained by consuming strawberries, watermelon, pink grapefruit, guava, and papaya. It is actually less desirable to eat raw tomatoes because cooking tomatoes or making tomato sauce release lycopene from storage sites and enhances the absorption process, as does dietary fat.

Including lycopene in a man's diet can act to lower his PSA. A phase II study found that whole tomato lycopene preventative supplementation reduced PSA significantly and maintained its effect on PSA over 1 year (39).

Of prospective dietary studies on lycopene, the largest and only study with multiple assessments of diet was conducted in the Health Professionals Follow-Up Study (HPFS). The HPFS first reported an inverse association between lycopene intake and PC. High intake of tomato-based products was associated with a 35% decreased risk of total PC and a 53% decreased risk of advanced stage PC (40).

Green Tea

In cultures where green tea is consumed often, incidence of and mortality from prostate cancer is significantly lower (41). A *Journal of Nutrition* report observed that the equivalent of six cups of green tea daily "significantly inhibits [prostate cancer] development and metastasis." However, most men will not drink six cups of green tea per day; therefore, supplementation with a concentrated extract appears to be an important aspect of herbal chemoprevention.

The antioxidant content of green tea is remarkable. Over 50 compounds with anti-inflammatory activity have been identified in this centuries-old beverage. Several targets for green tea compounds have been elucidated with regard to prostate cancer prevention and treatment including polyphenols, phytochemicals, and epigallocatechin-3-gallate (EGCG).

Polyphenols influence the down-regulation of ornithine carboxylase, which is overexpressed in patients with prostate cancer (42). Phytochemicals reduce concentrations of angiogenic vascular endothelial growth factor and reduce metastasis-related gene expression (matrix metalloproteinase [MMP]-2 and MMP-9) (43). EGCG inhibits the growth of both androgen-sensitive and androgen-insensitive prostate cancer in animal studies by inducing apoptosis and altering expression of regulatory proteins that are critical for cell survival. EGCG has also been shown to selectively inhibit cyclooxygenase (COX-2) in both hormone-sensitive and hormone-refractory human prostate cancer cells (44).

Pomegranate

Pomegranate is a rich source of polyphenolic compounds, including anthocyanins and hydrolyzable tannins, which have free-radical scavenging properties. It is reported that pomegranate contain higher antioxidant activity than green tea and red wine. The arils are excellent sources of dietary fiber, and the nutrients are entirely contained in this edible seed. Studies have also shown that anatomically discrete sections of the fruit act synergistically to exert antiproliferative and antimetastatic effects against PC cells (45).

A study on pomegranate juice at a single center during the course of 2 years showed that consuming pomegranate juice increases the mean PSA doubling time. This was in combination with corresponding laboratory effects on PC in vitro cell proliferation and apoptosis, as well as oxidative stress. The treatment was well tolerated, with no adverse effects reported. The results of this study are being further tested in an ongoing randomized, double-blinded, three-arm, placebo-controlled study (46).

Cranberry

Cranberry juice has long been consumed for the prevention of urinary tract infections, and research linked this property to the ability of cranberry proanthocyanidins (PACs) to inhibit adhesion of *Escherichia coli* bacteria to the genitourinary tract (47). Studies have also well documented the effects of PACs found in cranberries on MMP activity associated with prostate tumor metastasis, apoptosis in tumor cells, reduced ornithine decarboxylase activity, and anti-inflammatory activities such as inhibition of cyclooxygenases (48). These findings suggest a potential role for cranberry as part of a chemopreventive diet (49).

Saw Palmetto

Saw palmetto extract reduces the amount of dihydrotestosterone (DHT), a metabolically active form of testosterone, binding in the prostatic urethra. In vitro studies have reported that it weakly inhibits the action of 5-alpha reductase, the enzyme responsible for converting testosterone to DHT (50). In vivo studies have suggested that saw palmetto may protect against PC; however, there has been no evidence in humans regarding the association (51). One prospective cohort study of 35,171 men aged between 50 and 76 years found no association. However, it is of note that the dose and ratios of constituents varied widely among study participants (52).

Flaxseed

Increased inflammation is associated with high ratios of omega-6 to omega-3 fats. A recent investigation of the balance of these types of omega fats looked at supplementation of omega-3 fat and its impact on tumor growth. A preliminary study in patients with PC taking 30 g per day for approximately 1 month of ground flaxseed, which is high in omega-3 fats, showed a decreased rate of tumor growth (53).

Curcumin

Curcumin is a yellow pigment in the spice turmeric (also known as curry powder) and has been used for centuries as a treatment for inflammatory disease. The effects are not limited to the genitourinary system; curcumin has demonstrated profound impacts on neurological, cardiovascular, pulmonary, and metabolic diseases (54). A study at Columbia University found that curcumin is also involved in modulating proteins that suppress apoptosis and interfere with growth factors that promote cancer progression (55).

■ IMPACT OF VITAMINS, MINERALS, AND OTHER SUPPLEMENTS ON PROSTATE CANCER

Vitamin D and Calcium

Where sun exposure is low, prostate cancer rates increase (56). This ecologic data prompted a clinical study where 7 of 16 men with bony metastatic PC, which had been unresponsive to conventional treatment, were found to have evidence of vitamin D deficiency. All were given 2,000 IU of vitamin D per day for 12 weeks, and pain levels were recorded. Results included reduction of pain and evidence of increased strength (57).

Calcitriol, the hormonally active form of vitamin D, inhibits the growth and development in several cancers where inflammation has been implicated in the development and progression. Calcitriol inhibits the synthesis and actions of proinflammatory prostaglandins by several mechanisms, and these anti-inflammatory actions in PC cells contribute to its potential as a chemopreventive and therapeutic agent (58).

It is appropriate to measure 25-hydroxyvitamin D in patients to ensure that they are at an adequate level. Although normal range is 20 to 55 ng/mL, ideally vitamin D levels should not fall below 32 ng/mL and any level below 20 ng/mL is considered a severely deficient state (59).

Numerous studies, including the Cancer Prevention Study II Nutrition Cohort, have reported positive associations between high calcium intake and increased incidence of and increased mortality from prostate cancer (60). With the abundance of calcium supplementation in the United States, more studies are needed to evaluate these potentially increased risks.

Vitamin E and Selenium

The SELECT (SELenium and vitamin E Cancer prevention Trial) was conducted to assess the efficacy of selenium and vitamin E alone, and in combination, on the incidence of prostate cancer. This randomized, double-blind, placebo-controlled, 2 × 2 factorial design clinical trial found that neither selenium nor vitamin E reduced the incidence of prostate cancer after 7 years and that vitamin E was associated with a 17% increased risk of prostate cancer compared to placebo. The null result was surprising given the strong preclinical and clinical evidence suggesting chemopreventive activity of selenium (61).

Although the SELECT results are equivocal when examining the effect of vitamin E on the risk of prostate cancer, alpha-tocopherol, the most potent form of naturally occurring vitamin E, had been shown to decrease the risk of prostate cancer in smokers. Interestingly, subsequent follow-up of this same cohort showed no association of vitamin E with prostate cancer, blurring the validity of this association (62).

It is likely that only specific subpopulations may benefit from vitamin E and/or selenium supplementation. Therefore, future studies should consider the baseline status of the participants and age of the cohort, among other characteristics, to determine the role of vitamin E and selenium in PC prevention and treatment.

Fish Oil

Fish oil has a high content of long-chain omega-3 fatty acids such as DHA and EPA. These fats are abundant in fish, crustaceans, and some algae. Fish oil has been shown to induce cell apoptosis and decrease proliferation in several cancer cell lines, including prostate cancer. It decreases PSA doubling time, especially when combined with a decreased intake of omega-6 polyunsaturated fats and *trans* fats (63, 64). Consumption of fish three to four times a week has proven to lead to a significant reduction (up to 40%–44%) in the incidence of prostate cancer (65, 66). It is recommended that patients take a purified fish oil supplement, 1,000 to 3,000 mg daily.

Active Hexose Correlated Compound

A mushroom mycelium extract, active hexose correlated compound (AHCC), is a generic term used to describe a plant polysaccharide extracted from a liquid culture produced from the mycelia of shiitake (*Lentinula edodes*) mushrooms (67). In basic studies on AHCC, it has been reported that AHCC has immunostimulating activity, anticancer activity, and cancer-preventive actions, and can prevent side effects during cancer chemotherapy, among other functions. Administering AHCC to patients with prostate cancer may impede cancer progression (68).

A phase II multicentered clinical trial in which AHCC was administered to patients with early stage PC who were expectantly managed demonstrated a decrease in PSA value by more than 50% in only 1 of 74 patients (1.4%) indicating that AHCC is an ineffective treatment for reducing PSA values by 50% (67). However, regarding advanced metastatic PC, AHCC administration has been shown to result in an excellent serologic PSA response (69).

■ IMPACT OF ANTI-INFLAMMATORY AGENTS

Zyflamend

Zyflamend is an over-the-counter product composed of several herbs in regulated concentrations. The constituents have anti-inflammatory, antioxidant, antiangiogenic, and/or antiproliferative effects. A recent phase I clinical trial was performed to determine whether Zyflamend could influence the progression of biopsy-proven high-grade PIN to prostate cancer. The results yielded 60% of patients with benign tissue, 36% with high-grade PIN, and 14.3% who developed prostate cancer at the final 18-month biopsy. A statistically significant reduction in serum C-reactive protein and reduction in nuclear factor kappa-B staining were also observed in the biopsy tissue samples (70).

Ginger Root

Ginger root, the rhizome of the plant *Zingiber officinale*, has been an herbal medicine for centuries, used to treat nauseas, motion sickness, upper respiratory infections, and intestinal parasites. Modern investigators have discovered in this rhizome more than 20 phytochemicals that inhibit COX-2 (71). These constituents have potent antioxidant and anti-inflammatory activities.

A recent study showed that combining ginger extract with its constituents (in particular, 6-gingerol) resulted in significant augmentation of antiproliferative activity of GEs (72). These data generate compelling grounds for further evaluation of ginger root alone and in combination with individual ginger biophenols for prostate cancer management.

Resveratrol

Resveratrol is a polyphenol found in a variety of plants including berries, grapes, red wine, and peanuts. It has been found to have several anticancer properties such as inhibiting angiogenesis and induction of apoptosis (73, 74). It has also been found to inhibit androgen-induced cell growth in prostate cancer cell lines through interacting with the androgen receptor(75). Resveratrol has been found to be chemopreventive for several malignancies, but its androgen properties have made it a significant interest as an adjuvant treatment of low-grade prostate cancer. Studies in human subjects have shown that resveratrol has poor bioavailability(76), but its proven anticancer properties in several cell lines create ongoing interest to use resveratrol as a therapeutic agent and have increased the efforts to improve its bioavailability.

■ EXERCISE, MEDITATION, AND PROSTATE CANCER

Obesity has been strongly implicated as an independent risk factor for high-grade prostate cancer and prostate cancer mortality(77). Excess body fat alters estrogen and testosterone activity. Lower testosterone is associated with lower PSA at diagnosis(78). Regular exercise is clearly beneficial for overall health, but it especially has a positive impact on men with PC.

A sedentary lifestyle is an important risk factor for PC, and exercise is associated with a decreased PC prevalence(79). The molecular mechanisms involved in this process remain unknown, but a recent study demonstrated that reactive oxygen species generated by physical exercise are a key regulatory factor in prostate cancer prevention. Running is known to enhance the antioxidant defense system, thus reducing oxidative stress. Any decrease in oxidative stress induced by exercise may delay the development of prostate cancer(80).

Yoga is an excellent alternative for men who don't enjoy running. It is an excellent form of exercise that incorporates various stretches to enhance flexibility, blood flow, and may improve sexual function(81).

Mind–body interventions, particularly relaxation and meditation, are another modality that patients with PC should explore. Biomedical research has provided undeniable evidence of the interconnectedness of the mind and body. The field of psychoneuroimmunology has defined the role of stress in reducing effectiveness of the immune system in combating infection and growth of malignant tumors(82). By incorporating exercise and practicing meditation, one can effectively reduce the harmful effects of stress and improve quality of life.

■ SUMMARY

Dietary modification and physical activity interventions in men with early PC enjoy strong support in the published research. The interventions described in this chapter are beneficial for multiple body systems, including the endocrine, cardiovascular, immune, and nervous systems.

With the number of cancer survivors continually rising thanks to early detection and improved treatments, and with our increasing understanding of the benefits of nutritional and exercise interventions in early stage cancers, it is essential that an integrative approach be taken by urologist, primary care physicians, and most important, the patient.

Clinical research into the use of such therapies in early prostate cancer is on the rise. More of this kind of research is imperative for the creation of consistent and effective protocols for chemoprevention. Recommendations for standardization and dosages of herbal medicines are often difficult to determine because of the lack of this kind of research. Still, the benefits of herbal and nutritional chemoprevention appear to greatly outweigh any harm that could come to a patient, particularly in the earliest stages of detectable disease, where active surveillance or "watchful waiting" would be the most likely intervention.

■ REFERENCES

1. Group USCSW. *United States Cancer Statistics: 1999–2009 Incidence and Mortality Web-based Report*. Atlanta, GA; 2013. http://www.cdc.gov/uscs.
2. Auprich M, Augustin H, Budaus L, et al. A comparative performance analysis of total prostate-specific antigen, percentage free prostate-specific antigen, prostate-specific antigen velocity and urinary prostate cancer gene 3 in the first, second and third repeat prostate biopsy. *BJU Int*. 2012;109(11):1627–1635.
3. Loeb S, Berglund A, Stattin P. Population-based study of utilization and determinants of active surveillance and watchful waiting for low- and intermediate-risk prostate cancer. *J Urol*. 2013;190:1742–1749.
4. Howlader N, Noone AM, Krapcho M, et al., eds. *SEER Cancer Statistics Review, 1975–2009 (Vintage 2009 Populations)*. Bethesda, MD: National Cancer Institute; 2012.
5. Rullis I, Shaeffer JA, Lilien OM. Incidence of prostatic carcinoma in the elderly. *Urology*. 1975;6(3):295–297.
6. Sakr WA, Grignon DJ, Crissman JD, et al. High grade prostatic intraepithelial neoplasia (HGPIN) and prostatic adenocarcinoma between the ages of 20–69: an autopsy study of 249 cases. *In Vivo*. 1994;8(3):439–443.
7. Scardino PT. Early detection of prostate cancer. *Urol Clin North Am*. 1989;16(4):635–655.
8. *Survival Rates for Prostate Cancer*. Atlanda, GA: American Cancer Society; 2013. http://www.cancer.org/cancer/prostatecancer/detailedguide/prostate-cancer-survival-rates.
9. Derweesh IH, Kupelian PA, Zippe C, et al. Continuing trends in pathological stage migration in radical prostatectomy specimens. *Urol Oncol*. 2004;22(4):300–306.
10. Parkin DM, Bray F, Ferlay J, Pisani P. Global cancer statistics, 2002. *CA Cancer J Clin*. 2005;55(2):74–108.
11. Bruner DW, Moore D, Parlanti A, Dorgan J, Engstrom P. Relative risk of prostate cancer for men with affected relatives: systematic review and meta-analysis. *Int J Cancer*. 2003;107(5):797–803.
12. Hemminki K, Czene K. Age specific and attributable risks of familial prostate carcinoma from the family-cancer database. *Cancer*. 2002;95(6):1346–1353.
13. Whittemore AS, Wu AH, Kolonel LN, et al. Family history and prostate cancer risk in black, white, and Asian men in the United States and Canada. *Am J Epidemiol*. 1995;141(8):732–740.

14. Zeegers MP, Jellema A, Ostrer H. Empiric risk of prostate carcinoma for relatives of patients with prostate carcinoma: a meta-analysis. *Cancer.* 2003;97(8):1894–1903.
15. Johns LE, Houlston RS. A systematic review and meta-analysis of familial prostate cancer risk. *BJU Int.* 2003;91(9):789–794.
16. Gronberg H, Damber L, Damber JE. Familial prostate cancer in Sweden. A nationwide register cohort study. *Cancer.* 1996;77(1):138–143.
17. Nilsen TI, Vatten LJ. Anthropometry and prostate cancer risk: a prospective study of 22,248 Norwegian men. *Cancer Causes Control.* 1999;10(4):269–275.
18. Habel LA, Van Den Eeden SK, Friedman GD. Body size, age at shaving initiation, and prostate cancer in a large, multiracial cohort. *Prostate.* 2000;43(2):136–143.
19. Giovannucci E, Rimm EB, Stampfer MJ, Colditz GA, Willett WC. Height, body weight, and risk of prostate cancer. *Cancer Epidemiol Biomarkers Prevention.* 1997;6(8):557–563.
20. Calle EE, Rodriguez C, Walker-Thurmond K, Thun MJ. Overweight, obesity, and mortality from cancer in a prospectively studied cohort of U.S. adults. *N Engl J Med.* 2003;348(17):1625–1638.
21. Veierod MB, Laake P, Thelle DS. Dietary fat intake and risk of prostate cancer: a prospective study of 25,708 Norwegian men. *Int J Cancer.* 1997;73(5):634–638.
22. Gong Z, Neuhouser ML, Goodman PJ, et al. Obesity, diabetes, and risk of prostate cancer: results from the prostate cancer prevention trial. *Cancer Epidemiol Biomarkers Prev.* 2006;15(10):1977–1983.
23. MacInnis RJ, English DR. Body size and composition and prostate cancer risk: systematic review and meta-regression analysis. *Cancer Causes Control.* 2006;17(8):989–1003.
24. Figg WD II. How do you want your steak prepared? The impact of meat consumption and preparation on prostate cancer. *Cancer Biol Ther.* 2012;13(12):1141–1142.
25. Joshi AD, Corral R, Catsburg C, et al. Red meat and poultry, cooking practices, genetic susceptibility and risk of prostate cancer: results from a multiethnic case-control study. *Carcinogenesis.* 2012;33(11):2108–2118.
26. Major JM, Cross AJ, Watters JL, Hollenbeck AR, Graubard BI, Sinha R. Patterns of meat intake and risk of prostate cancer among African-Americans in a large prospective study. *Cancer Causes Control.* 2011;22(12):1691–1698.
27. Gu Z, Suburu J, Chen H, Chen YQ. Mechanisms of omega-3 polyunsaturated fatty acids in prostate cancer prevention. *Biomed Res Int.* 2013;2013:824563.
28. Chua ME, Sio MC, Sorongon MC, Morales ML Jr. The relevance of serum levels of long chain omega-3 polyunsaturated fatty acids and prostate cancer risk: a meta-analysis. *Can Urol Assoc J.* 2013;7(5-6):E333-E343.
29. Higdon JV, Delage B, Williams DE, Dashwood RH. Cruciferous vegetables and human cancer risk: epidemiologic evidence and mechanistic basis. *Pharmacol Res.* 2007;55(3):224–236.
30. Choi S, Lew KL, Xiao H, et al. D,L-Sulforaphane-induced cell death in human prostate cancer cells is regulated by inhibitor of apoptosis family proteins and Apaf-1. *Carcinogenesis.* 2007;28(1):151–162.
31. Garikapaty VP, Ashok BT, Chen YG, Mittelman A, Iatropoulos M, Tiwari RK. Anti-carcinogenic and anti-metastatic properties of indole-3-carbinol in prostate cancer. *Oncol Rep.* 2005;13(1):89–93.
32. Cohen JH, Kristal AR, Stanford JL. Fruit and vegetable intakes and prostate cancer risk. *J Natl Cancer Inst.* 2000;92(1):61–68.
33. Setlur SR, Mertz KD, Hoshida Y, et al. Estrogen-dependent signaling in a molecularly distinct subclass of aggressive prostate cancer. *J Natl Cancer Inst.* 2008;100(11):815–825.
34. Pendleton JM, Tan WW, Anai S, et al. Phase II trial of isoflavone in prostate-specific antigen recurrent prostate cancer after previous local therapy. *BMC Cancer.* 2008;8:132.
35. Yan L, Spitznagel EL. Meta-analysis of soy food and risk of prostate cancer in men. *Int J Cancer.* 2005;117(4):667–669.
36. Park SY, Murphy SP, Wilkens LR, Henderson BE, Kolonel LN; Multiethnic Cohort Study. Legume and isoflavone intake and prostate cancer risk: the Multiethnic Cohort Study. *Int J Cancer.* 2008;123(4):927–932.
37. Engelhardt PF, Riedl CR. Effects of one-year treatment with isoflavone extract from red clover on prostate, liver function, sexual function, and quality of life in men with elevated PSA levels and negative prostate biopsy findings. *Urology.* 2008;71(2):185– 190; discussion 90.
38. Wei MY, Giovannucci EL. Lycopene, tomato products, and prostate cancer incidence: a review and reassessment in the PSA screening era. *J Oncol.* 2012;2012:271063.
39. Barber NJ, Zhang X, Zhu G, et al. Lycopene inhibits DNA synthesis in primary prostate epithelial cells in vitro and its administration is associated with a reduced prostate-specific antigen velocity in a phase II clinical study. *Prostate Cancer Prostatic Dis.* 2006;9(4):407–413.
40. Ilic D, Forbes KM, Hassed C. Lycopene for the prevention of prostate cancer. *Cochrane Database Syst Rev.* 2011;(11):CD008007.
41. Kurahashi N, Sasazuki S, Iwasaki M, Inoue M, Tsugane S, Group JS. Green tea consumption and prostate cancer risk in Japanese men: a prospective study. *Am J Epidemiol.* 2008;167(1):71–77.
42. Adhami VM, Ahmad N, Mukhtar H. Molecular targets for green tea in prostate cancer prevention. *J Nutr.* 2003;133(7 suppl):2417S-2424S.
43. Pezzato E, Sartor L, Dell'Aica I, et al. Prostate carcinoma and green tea: PSA-triggered basement membrane degradation and MMP-2 activation are inhibited by (-)epigallocatechin-3-gallate. *Int J Cancer.* 2004;112(5):787–792.
44. Stuart EC, Scandlyn MJ, Rosengren RJ. Role of epigallocatechin gallate (EGCG) in the treatment of breast and prostate cancer. *Life Sci.* 2006;79(25):2329–2336.
45. Kroeger N, Belldegrun AS, Pantuck AJ. Pomegranate extracts in the management of Men's urologic health: scientific rationale and preclinical and clinical data. *Evid Based Complement Alternat Med.* 2013;2013:701434.
46. Pantuck AJ, Leppert JT, Zomorodian N, et al. Phase II study of pomegranate juice for men with rising prostate-specific antigen following surgery or radiation for prostate cancer. *Clin Cancer Res.* 2006;12(13):4018–4026.
47. Howell AB, Vorsa N, Der Marderosian A, Foo LY. Inhibition of the adherence of P-fimbriated *Escherichia coli* to uroepithelial-cell surfaces by proanthocyanidin extracts from cranberries. *N Eng J Med.* 1998;339(15):1085–1086.
48. Deziel BA, Patel K, Neto C, Gottschall-Pass K, Hurta RA. Proanthocyanidins from the American Cranberry (*Vaccinium macrocarpon*) inhibit matrix metalloproteinase-2 and matrix metalloproteinase-9 activity in human prostate cancer cells via alterations in multiple cellular signalling pathways. *J Cell Biochem.* 2010;111(3):742–754.
49. Neto CC. Cranberry and its phytochemicals: a review of in vitro anticancer studies. *J Nutr.* 2007;137(1 suppl):186S-193S.
50. Habib FK, Ross M, Ho CK, Lyons V, Chapman K. Serenoa repens (Permixon) inhibits the 5alpha-reductase activity of human prostate cancer cell lines without interfering with PSA expression. *Int J Cancer.* 2005;114(2):190–194.
51. Yang Y, Ikezoe T, Zheng Z, Taguchi H, Koeffler HP, Zhu WG. Saw Palmetto induces growth arrest and apoptosis of androgen-dependent prostate cancer LNPC cells via inactivation of STAT 3 and androgen receptor signaling. *Int J Oncol.* 2007;31(3):593–600.
52. Bonnar-Pizzorno RM, Littman AJ, Kestin M, White E. Saw palmetto supplement use and prostate cancer risk. *Nutr Cancer.* 2006;55(1):21–27.
53. Demark-Wahnefried W, Polascik TJ, George SL, et al. Flaxseed supplementation (not dietary fat restriction) reduces prostate cancer proliferation rates in men presurgery. *Cancer Epidemiol Biomarkers Prev.* 2008;17(12):3577–3587.

54. Aggarwal BB, Sung B. Pharmacological basis for the role of curcumin in chronic diseases: an age-old spice with modern targets. *Trends Pharmacol Sci.* 2009;30(2):85–94.
55. Dorai T, Cao YC, Dorai B, Buttyan R, Katz AE. Therapeutic potential of curcumin in human prostate cancer. III. Curcumin inhibits proliferation, induces apoptosis, and inhibits angiogenesis of LNPC prostate cancer cells in vivo. *Prostate.* 2001;47(4):293–303.
56. John EM, Koo J, Schwartz GG. Sun exposure and prostate cancer risk: evidence for a protective effect of early-life exposure. *Cancer Epidemiol Biomarkers Prev.* 2007;16(6):1283–1286.
57. Van Veldhuizen PJ, Taylor SA, Williamson S, Drees BM. Treatment of vitamin D deficiency in patients with metastatic prostate cancer may improve bone pain and muscle strength. *J Urol.* 2000;163(1):187–190.
58. Krishnan AV, Moreno J, Nonn L, Swami S, Peehl DM, Feldman D. Calcitriol as a chemopreventive and therapeutic agent in prostate cancer: role of anti-inflammatory activity. *J Bone Miner Res.* 2007;22(suppl 2):V74–V80.
59. Holick MF. Calcium and vitamin D. Diagnostics and therapeutics. *Clin Lab Med.* 2000;20(3):569–590.
60. Skinner HG, Schwartz GG. Serum calcium and incident and fatal prostate cancer in the National Health and Nutrition Examination Survey. *Cancer Epidemiol Biomarkers Prev.* 2008;17(9):2302–2305.
61. Klein EA, Thompson IM, Lippman SM, et al. SELECT: the selenium and vitamin E cancer prevention trial. *Urolo Oncol.* 2003;21(1):59–65.
62. Heinonen OP, Albanes D, Virtamo J, et al. Prostate cancer and supplementation with alpha-tocopherol and beta-carotene: incidence and mortality in a controlled trial. *J Natl Cancer Inst.* 1998;90(6):440–446.
63. Kobayashi N, Barnard RJ, Henning SM, et al. Effect of altering dietary omega-6/omega-3 fatty acid ratios on prostate cancer membrane composition, cyclooxygenase-2, and prostaglandin E2. *Clin Cancer Res.* 2006;12(15):4662–4670.
64. Kelavkar UP, Hutzley J, Dhir R, Kim P, Allen KG, McHugh K. Prostate tumor growth and recurrence can be modulated by the omega-6:omega-3 ratio in diet: athymic mouse xenograft model simulating radical prostatectomy. *Neoplasia.* 2006;8(2):112–124.
65. Norrish AE, Skeaff CM, Arribas GL, Sharpe SJ, Jackson RT. Prostate cancer risk and consumption of fish oils: a dietary biomarker-based case-control study. *Br J Cancer.* 1999;81(7):1238–1242.
66. Augustsson K, Michaud DS, Rimm EB, et al. A prospective study of intake of fish and marine fatty acids and prostate cancer. *Cancer Epidemiol Biomarkers Prev.* 2003;12(1):64–67.
67. Sumiyoshi Y, Hashine K, Kakehi Y, et al. Dietary administration of mushroom mycelium extracts in patients with early stage prostate cancers managed expectantly: a phase II study. *Jpn J Clini Oncol.* 2010;40(10):967–972.
68. deVere White RW, Hackman RM, Soares SE, Beckett LA, Sun B. Effects of a mushroom mycelium extract on the treatment of prostate cancer. *Urology.* 2002;60(4):640–644.
69. Turner J, Chaudhary U. Dramatic prostate-specific antigen response with activated hemicellulose compound in metastatic castration-resistant prostate cancer. *Anticancer Drugs.* 2009;20(3):215–216.
70. Capodice JL, Gorroochurn P, Cammack AS, et al. Zyflamend in men with high-grade prostatic intraepithelial neoplasia: results of a phase I clinical trial. *J Soc Integr Oncol.* 2009;7(2):43–51.
71. Shukla Y, Singh M. Cancer preventive properties of ginger: a brief review. *Food Chem Toxicol.* 2007;45(5):683–690.
72. Brahmbhatt M, Gundala SR, Asif G, Shamsi SA, Aneja R. Ginger phytochemicals exhibit synergy to inhibit prostate cancer cell proliferation. *Nutr Cancer.* 2013;65(2):263–272.
73. Aggarwal BB, Bhardwaj A, Aggarwal RS, Seeram NP, Shishodia S, Takada Y. Role of resveratrol in prevention and therapy of cancer: preclinical and clinical studies. *Anticancer Res.* 2004;24(5A):2783–2840.
74. Shukla Y, Singh R. Resveratrol and cellular mechanisms of cancer prevention. *Ann N Y Acad Sci.* 2011;1215:1–8.
75. Mitchell SH, Zhu W, Young CY. Resveratrol inhibits the expression and function of the androgen receptor in LNPC prostate cancer cells. *Cancer Res.* 1999;59(23):5892–5895.
76. Subramanian L, Youssef S, Bhattacharya S, Kenealey J, Polans AS, van Ginkel PR. Resveratrol: challenges in translation to the clinic—a critical discussion. *Clin Cancer Res.* 2010;16(24):5942–5948.
77. Zadra G, Photopoulos C, Loda M. The fat side of prostate cancer. *Biochim Biophys Acta.* 2013;1831:1518–1532.
78. Tymchuk CN, Tessler SB, Aronson WJ, Barnard RJ. Effects of diet and exercise on insulin, sex hormone-binding globulin, and prostate-specific antigen. *Nutr Cancer.* 1998;31(2):127–131.
79. Amling CL. Relationship between obesity and prostate cancer. *Curr Opin Urol.* 2005;15(3):167–171.
80. Rebillard A, Lefeuvre-Orfila L, Gueritat J, Cillard J. Prostate cancer and physical activity: adaptive response to oxidative stress. *Free Radic Biol Med.* 2013;60:115–124.
81. Mishra SI, Scherer RW, Snyder C, Geigle PM, Berlanstein DR, Topaloglu O. Exercise interventions on health-related quality of life for people with cancer during active treatment. *Cochrane Database Syst Rev.* 2012;8:CD008465.
82. Coker KH. Meditation and prostate cancer: integrating a mind/body intervention with traditional therapies. *Semin Urol Oncol.* 1999;17(2):111–118.

9.1 Traditional Radical Prostatectomy

ZACHARY L. SMITH
THOMAS J. GUZZO

INTRODUCTION

Radical prostatectomy for the treatment of prostate cancer was first performed by Young in 1904 (1). The operation was performed via a perineal approach that remained the standard for many decades. The first radical retropubic prostatectomy (RRP) was performed by Terence Millin in 1947 (2). There were few advances in surgical technique until 1979 when Reiner and Walsh described Santorini's plexus of the dorsal vein, now typically referred to as the dorsal venous complex (DVC), allowing for drastically reduced blood loss and an overall safer operation (3). Over the next several years, there were many discoveries that continued to improve the operation, such as the description of the striated urethral sphincter as well as the neurovascular bundles (NVBs) (4, 5). It was shortly after these discoveries that the modern-day RRP was first performed—referred to as the *anatomical radical prostatectomy*—incorporating all of the knowledge of the anatomy of the male pelvis and applying this for optimal outcomes in cancer eradication and preservation of continence and potency (6).

Since the advent of the modern RRP, it has remained the gold-standard therapy for clinically localized prostate cancer. Recent improvements in the operation have primarily focused on minimally invasive techniques. In fact, robotic-assisted laparoscopic radical prostatectomy (RARP) is now the most common surgical approach used in the United States (7). However, multiple systematic reviews have failed to provide sufficient data to support any particular modality as having superior oncological or functional outcomes (8, 9). As a result, many urologists continue to offer RRP to their patients as an excellent option for definitive treatment of their prostate cancer.

ANATOMY AND SURGICAL TECHNIQUE

RRP can be performed with most standard laparotomy instrument sets, having very few special requirements. Some institutions prefer spinal or epidural anesthesia over general anesthesia for this procedure because there has been suggestion that this approach is associated with less blood loss and a lower frequency of thromboembolic events (10, 11). After induction of appropriate anesthesia, an 8- to 10-cm incision is made in the midline from the pubis toward the umbilicus. The rectus muscles are separated at the midline, and the underlying tissues and fascia are dissected in an extraperitoneal fashion to expose the space of Retzius. In most cases, a bilateral pelvic lymph node dissection (PLND) is carried out. The extent of the dissection is debated, with routine extended PLND being reserved for patients with high-risk disease in most instances. In most patients, removal of the nodes overlying and beneath the external iliac vein will suffice. It is imperative that the obturator nerve be identified during this portion of the procedure to avoid debilitating injury.

A malleable retractor or a sponge stick is used to superiorly displace the bladder and peritoneum. To expose the prostate, the endopelvic fascia must be incised and puboprostatic ligaments divided. Care should be taken to avoid injuring the superficial branch of the DVC. After adequate exposure of the anterior surface of the prostate, the DVC must be ligated and divided. This is done in many different ways, including en bloc suture ligation, individual vessel suture ligation, or en bloc stapling. Most commonly, sutures are used to ligate the DVC proximally and distally before sharp division. Appropriate control of the DVC is paramount as it allows for direct visualization of the apex of the prostate, which is critical to oncologic and functional outcomes.

Attention is then turned to preservation of the NVBs bilaterally. This is possible in the majority of men who are surgical candidates (12). To do this, the lateral pelvic fascia must be separated, gently removing the levator fascia and NVB from the prostate and leaving the prostatic fascia attached. If nodularity is palpable in the lateral pelvic fascia or if the NVB is completely fixed to the prostate, this suggests extracapsular disease and the NVB should be excised on that side.

After adequate control of the DVC as described earlier, the junction of the urethra and the apex of the prostate should be well exposed. This can be then isolated and transected anteriorly, exposing the lumen of the urethra and the foley catheter. Three to five sutures are then placed through the urethral stump and secured individually and not tied down. The posterior urethra is divided, and the remaining circumferential sutures are placed in the urethra. Dissection is continued posteriorly, freeing the prostate from the rectum. The lateral pedicles should be divided at this point to prevent any bleeding during excision of the seminal vesicles.

After mobilizing the entire prostate, the anterior bladder neck is incised at the prostatovesicular junction. The foley catheter is looped around the body of the prostate and used to apply traction. The bladder neck incision is widened with studious attention paid to vessels in the inferior vesical pedicles. When dividing the posterior bladder neck, special observation must be paid to the ureteral orifices as the trigone can present in varying ways at this region. Ureteral orifice visualization can be particularly challenging if the patient has a large intravesical median lobe. Intravenous methylene blue or Indigo Carmine® may be administered to aid in visualization of the ureteral orifices. Once the bladder neck has been completely divided, the vas deferentia may be ligated and divided and the seminal vesicle dissection can be completed. Care should be taken to not injure the pelvic plexus during this time, which is intimately associated with the lateral aspects of the seminal vesicles. After completion of this, the specimen is ready for removal from the surgical field.

The bladder neck should be inspected for shape and diameter of its opening. Particularly in patients with large prostatic median lobes, reconstruction of the bladder neck may be required to allow for a proper fit during anastomosis to the urethra. The urethral sutures are passed into the bladder neck but not tied down. The final Foley catheter is then placed. Once the Foley catheter is in good position in the bladder and the balloon is inflated, all anastomotic sutures are then tied down circumferentially. The catheter is irrigated to check for any anastomotic leaks, and a suction drain is typically placed in the pelvis. The abdomen is then closed in standard surgical fashion, thus concluding the operation.

Postoperatively, the Foley catheter is left in place for 7 to 14 days depending on surgeon preference and satisfaction with the anastomosis. A voiding cystourethrogram (VCUG) may be performed prior to Foley catheter removal to assess for any anastomotic leaks. This practice is based on surgeon preference or clinical suspicion, in such cases as increased output of the pelvic suction drain. If an anastomotic leak is found on a VCUG, the Foley catheter is left in place for an extended duration until resolution, which is determined by repeat VCUG.

■ OUTCOMES AND COMPLICATIONS

When analyzing the results of RRP, the often mentioned "trifecta" of postoperative outcomes consists of cancer control (prostate-specific antigen [PSA] detectability), continence, and potency (13). There has been improvement across the field in most of these variables, likely owing to improvements in surgical technique as well as the drastic stage migration seen over the last two decades, primarily due to routine PSA screening (14). There is now a much higher proportion of patients being diagnosed with prostate cancer, while their disease is still at a low-risk stage. Early detection has helped to make RRP an even more ideal choice for definitive treatment with curative intent.

Cancer Control

RRP has been shown in multiple large series to have a 15-year cancer-specific survival (CSS) of greater than 87% (15–20). Most of these data come from high-volume centers and reflect the importance of a proficient surgical team. Also, large databases of these institutions have allowed us to learn a great deal about long-term oncologic outcomes. Table 9.1.1 summarizes the long-term outcome data from a selection of such series.

Eggener et al. showed in their series of 23,910 patients that the outcomes of RRP are quite good, but stratification by disease stage is highly impactful on the outcome (16). This study showed that the 15-year prostate cancer–specific mortality (PCSM) for pathological Gleason score ≤6, 7, and 8 to 10 was 0.2% to 1.2%, 4.2% to 11%, and 26% to 37%, respectively. When stratified by other pathological characteristics, the 15-year PCSM risk was 0.8% to 1.5%, 2.9% to 10%, 15% to 27%, and 22% to 30% for organ-confined disease, extraprostatic extension, seminal vesicle invasion, and lymph node metastasis, respectively.

Walsh and coworkers recently published long-term follow-up data on his 30-year history of performing the anatomical RRP (20). This single-surgeon series consisted of 4,478 men who underwent the operation between 1982 and 2011. This demonstrated a CSS of 97%, 94%, 90%, and 86% at 10, 15, 20, and 25 years, respectively. Biochemical recurrence-free survival for these same intervals was 82%, 78%, 74%, and 68%, respectively.

The above figures represent the results of experienced and skilled surgeons; however, with proper technique, these results can be extrapolated to the general public at large. In addition, the advantage of RRP over observation has now been substantiated in a randomized trial by the Scandinavian Prostate Cancer Study Group

Table 9.1.1 Oncologic outcomes following radical retropubic prostatectomy

		OS (%)		CSS (%)		bRFS (%)		MFS (%)	
Author (*Database*)	No. of Patients	10 y	15 y	10 y	15 y	10 y	15 y	10 y	15 y
Han et al. (17) *(JHU)*	2,091	—	—	96	89	72	61	89	81
Roehl et al. (21) *(W. Catalona [WUSTL])*	3,478	83	—	97	—	68	—	—	—
Bianco et al. (18) *(P. Scardino [MSKCC & Baylor])*	1,746	89	67	95	89	77	75	—	—
Boorjian et al. (22) *(Mayo Clinic)*[a]	1,238	77	—	92	—	—	—	85	—
Lewinshtein et al. (19) *(Virginia Mason)*	459	77	61	94	87	66	66	93	90
Mullins et al. (20) *(P. Walsh [JHU])*	4,478	—	—	97	94	82	78	94	92

[a]NCCN high-risk disease patients only.

Abbreviations: OS, overall survival; CSS, cancer-specific survival; bRFS, biochemical recurrence-free survival; MFS, metastasis-free survival; JHU, Johns Hopkins University; WUSTL, Washington University in St Louis; MSKCC, Memorial Sloan Kettering Cancer Center.

Number 4 (SPCG-4). This trial reported the advantage for patients undergoing RRP over watchful waiting, showing a 50% improvement in metastasis-free survival, CSS, and overall survival at 15 years (23). The SPCG-4 investigators also found the number needed to treat to avert one death as 15 overall and 7 for men younger than 65 years. However, the vast majority of cancers in the SPCG-4 study were not detected by PSA screening, which in turn limits our ability to generalize these findings to a more contemporary population.

Continence

Urinary incontinence represents a significant quality-of-life burden following RRP. Incontinence is usually secondary to intrinsic striated urethral sphincter deficiency. If a man has a poorly developed or weakened sphincter, this may be exaggerated after surgery as stress urinary incontinence. However, the principal cause is likely damage to the sphincter during dissection of the prostate apex and/or during ligation of the DVC.

The reported incidence of urinary incontinence varies in the literature due to the inconsistency in rating the degree of urine leakage. A meta-analysis of 30 studies from high-volume centers found the weighted mean continence rate at 12 months to be 79% (24). Walsh et al. found this incidence to be 93% in his series (25). Looking past the first year postoperatively, a large population-based study found that only 8.4% of men had either frequent urinary leakage or no control at 24 months follow-up (26). Unfortunately, in addition to the limitations posed by inconsistent *reporting* of the degree of urine leakage, there is also inconsistency in the means of *measuring* the amount of leakage. This is done by subjective patient reporting in most studies, while less often this is objectively obtained via pad weight.

Potency

There are multiple factors that contribute to erectile function following RRP including patient age, preoperative function, and the quality of NVB preservation at the time of surgery. A sampling of high-volume centers reported the 12-month weighted mean potency rates for patients who underwent unilateral or bilateral nerve sparing as 43.1% and 60.6%, respectively (24). The Johns Hopkins University group assessed recovery of sexual function via a third-party validated questionnaire (27). These rates, with or without sildenafil administration, were 42%, 49%, and 73% at 3, 6, and 12 months follow-up, respectively.

Different methods of penile rehabilitation have been described. It has been common practice for many years to recommend scheduled (nightly or every other day) phosphodiesterase type 5 (PDE5) inhibitor dosing to facilitate return of normal blood circulation to the penis. However, there have been two randomized trials that have supported on-demand dosing of PDE5 inhibitors as the most efficacious route to the recovery of sexual function (28, 29).

Other Complications

RRP may be associated with the same postoperative complications as any major abdominopelvic surgery. This includes delayed bleeding, thromboembolic events, wound infections, and injury to the surrounding organs. However, there are some risks that are unique to RRP, which are worthy of mention.

Bladder neck contracture (BNC) occurs in 0.5% to 10% of patients after RRP (30). This is believed to occur secondary to poor coaptation of the mucosal surfaces of the urethra and bladder during the anastomosis or from a prolonged anastomotic leak. These may occur secondary to failure to evert the mucosa of the urethra and bladder, poorly tied anastomotic sutures, disruption due to traumatic Foley catheter manipulation, or displacement secondary to postoperative hematoma. Fortunately, a BNC can be typically treated successfully with endoscopic management via incision or dilation. Rarely, a BNC can represent a severe process and can result in a recurrent or refractory narrowing of the anastomosis. In these situations, a more radical procedure of the bladder neck may be required to return patency. Unfortunately, this often results in poorer outcomes for the patient's continence.

As with any operation of the urinary tract, there is a risk of urine leakage and formation of a urinoma. These are often handled conservatively; however, if they become large and cause the patient discomfort or if they become infected, they may require percutaneous drainage. In addition, the search for a continuous source of the urine leakage must be investigated to assure appropriate resolution. Similar to a urinoma, patients may experience formation of a lymphocele secondary to the PLND. These are often treated with a similar algorithm as urinomas; however, these less often require any intervention. Typically, lymphoceles are only drained if the patient is symptomatic.

OTHER CONSIDERATIONS

A presumed easier postoperative recovery is one of the primary attractants to RARP for patients; however, there are some risks to RARP that do not exist with RRP. For example, the transperitoneal approach predisposes patients to a greater risk of bowel injury and postoperative intra-abdominal adhesions. In fact, compared with RRP, RARP is associated with a higher proportion of deviations from the standard postoperative pathway, primarily due to ileus (1.9% incidence with RARP, 0.28% with RRP; $P < .001$) (31).

Unfortunately, some patients experience recurrence of their disease following RRP, despite appropriate patient selection and good surgical technique. A recent study examined patients who ultimately developed castrate-resistant prostate cancer (CRPC) and explored if there were any eventual palliative benefits to the specific primary treatment they received (32). At the time of diagnosis of CRPC or metastatic disease, patients who had initially undergone RRP showed a significantly lower level of local complications compared with those who underwent radiation therapy as their primary treatment (20.0% vs. 46.7%; $P = .007$). The most common local complications seen were bladder outlet and ureteric obstruction.

CONCLUSIONS

RRP has continued to exist as one of the principal treatment options for patients with clinically localized prostate cancer. Advances in technique and technology alike have afforded the operation improvements in its perioperative morbidity as well as long-term outcomes. For patients who desire treatment with curative intent and have a good life expectancy, RRP remains the first-line treatment for management of their prostate cancer.

REFERENCES

1. Young HH. VIII. Conservative perineal prostatectomy: the results of two years' experience and report of seventy-five cases. *Ann Surg.* 1905;41:549–557.
2. Millin T. Retropubic prostatectomy. *J Urol.* 1948;59:267–280.
3. Reiner WG, Walsh PC. An anatomical approach to the surgical management of the dorsal vein and Santorini's plexus during radical retropubic surgery. *J Urol.* 1979;121:198–200.
4. Oelrich TM. The urethral sphincter muscle in the male. *Am J Anat.* 1980;158:229–246.
5. Walsh PC, Donker PJ. Impotence following radical prostatectomy: insight into etiology and prevention. *J Urol.* 1982;128:492–497.
6. Walsh PC, Lepor H, Eggleston JC. Radical prostatectomy with preservation of sexual function: anatomical and pathological considerations. *Prostate.* 1983;4:473–485.
7. Yates DR, Vaessen C, Roupret M. From Leonardo to da Vinci: the history of robot-assisted surgery in urology. *BJU Int.* 2011;108:1708–1713; discussion 1714.
8. Ficarra V, Novara G, Artibani W, et al. Retropubic, laparoscopic, and robot-assisted radical prostatectomy: a systematic review and cumulative analysis of comparative studies. *Eur Urol.* 2009;55:1037–1063.
9. Finkelstein J, Eckersberger E, Sadri H, Taneja SS, Lepor H, Djavan B. Open versus laparoscopic versus robot-assisted laparoscopic prostatectomy: the European and US experience. *Rev Urol.* 2010;12:35–43.
10. Peters CA, Walsh PC. Blood transfusion and anesthetic practices in radical retropubic prostatectomy. *J Urol.* 1985;134:81–83.
11. Shir Y, Raja SN, Frank SM, Brendler CB. Intraoperative blood loss during radical retropubic prostatectomy: epidural versus general anesthesia. *Urology.* 1995;45:993–999.
12. Walsh PC. Nerve grafts are rarely necessary and are unlikely to improve sexual function in men undergoing anatomic radical prostatectomy. *Urology.* 2001;57:1020–1024.
13. Borregales LD, Berg WT, Tal O, et al. 'Trifecta' after radical prostatectomy: is there a standard definition? *BJU Int.* 2013;112:60–67.
14. Han M, Partin AW, Chan DY, Walsh PC. An evaluation of the decreasing incidence of positive surgical margins in a large retropubic prostatectomy series. *J Urol.* 2004;171:23–26.
15. Stephenson AJ, Kattan MW, Eastham JA, et al. Prostate cancer-specific mortality after radical prostatectomy for patients treated in the prostate-specific antigen era. *J Clin Oncol.* 2009;27:4300–4305.
16. Eggener SE, Scardino PT, Walsh PC, et al. Predicting 15-year prostate cancer specific mortality after radical prostatectomy. *J Urol.* 2011;185:869–875.
17. Han M, Partin AW, Zahurak M, et al. Biochemical (prostate specific antigen) recurrence probability following radical prostatectomy for clinically localized prostate cancer. *J Urol.* 2003;169:517.
18. Bianco FJ Jr, Scardino PT, Eastham JA. Radical prostatectomy: long-term cancer control and recovery of sexual and urinary function ("trifecta"). *Urology.* 2005;66:83.
19. Lewinshtein D, Teng B, Valencia A, et al. The association between pre-operative PSA and prostate cancer-specific mortality in patients with long-term follow-up after radical prostatectomy. *Prostate.* 2012;72:24.
20. Mullins JK, Feng Z, Trock BJ, Epstein JI, Walsh PC, Loeb S. The impact of anatomical radical retropubic prostatectomy on cancer control: the 30-year anniversary. *J Urol.* 2012;188:2219–2224.

21. Roehl KA, Han M, Ramos CG, et al. Cancer progression and survival rates following anatomical radical retropubic prostatectomy in 3,478 consecutive patients: long-term results. *J Urol.* 2004;172:910.
22. Boorjian SA, Karnes RJ, Viterbo R, et al. Long-term survival after radical prostatectomy versus external-beam radiotherapy for patients with high risk prostate cancer. *Cancer.* 2011;117:2883.
23. Bill-Axelson A, Holmberg L, Ruutu M, et al. Radical prostatectomy versus watchful waiting in early prostate cancer. *N Engl J Med.* 2011;364:1708–1717.
24. Coelho RF, Rocco B, Patel MB, et al. Retropubic, laparoscopic, and robot-assisted radical prostatectomy: a critical review of outcomes reported by high-volume centers. *J Endourol.* 2010;24:2003–2015.
25. Walsh PC, Marschke P, Ricker D, Burnett AL. Patient-reported urinary continence and sexual function after anatomic radical prostatectomy. *Urology.* 2000;55:58–61.
26. Stanford JL, Feng Z, Hamilton AS, et al. Urinary and sexual function after radical prostatectomy for clinically localized prostate cancer: the Prostate Cancer Outcomes Study. *JAMA.* 2000;283:354–360.
27. Parsons JK, Marschke P, Maples P, Walsh PC. Effect of methylprednisolone on return of sexual function after nerve-sparing radical retropubic prostatectomy. *Urology.* 2004;64:987–990.
28. Montorsi F, Brock G, Lee J, et al. Effect of nightly versus on-demand vardenafil on recovery of erectile function in men following bilateral nerve-sparing radical prostatectomy. *Eur Urol.* 2008;54:924–931.
29. Pavlovich CP, Mettee LZ, Su LM, Jarow JP, Trock BJ. Nightly sildenafil is unnecessary after minimally invasive nerve-sparing radical prostatectomy: on demand sildenafil provides equivalent restoration of erectile function. *J Urol.* 2009;181:485.
30. Schaeffer EM, Partin AW, Lepor H, Walsh PC. Radical retropubic and perineal prostatectomy. In: Wein AJ, Kavoussi LR, Novick AC, Partin AW, Peters CA, eds. *Campbell-Walsh Urology.* 10th ed. Philadelphia, PA: Elsevier Saunders; 2012.
31. Pierorazio PM, Mullins JK, Ross AE, et al. Trends in immediate perioperative morbidity and delay in discharge after open and minimally invasive radical prostatectomy (RP): a 20-year institutional experience. *BJU Int.* 2013;112:45–53.
32. Won AC, Gurney H, Marx G, De Souza P, Patel MI. Primary treatment of the prostate improves local palliation in men who ultimately develop castrate-resistant prostate cancer. *BJU Int.* 2013;112:E250–E255.

9.2 Laparoscopic Radical Prostatectomy: Techniques and Complications

FERNANDO PABLO SECIN

KARIM TOUIJER

■ SUMMARY

Laparoscopic radical prostatectomy (LRP) has gained increasing importance in the laparoscopic urologic oncology field and became an established treatment for localized prostate cancer. The indications for LRP are the same as those for the open technique. The advantages of the laparoscopic approach are a magnified view of the anatomic structures and a decreased venous bleeding in the surgical field allowing an accurate dissection of the prostate and neurovascular bundles (NVBs). The LRP technique is well standardized. Five trocars are used; the patient is placed in the Trendelenburg position. The sequential steps of the operation are dissection of the seminal vesicles (SVs), a direct approach, after incising the peritoneum above Douglas' cul-de-sac; creation of a space between the rectum and prostate behind Denonvilliers' fascia (they can also be dissected after opening the posterior bladder neck [PBN]), release of the bladder to approach the space of Retzius; opening of the endopelvic fascia and intracorporeal ligature of the dorsal vascular complex (DVC); dissection of the prostate from the bladder, by close dissection of the bladder neck; control of the pedicles and dissection of the NVB; sectioning of the urethra and removal of the prostate in a bag; urethrovesical anastomosis is performed with interrupted running of intracorporeal sutures; Foley catheter installation; and placement of an aspiration drain and closure. Knowledge of the prostatic anatomy, advanced laparoscopic skills, and expertise in surgical oncology are essential to provide optimal oncologic outcomes while maintaining the highest standards of life quality.

■ INTRODUCTION

LRP has gained an increasing importance in the laparoscopic urologic oncology field and has become an established treatment for localized prostate cancer. The initial report of LRP by Schuessler et al. was of nine cases performed through a transperitoneal approach (1). Shortly thereafter, a single case of a LRP through an extraperitoneal approach was reported (2). However, in the largest initial series originating from France, the transperitoneal approach was used (3–9). With accrued experience and worldwide use, modifications in the approach and the instrumentation used were introduced (10–16). This chapter describes the antegrade transperitoneal LRP initially described by Prof. Dr. Bertrand Guillonneau in France, a technique he subsequently improved and developed at Memorial Sloan Kettering Cancer Center, and reviews its potential complications.

■ PATIENT SELECTION AND PREOPERATIVE PREPARATION

The indications for LRP are the same as those for the open technique (17). However, similarly to the open approach, the surgeon often faces different situations that might make the laparoscopic approach more technically challenging. These include obese patients, patients with a large prostate gland, patients whose prostates have a large median lobe, presence of accessory vessels, patients with a narrow deep pelvis, those with a history of abdominal/pelvic surgery or pelvic fracture, and those with previous radiotherapy to the pelvis.

No bowel or rectal preparation is needed, but a fleet enema is often recommended particularly in patients who had prior prostate radiotherapy. A single dose of a first-generation cephalosporin is administrated prior to surgery as antibiotic prophylaxis (18, 19).

Venous thromboembolic prophylaxis is accomplished by administering low-molecular-weight heparin subcutaneously before the operation according to the patient's risk of deep venous thrombosis. Patients continue to receive this daily dose until they are discharged (20, 21). Pneumatic compression stockings are also used during the surgery, and they are discontinued when the patient resumes ambulation (22, 23).

■ RATIONALE FOR TRANSPERITONEAL APPROACH

Both transperitoneal and preperitoneal prostatectomy techniques can be performed (24,25). The main advantages of the transperitoneal approach are greater mobilization of the bladder, which allows a tension-free anastomosis, more working space, and a more meticulous dissection of the SVs. It is our belief that early dissection of the SV can minimize damage to the pelvic plexus, which is particularly important when a nerve-sparing procedure is planned.

The transperitoneal approach allows faster placement of the trocars. However, the preperitoneal approach eliminates the time associated with the transperitoneal bladder dissection. The preperitoneal method may also reduce even further the minimal but real risk of bladder injury, given that the space of Retzius is developed initially. In addition, once performed, there is little concern regarding visceral injury.

The bowel is in the operative field with the transperitoneal approach, and, thus, a steeper Trendelenburg position is required to move the bowel out of the pelvic cavity, at least during the initial step, when dissection of the SV is considered.

In the preperitoneal approach, the peritoneum isolates the operative field from the abdominal cavity. This method is advantageous, as bleeding, when encountered, does not contact the bowel, thus avoiding reflex ileus. Also, a non-watertight urethrovesical anastomosis does not result in urinary ascites with its associated complications. However, the transperitoneal approach allows a more extensive lymph node (LN) dissection when clinically indicated.

It is our experience that the transperitoneal approach does not prevent the patient from receiving adjuvant radiation therapy if required, as all pelvic structures are repositioned to their preoperative anatomical locations. The small bowel does not get interposed between the pubic bone and the bladder postoperatively.

There is a widespread belief that minimally invasive prostatectomy should mimic what is done in open surgery. Actually, the extraperitoneal laparoscopic technique is expected to improve on the open prostatectomy technique given its much better visualization and working room.

■ THE INSTRUMENTS

The quality of the optical chain (camera and monitor) is important, especially late in the procedure when the anatomical constraints of the deep pelvis limit the quality of the images. The monitors can either be flat liquid crystal display panels or conventional cathode ray tube (CRT). The quality of the conventional CRT in terms of color, resolution, brightness, and viewing angle is superior and is our preference.

We perform the LRP with mostly reusable material: two axial long prehension forceps, bipolar forceps (one thin, one flat, and one triangular), laparoscopic scissors, three 5.5 × 55-mm trocars, one 5.5 × 55-mm trocar with a lateral insufflation valve, one 10-mm Trocar, two straight needle holders, one 24-French Heggar rectal bougie n° and a 20-Frenc Béniqué urethral sound. The only disposable material is a 10-mm bag to remove the specimen and a 5-mm suction cannula (can also be reusable). In obese patients, we use longer trocars (5.5 × 70 mm).

■ SURGICAL TECHNIQUE

Transperitoneal pneumoperitoneum is made with the patient in the flat position and set at an intra-abdominal pressure of 12 mmHg. A 10-mm trocar is then inserted into the umbilicus for passage of the 0° laparoscope. Next, the patient is positioned in Trendelenburg, so that small bowel and the sigmoid colon mobilize cephalad to facilitate access to the pelvic region. The height and tilt of the operating table is adjusted to the surgeon's preference. Four 5-mm trocars are inserted: one into the left iliac fossa, one into the midline halfway between the umbilicus and the pubis, one at the level of the umbilicus in the right pararectal line, and the last in the right iliac fossa at McBurney's point (Figure 9.2.1). Standardized steps are classically described.

Pelvic Lymph Node Dissection

The rationale for performing the pelvic lymph node dissection (PLND) at the beginning of the surgery is that anatomic landmarks are unaltered. In addition, the field

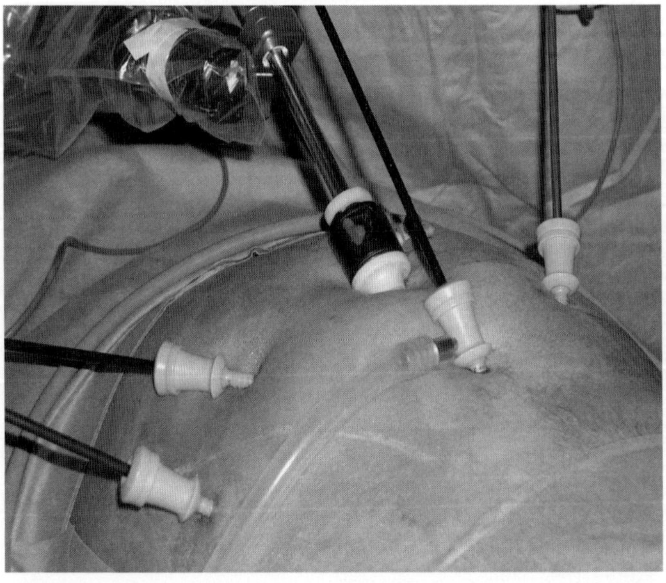

FIGURE 9.2.1 Disposition of trocars in the abdomen.

is completely bloodless at the start, allowing optimal visualization and possibly maximum preservation of the obturator neurovascular structures. It might also minimize the risk of ureteral injury.

The routine borders of the laparoscopic PLND have been the external iliac vein laterally, the medial umbilical ligament medially, the obturator nerve posteriorly, the Cooper ligament distally, and the bifurcation of the iliac vein proximally. The average number of LNs removed with this technique was nine as per a recent prospective study by Touijer et al. (26). After we switched to a more extended PLND, the median nodal count increased to 14 ($P < .001$). Among patients with a risk of lymph node metastases (LNM) >1.5% as predicted by the Partin tables (27), the incidence of LNM increased from 4.1% to 15.4% with this extended PLND technique. Thus, extended PLND is routinely performed on all patients unless contraindicated. The borders of the extended PLND are the medial aspect of the external iliac artery laterally, the lateral aspect of the medial umbilical ligament medially, the pelvic floor posteriorly, the pubic ramus covered by the Cooper ligament distally, and the bifurcation of the iliac vein and crossing of the ureter over the iliac vessels proximally. Thus, the lymphatic chains and nodes of the obturator and hypogastric arteries and veins, as well as those corresponding to the external iliac veins, are removed. This extent of PLND can only be achieved through a transperitoneal approach (28).

First Step: Posterior Approach to the Seminal Vesicles

On occasion, the sigmoid colon needs to be mobilized from the parietal peritoneal fold to allow its complete mobilization out of the pouch of Douglas and eventually expose the left iliac vessels if a LN dissection is to be performed. Once mobilized, the sigmoid colon may be held gently by the assistant with the suction canula, retracting the rectum superiorly, which facilitates access to the SV dissection (Figure 9.2.2). A 4- to 5-cm horizontal incision is made approximately 2 cm above the cul de sac on the anterior aspect of the pouch of Douglas. The dissection should then follow the inferior peritoneal flap. After coagulation of the few subperitoneal vessels, the dissection continues into an avascular plane.

Once the sheath of the fascia upholstering the SV complex is identified, the outlines of the SVs and vasa deferentia (VD) are visible. This sheath of this fascia is transversally incised allowing clear identification of the VD. The vas is dissected a few centimeters from the ampulla and coagulated with bipolar forceps or clipped and then transected. The deferential artery runs between the vas and the SV and will not be visible until the vas is sectioned. This artery is large and can cause serious intra- and postoperative bleeding, so careful control is mandatory. Division of the vas and deferential artery allows access to the SV just

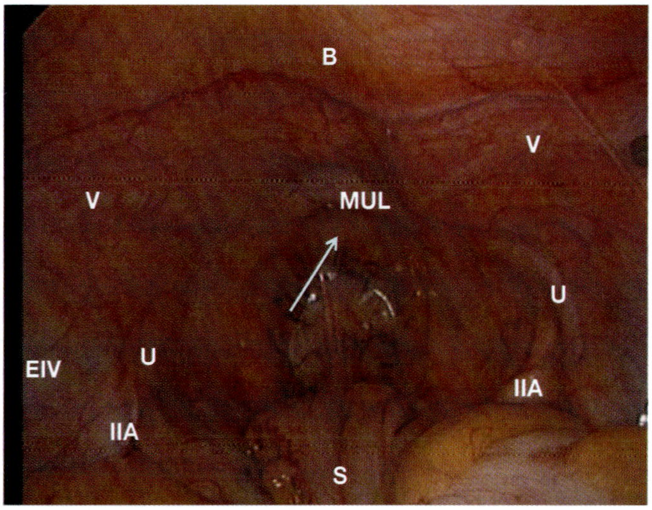

FIGURE 9.2.2 Laparoscopic anatomy of the pelvic cavity. U, ureter; IIA, Internal iliac artery; EIV, external iliac vessels; B, bladder; MUL, median umbilical ligament; V, vas deferens; S, sigmoid colon. Arrow shows the point of access to seminal vesicle dissection.

behind. The assistant's grasping of the prostatic end of the vas facilitates exposure of the posterior aspect of the SV. The dissection of the SV should be carried out following a plane along its surface to avoid thermal damage to any surrounding neurological structures.

The posterior aspect of the SV is usually nonvascularized and can be easily freed from Denonvilliers' fascia. The anterior aspect of the SV, the one in contact with the bladder, is usually the plane where one to three arteries penetrate the gland.

The dissection of the tip of the SV exposes one or two arteries that must be controlled and sectioned to free the SV completely. Failure to selectively control any of these SV arteries may cause significant postoperative hemorrhage.

Once the first SV is dissected (usually the right one), the assistant should retract the previously dissected and transected vas to bring the contralateral VD to the midline and facilitate its dissection. The same surgical strategy for the dissection of the VD and the SV is applied to the contralateral side. The assistant retracts both VD upward with a grasper introduced through the suprapubic port to tent Denonvilliers' fascia. The Denonvilliers' fascia is then incised horizontally 1 cm in the midline, where it reflects between the prostatic base and the posterior surface of the SV to expose the prerectal fat (Figure 9.2.3). This maneuver simplifies the subsequent location of the medial limit of the NVBs, as it detaches the prostate from the rectum and prostatic pedicles. No further attempt should be made to develop a plane between the prostate and the rectum posteriorly toward the prostatic apex.

The posterior approach to the SV constitutes the dissection of choice because it allows a delicate dissection of the SV, minimizing the risk of injuring the inferior hypogastric plexus and the cavernous nerves, and it improves the mobilization of the bladder neck at the moment of the

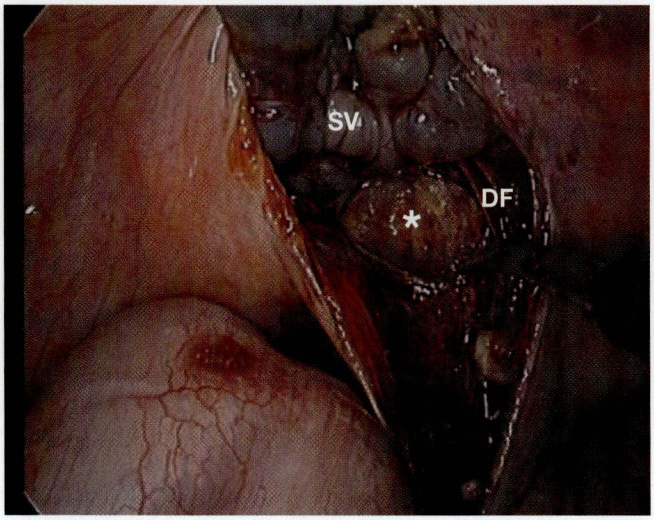

FIGURE 9.2.3 Posterior access to the seminal vesicles (SV) and opening of Denonvilliers' fascia (DF), exposing prerectal fat.

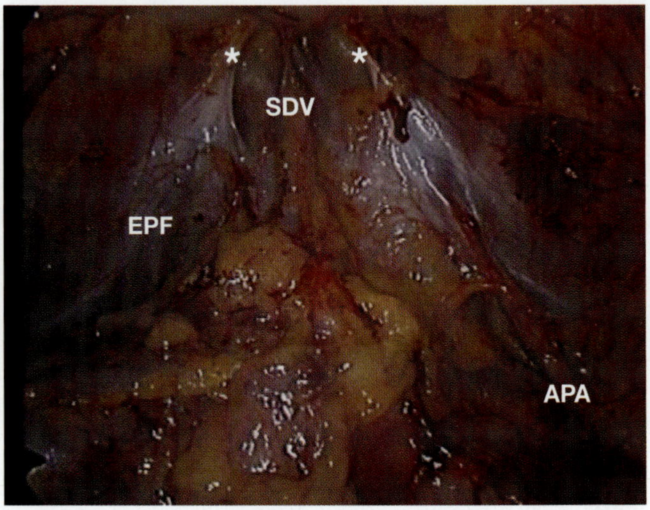

FIGURE 9.2.4 Endopelvic fascia and puboprostatic ligaments. SDV, superficial dorsal vein; EPF, endopelvic fascia; *, puboprostatic ligaments; APA, accessory pudendal artery.

posterior bladder neck dissection. However, an anterior approach to the SV is recommended when the patient has a large median lobe (29) or is already impotent. In addition, unclear anatomy or difficulty in identifying the SV or VD should prompt the surgeon to approach the SV anteriorly, after opening of the posterior bladder neck.

Second Step: Anterior Approach of the Prostate

The dissection of the retropubic space is performed applying an urachal sparing technique, in which both the urachus and the medial umbilical ligaments are spared (30). The technique consists of incising the anterior parietal peritoneum lateral to the medial umbilical ligaments, allowing access to the retropubic space by developing the embryologic coalescence plane between the urachus and the anterior primitive parietal peritoneum, and locating the initial point of access between the medial and the lateral umbilical ligaments (peritoneal fold on the inferior epigastric vessels) anterior to the VD; posteriorly, the dissection is carried out up to the crossing of the VD with the umbilical ligaments. Developing the prevesical and retropubic spaces spares both the urachus and the medial umbilical ligaments. It is essential to free the bladder wall from its lateral and anterior attachments to create a large working space and to permit a tension-free vesicourethral anastomosis at the end of the operation. The fat of the retropubic space must be swept laterally to expose clearly the internal obturator muscles, the endopelvic fascia, and the puboprostatic ligaments (Figure 9.2.4). Once the superficial dorsal vein is transected, the fat covering the endopelvic fascia can be easily swept off.

The entire endopelvic fascia is incised laterally on its line of reflection, starting at the level of the base of the prostate and extending anteriorly toward the apex, exposing the levator ani muscle. We identify one or more accessory pudendal arteries (APAs) during dissection of either the endopelvic fascia or the puboprostatic ligaments in 25% of cases. This APA should be preserved, since, instead of penetrating into the prostate, it continues parallel to the DVC toward the anterior perineum, and it may have an impact on recovery of potency in patients undergoing nerve sparing surgery (31–34).

The DVC is then ligated with a 2–0 polyglactin suture on an SH needle. Depending on the size of the plexus, a second separate suture or a "figure of 8" stitch may be placed to make the ligation more secure. In the case of bleeding from the DVC, it is useless to try to control it with any kind of fulguration. Instead, the intra-abdominal pressure can be transiently raised up to 20 mmHg while the definitive ligature is placed.

Transection of the complex is not required at this point as it will only cause useless bleeding. This step will be performed later in the operation. Actually, the whole sectioning and suture of the DVC is sometimes carried out at the time of apical dissection, especially in the presence of APAs.

A stitch to prevent back bleeding from the preprostatic veins is placed on the anterior aspect of the prostate. This stitch may be of help during the bladder neck dissection by decreasing the back flow coming from the transected veins on the prostatic side.

Between May and December 2005, 100 consecutive patients who underwent transperitoneal urachal-sparing LRP were prospectively evaluated for technique feasibility, intraoperative quality of the anastomosis, length of catheterization, and postoperative complications. We found sparing of the urachus and medial umbilical ligaments saves time, avoids the risk of bleeding from both the urachus and the umbilical ligaments, and keeps the bladder out of the field during the dissection of the bladder neck (35). Furthermore, this approach neither added noticeable tension to the urethrovesical anastomosis nor increased the morbidity of the procedure. In comparison to the extraperitoneal approach, it offers a wider working space and a tension-free urethrovesical anastomosis and allows for an extended PLND. In addition, incision of the urachus and the umbilical ligaments was never necessary to complete the LRP. The median time to catheter removal remained unchanged (7 days). However, urachal-sparing LRP will not prevent uroperitoneum or intraperitoneal bleeding if a urinary leak or a surgical field hemorrhage occurs.

Third Step: Bladder Neck Dissection

This step is often felt to be difficult since the anatomical landmarks are not as well defined as in other phases of the surgery. The place where the bladder neck should be dissected is exactly where the fat becomes adherent to the anterior bladder wall. For this area to be recognized, the anterior prevesical fat must be swept off superiorly until it becomes more adherent to the detrusor. This causes a faint outline at the prostatovesical junction, at the exact location where it should be opened. It is generally easy to develop the plane of dissection between bladder and prostate with sharp and blunt dissection. The vesical end of the prostatic urethra is identified by a sudden change in the orientation of the muscular fibers, which become longitudinal rather than circular or plexiform. The bladder is emptied again and the catheter balloon deflated.

The bladder neck is incised transversally, and the tip of the Foley catheter is pulled upward with a grasper inserted through the suprapubic port. The assistant pulls this grasper and at the same time places tension by pulling the Foley catheter to tent and lift up the prostate and expose the PBN wall. The entire thickness of the PBN wall is then incised. This is a step where the dissecting pace should be reduced as this is a highly vascularized area, and discrete coagulation alternating the use of the tip of the scissors and the bipolar forceps is needed. The ureteral orifices may be close to the edge of the bladder and their location should always be checked, especially when a median lobe is present, as the bladder mucosa may need to be incised closer to the ureteral orifices to achieve a safe oncologic margin.

The correct plane of dissection leads to the recognition of longitudinal muscular fibers tented between the prostate base and the posterior layer of the detrusor at the bladder neck. This fibromuscular tissue should be incised to gain access to the previously dissected vasa and the SVs. The VD and SV (which were previously dissected) are then simply brought forward. This maneuver leaves both prostatic pedicles and the edges of the bladder neck lateral to the SVs.

Many reports on LRP state that incision of the "anterior layer of Denonvilliers fascia" is needed to access the SV and VD during dissection of the PBN (11, 14, 15, 36–41), which is inconsistent with the accepted anatomic description of Denonvilliers fascia (42–45).

We replicated the laparoscopic anterior and PBN dissection on 5 fresh cystoprostatectomy specimens and on 20 additional prostatectomy specimens, and biopsied the identified components of the PBN for histologic evaluation by 2 specialized uropathologists. After incising the mucosa of the PBN, we identified an intimate fusion of two tissue layers that needed to be cut into to gain access to the SV and VD. The inner layer was composed of longitudinally disposed smooth muscle fibers in all patients, in continuation with the outer longitudinal fibers of the detrusor. The outer layer was composed of fibroadipose tissue, in continuation with the adventitia of the bladder. We did not find Denonvilliers fascia interposed between the posterior bladder wall and the SV. We concluded that there had been an anatomic misinterpretation, and those longitudinal muscle fibers correspond to the median fascicle of the dorsal muscle bundle of the outer longitudinal layer of the bladder. In addition, they constitute a critical anatomic landmark to guide the surgeon into the correct plane of dissection of the SV and VD (46–48).

Because dissection of the PBN is one of the crucial and difficult steps of LRP, we systematically try to identify these fibers to ascertain the correct plane of dissection, particularly in difficult scenarios, for example, salvage prostatectomy or in patients with benign prostatic hyperplasia, large median lobes, or prior transurethral resection of the prostate. Recognition of the longitudinal muscle fibers represents a pivotal component of a PBN dissection properly done. Incision of these fibers not only provides safe access to both the SV and VD but also helps the surgeon to stay away from the base of the prostate and minimize the possibility of a positive surgical margin (PSM) at this location. This will subsequently facilitate identification and control of the prostatic pedicles as well as adequate dissection of the NVB.

Fourth Step: Control of the Prostatic Pedicles and Dissection of the NVB

Once the edges of the bladder neck are dissected, lateral to the SV, the entire tissue is composed of prostatic pedicle first and the NVB posteriorly. The prostatic pedicle should be taken down with meticulous coagulation with thin bipolar (the so-called nano bipolars) or controlled with clips. This procedure is facilitated by anterior traction on the SVs. Dissection of the NVB can be performed at variable distances from the prostate. The amount of periprostatic tissue removed with the specimen will depend on the characteristics of the tumor, its location and Gleason score, magnetic resonance imaging (MRI) results, and digital rectal examination (DRE).

Keeping this in mind, there are three surgical methods to dissect the NVB (Figure 9.2.5). First, an intrafascial technique where the NVB is completely preserved, as the dissection is carried out between the prostate gland and the prostatic fascia (Figure 9.2.6). Second, an interfascial technique where the NVB dissection is performed lateral to the prostatic fascia but sparing as much NVB as possible. Finally, the extrafascial dissection takes place lateral to the NVB.

The type of NVB dissection (intrafascial, interfascial, or extrafascial) (49) is currently tailored to the side-specific characteristics of the tumor, based on results of 14-core biopsy labeled according to the location, the rectal examination, serum prostate-specific antigen (PSA), and evidence of extracapsular extension (ECE) on endorectal coil MRI.

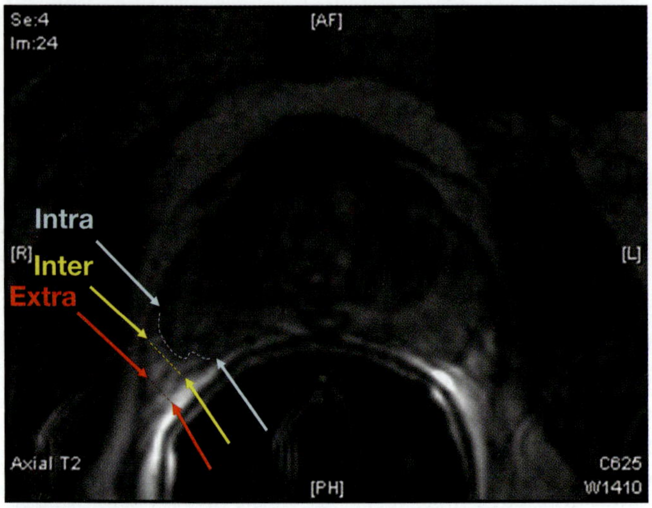

FIGURE 9.2.5 Planes of neurovascular bundle dissection. Extra, extrafascial; Inter, interfascial; Intra, intrafascial.

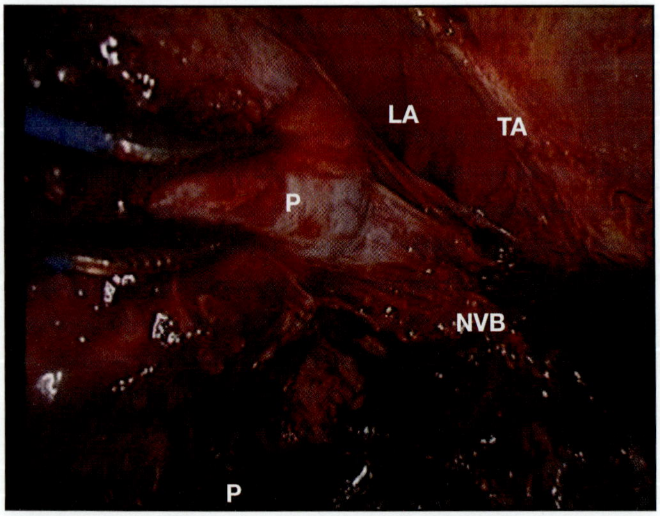

FIGURE 9.2.6 Intrafascial dissection of the right NVB. P, prostate; LA, levator ani; TA, tendinous arch of the pelvis; NVB: neurovascular bundle.

As a general rule, an intrafascial dissection is currently performed in patients with prostate sides with no palpable nodules and a negative ipsilateral biopsy. However, a prostate side with a single-positive biopsy with Gleason 3 + 3 or 3 + 4 compromising a medial core without signs of ECE may be suitable for an intrafascial dissection. Based on oncology safety grounds, the intrafascial dissection of the NVB is limited to the posterolateral aspect of the prostate; Denonvilliers' fascia is always left covering the posterior aspect of the prostate, and the prostatic fascia always remains covering the anterolateral face of the gland. These criteria should be taken as a general guideline and not as a strict rule.

In a recent study of preoperative and intraoperative risk factors for side-specific PSMs in LRP, we found that sparing of NVBs (intrafascial technique) was not a risk factor for positive margins in adequately selected patients. Elevated serum PSA (>10 ng/mL), small glands (<30 g), biopsy Gleason scores of 7, or bulky disease as indicated by high percentage of tumor on biopsy cores were independent predictors of side-specific PSMs. Preoperative use of MRI and clinical stage were neither protective nor risk factors. The side-specific PSM rate was 7%, and the overall unadjusted PSM rates decreased from 17% to 9% over time (50).

Fifth Step: Apical Dissection of the Prostate

At this point in the operation, the prostate is anchored by four definite structures: the DVC, the urethra, the distal attachments of the Denonvilliers' fascia to the rectourethralis muscle, and the distal third of both NVBs.

In sequence, we first section the (sometimes already ligated) DVC. The DVC is incised until an avascular plane of dissection between the DVC and the urethra is developed. A Béniqué sound is introduced to help identify the urethra by improving the tactile perception of its limits. Next, we complete the dissection of the distal third of the neurovascular bundles. During this step, excessive traction on the prostate should be avoided so as not to stretch the urethra and the sphincteric complex (Figure 9.2.7).

Then, once the NVBs have been dissected from the apex, the distal attachments of Denonvilliers' fascia are incised on both sides. It is individualized at the apex and dissected from the posterior aspect of the urethra. Finally, after the prostate has been freed from all these structures, it will be left hanging from the urethra and is incised with cold scissors. In agreement with other authors (51), we observed that sectioning the urethra after dissection of the apex decreases the incidence of positive apical margins.

Extensive dissection or skeletonization of the urethra should be avoided as it may be the chief mechanism contributing to postoperative urinary incontinence. The puboprostatic ligaments should be incised closer to the prostate

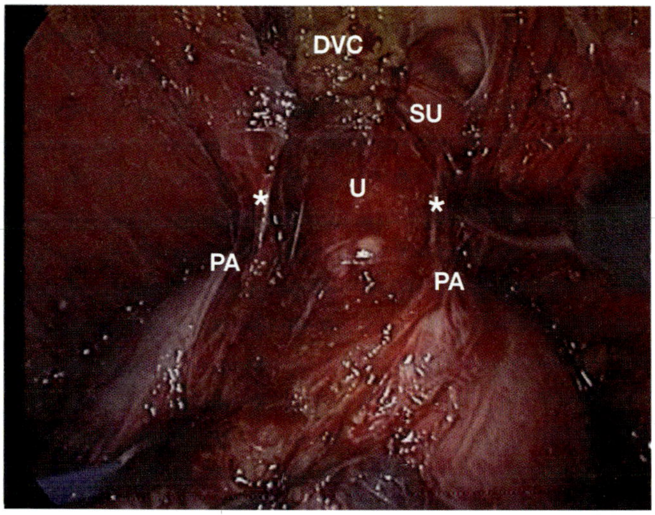

FIGURE 9.2.7 Apical dissection of the prostate. U, urethra; PA, prostate ápex; *, pillars of the urethra; SU, sphincteric complex; DVC, dorsal vascular complex.

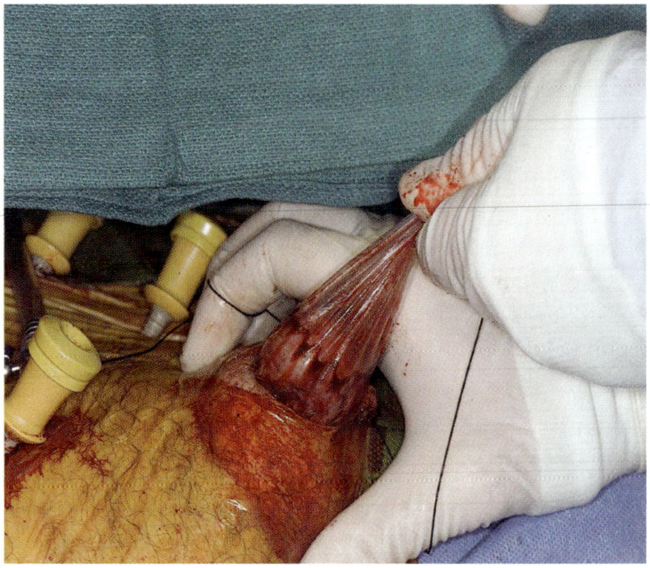

FIGURE 9.2.8 Prostate extraction in a bag through an extension of the umbilical incision.

gland than to the pubic bone to minimize any damage to the anchoring system of the urethra to the posterior aspect of the pubic bone.

Once the specimen is free, a 5-mm scope is inserted through a lateral port and the gland is placed into the 10-mm laparoscopic bag. The umbilical incision is extended at the midline according to the size of the gland and the specimen is extracted (Figure 9.2.8). The gland is macroscopically examined for the presence of induration, nodularity, or an area suspicious for positive margin that could require confirmation by frozen section examination. When in doubt of a PSM, we recommend submitting the entire gland for pathologic evaluation, tagging the suspicious areas with a 6–0 stitch. Evaluation of a possible positive margin should not be done from a second sample of tissue taken from the prostatic bed. In the event of a pathologic confirmation of a PSM, additional tissue is to be resected.

The umbilical fascia is carefully closed with two running 0 sutures starting at each edge and tightened (not tied) around a 10-mm trocar. Then the abdomen is re-insufflated. The pelvis is inspected and any clots are aspirated, and the pelvis is irrigated with saline at 37°C temperature. Hemostasis is confirmed. Always include inspection of the SV lodge, the prostatic pedicles, and the NVBs, as these are the most frequent locations of bleeding.

Sixth Step: Urethrovesical Anastomosis

We never evert the bladder mucosa and we do not reconstruct a large bladder neck opening before the anastomosis is done. An anterior tennis racquet is usually performed at the end if needed. In 350 cases followed prospectively, we found only one case of bladder neck contracture (BNC) secondary to a pelvic hematoma.

When the anastomosis is performed with interrupted sutures, approximately 10 interrupted stitches of 3–0 polyglactin suture with a 18-mm half circle needle are used. All knots are tied intracorporally. The Béniqué sound not only helps to guide the needle into the urethral lumen but also to take the full thickness of the urethral wall with the stitch.

The three first sutures are placed posteriorly at 5, 6, and 7 o'clock, going inside-out on the urethra and outside-in on the bladder neck. The 5 o'clock stitch goes inside-out on the urethra (right hand, forehand) and outside-in on the bladder (right hand, forehand); the 6 and 7 o'clock stitches go inside-out on the urethra (right hand, forehand) and outside-in on the bladder (left hand, forehand). Therefore, these stitches are tied intraluminally, and in our experience, this has not been associated with calcifications, lithiasis, or BNC.

Four other sutures are symmetrically placed at 4 and 8, then 2 and 10 o'clock, and tied outside the lumen. The sutures at 4 and 2 o'clock go outside-in on the bladder (right hand, forehand) and inside-out on the urethra (left hand, backhand). The sutures at 8 and 10 o'clock go outside-in on the bladder (left hand, forehand) and inside-out on the urethra (right hand, backhand).

Three final anterior stitches are placed at 11, 12, and 1 o'clock, symmetrically to the posterior stitches. The 11 and 12 o'clock stitches go outside-in on the urethra (right hand, forehand) and inside-out on the bladder (right hand, forehand), whereas the 1 o'clock stitch goes outside-in on the urethra (right hand, forehand) and inside-out on the bladder (left hand, forehand). Once the stitches are tied, the Foley catheter is inserted. The bladder is filled with 180 mL of saline to check for water tightness of the anastomosis and confirm the correct position of the catheter. Finally, the balloon is inflated with 10 mL of sterile water.

The urethrovesical anastomosis can also be accomplished with a running suture, which may be less demanding but which may theoretically reduce the lumen of the anastomosis (52). The reader is referred to this citation for technical details.

Seventh Step: Completing the Operation and Drainage

The abdominal pressure is lowered to 5 mmHg, to check for venous bleeding. One or two suction drains are placed, one anteriorly in the retropubic space and one posteriorly, between the rectum and the bladder in case the SV had been dissected with a posterior approach. The 5-mm trocars are removed under visual control, and the parietal orifices are checked to exclude any vascular injury, particularly of the epigastric vessels. At the end, the two running sutures are tied together to close the fascial layer of the umbilical incision. A 4–0 running subcuticular Poliglecaprone is used in all port incisions.

■ POSTOPERATIVE CARE

For pain management, patients are initially given morphine sulfate in the recovery room 2 to 5 mg intravenously (IV) q2 hours as needed + Ketorolac 15 mg IV q6 hours for a maximum of six doses. When patients can tolerate fluids orally, Oxycodone 5 mg with acetaminophen 325 mg replaces the previous medications. Patients are requested to ambulate with assistance on the night of the surgery and then without it the following day until discharge. Patients are given clear fluids 6 hours after surgery and a light breakfast the following morning. Diet is progressed to regular if adequately tolerated.

The Foley catheter is removed after postoperative day 7. Cystograms are not routinely performed. Kegel exercises are started 3 days after catheter removal (53–55).

Patients usually start passing flatus on postoperative day 2 and have their first bowel movement on postoperative day 3. It is recommended that they avoid abundant meals until after they start moving bowels. Drinking fluids is encouraged while patients have the Foley catheter in place; however, fluid may be decreased to what they normally drink after the Foley catheter is removed.

Full exercise, including sexual activity, may be resumed 3 weeks after surgery (56–58).

■ COMPLICATIONS AND MANAGEMENT (59)

Intraoperative Complications

Bleeding From the DVC

Although laparoscopy allows a clear vision of the apex, and the pneumoperitoneum provides a tamponade effect, bleeding from the DVC can be significant and may affect the remainder of the operation due to impaired visibility. A meticulous, not extensive though, apical dissection defining the principal anatomical elements around the DVC is essential to preventing unnecessary hemorrhage. When the ligating suture is loose, placed too proximal, or cut during the transection of the DVC, bleeding can be controlled by increasing the pneumoperitoneum pressure up to 20 mmHg, by clamping the DVC with a grasper, or simply by having the assistant compress the DVC against the pubic bone with the Benique sound. This allows a tamponade effect while the surgeon is calmly preparing a second ligating suture. Once tied, the DVC stitch can be anchored to the periosteum of the pubic symphysis.

Bladder Injury

The bladder is more likely to be inadvertently damaged at three different times during transperitoneal LRP. First, during the posterior dissection of the SV, dissection in fatty tissue should alert the surgeon of a plane either too close to the bladder or too close to the rectum. Second, during the development of the retropubic space, any excessive bleeding should alert the surgeon of a dissection too close to the bladder. Third, during the dissection of the PBN, the area at risk is the trigone and retrotrigonal bladder wall. On identification, the surgeon should verify the integrity of the ureters and ureteral orifices and repair the bladder with resorbable suture.

Rectal Injury

Rectal injuries most frequently occur during prostate dissection at the apex. They may result from a direct cut into the rectal wall or from a microperforation secondary to thermal injury due to excessive cauterization on the rectal wall surface (60). The risk of rectal injury increases when there is a substantial amount of periprostatic inflammatory reaction, prior prostate surgery or radiation, a large volume gland with a narrow pelvis, extrafascial NVB dissection, and surgeon inexperience. Intraoperative rectal examination with the finger, rectal bougie, or the water test (filling the pelvis with saline and air insufflation through the rectum) might help prevent or identify rectal injuries while incising Denonvilliers' fascia and dissecting the posterior surface of the prostate.

If an incision on the rectal wall is recognized, it is generally accepted that the defect can be sutured primarily with two layers of interrupted 2–0 silk after débridement of any devitalized tissue if no gross fecal soiling is observed. Interposition of an omental flap or pararectal fat flap is not routinely necessary. However, in face of a large, devitalized rectal laceration or of gross soiling, a temporary diverting colostomy is advisable.

Microperforations of the rectal wall often go unrecognized until after the Foley catheter is removed and is manifested by a rectourethral fistula. The first therapeutic option is to reinsert the Foley catheter until the fistula heals spontaneously. If this conservative method fails, elective surgical approach of the rectourethral fistula should be considered. Needless to say, prevention is the mainstay of therapy.

Ureter Injury

An injury to the ureter can occur during the dissection of the SV by mistakenly sectioning the ureter instead of the VD, by an inadvertent thermal injury, or injury of the ureteral orifice during dissection of the PBN. When the injury is not identified intraoperatively, a persistent urine leakage or uroperitoneum with a watertight anastomosis suggests the diagnosis. Ureteral reimplantation is the treatment of choice. Another reported ureteral complication is a postoperative anuria caused by incorporation of the ureteral orifices in the urethrovesical anastomotic sutures. If identified while the patient is in hospital, the anastomosis should be redone laparoscopically.

Epigastric Artery Injury

Because of anatomy, the epigastrics are more frequently injured while placing the right paramedian port. Bleeding around the trocar, either internally or externally, suggests a vessel injury. Placement of the port lateral to the rectus abdominis muscle is safer. Venous injury can be managed successfully by tamponade, whereas arterial injury requires surgical hemostasis using the Reverdin or the Carter-Thomason needle. As a fundamental rule of laparoscopic surgery, all the trocars should be removed under direct vision with decreased abdominal pressure.

Postoperative Complications

Urine Leakage

An increased and prolonged urine output from the pelvic drain suggests the diagnosis. In the majority of cases, the left posterior aspect of the anastomosis may not be watertight and is managed conservatively by prolonging both bladder and pelvic drainage. If the leak persists despite a conservative treatment, a ureteral injury or an eversion of the ureteral orifice outside of the anastomosis needs to be ruled out.

On occasions, the urinary leak may be diagnosed after the catheter is removed. In patients with transperitoneal radical prostatectomy, the sudden onset of sharp abdominal pain during or immediately after urination is a urinary leak until proven otherwise. The treatment consists of reinsertion of the catheter and reassessment of the anastomosis by a retrograde cystogram at a later date to ascertain a complete healing of the anastomosis. We advocate obtaining a urinalysis before any manipulation to identify and treat any urinary tract infection and limit the risk of uroperitonitis.

Small Bowel Injury

The small bowel can be injured either early in the operation during trocar placement or by thermal injury during prostate dissection. A missed bowel injury will manifest by ileus, increased abdominal pain, and decreased white blood cell counts with or without signs of systemic infection. Prompt computed tomography scan imaging with oral contrast may lead to the diagnosis. Therapy requires a re-exploration, which can be done laparoscopically.

Nerve Compression and Compartment Syndrome

Ulnar and brachial neurapraxia have been reported following LRP and have resulted in a transient paresis. This type of complication is related to patient positioning. One way to prevent it is by avoiding narrow OR tables so that the operating surgeon does not inadvertently lean on the patient's arm.

We prefer the low lithotomy position because it allows easy access to the rectum if needed. However, lithotomy position for long periods of time may lead to compartment syndrome, a potential complication that should always be ruled out postoperatively. Overtightness of the calves by the sequential compressive devices and stirrups might contribute to this syndrome. Distal pulses should always be assessed pre- and postoperatively as well as distal capillary refill at the nail beds, as it usually precedes cessation of arterial flow. Myoglobinuria, electrolyte disturbances, disorders of acid–base balance, and serum CK values of over 2,000 U/L after surgery may be considered a warning sign in ventilated and sedated patients, in whom early clinical symptoms of compartment syndrome, such as pain and paresthesias, cannot be ascertained (61). The treatment is emergent fasciotomy of the muscular groups involved.

Obturator nerve neurapraxia is usually associated with PLND. It is manifested by different degrees of postoperative throbbing, unrelenting leg pain, and weakness. Abducting capacity of the leg is markedly diminished and more frequently takes place on the left side due to the greater difficulty of the PLND on this side (62,63).

In the presence of postoperative leg pain, think first of acute compartment syndrome, particularly if symptoms are bilateral, outside the abductor muscle territory, and in a patient in whom PLND had not been performed.

■ CONCLUSIONS

LRP was introduced almost 20 years ago for the surgical treatment of localized prostate cancer. Since its inception, the technique, however challenging, has undergone continuous refinements that make it today a feasible, reproducible, and teachable operation practiced by urologists worldwide, particularly in countries where the cost constraints of the robotic assistance makes it unavailable. The advantages of the laparoscopic approach are a magnified view of the anatomic structures and decreased venous bleeding in the surgical field to allow an accurate dissection of the prostate and NVB. These advantages should translate to better outcomes, in terms of cancer control and functional results.

■ REFERENCES

1. Schuessler WW, Schulam PG, Clayman RV, Kavoussi LR. Laparoscopic radical prostatectomy: initial short-term experience. *Urology.* 1997;50:854–857.
2. Raboy A, Ferzli G, Albert P. Initial experience with extraperitoneal endoscopic radical retropubic prostatectomy. *Urology.* 1997;50:849–853.
3. Guillonneau B, Cathelineau X, Barret E, Rozet F, Vallancien G. Laparoscopic radical prostatectomy. Preliminary evaluation after 28 interventions. *Presse Med.* 1998;27:1570–1574.
4. Guillonneau B, Cathelineau X, Barret E, Rozet F, Vallancien G. Laparoscopic radical prostatectomy: technical and early oncological assessment of 40 operations. *Eur Urol.* 1999;36:14–20.
5. GuillonneauB,CathelineauX,DoubletJD,BaumertH,VallancienG. Laparoscopic radical prostatectomy: assessment after 550 procedures. *Crit Rev Oncol Hematol.* 2002;43:123–133.
6. Guillonneau B, Cathelineau X, Doublet JD, Vallancien G. Laparoscopic radical prostatectomy: the lessons learned. *J Endourol.* 2001;15:441–445; discussion 447–448.
7. Guillonneau B, el-Fettouh H, Baumert H, et al. Laparoscopic radical prostatectomy: oncological evaluation after 1,000 cases a Montsouris Institute. *J Urol.* 2003;169:1261–1266.
8. Guillonneau B, Rozet F, Barret E, Cathelineau X, Vallancien G. Laparoscopic radical prostatectomy: assessment after 240 procedures. *Urol Clin North Am.* 2001;28:189–202.
9. Vallancien G, Guillonneau B, Cathelineau X, Baumert H, Doublet JD. Localized prostatic cancer: treatment with laparoscopic radical prostatectomy: study with 841 cases. *Bull Acad Natl Med.* 2002;186:117–123; discussion 123–114.
10. Bollens R, Vanden Bossche M, Roumeguere T, et al. Extraperitoneal laparoscopic radical prostatectomy. Results after 50 cases. *Eur Urol.* 2001;40:65–69.
11. Dubernard P, Benchetrit S, Chaffange P, Hamza T, Van Box Som P. [Retrograde extraperitoneal laparoscopic prostatectomy (R.E.I.P). Simplified technique (based on a series of 143 cases]. *Prog Urol.* 2003;13:163–174.
12. Hoznek A, Antiphon P, Borkowski T, et al. Assessment of surgical technique and perioperative morbidity associated with extraperitoneal versus transperitoneal laparoscopic radical prostatectomy. *Urology.* 2003;61:617–622.
13. Rassweiler J, Marrero R, Hammady A, Erdogru T, Teber D, Frede T. Transperitoneal laparoscopic radical prostatectomy: ascending technique. *J Endourol.* 2004;18:593–599; discussion 599–600.
14. Rassweiler J, Sentker L, Seemann O, Hatzinger M, Rumpelt HJ. Laparoscopic radical prostatectomy with the Heilbronn technique: an analysis of the first 180 cases. *J Urol.* 2001;166:2101–2108.
15. Stolzenburg JU, Do M, Pfeiffer H, Konig F, Aedtner B, Dorschner W. The endoscopic extraperitoneal radical prostatectomy (EERPE): technique and initial experience. *World J Urol.* 2002;20:48–55.
16. Stolzenburg JU, Do M, Rabenalt R, et al. Endoscopic extraperitoneal radical prostatectomy: initial experience after 70 procedures. *J Urol.* 2003;169:2066–2071.
17. Touijer AK, Guillonneau B. Laparoscopic radical prostatectomy. *Urol Oncol.* 2004;22:133–138.
18. Dellinger EP, Gross PA, Barrett TL, et al. Quality standard for antimicrobial prophylaxis in surgical procedures. The Infectious Diseases Society of America. *Infect Control Hosp Epidemiol.* 1994;15:182–188.
19. Waddell TK, Rotstein OD. Antimicrobial prophylaxis in surgery. Committee on Antimicrobial Agents. *Can Infect Dis Soc.* 1994;151:925–931.
20. Colwell CW Jr. Dosing and timing of low-molecular-weight heparin thromboprophylaxis in total hip arthroplasty. *Orthopedics.* 2003;26:1155–1161; quiz 1162–1153.
21. Howard PA. Dalteparin: a low-molecular-weight heparin. *Ann Pharmacother.* 1997;31:192–203.
22. Secin FP, Jiborn T, Bjartell AS, et al. Multi-institutional study of symptomatic deep venous thrombosis and pulmonary embolism in prostate cancer patients undergoing laparoscopic or robot-assisted laparoscopic radical prostatectomy. *Eur Urol.* 2008;53(1):134–145.
23. Beebe DS, McNevin MP, Crain JM, et al. Evidence of venous stasis after abdominal insufflation for laparoscopic cholecystectomy. *Surg Gynecol Obstet.* 1993;176:443–447.
24. Cathelineau X, Cahill D, Widmer H, et al. Transperitoneal or extraperitoneal approach for laparoscopic radical prostatectomy: a false debate over a real challenge. *J Urol.* 2004;171:714–716.
25. Joseph JV, Patel HR. Transperitoneal or extraperitoneal approach for laparoscopic radical prostatectomy: a false debate over a real challenge. *J Urol.* 2004;172:1545.
26. Touijer AK, Rabbani F, Romero Otero J, Secin FP, Guillonneau B. Extended versus limited laparoscopic pelvic lymph node dissection for prostate cancer: the value of Partin tables in selection of the need for and the extent of dissection. *J Endourol.* 2006;20(suppl 1): A156, Abstract MP9–22.
27. Partin AW, Mangold LA, Lamm DM, Walsh PC, Epstein JI, Pearson JD. Contemporary update of prostate cancer staging nomograms (Partin tables) for the new millennium. *Urology.* 2001;58:843–848.
28. Touijer K, Rabbani F, Otero JR, et al. Standard vs limited pelvic lymph node dissection for prostate cancer in patients with a predicted probability of nodal metastasis greater than 1%. *J Urol.* 2007;178(1):120–124.
29. Secin FP, Karanikolas N, Touijer K, Guillonneau B. How to manage a large median lobe during laparoscopic radical prostatectomy (video). American Urological Association meeting; 2005; San Antonio, TX.
30. Secin FP, Bianco FJ, KaranikolasN, Touijer AK, Guillonneau B. Urachal sparing laparoscopic radical prostatectomy (video). European Congress of Urology; 2006; Paris, France.
31. Secin FP, Karanikolas N, Touijer AK, Salamanca JI, Vickers AJ, Guillonneau B. Anatomy of accessory pudendal arteries in laparoscopic radical prostatectomy. *J Urol.* 2005;174(2):523–526.

32. Secin FP, Touijer K, Mulhall J, Guillonneau B. Anatomy and preservation of accessory pudendal arteries in laparoscopic radical prostatectomy. *Eur Urol.* 2007;51(5):1229–1235.
33. Secin FP, Karanikolas N, Kuroiwa K, Vickers A, Touijer K, Guillonneau B. Preservation of accessory pudendal arteries during laparoscopic radical prostatectomy and the impact on surgical margins. *Eur Urol.* 2005;48(5):786–792.
34. Mulhall JP, Secin FP, Guillonneau B. Artery-sparing radical prostatectomy: myth or reality? *J Urol.* 2008;179(3):827–831.
35. Secin FP, Touijer K, Karanikolas N, Raj GV, Guillonneau B. Laparoscopic radical prostatectomy: lessons learned in surgical technique. *Eur Urol Suppl.* 2006;5:942–949.
36. Guillonneau B, Vallancien G. Laparoscopic radical prostatectomy: the Montsouris tecnique. *J Urol.* 2000;163:1643–1649.
37. Menon M, Shrivastava A, Kaul S, Bhandari A, Sarle R, Hemal A. V342: a quest for better nerve preservation in Vattikuti Institute Prostatectomy (VIP): the veil of Aphrodite. *J Urol.* 2005.
38. Menon M, Tewari A, Peabody J. Vattikuti Institute prostatectomy: technique. *J Urol.* 2003;169:2289–2292.
39. Tewari A, Menon M. Vattikuti institute prostatectomy: surgical technique and current results. *Curr Urol Rep.* 2003;4:119–123.
40. Tse E, Knaus R. Laparoscopic radical prostatectomy—results of 200 consecutive cases in a Canadian medical institution. *Can J Urol.* 2004;11:2172–2185.
41. Rozet F, Galiano M, Cathelineau X, Barret E, Cathala N, Vallancien G. Extraperitoneal laparoscopic radical prostatectomy: a prospective evaluation of 600 cases. *J Urol.* 2005;174:908–911.
42. Denonvilliers CP. Propositions et observation d'anatomie, de physiologie at de pathologie. *These De l'Ecole De Medicine.* 1837;285:23.
43. Lindsey I, Guy RJ, Warren BF, Mortensen NJ. Anatomy of Denonvilliers' fascia and pelvic nerves, impotence, and implications for the colorectal surgeon. *Br J Surg.* 2000;87:1288–1299.
44. Lindsey I, Warren BF, Mortensen NJ. Denonvilliers' fascia lies anterior to the fascia propria and rectal dissection plane in total mesorectal excision. *Dis Colon Rectum.* 2005;48:37–42.
45. van Ophoven A, Roth S. The anatomy and embryological origins of the fascia of Denonvilliers: a medico-historical debate. *J Urol.* 1997;157:3–9.
46. Secin FP, Touijer AK, Karanikolas N, et al. The vesicoprostatic muscle: a critical landmark during dissection of the posterior bladder neck in laparoscopic radical prostatectomy (video). American Urological Association Meeting; 2006; Atlanta, GA.
47. Gil Vernet S. *Morphology and Function of Vesico-Prostatourethral Musculature.* 1968 ed. Treviso, Italy: Edizioni di Urologia; 1968.
48. Secin FP, Karanikolas N, Gopalan A, et al. The Anterior Layer of Dennonvilliers' Fascia: a common misunderstanding in laparoscopic radical prostatectomy. *J Urol.* 2007;177(2):521–525.
49. Stolzenburg JU, Kallidonis P, Do M, et al. A comparison of outcomes for interfascial and intrafascial nerve-sparing radical prostatectomy. *Urology.* 2010;76(3):743–748.
50. Secin FP, Serio A, Bianco FJ Jr, et al. Preoperative and intraoperative risk factors for side-specific positive surgical margins in laparoscopic radical prostatectomy for prostate cancer. *Eur Urol.* 2007;51(3):764–771.
51. Katz R, Salomon L, Hoznek A, de la Taille A, Antiphon P, Abbou CC. Positive surgical margins in laparoscopic radical prostatectomy: the impact of apical dissection, bladder neck remodeling and nerve preservation. *J Urol.* 2003;169:2049–2052.
52. Van Velthoven RF, Ahlering TE, Peltier A, Skarecky DW, Clayman RV. Technique for laparoscopic running urethrovesical anastomosis: the single knot method. *Urology.* 2003;61(4):699–702.
53. Hunter KF, Moore KN, Cody DJ, Glazener CM. Conservative management for postprostatectomy urinary incontinence. *Cochrane Database Syst Rev.* 2004;2:CD001843.
54. Moul JW. Pelvic muscle rehabilitation in males following prostatectomy. *Urol Nurs.* 1998;18:296–301.
55. Van Kampen M, De Weerdt W, Van Poppel H, De Ridder D, Feys H, Baert L. Effect of pelvic-floor re-education on duration and degree of incontinence after radical prostatectomy: a randomised controlled trial. *Lancet.* 2000;355:98–102.
56. Raina R, Lakin MM, Agarwal A, et al. Long-term effect of sildenafil citrate on erectile dysfunction after radical prostatectomy: 3-year follow-up. *Urology.* 2003;62:110–115.
57. Zippe CD, Kedia AW, Kedia K, Nelson DR, Agarwal A. Treatment of erectile dysfunction after radical prostatectomy with sildenafil citrate (Viagra). *Urology.* 1998;52:963–966.
58. Zippe CD, Raina R, Thukral M, Lakin MM, Klein EA, Agarwal A. Management of erectile dysfunction following radical prostatectomy. *Curr Urol Rep.* 2001;2:495–503.
59. Guillonneau B, Rozet F, Cathelineau X, et al. Perioperative complications of laparoscopic radical prostatectomy: the Montsouris 3-year experience. *J Urol.* 2002;167:51–56.
60. Guillonneau B, Gupta R, El Fettouh H, Cathelineau X, Baumert H, Vallancien G. Laparoscopic management of rectal injury during laparoscopic radical prostatectomy. *J Urol.* 2003;169:1694–1696.
61. Lampert R, Weih EH, Breucking E, Kirchhoff S, Lazica B, Lang K. Postoperative bilateral compartment syndrome resulting from prolonged urological surgery in lithotomy position. Serum creatine kinase activity (CK) as a warning signal in sedated, artificially respirated patients. *Anaesthesist.* 1995;44:43–47.
62. Arai Y, Egawa S, Terachi T, et al. Morbidity of laparoscopic radical prostatectomy: summary of early multi-institutional experience in Japan. *Int J Urol.* 2003;10:430–434.
63. Spaliviero M, Steinberg AP, Kaouk JH, Desai MM, Hammert WC, Gill IS. Laparoscopic injury and repair of obturator nerve during radical prostatectomy. *Urology.* 2004;64:1030.

9.3 Robotic Radical Prostatectomy: The Thomas Jefferson University Experience

COSTAS D. LALLAS
EDOUARD J. TRABULSI

Radical prostatectomy for the treatment of clinically localized and locally advanced prostate cancer has undergone a significant and controversial transformation in the last 10 to 15 years. At the crux of the controversy is a surgical technique that has all but replaced the gold-standard, radical retropubic prostatectomy (RRP); that technique is robotic-assisted radical prostatectomy (RARP). From a temporal standpoint, RARP came into existence just after laparoscopic radical prostatectomy (LRP), the first attempt at minimally invasive prostatectomy that had some popularity in the 1990s but is now essentially obsolete in the United States, having been supplanted by RARP. Part of the reason for this occurrence is the technical difficulty and irreproducibility of good outcomes with LRP, both of which have been achieved by its successor. Other advantages of RARP over LRP include a more ergonometric setup that is less taxing to the surgeon; more degrees of freedom of motion enabled by wristed instruments that offer finer dissection and more accurate movements in the tight male pelvis; nonparadoxical movements that make the operation easier to learn and certainly easier to teach to trainees; and more advanced optics, being three dimensional, magnified, and high definition.

Critics of RARP cite the lack of tactile feedback in robotic surgery that is inherent in open, and to a lesser degree, in a laparoscopic surgery. This would certainly be an issue for palpable tumors in patients with clinical T3 or bulky disease. In addition, no one has yet been able to completely explain away the increased cost associated with robotic surgery over the more traditional forms of surgery, namely open and laparoscopic. According to a *Perspective* article in the *New England Journal of Medicine*, across 20 types of surgery, the additional variable cost of using a robot-assisted procedure was about $1,600 or about 6% of the cost of the procedure in 2007. When the amortized cost of the robot itself was included, the additional total cost of using a robot-assisted procedure rose to about $3,200 or about 13% of the cost of these procedures (1). Although this would appear to be sufficient deterrent against the widespread use of this technology, in reality it has not changed the continued increased growth rate of Intuitive Surgical, Inc., the company that manufactures the daVinci® surgical system, its only product and the only robotic surgical system in commercial existence at the time of the writing of this chapter. Intuitive Surgical claims that more men in the United States choose RARP over LRP and standard open radical prostatectomy for the treatment of their prostate cancer, with an estimate of 80% of all radical prostatectomies having been performed with robotic assistance in the last calendar year (2).

At our institution, the vast majority (85%–90%) of all radical prostatectomies performed for clinically localized or locally advanced prostate cancer are RARP with the remainder being RRP. It is surgeon's preference when considering which technique to perform, although many of our RRP candidates had been excluded from consideration for RARP for a variety of reasons. Our current absolute contraindications for RARP include morbid obesity (body mass index >55), extensive prior intra-abdominal surgeries, or bulky disease. Most of these patients are treated with RRP or primary radiotherapy. With regard to the last mentioned contraindication, namely bulky disease, we believe that the ability to feel cancer-related induration during surgery may benefit these patients from an oncologic standpoint, and we will obtain pelvic magnetic resonance imaging (MRI) on those patients who we consider to be at risk for gross extracapsular extension. If that MRI demonstrates findings consistent with bulky locally advanced disease, we will recommend these patients for open RRP as the primary surgical consideration.

Our evaluation for newly diagnosed prostate cancer patients closely follows National Comprehensive Cancer Network guidelines, with a bone scan performed for staging for intermediate- and high-risk disease. As mentioned in the previous section, a pelvic MRI is obtained on patients who are believed to be at risk for locally invasive, bulky disease and in whom a RARP may thus not be appropriate. For those patients who are to undergo a RARP, a cystoscopy is performed preoperatively to evaluate for urethral strictures, a hypertrophic median lobe, bladder mucosal abnormalities, and the proximity of the ureteral orifices to the bladder neck.

■ PROCEDURE

Pneumoperitoneum is established up to a pressure of 15 mmHg with a Veress needle through a vertical incision approximately 1 to 2 cm supraumbilically in the midline, and the first trocar (12 mm) is placed at this point; this is the camera port. Next, four working ports (3 8-mm robotic ports and an additional 12-mm assistant port in the right lower quadrant) are placed along a semilunar arc that extends 15 to 16 mm from a focal point at the center of the pubic symphysis. A final 5-mm assistant port is placed in the right upper quadrant about 5 to 6 cm cephalad from the 8-mm right periumbilical robotic port in the same longitudinal plane. Prior to docking the robot, the patient is placed in a steep Trendelenburg position. Once the robot is docked, instruments are inserted. We use a 0° lens, monopolar cautery shears, bipolar forceps, and a grasping forceps for the entire procedure. Needle drivers are inserted for the appropriate portions of the case. RARP is performed exclusively through a transperitoneal approach at our institution.

When we described our technique in the past, we mentioned selectively starting the procedure through an approach posterior to the bladder at the level of the ampullae of the vasa deferentia and the seminal vesicles for patients on whom we believed that the posterior bladder neck dissection may be complicated, such as with very large or very small prostates, a large median lobe, or in patients who had undergone prior bladder neck procedures, such as a transurethral resection of the prostate (3). We believe that this initial posterior dissection, by mobilizing the rectum posteriorly at the onset of the procedure, assists the surgeon in disarticulating the posterior bladder neck in the appropriate plane. This initial posterior dissection also ensures efficient and complete dissection of the seminal vesicles, with the potential benefit of less traction and dissection near the more laterally located neurovascular bundles. Since this time, we have adopted an initial posterior approach for all of our RARP procedures. Not only does this help to manage one of the more stressful portions of the case, particularly at a teaching institution, but also there is hypothetical benefit when it comes to nerve sparing, taking into account that the neurovascular bundle that controls erections courses along the tip of the seminal vesicle prior to diving into the posterolateral groove along the longitudinal axis of the prostate (4).

Although not all surgeons have adopted the posterior approach at the onset of RARP, there are remarkable similarities in technique for the remainder of the case, culminating in the anastomosis, in which the Van Velthoven one knot, two suture method, has gained essentially unanimous adaptation. Two reasons for uniformity in technique for RARP are undoubtedly the reproducibility and advancement in teaching media. Because of the visual nature of this procedure and the fact that a robotic surgery can be readily digitally captured and uploaded, the evolution of technique can take a much more rapid pace, converging on the most efficacious methods. A learning surgeon need not go any further than his home or office computer to study and perfect RARP.

In order, starting from the posterior approach, our technique of RARP flows through the following surgical steps: takedown of the bladder by incising bilateral medial umbilical ligaments and the urachus; removal of fat overlying the prostate; incision of the bilateral endopelvic fascia with division of bilateral puboprostatic ligaments; dissection of the anterior bladder neck (*anterior peel*) to open the bladder and utilization of the Foley catheter for upward traction to facilitate dissection of the posterior bladder neck; exposure and anterior traction of the previously dissected vasa deferentia and seminal vesicles; incision of Denonvilliers' fascia and isolation of the prostatic pedicles and neurovascular bundles; ligation of the prostatic pedicles and accomplishment of degree of nerve-sparing based on patient and tumor parameters; ligation and division of the dorsal venous complex (DVC) with subsequent division of the urethra and rectourethralis tissue; pelvic lymph node dissection with template based on risk stratification of patient; running vesicourethral anastomosis based on the technique described by Van Velthoven (3).

■ OUTCOMES

There are a couple noteworthy alterations in our technique that we have employed in response to systematic subanalyses of our outcomes and equipment modifications by both the manufacturers of the robotic surgical system and surgical technologies in general. In 2007, we evaluated our positive surgical margin (PSM) outcomes in our first 200 RARP cases. When focusing on organ-confined (pT2) disease, we noted a PSM incidence of 10%, which at the time was consistent with other reports in the literature for all approaches to radical prostatectomy. When inspecting our PSMs more closely, however, we noted that 60% of those PSM in pT2 disease were apical. In response to that, we undertook the following alterations to our technique in apical dissection: (1) in distinction to ligating the DVC at the beginning of the operation, after division of the endopelvic fascia, we started to do so at the end of the operation, after dividing the pedicles and dissecting free the neurovascular bundles. In doing such, we felt that we were visualizing the DVC more completely and obtaining a cleaner ligation without including incidental apical tissue; and (2) we left a small (1–2 mm) cuff of distal urethra on the apex of the prostate when dividing as opposed to dividing flush with the urethroprostatic junction. The 100 cases after these alterations saw our pT2 PSM rate drop significantly to 6%, with 35% being located apically.

The next alteration to our technique was our method of nerve sparing. Although there are several vessel sealant technologies that are available to the surgeon on the robotic platform and to the assistant surgeon at the bedside, and all of these technologies can readily secure the prostatic pedicles with minimal thermal spread to the adjacent neurovascular bundles, we have gone back to the tenets of nerve sparing that we learned in open prostatectomy, namely no thermal energy around the neurovascular bundles with minimal traction and manipulation of the tissue. The robotic Hem-o-lok® clip applier has well lended itself to this approach, and we (5) regularly employ these clips to our patients who receive a bilateral nerve sparing procedure. Accordingly, our potency rate, defined as an ability to have sexual intercourse, in men who had unaffected preoperative erections and who received a bilateral nerve sparing procedure, is 80% to 85% when evaluated at 1 year post-RARP. The corresponding continence rate in these men is approximately 95%; both of these rates compare very favorably with what has been reported the radical prostatectomy literature, regardless of the surgical approach (6).

A relatively new innovation in surgical equipment that we, like others, have started to utilize in our urethrovesical anastomosis is the barbed suture. We find that utilization of this suture type keeps a constant back tension on the already completed anastomosis, allowing us to use both of our working instruments to place upcoming sutures. This effectively converts this portion of the operation from a one-handed procedure to a more coordinated two-handed procedure. This not only improves the quality of the anastomosis but also speeds this part of the operation.

Robotic technology has indeed radically impacted the surgical management of prostate cancer. One of the most impressive facts, however, is that the technology is still in its relative infancy, with the first RARP only performed within the last 13 years. In analyzing the rapid adoption of the technology and evolution of RARP, coupled with the constant changes and improvement of both robotic and surgical technologies in general, it is exciting to imagine what the future will hold.

■ REFERENCES

1. Barbash GI, Glied SA. New technology and health care costs—the case of robot-assisted surgery. *N Engl J Med.* 2007;363:701–704.
2. *Intuitive Surgical, Inc. daVinci Surgery: Urology.* http://www.intuitivesurgical.com/specialties/urology/. Updated January 1, 2013. Accessed June 25, 2013.
3. Lallas CD, Trabulsi EJ. Laparoscopic and robotic radical prostatectomy. In: Keane TE, Graham SD, eds. *Glenn's Urologic Surgery.* Philadelphia, PA: Lippincott Williams and Wilkins; 2010:867–878.
4. Takenaka A, Leung RA, Fujisawa M, et al. Anatomy of autonomic nerve component in the male pelvis: the new concept from a perspective for robotic nerve sparing radical prostatectomy. *World J Urol.* 2006;24(2):136–143.
5. Zorn KC, Trinh QD, Jeldres C, et al. Prospective randomized trial of barbed polyglyconate suture to facilitate vesico-urethral anastomosis during robot-assisted radical prostatectomy: time reduction and cost benefit. *BJU Int.* 2012;109(10):1526–1532.
6. Trabulsi EJ, Zola JC, Gomella LG, et al. Transition from pure laparoscopic to robotic-assisted radical prostatectomy: a single surgeon institutional evolution. *Urol Oncol.* 2010;28(1):81–85.

9.4 Surgical Training, Digital Capture, Virtual Reality, and the Future of Radical Prostatectomy

COSTAS D. LALLAS

Inherent in the argument of which method of radical prostatectomy will stand the test of time, radical retropubic prostatectomy (RRP) or robotic-assisted radical prostatectomy (RARP), is training: Many posit that because RARP is a predominantly visual operation and because every movement that a surgeon makes during the operation is projected onto a screen for all to see, that it is easier to teach. Indeed, the relative extinction of RRP will not occur while this current generation of experienced open prostatectomists continues to make its case, but the newer generations of urologists leave their training programs having been overwhelmingly instructed how to surgically treat clinically localized and locally advanced prostate cancer with robotic assistance. In short, if the vast majority of domestic trainees are most comfortable treating prostate cancer surgically with RARP, eventually this will be the new gold standard, with RRP reserved for patients not fit for RARP. An article evaluating the centralization of radical prostatectomy queried the Nationwide Inpatient Sample, which revealed that 586,429 men underwent radical prostatectomy in the United States from 2000 to 2008. During this time period, there was a 74% increase in the total number of radical prostatectomies performed along with a 19% decrease in the number of hospitals performing radical prostatectomy, resulting in a statistically significant increase in annual hospital radical prostatectomy volume. On multivariate analysis, higher radical prostatectomy hospital volume was associated with the year of the surgery, teaching status, large bed size, urban location, and presence of a robot at the institution (1). What are the training advantages that are available to the robotic surgeon that facilitate teaching the procedure and how does this compare to its open counterpart?

In the classic RRP Halstedian model of surgical instruction, the assistant standing directly across from the primary surgeon was the only individual in the room who stood a chance to observe, much less learn the procedure, especially given the exposure of the prostate deep within the male pelvis. Other than this hands-on experience, you were left to your own devices with textbooks, manuscripts, and surgical atlases. The irony is that with the advent of minimally invasive surgery came the concept of the learning curve, or the number of procedures that must be performed by a surgeon prior to becoming competent at the procedure. For RARP, that number is debatable but has been projected to be as low as 20 cases and as high as 1,000 (2); no one has defined a learning curve threshold for RRP. Although this may be in part a byproduct of the recent emphasis placed on surgical training, medical errors, and competency, it also underscores the variability seen among trainees in learning RRP. In fact, because of the visual nature of RARP, there is a much more linear relationship between number of cases and surgical proficiency. Related to this fact, there are visual-based training devices that are available to the robotic surgeon that make teaching more effective.

■ DUAL CONSOLE

In 2009, Intuitive Surgical, Inc., introduced their newest model of the daVinci® robotic surgical system, the Si. From this platform, which remains in place today, the company has launched many of their new instrumentations and improvements. One of these innovations is the dual console: the ability to attach two working consoles to the daVinci® tower, allowing two surgeons to be actively involved in the operation. Both surgeons have the same three-dimensional view of the operation, and both can control any or all of the working instruments at any given time, which is accomplished with the push of a button. The surgeon in the nonoperating console can use his hand-controlled joysticks to direct virtual indicators that are projected into the working console and on the external viewing screens to point out anatomy, tissue planes, and so on. When a teaching surgeon sits in the second console, he is transformed from a passive instructor attempting to decipher anatomic detail from a two-dimensional monitor to an active participant who sees what the trainee sees and teaches in a more effective manner. Moreover, when he feels like the trainee is not progressing, he can easily take over the operation much in the manner of a driving instructor in a car fitted with dual driving apparatus. He can do so without breaking scrub, moving the trainee off of the console, and waiting for the new assistant to take the surgeon's place; thus, the flow of the operation is not broken for the sake of instruction. In addition, if the opportunity arises, the two surgeons can operate in concert, with one controlling the two main working instruments and the other on the third, using it for real-time intervention as opposed to passive retraction. Such collaborative robotic surgery, although not yet gaining widespread utilization, has tremendous potential.

Remarkably, there are no articles in the literature that have been published at the time of the writing of this chapter citing the value of the dual console; although at the sectional meeting of the Society of Urologic Robotic Surgeons at this year's American Urologic Association annual meeting, many surgeons from teaching institutions touted its role in their operating rooms. However, one overriding complaint was that, although it does have significant advantages as a teaching tool, it adds another approximately half-million dollars to the cost of the purchase of a new system. This fact alone may prevent its widespread adoption, although in the opinion of these investigators, it should be a sine qua non in the operating room of a teaching institution.

■ DIGITAL CAPTURE, DUPLICATION, AND THE INTERNET

By virtue of being a visual operation, any RARP procedure can be easily digitally captured and immortalized onto a variety of media. Although there are circulating videos of RRP, theses cannot compare to the extensive, unadulterated recordings accomplished with RARP, no matter how creative the camera placement. The benefits of such recordings are innumerable. From an individual standpoint, a surgeon can review a case that was performed to learn a step, view a complication, or alter a technique. One document in the literature reports the ability to improve pT2 surgical margin rates through reviewing video documentation in laparoscopic prostatectomy. In this report, 240 consecutive patients who underwent this operation had the procedure recorded. After review of the pathology and margin status, the authors were able to go back and review the videos, identify the critical maneuvers, and alter their technique to cut their positive margin rate in half (3).

From an educational standpoint, these videos can be readily made available to trainees for systematic review. If the trainee is looking for a newer technique or method of surgery, wanting to see how an expert in the procedure may handle difficult anatomy or clinical situations, or just curious, they need not go any further than their own computer, where they may have a publically circulated compact disc/DVD or Internet connection. Public domains such as YouTube® (www.youtube.com) and more private domains that require a login, such as the daVinci® Surgery Online Community (www.davincisurgerycommunity.com) contain multiple full-length RARP videos free of cost that have been uploaded by surgeons around the world. A final source is peer-review journals, which have long realized the value of circulating visual media under the auspices of their journal name. For example, the *Journal of Endourology* has an online peer-reviewed complement, *Videourology*®, that offers high-caliber video demonstrations of the latest cutting-edge robotic and laparoscopic surgical techniques with online access available with a subscription.

These extensive learning opportunities that are available for RARP have no comparison in the open counterpart and will continue to increase with time. It is conceivable that a trainee, when learning RARP, can visually research the procedure, placing them much higher on the learning curve with the endpoint being autonomous surgical proficiency.

■ VIRTUAL REALITY SIMULATION

One of the products of the rapidly evolving field of robotic surgery, which is under external pressures from the public and lawmakers alike for patient safety, has been the development and promotion of simulation. *Simulation* is a broad-based term that incorporates standardized teaching and assessment tools designed to replicate a realistic environment where trainees are forced to act upon a variety of scenarios so that their performance during the actual event is more constant, controlled, and automatic. Very much in the vein of aviation and military simulation, surgical simulation is part of a comprehensive curriculum that is required for a surgeon to practice as a board-certified practitioner.

Virtual reality (VR) simulation is the natural evolution of these requirements combined with technology; it is perfectly matched to the robotic platform. Currently, there are multiple VR simulators available on the market, with all offering stand-alone hardware that is independent of an operating room, a vision monitor that allows a user or tutor to observe and critique the procedure, and minimal cost of operation as no consumables or disposables are required. All also offer a variety of skill sets and performance metrics for the trainee that help to hone particular tasks that are required in robotic surgery, such as camera and arm movement and coordination. There are also several validation studies available for each of these VR simulation systems evaluating their ability to replicate robotic surgery and demonstrate improvement in the trainee (4).

Although no one doubts the benefit of VR simulation for the novice robotic surgeon, VR simulation for robotic surgery falls short in the intermediate and advanced levels. Most validation studies fail to demonstrate construct validity at these levels and it is thus believed that VR simulation for robotic surgery is still in its infancy. One major hurdle is the development of procedural-based programs, as opposed to cartoonish skill sets. In fact, the amount of research and funding required for the development of such software is daunting, but it is tantalizing to imagine the future of this technology in teaching RARP. The intermediate surgeon who is fine-tuning technique is able to draw upon a host of preloaded methods of a particular step of the procedure, and the advanced surgeon is being able to overlay an anatomic three-dimensional representation of the patient's anatomy into a VR surgery, thus being able to operate on the patient before sitting down in the operating room.

The future of radical prostatectomy must be considered in light of the training methods involved in teaching the surgery. In the information age, a procedure well matched to the educational media available and universally utilized will likely prevail.

■ REFERENCES

1. Anderson CB, Penson DF, Ni S, et al. Centralization of radical prostatectomy in the United States. *J Urol.* 2013;189(2):500–506.
2. Secin FP. The learning curve of robotic assisted laparoscopic radical prostatectomy: what is the evidence? *Arch Esp Urol.* 2011;64(8):830–838.
3. Touijer K, Kuroiwa K, Saranchuk JW, et al. Quality improvement in laparoscopic radical prostatectomy for pT2 prostate cancer: impact of video documentation review on positive surgical margin. *J Urol.* 2005;173(3):765–768.
4. Lallas CD, Davis JW; Members of the Society of Urologic Robotic Surgeons. Robotic surgery training with commercially available simulation systems in 2011: a current review and practice pattern survey from the society of urologic robotic surgeons. *J Endourol* 2012;26(3):283–293.

10.1.1 External Beam Radiation Therapy: Conventional Fractionation

DAVID E. GREENE

RICHARD K. VALICENTI

INTRODUCTION

Prostate cancer is the most common cancer in males and their second most common cause of cancer death. Extrapolating from data gathered between 2005 and 2007, U.S. men have a 16.2% lifetime risk of being diagnosed with prostate cancer. Roughly 70% of these patients will present with organ-confined disease, with the majority, in the prostate-specific antigen (PSA) era, presenting with localized, low-risk prostate cancer (1,2).

Risk stratification into low-risk, intermediate-risk, and high-risk prognostic groups is based on PSA, clinical tumor stage, and Gleason score, and dictates appropriate initial management options. Based on the work by D'Amico et al., the following inclusion criteria are most commonly used to define the prognostic groups: Low-risk includes stage T1c to T2a tumors and PSA ≤ 10 ng/mL and Gleason score ≤6; intermediate-risk includes those with stage T2b to T2c tumors, and/or PSA > 10 but ≤20 ng/mL, and/or Gleason score 7; and high-risk includes stage T3 to T4 tumors, and/or PSA > 20 ng/mL, and/or Gleason score 8 to 10 (3). Low-risk prostate cancer correlates with American Joint Committee on Cancer 7th edition Group I (4). Models incorporating the percentage of positive prostate biopsy cores, the pretreatment PSA velocity, the presence or absence of perineural invasion observed on biopsy, the T-stage, and the patient's age provide further prognostic information when selecting the most appropriate treatment strategy for individual patients (5–7). Significant debate continues with regard to the treatment of low-risk prostate cancer and centers around the necessity of treatment, the selection of treatment strategy, and the cost of treatment to patients and society as a whole. This debate is addressed elsewhere in the textbook and is beyond the scope of this chapter, which has its focus on external beam radiation therapy (EBRT) for men diagnosed with prostate cancer in the low-risk category.

PRETREATMENT EVALUATION OF THE LOW-RISK PATIENT

In addition to routine history and physical examination including a digital rectal examination, serum PSA, transrectal ultrasound, and serum testosterone should be obtained. Consensus guidelines from the American Urological Association (AUA), American College of Radiology (ACR), and National Comprehensive Cancer Network (NCCN) discourage routine radiographic and scintigraphic staging for low-risk patients (8–10). Imaging of the pelvis using Computed Tomography (CT) or Magnetic Resonance Imaging (MRI) may be obtained to assist in the evaluation of the size of the prostate gland, the extent and location of the primary tumor, and radiation treatment planning. The risk of pelvic lymph node involvement in localized, low-risk prostate cancer is reported to be 1% to 5%, and the likelihood of bone metastases is negligible in men with low-risk prostate cancer (11,12). Therefore, bone scan is only appropriate for those low-risk patients in whom there is high suspicion for metastatic disease based on clinical findings or for those patients in whom osteopenia, osteoporosis, or osteoarthritis is suspected to establish a baseline prior to RT. CT staging is generally not recommended for the evaluation of pelvic nodal involvement in men with PSA < 25 ng/mL, and even at these levels it has relatively poor sensitivity (13,14).

Although CT-based imaging of the pelvis is the current standard for radiation treatment planning, T2-weighted endorectal MRI provides superior soft tissue resolution to delineate the anatomy of the prostate, seminal vesicles, neurovascular bundles, and pelvic floor (15). An MRI offers the ability to detect disease within and adjacent to the prostate gland that is not as easily visualized on CT (16–18). CT images used for treatment planning were found in a study from University of California San Francisco (UCSF) to correlate with an average 32% increase versus MRI in resulting prostate volume definition. An MRI, if obtained, can be fused to treatment planning CTs, allowing improved accuracy in contour definition of target and normal tissue volumes (19–21). This may result in improved clinical outcomes by decreasing normal tissue toxicity and allowing for tumor-directed boost therapy. Although these theoretical advantages are clear, the clinical necessity of MRI for planning has not yet been established (22). MRI-, magnetic resonance spectroscopy–, and radiolabeled choline–based positron emission tomography may additionally have a role in the evaluation of tumor response to EBRT (23–25).

■ CLINICAL TRIALS

The rationale driving the current standard of EBRT for low-risk prostate cancer is predicated on the results of several prospective randomized controlled trials and single-institution reports. The most significant improvements in disease control and reductions in toxicity for low-risk patients have been observed with dose-escalated, image-guided, intensity-modulated radiation therapy (IMRT).

The dose escalation trials established that high-dose radiation therapy (RT) delivered through conformal technique (78–81 Gy delivered to the prostate) is well tolerated and results in significant improvement in freedom from biochemical failure and disease-free survival versus conventional dose (64–70 Gy) regimens for men with low-risk prostate cancer, although it has not been shown to confer an overall survival advantage (26–33).

■ DOSE ESCALATION

Prior to the advent of three-dimensional conformal radiation therapy (3DCRT), 70 Gy was established as the maximal tolerable dose due to limitations conferred by rectal and bladder toxicity (34, 35). With improved dose conformality, the ability to safely deliver higher doses to the prostate was established, and resultant improvements, especially in biochemical progression-free survival, were seen. As technological innovations have allowed improvement in treatment planning algorithms, beam targeting, and target confirmation through image guidance and the use of implanted fiducial markers or radio beacons, the amount of normal tissue irradiated, and thus of treatment-related toxicity, has been significantly reduced.

■ MD ANDERSON CANCER CENTER 93-002

This trial evaluated the effect of dose escalation from 70 to 78 Gy on freedom from failure and was among the first to include biochemical (PSA) freedom from failure as an endpoint. Between 1993 and 1998, 301 patients with stage T1 to T3, including 61 low-risk patients, were randomized to receive 70 or 78 Gy via EBRT to the prostate gland. All patients received an initial 46 Gy in 2 Gy daily fractions via a four-field box technique. Following delivery of 46 Gy, each group received a 3DCRT boost commensurate with their remaining prescribed total dose, such that the conventional dose arm received an additional 24 Gy via a four-field technique, and the high-dose arm received a 32 Gy boost via a six-field technique. At 8 years follow-up, freedom from biochemical failure favored the 78 Gy arm, 59% versus 78% ($P = .04$) (29, 31).

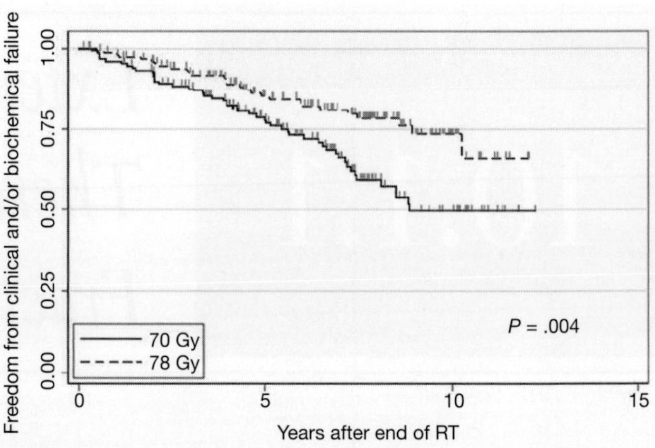

FIGURE 10.1.1.1 Report of the long term outcomes of the randomized dose escalation trials demonstrates improvement in freedom from biochemical failure for men treated with 78 Gy when compared with those treated to 70 Gy.
Source: From Ref. (29). Kuban DA, Tucker SL, Dong L, et al. Long-term results of the M. D. Anderson randomized dose-escalation trial for prostate cancer. *Int J Radiat Oncol Biol Phys*. 2008;70:67–74.

Notably, the rate of Radiation Therapy Oncology Group (RTOG) grade 2 or greater rectal toxicity was 14% higher in the 78 Gy arm and was found to correlate with the volume of rectum receiving greater than or equal to 70 Gy (29) (Figure 10.1.1.1).

■ PROTON RADIATION ONCOLOGY GROUP 95-09

This trial evaluated the effect of dose escalation from 70.2 to 79.2 GyE on local failure, biochemical failure, and overall survival in patients with localized prostate cancer. Three hundred and ninety-three patients with stage T1b to T2b prostate cancer and PSA levels <15 ng/mL were randomized to receive external beam radiation to a total dose of either 70.2 or 79.2 GyE delivered via conformal photon therapy with conformal proton boost. The prostate gland plus a 12- to 15-mm margin received a conformal proton dose of 19.8 or 28.8 GyE in 1.8-GyE fractions. Subsequent to initial proton treatment, all patients received 50.4 Gy to the prostate gland and seminal vesicles, plus a 10-mm margin, via a conformal four-field technique. At 10-year follow-up, biochemical failure rates were halved from 32.3% for the conventional dose arm to 16.7% for the dose-escalated arm. High-dose therapy conferred improved outcomes in all risk groups, although this was only statistically significant for those with low-risk disease (58% of the cohort) in which 28.2% of those receiving conventional dose failed versus 7.1% of those receiving high dose ($P = .0001$). No significant difference in acute or late toxicity was noted between the two arms (32) (Figures 10.1.1.2 and 10.1.1.3).

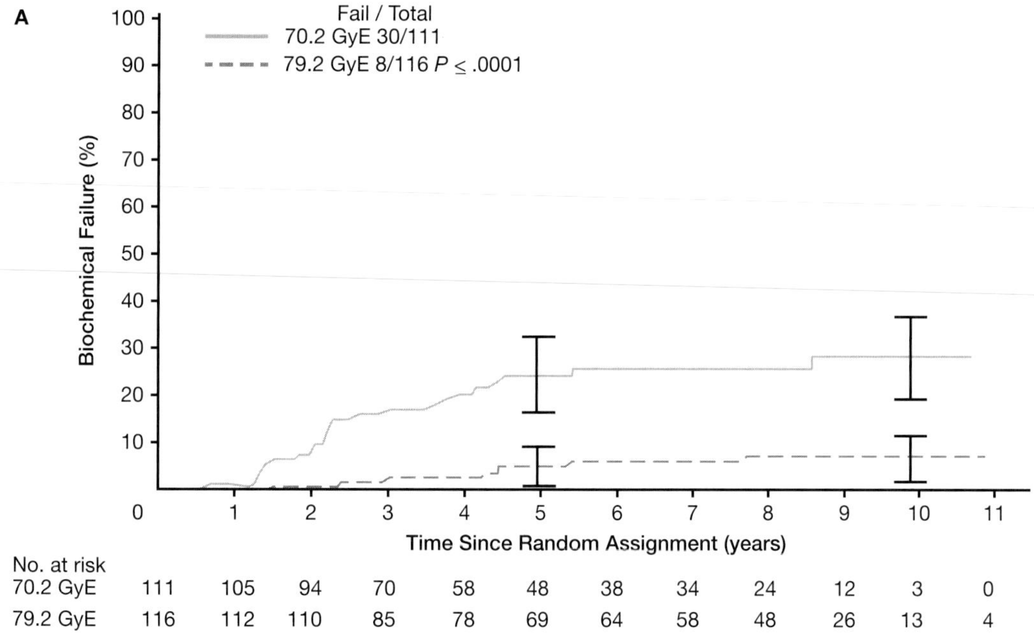

FIGURE 10.1.1.2 At 10-year follow-up, biochemical failure rates were significantly lower than those reported for the dose-escalated arm.
Source: From Ref. (32). Zietman AL, Bae K, Slater JD, et al. Randomized trial comparing conventional-dose with high-dose conformal radiation therapy in early-stage adenocarcinoma of the prostate: long-term results from proton radiation oncology group/american college of radiology 95-09. *J Clin Oncol.* 2010;28:1106–1111.

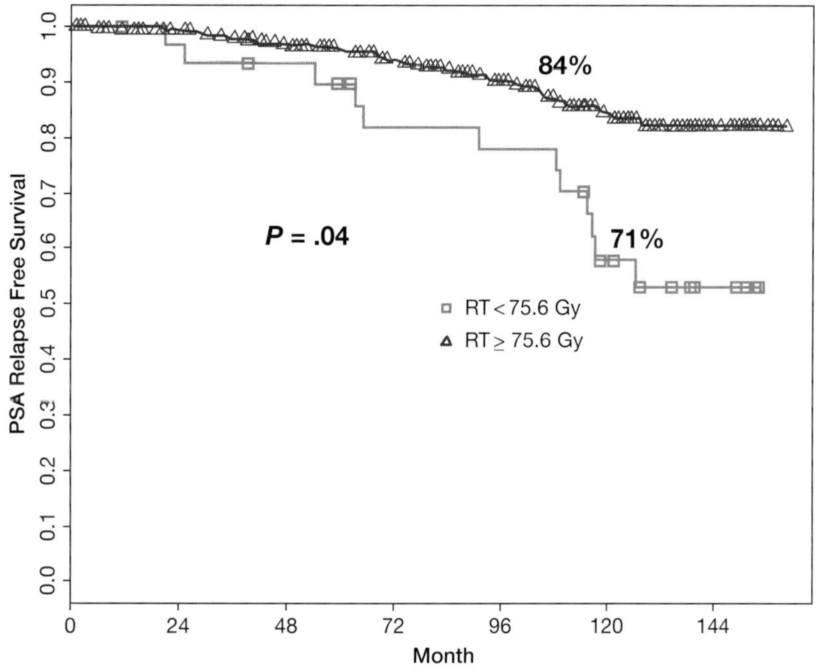

FIGURE 10.1.1.3 Doses greater than 75.6 Gy conferred a 13% improvement in PSA relapse free survival.
Source: From Ref. (36). Zelefsky MJ, Pei X, Chou JF, et al. Dose escalation for prostate cancer radiotherapy: predictors of long-term biochemical tumor control and distant metastases-free survival outcomes. *Eur Urol.* 2011;60:1133–1139.

■ DUTCH TRIAL CKTO 6910

This trial was conducted to evaluate the effect of dose escalation from 68 to 78 Gy on freedom from failure. To that end, 669 patients with stage T1b-4 prostate cancer at four institutions in the Netherlands were randomized to receive either 68 or 78 Gy via a 3DCRT technique. The clinical target volume (CTV) included the prostate plus or minus the seminal vesicles depending on assessed risk for seminal vesicle involvement based on the Partin method. Planning target volume (PTV) included a 10-mm expansion for the initial 68 Gy for all patients, followed by an additional 10 Gy with 5-mm expansion, except 0 mm toward the rectum, for patients receiving 78 Gy. In two institutions, neoadjuvant hormone therapy was prescribed for some, mostly high-risk patients. The study was not statistically powered to detect a difference due to the addition or withholding of hormonal therapy. With 4 years follow-up, the freedom from biochemical failure was 64% in the high-dose arm versus 54% in the low-dose arm (P = .02). There was no significant difference in overall survival between the treatment arms. At 6 years, there was a nonsignificant trend for improved freedom from failure 84% versus 80% favoring dose escalation for low-risk patients (P = .57) (37).

At 70 months follow-up, the 7-year biochemical control rates continued to favor the high-dose arm 56% versus 45%, P = .03. The cumulative incidence of late grade 2 or greater gastrointestinal (GI) toxicity manifested by rectal bleeding and incontinence was increased in the 78-Gy arm compared with the 68-Gy arm (35% vs. 25% at 7 years; P = .04) (38).

■ MRC RT01 TRIAL

This trial sought to evaluate whether neoadjuvant hormonal therapy combined with dose-escalated radiotherapy (74 vs. 64 Gy) would improve cancer control as measured by biochemical progression-free survival, freedom from local progression, metastasis-free survival, and overall survival, without a prohibitive increase in treatment-associated toxicity when compared with neoadjuvant hormonal therapy followed by standard dose radiotherapy. This is the largest randomized prospective dose escalation trial and the only one to prescribe neoadjuvant hormonal therapy uniformly to all patients. Eight hundred and forty-three men with stage T1b to T3a, N0, M0 prostate cancer, and serum PSA of <50 ng/mL first received between 3 and 6 months of neoadjuvant hormonal therapy and were randomly assigned to receive either 64 Gy over 32 fractions in 6.5 weeks or an 74 Gy over 37 fractions in 7.5 weeks.

The gross tumor volume (GTV) for all patients included the prostate gland and all or a portion of the seminal vesicles depending on the risk group. In low-risk patients, GTV included the base of the seminal vesicles, and in intermediate- and high-risk patients, GTV included all of the seminal vesicles. A 5-mm expansion was made from GTV to CTV, and a subsequent 5-mm to 1-cm expansion from CTV was made to PTV. Biochemical progression-free survival at 5 years (63 months average) favored the dose-escalated patients across all risk groups, 71% versus 60% (P = .0007), and in the intermediate-risk group by 9% (79% vs. 70%). There was no observed difference in freedom from local progression or overall survival. There was an increased incidence of late GI toxicity and genitourinary (GU) toxicity in the 74-Gy arm (28).

■ GENITOURINARY TUMOR GROUP (GETUG)

Three hundred and six patients were randomized to receive 70 or 80 Gy via a 3DCRT technique. At median follow-up of 61 months, a 10% benefit favoring the high-dose arm was reported. Although GETUG did not conduct formal risk group stratification, the reported results demonstrated no benefit to dose escalation in patients with initial Prostate Specific Antigen (iPSA) < 15 ng/mL, which leads some to infer that there was no benefit to dose escalation in the low-risk cohort. As prostate cancer, and in particular low-risk prostate cancer, tends to have a protracted natural history, more mature data may yet reveal a benefit (39).

As a group, these trials demonstrated a benefit for dose-escalated RT for low-risk prostate cancer in terms of biochemical freedom from failure and local control, but failed to demonstrate an improvement in overall survival. Viani et al. published a meta-analysis of the dose escalation studies, found a significant reduction in risk of biochemical failure for low-risk patients with high-dose radiation, and concluded that dose-escalated radiation should be offered without regard to risk group (40,41). Table 10.1.1.1 summarizes the outcomes of the dose escalation trials. Overall,

■ Table 10.1.1.1 Dose escalation trials

Study	Number of Patients	Risk Groups	Dose Levels	Outcome	*P* Value
MDACC 93-002	301	LR: 61 IR: 139 HR: 101	78 Gy 70 Gy	8-yr bNED 78% 8-yr bNED 59%	P = .004
PROG 95-09	392	LR: 227 IR: 129 HR: 33	79.2 GyE 70 GyE	5-yr bNED 80% 5-yr bNED 61%	P < .001
NCI CKTO	664	LR: 120 IR: 182 HR: 362	78 Gy 68 Gy	5-yr FFF 64% 5-yr FFF 54%	P = .01
MRC RT 01	843	LR: 204 IR: 264 HR: 362	NHT + 74 Gy NHT + 64 Gy	5-yr bPFS 71% 5-yr bPFS 60%	P = .0007

Abbreviations: bNED, biochemically without evidence of disease; bPFS, biochemical progression free survival; FFF, freedom from failure; HR, high risk; IR, intermediate risk; LR, low risk; NHT, neoadjuvant hormonal therapy.

GI and GU toxicity in the high-dose arms were increased versus conventional dose arms with the exception of those treated with protons. A caveat is that these trials were conducted prior to the advent of or did not allow IMRT, which has permitted substantial improvements in the conformality of delivered doses and resultant reduction in normal tissue dose profiles and toxicity.

IMRT AND IGRT

The results of RTOG 0126 provide a prospective evaluation of toxicity outcomes for dose escalation to 79.2 versus 70.2 Gy delivered via 3DCRT or IMRT techniques for localized prostate cancer patients. An interim analysis of toxicity was presented by Michalski at the plenary session of American Society for Radiation Oncology (ASTRO) in 2011. Of the 748 patients randomized to 79.2 Gy, 491 received 3DCRT and 257 received IMRT. At a median follow-up of 4.6 and 3.5 years, respectively, there was a statistically significant reduction in acute GU and GI toxicity favoring IMRT, as well as a trend for reduction in late GI side effects. Notably, even when high-dose constraints to the rectum were met, IMRT was associated with significantly less toxicity than 3DCRT (42).

The historical rates of grade 2+ GI toxicity in the dose escalation trials ranged from 20% to 35%, which, as detailed below, is a significant improvement when compared with 2D conventional planning. The advent of IMRT allowed for significant reduction in the volume of rectum and bladder receiving intermediate and high doses versus 3DCRT, resulting in dramatically decreased grade 2 GI and GU toxicity, and near absence of grade 3 toxicity (43,44).

Image-guided radiation therapy (IGRT) has allowed for further improvements in early and late toxicity for patients undergoing EBRT. This is secondary to decreased uncertainty regarding interfraction organ motion and set-up error, allowing reduction in PTV margins and therefore reduction of the volume of normal tissue receiving high and intermediate doses of radiation

Zelefsky and Spratt have reported long-term GI and GU toxicity profiles of men receiving high-dose RT with and without IMRT and with and without image guidance at Memorial Sloan Kettering Cancer Center (MSKCC), demonstrating a clear benefit to IMRT and IGRT (Figures 10.1.1.4 and 10.1.1.5).

With regard to oncologic outcomes, single-institution reports of IMRT results have been excellent. Zelefsky et al. reported the results of 275 low-risk patients treated to 81 Gy at MSKCC. At 3 years, biochemical failure was reported at 8%; at 7-year median follow-up, Biochemical Failure (BF) was 15%; and at 10 years, actuarial failure was 19%. The results of the low-risk and very low-risk cohort of a total of 1,002 patients treated to 86.4 Gy with IMRT had a 5-year actuarial failure rate of 2.3% by ASTRO definition (Figure 10.1.1.6) (43).

HYPOFRACTIONATION AND SBRT

Hypofractionation for the treatment of prostate cancer has recently experienced renewed interest based on radiobiological properties of prostate tumor cells and resultant theoretical improvements in the therapeutic ratio with increased fraction sizes. Although most tumors have alpha/beta ratios around 8, prostate cancer cells are postulated to have an alpha/beta ratio of 2. As the rectum is the major dose-limiting structure for the delivery of radiation to the prostate and has a higher alpha/beta ratio estimated

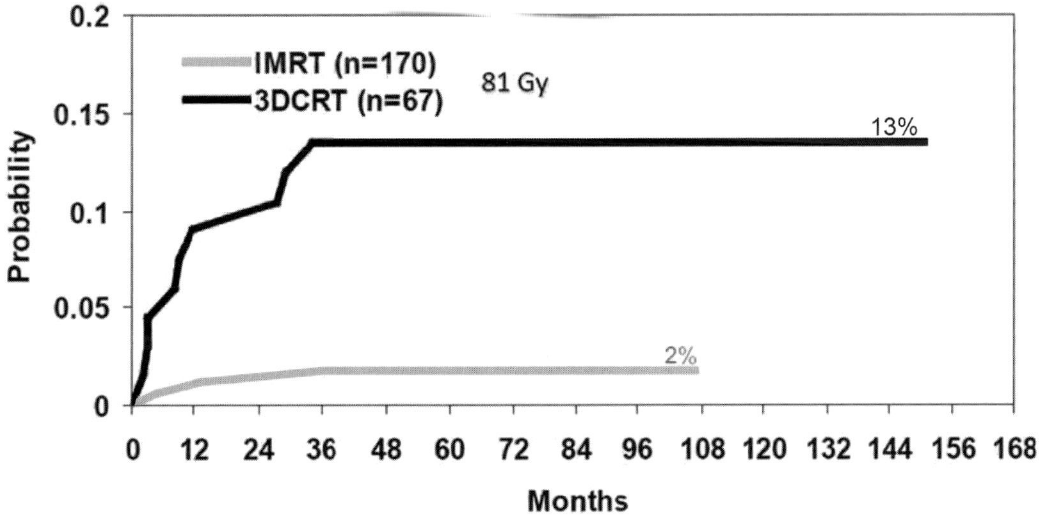

FIGURE 10.1.1.4 Late grade 2 GI toxicity.
Source: From Ref. (44). Zelefsky MJ, Chan H, Hunt M, Yamada Y, Shippy AM, Amols H. Long-term outcome of high dose intensity modulated radiation therapy for patients with clinically localized prostate cancer. *J Urol.* 2006;176:1415–1419.

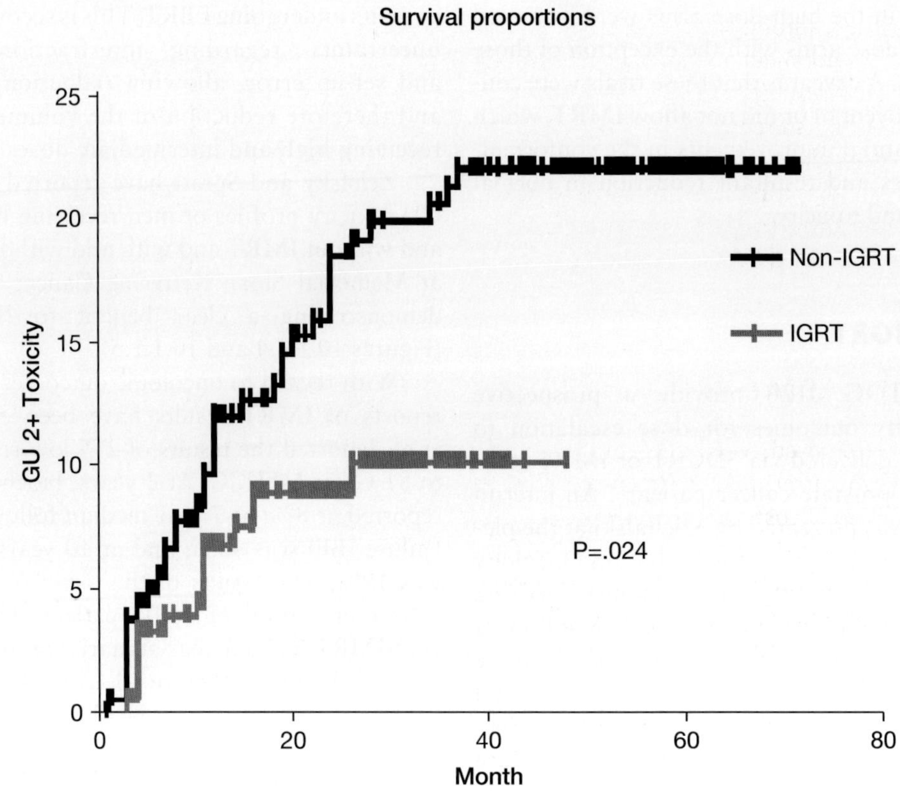

FIGURE 10.1.1.5 Actuarial grade 2+ urinary toxicity in patients treated to 86.4 Gy.
Source: From Ref. (43). Spratt DE, Pei X, Yamada J, Kollmeier MA, Cox B, Zelefsky MJ. Long-term survival and toxicity in patients treated with high-dose intensity modulated radiation therapy for localized prostate cancer. *Int J Radiat Oncol Biol Phys.* 2013;85:686–692.

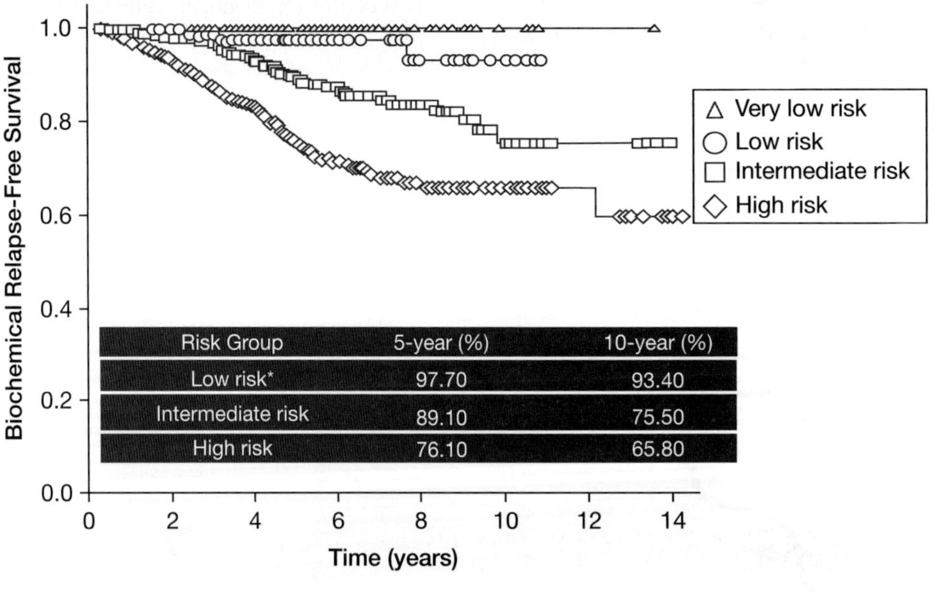

FIGURE 10.1.1.6 The data in the figure demonstrate the ability of IMRT to allow dose escalation without increased acute toxicity or decrement in oncologic efficacy.
Source: From Ref. (43). Spratt DE, Pei X, Yamada J, Kollmeier MA, Cox B, Zelefsky MJ. Long-term survival and toxicity in patients treated with high-dose intensity modulated radiation therapy for localized prostate cancer. *Int J Radiat Oncol Biol Phys.* 2013;85:686–692.

at 4 to 6, it follows that hypofractionation should permit greater tumor killing without an attendant increase in the incidence of late toxicity (45,46). Several randomized and nonrandomized trials have demonstrated the feasibility, tolerability, and noninferiority of hypofractionated regimens (28,47–49).

In a representative single-institution series from the Cleveland Clinic, 770 patients received 70 Gy over 28 fractions via an IMRT technique. At 45 months median follow-up, biochemical control rates in low-, intermediate-, and high-risk patients were 94%, 83%, and 72%, respectively. There was no increase in acute or late GI or GU toxicity (48).

Based on the same radiobiological principles, and in concert with the development of emerging technologies and patient preferences, limited initial single-institution experiences with stereotactic body radiation therapy (SBRT) and high-dose rate (HDR) monotherapy approaches to extreme hypofractionation have shown promising results but require further evaluation (50–55). Oncologic outcomes of selected SBRT studies are summarized in Table 10.1.1.2.

TOXICITY OF RADIATION THERAPY

RT is generally well tolerated, with certain prognostic factors such as prior transurethral resection of prostate, pretreatment International Prostate Symptom Score, AUA score, anticoagulant use, inflammatory bowel disease, and radiation technique predicting an increased propensity to develop complications. Commonly reported acute symptoms include urinary frequency, urgency, nocturia, diarrhea, and tenesmus. These symptoms are usually well controlled with supportive care, alpha blockers, loperamide, and steroid suppositories and resolve shortly after completion of therapy. Urethral strictures, hematuria, hematochezia, proctitis, and incontinence occur infrequently at 1 to 3 years posttreatment. Urethral dilatation, argon plasma laser coagulation, formalin therapy, and hyperbaric oxygen have been reported as effective treatments for these late toxicities. Improvements in toxicity profiles have been demonstrated for advances in RT technologies and are summarized below.

Toxicity of Conventional 2D planning

Over a thousand patients treated on RTOG trials 7506 and 7706 were followed up for a minimum of 7 years and had a reported incidence of ≥grade 3 bowel complications of 3.3% and a reported incidence of grade 3 or greater urinary complications in 7.7% of patients. These trials established 70 Gy as the maximal tolerable dose prior to the advent of conformal planning techniques (35).

Toxicity of 3DCRT

RTOG 9406 evaluated the development of grade 3 or greater GI or GU toxicity in five dose levels from 68.4 to 79.2 Gy delivered via a 3DCRT technique. Group 1 patients had no elective seminal vesicle irradiation. Group 2 patients received treatment of the prostate and seminal vesicles for 54 to 55.8 Gy followed by prostate boost. Rates of grade 2 or greater GI toxicity rates were 9%, 7%, 11%, 10%, and 25% for group 1 and 13%, 9%, 14%, 16%, and 26% for group 2 at 68.4 in 1.8 Gy/fx, 73.8 Gy in 1.8 Gy/fx, 79.2 Gy in 1.8 Gy/fx, 74.0 Gy in 2.0 Gy/fx, and 78.0 Gy in 2.0 Gy/fx, respectively. The incidence of grade 2 or greater GU toxicity were 24%, 22%, 18%, 29%, and 23% for group 1 and 19%, 16%, 21%, 21%, and 28% for group 2. This trial demonstrated the reduction in toxicity, particularly in grade 3 or greater toxicity, despite radiation doses that were more than 10 Gy higher when conformal techniques were used (61).

Toxicity of IMRT

Similar to the improvements seen with the advent of 3DCRT versus conventionally planned two-dimensional radiation therapy (2DRT), IMRT techniques have allowed the same or higher radiation doses to be delivered with a reduction in grade 2 and grade 3 urinary and rectal complications. As detailed by Zelefsky et al., 561 patients treated with IMRT at MSKCC to 81 Gy had an 8-year likelihood of developing grade 2 rectal toxicity of 1.6%. Eight-year grade 2 or 3 urinary toxicity rates were 9% and 3%, respectively (44).

Toxicity of Hypofractionation/SBRT

Although data from prospective trials currently underway will provide greater insight into toxicity profiles of hypofractionation and SBRT, the available data suggest acceptable toxicity levels. Data are summarized in Table 10.1.1.3.

Table 10.1.1.2 Summary of oncologic outcomes of hypofractionation studies

Study	Number of Patients	Dose/Fx	Fx	Total Dose (Gy)	Median F/u (mo)	PSA Control (%)
Virginia Mason (2010)	40	6.7	5	33.5	41	90
Stanford (2009)	41	7.25	5	36.25	33	100
Naples (2009)	112	7–7.25	5	35–36	24	99
Winthrop (2010)	304	7–7.25	5	35–36	30	99
Boike (2011)	45	9–10 Gy	5	45–50	30	100
Georgetown (2013)	100	7–7.25	5	35–36	27	99

Abbreviation: PSA, prostate-specific antigen.
Source: From Refs. (52, 55–60).

Table 10.1.1.3 Summary of late GI and GU toxicity outcomes of hypofractionation studies

Study	Dose (Gy)	Median F/u (mo)	Late GI Toxicity	Late GU Toxicity
King et al. (64)	36.25	33	48% G1–G2	65% G1–G2; 5% G3
Katz et al. (57)	35	30	9% G1/G2	9% G1/G2 0.5% G3
Bolzicco et al. (62)	35	20	2.2% G2	9% G1/G2 2.2% G3
Freeman and King (63)	36.25	60	15.5% G1–G2	32% G1/G2 2.5% G3
King et al. (65)	36.25	32	16% G1–G2	28% G1/G2 3.5% G3

Abbreviations: GI, gastrointestinal; GU, genitourinary.
Source: From Refs. (57,62–66).

SECOND MALIGNANCIES

RT is known generally to be associated with an increased risk for the development of second primary cancers within the radiation field. This is particularly true for young patients with long posttreatment survival. For prostate cancer patients, particularly in the era of modern RT techniques, the increased risk of second primary cancer is not yet known. A matched pair retrospective study comparing 2,120 patients receiving RT at a single institution on a 1:1 basis with surgical patients according to age and follow-up time was recently reported. RT techniques consisted of conventional or two-dimensional RT (36%), three-dimensional conformal RT, and/or intensity-modulated RT (29%), brachytherapy (16%), and a combination of 2DRT and Brachytherapy (BT) (19%).

They found that the overall risk of developing a second primary cancer was not significantly different between the matched pair (hazard ratio [HR] 1.14, 95% confidence interval [CI] 0.94–1.39). In addition, they noted that the risk became significant >5 years (HR 1.86, 95% CI 1.36–2.55) or >10 years after RT (HR 4.94, 95% CI 2.18–11.2). The most significant sites of increased risk were bladder, lymphoproliferative, and sarcoma. Of the different RT techniques, only 2DRT was associated with a significantly higher risk (HR 1.76, 95% CI 1.32–2.35), but not BT boost (HR 0.83, 95% CI 0.50–1.38), 3DCRT/IMRT (HR 0.81, 95% CI 0.55–1.21), or BT (HR 0.53, 95% CI 0.28–1.01) (67).

CONCLUSIONS

Evidence supports that patients with low-risk prostate cancer have a benefit in biochemical freedom from failure when treated with dose-escalated RT (78–81 Gy) versus conventional dose RT. Hypofractionation may also confer equivalent or improved outcomes, in this case with shorter treatment times and at lower cost, but requires further evaluation. A multitude of modern therapeutic modalities exist that can technically deliver highly conformal radiation to the prostate, but phase III evidence is lacking to demonstrate superiority of one technique compared with another. The use of radiotherapy technologies should be based on prospective assessment of quality of life and modeling of cost-effectiveness.

Emerging therapeutic modalities such as stereotactic body RT are promising areas of future investigation, especially given confirmatory evidence regarding the alpha/beta ratio in prostate cancer. Highly conformal treatment delivery techniques, improved intratreatment evaluation, and improved pretreatment target localization and registration have significantly decreased the incidence of serious toxicity secondary to RT.

REFERENCES

1. Jemal A, Siegel R, Xu J, Ward E. Cancer statistics, 2010. *CA Cancer J Clin.* 2010;60:277–300.
2. Siegel R, Naishadham D, Jemal A. Cancer statistics, 2012. *CA Cancer J Clin.* 2012;62:10–29.
3. D'Amico AV, Whittington R, Malkowicz SB, et al. Biochemical outcome after radical prostatectomy, external beam radiation therapy, or interstitial radiation therapy for clinically localized prostate cancer. *JAMA.* 1998;280:969–974.
4. Edge SB. *American Joint Committee on Cancer. AJCC Cancer Staging Manual.* New York, NY: Springer; 2010.
5. Briganti A, Chun FK, Hutterer GC, et al. Systematic assessment of the ability of the number and percentage of positive biopsy cores to predict pathologic stage and biochemical recurrence after radical prostatectomy. *Eur Urol.* 2007;52:733–743.
6. D'Amico AV, Renshaw AA, Cote K, et al. Impact of the percentage of positive prostate cores on prostate cancer-specific mortality for patients with low or favorable intermediate-risk disease. *J Clin Oncol.* 2004;22:3726–3732.
7. D'Amico AV, Renshaw AA, Sussman B, Chen MH. Pretreatment PSA velocity and risk of death from prostate cancer following external beam radiation therapy. *JAMA.* 2005;294:440–447.
8. Amis ES Jr, Bigongiari LR, Bluth EI, et al. Post-treatment follow-up of prostate cancer. American College of Radiology. ACR Appropriateness Criteria. *Radiology.* 2000;215(suppl):773–778.
9. Greene KL, Albertsen PC, Babaian RJ, et al. Prostate specific antigen best practice statement: 2009 update. *J Urol.* 2009;182:2232–2241.

10. Mohler J, Bahnson RR, Boston B, et al. NCCN clinical practice guidelines in oncology: prostate cancer. *J Natl Compr Canc Netw.* 2010;8:162–200.
11. Abuzallouf S, Dayes I, Lukka H. Baseline staging of newly diagnosed prostate cancer: a summary of the literature. *J Urol.* 2004;171:2122–2127.
12. Heidenreich A, Varga Z, Von Knobloc.R. Extended pelvic lymphadenectomy in patients undergoing radical prostatectomy: high incidence of lymph node metastasis. *J Urol.* 2002;167:1681–1686.
13. Chybowski FM, Keller JJ, Bergstralh EJ, Oesterling JE. Predicting radionuclide bone scan findings in patients with newly diagnosed, untreated prostat. cancer: prostate specific antigen is superior to all other clinical parameters. *J Urol.* 1991;145:313–318.
14. Eberhardt SC, Carter S, Casalino DD, et al. ACR Appropriateness criteria prostate cancer—pretreatment detection, staging, and surveillance. *J Am Coll Radiol.* 2013;10:83–92.
15. Reinsberg SA, Payne GS, Riches SF, et al. Combined use of diffusion-weighted MRI and 1H MR spectroscopy to increase accuracy in prostate cancer detection. *Am J Roentgenol.* 2007;188:91–98.
16. Haider MA, van der Kwast TH, Tanguay J, et al. Combined T2-weighted and diffusion-weighted MRI for localization of prostate cancer. *Am J Roentgenol.* 2007;189:323–328.
17. Flanigan RC, McKay TC, Olson M, Shankey TV, Pyle J, Waters WB. Limited efficacy of preoperative computed tomographic scanning for the evaluation of lymph node metastasis in patients before radical prostatectomy. *Urology.* 1996;48:428–432.
18. Heesakkers RA, Hovels AM, Jager GJ, et al. MRI with a lymph-node-specific contrast agent as an alternative to CT scan and lymph-node dissection in patients with prostate cancer: a prospective multicohort study. *Lancet Oncol.* 2008;9:850–856.
19. Kagawa K, Lee WR, Schultheiss TE, Hunt MA, Shaer AH, Hanks GE. Initial clinical assessment of CT-MRI image fusion software in localization of the prostate for 3D conformal radiation therapy. *Int J Radiat Oncol Biol Phys.* 1997;38:319–325.
20. Rasch C, Barillot I, Remeijer P, Touw A, van Herk M, Lebesque JV. Definition of the prostate in CT and MRI: a multi-observer study. *Int J Radiat Oncol Biol Phys.* 1999;43:57–66.
21. Roach MIII, Faillace-Akazawa P, Malfatti C, Holland J, Hricak H. Prostate volumes defined by magnetic resonance imaging and computerized tomographic scans for three-dimensional conformal radiotherapy. *Int J Radiat Oncol Biol Phys.* 1996;35:1011–1018.
22. Villeirs GM, De Meerleer GO. Magnetic resonance imaging (MRI) anatomy of the prostate and application of MRI in radiotherapy planning. *Eur J Radiol.* 2007;63:361–368.
23. Mazaheri Y, Shukla-Dave A, Muellner A, Hricak H. MRI of the prostate: clinical relevance and emerging applications. *J Magn Reson Imaging.*2011;33:258–274.
24. Pickett B, Kurhanewicz J, Coakley F, Shinohara K, Fein B, Roach MIII. Use of MRI and spectroscopy in evaluation of external beam radiotherapy for prostate cancer. *Int J Radiat Oncol Biol Phys.* 2004;60:1047–1055.
25. Pucar D, Shukla-Dave A, Hricak H, et al. Prostate cancer: correlation of MR imaging and MR spectroscopy with pathologic findings after radiation therapy-initial experience. *Radiology.* 2005;236:545–553.
26. Al-Mamgani A, Heemsbergen WD, Levendag PC, Lebesque JV. Subgroup analysis of patients with localized prostate cancer treated within the Dutch-randomized dose escalation trial. *Radiother Oncol.* 2010;96:13–18.
27. Al-Mamgani A, van Putten WL, Heemsbergen WD, et al. Update of Dutch multicenter dose-escalation trial of radiotherapy for localized prostate cancer. *Int J Radiat Oncol Biol Phys.* 2008;72:980–988.
28. Dearnaley DP, Sydes MR, Graham JD, et al. Escalated-dose versus standard-dose conformal radiotherapy in prostate cancer: first results from the MRC RT01 randomised controlled trial. *Lancet Oncol.* 2007;8:475–487.
29. Kuban DA, Tucker SL, Dong L, et al. Long-term results of the M. D. Anderson randomized dose-escalation trial for prostate cancer. *Int J Radiat Oncol Biol Phys.* 2008;70:67–74.
30. Peeters ST, Heemsbergen WD, Koper PC, et al. Dose-response in radiotherapy for localized prostate cancer: results of the Dutch multicenter randomized phase III trial comparing 68 Gy of radiotherapy with 78 Gy. *J Clin Oncol.* 2006;24:1990–1996.
31. Pollack A, Zagars GK, Starkschall G, et al. Prostate cancer radiation dose response: results of the M. D. Anderson phase III randomized trial. *Int J Radiat Oncol Biol Phys.* 2002;53:1097–1105.
32. Zietman AL, Bae K, Slater JD, et al. Randomized trial comparing conventional-dose with high-dose conformal radiation therapy in early-stage adenocarcinoma of the prostate: long-term results from proton radiation oncology group/american college of radiology 95-09. *J Clin Oncol.* 2010;28:1106–1111.
33. Zietman AL, DeSilvio ML, Slater JD, et al. Comparison of conventional-dose vs high-dose conformal radiation therapy in clinically localized adenocarcinoma of the prostate: a randomized controlled trial. *JAMA.* 2005;294:1233–1239.
34. Lawton CA, Won M, Pilepich MV, et al. Long-term treatment sequelae following external beam irradiation for adenocarcinoma of the prostate: analysis of RTOG studies 7506 and 7706. *Int J Radiat Oncol Biol Phys.* 1991;21:935–939.
35. Pilepich MV, Asbell SO, Krall JM, et al. Correlation of radiotherapeutic parameters and treatment related morbidity—analysis of RTOG Study 77-06. *Int J Radiat Oncol Biol Phys.* 1987;13:1007–1012.
36. Zelefsky MJ, Pei X, Chou JF, et al. Dose escalation for prostate cancer radiotherapy: predictors of long-term biochemical tumor control and distant metastases-free survival outcomes. *Eur Urol.* 2011;60:1133–1139.
37. Heemsbergen WD, Hoogeman MS, Witte MG, Peeters ST, Incrocci L, Lebesque JV. Increased risk of biochemical and clinical failure for prostate patients with a large rectum at radiotherapy planning: results from the Dutch trial of 68 GY versus 78 Gy. *Int J Radiat Oncol Biol Phys.* 2007;67:1418–1424.
38. Al-Mamgani A, Heemsbergen WD, Peeters ST, Lebesque JV. Role of intensity-modulated radiotherapy in reducing toxicity in dose escalation for localized prostate cancer. *Int J Radiat Oncol Biol Phys.* 2009;73:685–691.
39. Beckendorf V, Guerif S, Le Prise E, et al. 70 Gy versus 80 Gy in localized prostate cancer: 5-year results of GETUG 06 randomized trial. *Int J Radiat Oncol Biol Phys.* 2011;80:1056–1063.
40. Viani GA, da Silva LG, Stefano EJ. High-dose conformal radiotherapy reduces prostate cancer-specific mortality: results of a meta-analysis. *Int J Radiat Oncol Biol Phys.* 2012;83:e619–e625.
41. Viani GA, Stefano EJ, Afonso SL. Higher-than-conventional radiation doses in localized prostate cancer treatment: a meta-analysis of randomized, controlled trials. *Int J Radiat Oncol Biol Phys.* 2009;74:1405–1418.
42. Michalski JM, Yan Y, Watkins-Bruner D, et al. Preliminary toxicity analysis of 3-dimensional conformal radiation therapy versus intensity modulated radiation therapy on the high-dose arm of the Radiation Therapy Oncology Group 0126 prostate cancer trial. *Int J Radiat Oncol Biol Phys.* 2013;87:932–938.
43. Spratt DE, Pei X, Yamada J, Kollmeier MA, Cox B, Zelefsky MJ. Long-term survival and toxicity in patients treated with high-dose intensity modulated radiation therapy for localized prostate cancer. *Int J Radiat Oncol Biol Phys.* 2013;85:686–692.
44. Zelefsky MJ, Chan H, Hunt M, Yamada Y, Shippy AM, Amols H. Long-term outcome of high dose intensity modulated radiation therapy for patients with clinically localized prostate cancer. *J Urol.* 2006;176:1415–1419.
45. Brenner DJ, Martinez AA, Edmundson GK, Mitchell C, Thames HD, Armour EP. Direct evidence that prostate tumors show high sensitivity to fractionation (low alpha/beta ratio), similar to late-responding normal tissue. *Int J Radiat Oncol Biol Phys.* 2002;52:6–13.

46. Fowler JF, Ritter MA, Chappell RJ, Brenner DJ. What hypofractionated protocols should be tested for prostate cancer? *Int J Radiat Oncol Biol Phys.* 2003;56:1093–1104.
47. Konski A, Speier W, Hanlon A, Beck JR, Pollack A. Is proton beam therapy cost effective in the treatment of adenocarcinoma of the prostate? *J Clin Oncol.* 2007;25:3603–3608.
48. Kupelian P, Willoughby T, Mahadevan A, et al. Multi-institutional clinical experience with the Calypso System in localization and continuous, real-time monitoring of the prostate gland during external radiotherapy. *Int J Radiat Oncol Biol Phys.* 2007;67:1088–1098.
49. Norkus D, Miller A, Kurtinaitis J, et al. A randomized trial comparing hypofractionated and conventionally fractionated three-dimensional external-beam radiotherapy for localized prostate adenocarcinoma: a report on acute toxicity. *Strahlenther Onkol.* 2009;185:715–721.
50. Allen AM, Pawlicki T, Dong L, et al. An evidence based review of proton beam therapy: the report of ASTRO's emerging technology committee. *RadiotherOncol.* 2012;103:8–11.
51. Aluwini S, van Rooij P, Hoogeman M, et al. CyberKnife stereotactic radiotherapy as monotherapy for low- to intermediate-stage prostate cancer: early experience, feasibility, and tolerance. *J Endourol.* 2010;24:865–869.
52. Boike TP, Lotan Y, Cho LC, et al. Phase I dose-escalation study of stereotactic body radiation therapy for low- and intermediate-risk prostate cancer. *J Clin Oncol.* 2011;29:2020–2026.
53. Buyyounouski MK, Price RA Jr, Harris EE, et al. Stereotactic body radiotherapy for primary management of early-stage, low- to intermediate-risk prostate cancer: report of the American Society for Therapeutic Radiology and Oncology Emerging Technology Committee. *Int J Radiat Oncol Biol Phys.* 2010;76:1297–1304.
54. Macias V, Biete A. Hypofractionated radiotherapy for localised prostate cancer. Review of clinical trials. *Clin Transl Oncol* 2009; 11:437–445.
55. Madsen BL, Hsi RA, Pham HT, Fowler JF, Esagui L, Corman J. Stereotactic hypofractionated accurate radiotherapy of the prostate (SHARP), 33.5 Gy in five fractions for localized disease: first clinical trial results. *Int J Radiat Oncol Biol Phys.* 2007;67:1099–1105.
56. Chen LN, Suy S, Uhm S, et al. Stereotactic body radiation therapy (SBRT) for clinically localized prostate cancer: the Georgetown University experience. *Radiat Oncol.* 2013;8:58.
57. Katz AJ, Santoro M, Ashley R, Diblasio F, Witten M. Stereotactic body radiotherapy for organ-confined prostate cancer. *BMC Urol.* 2010;10:1.
58. King CR, Brooks JD, Gill H, Pawlicki T, Cotrutz C, Presti JC Jr. Stereotactic body radiotherapy for localized prostate cancer: interim results of a prospective phase II clinical trial. *Int J Radiat Oncol Biol Phys.* 2009;73:1043–1048.
59. King CR, Brooks JD, Gill H, Presti JC Jr. Long-term outcomes from a prospective trial of stereotactic body radiotherapy for low-risk prostate cancer. *Int J Radiat Oncol Biol Phys.* 2012;82:877–882.
60. King CR, Freeman D, Kaplan I, et al. Stereotactic body radiotherapy for localized prostate cancer: pooled analysis from a multi-institutional consortium of prospective phase II trials. *Radiother Oncol.* 2013;109:217–221.
61. Michalski JM, Bae K, Roach M, et al. Long-term toxicity following 3D conformal radiation therapy for prostate cancer from the RTOG 9406 phase I/II dose escalation study. *Int J Radiat Oncol Biol Phys.* 2010;76:14–22.
62. Bolzicco G, Favretto MS, Satariano N, Scremin E, Tambone C, Tasca A. A single-center study of 100 consecutive patients with localized prostate cancer treated with stereotactic body radiotherapy. *BMC Urol.* 2013;13:49.
63. Freeman DE, King CR. Stereotactic body radiotherapy for low-risk prostate cancer: five-year outcomes. *Radiat Oncol.* 2011;6:3.
64. King CR, Brooks JD, Gill H, Pawlicki T, Cotrutz C, Presti JC Jr. Stereotactic body radiotherapy for localized prostate cancer: interim results of a prospective phase II clinical trial. *Int J Radiat Oncol Biol Phys.* 2009;73:1043–1048.
65. King CR, Collins S, Fuller D, et al. Health-related quality of life after stereotactic body radiation therapy for localized prostate cancer: results from a multi-institutional consortium of prospective trials. *Int J Radiat Oncol Biol Phys.* 2013;87:939–945.
66. Tambone C, Tasca A, Guglielmi R. Image-guided stereotactic body radiation therapy for clinically localized prostate cancer: preliminary clinical results. *Technol Cancer Res Treat.* 2010;9:473–477.
67. Huang J, Kestin LL, Ye H, Wallace M, Martinez AA, Vicini FA. Analysis of second malignancies after modern radiotherapy versus prostatectomy for localized prostate cancer. *Radiother Oncol.* 2011;98:81–86.

10.1.2 Hypofractionated Radiation Therapy for Localized Prostate Cancer

NICHOLAS G. ZAORSKY

ROBERT B. DEN

■ OVERVIEW

Dose-escalated conventionally fractionated external beam radiation therapy (EBRT; a single 1.8–2.0 Gy fraction, delivered in approximately 15 minutes per day, 5 days per week, for 8–9 weeks, to a total dose of 76–80 Gy) is an established treatment modality for men in all disease risk groups. Emerging evidence from experimental and clinical studies from the year 2001 suggested that the α/β ratio for prostate cancer may be as low as 1.5 Gy, which has prompted investigators around the world to explore moderately hypofractionated radiation therapy (HFRT; 2.1–3.5 Gy/fraction, for approximately 15 minutes per day, 5 days per week, for about 4 weeks, to a total dose of ~52–72 Gy). This chapter reviews the impetus and the current clinical evidence supporting moderate hypofractionated EBRT for prostate cancer. Although HFRT has many theoretical advantages, there is no clear evidence from prospective, randomized, controlled trials showing that hypofractionated schedules have improved outcomes or lower toxicity than conventionally fractionated regimens.

■ BACKGROUND TO DOSE-ESCALATED CONVENTIONALLY FRACTIONATED RADIATION THERAPY

Prostate cancer is the second most prevalent solid tumor diagnosed in men of the United States and Western Europe (1). Given the widespread utilization of prostate-specific antigen (PSA) testing, most contemporary prostate cancer patients present with localized disease (clinical stage T1–T2). For these patients, EBRT is a popular treatment option. In the mid-1990s, the most commonly used method to deliver EBRT was a four-field technique (i.e., two beams aimed in the anteroposterior axis and two in the left–right lateral axis). At the time, there was no consistent agreement on the optimal dose of fractionation regimen used for treatment (2). Nondose-escalated conventionally fractionated radiation therapy (non-DE-CFRT; a single 1.8–2.0 Gy fraction lasting 15 minutes per day, 5 days per week) schedules were typically administered over 6 to 7 weeks with doses of 60 to 70 Gy (3).

By the turn of the century, DE-CFRT (a single 1.8–2.0 Gy fraction, delivered in approximately 15 minutes per day, 5 days per week, for 8–9 weeks, to a total dose of 76–80 Gy) gained popularity as it was shown in multiple randomized controlled trials (RCTs) to improve rates of tumor control and decrease cancer-specific mortality (4–8). The rationale behind the efficacy of DE-CFRT was that it provided a homogenous dose distribution to the prostate and surrounding tissues (e.g., pelvic lymph nodes), which potentially harbor micrometastases.

■ RATIONALE BEHIND HYPOFRACTIONATED RADIATION THERAPY

HFRT (2.1–3.5 Gy/fraction, for about 15 minutes per day, 5 days per week, for about 4 weeks) is theoretically advantageous compared to DE-CFRT for three reasons. First, radiobiological models in 2001 suggested that the use of higher doses per fraction would improve killing of prostate cancer cells and minimize toxicity to the surrounding tissues. Second, the patient would benefit from a shorter overall treatment time (8 weeks of DE-CFRT vs. 4 weeks of HFRT). Third, HFRT is theorized to be more cost efficient.

Radiobiology

CFRT is theorized to kill prostate cancer cells though the "3 Rs" of radiation therapy (RT): (1) reoxygenation (allowing more cells to become oxic, which makes RT more effective); (2) redistribution (allowing for tumor cells to cycle into more radiosensitive phases of the cell cycle); and (3) repair (allowing normal cells to repair sublethal damage). As the total RT dose delivered increases, the number of surviving cancer cells decreases. However, the advantages of dose escalation are countered by the damage to surrounding normal tissues.

An α/β ratio estimates the effects of radiation on tissues. The α/β ratio is generally believed to be >10 Gy for early-responding tissue (e.g., skin, mucosa, and most tumors) and 3 to 5 Gy for late-responding tissue (e.g., connective tissues, muscles), where genitourinary (GU) and gastrointestinal (GI) toxicity occur. The α/β ratio is used in the calculation of the biologically equivalent dose (BED):

$$BED = (nd[1 + d/(\alpha/\beta)])$$

where n is the number of radiation fractions and d is the fraction size.

Hypothesis-generating reports in 2001 suggested that prostate cancer cells had a relatively low α/β ratio of ~1.5 Gy, implying that the cells were more sensitive to large fraction doses (9). In addition, calculation models with an α/β ratio of 1.5 Gy showed that a prolonged course of RT (i.e., from CFRT) was disadvantageous. First, dose escalation is necessary to offset accelerated cancer cell repopulation (10). Second, given the lower α/β ratio for prostate cancer than late-responding tissues, there would be potential for therapeutic gain and minimized toxicity to surrounding tissues with larger fraction sizes (11, 12).

Notably, not all trials assumed that the argument of a low α/β ratio for prostate cancer in their methodology. The "initial" (i.e., pre-2001) HFRT versus CFRT trials (13–15) had no assumptions about the α/β ratio and used non-DE-CFRT. Although there has been controversy in calculating the accurate α/β ratio for prostate cancer (16), investigators of HFRT trials after 2001 (i.e., "modern" trials) (17–22) tried to maintain a high BED (at an α/β ratio of 1.5) to kill prostate cancer cells while minimizing the BED (at α/β ratios of 3–10) for toxicity. The BED curves for α/β ratios of 1.5 to 10 Gy for CFRT (to a total dose of 66 and 78 Gy), initial HFRT trials, and modern HFRT trials included in this chapter are juxtaposed in Figure 10.1.2.1.

Patient Perspective

The 8 weeks of DE-CFRT is inconvenient to men who live far from RT centers or are unable to travel, and it is the most frequently patient-cited disadvantage of DE-CFRT and a major cause of patient nonadherence (23). Considering the travel time and automobile expenses, the shorter course of HFRT may save each man an average of $1,900 in out-of-pocket expenses (24). Thus, a man would appreciate the HFRT schedule compared to DE-CFRT.

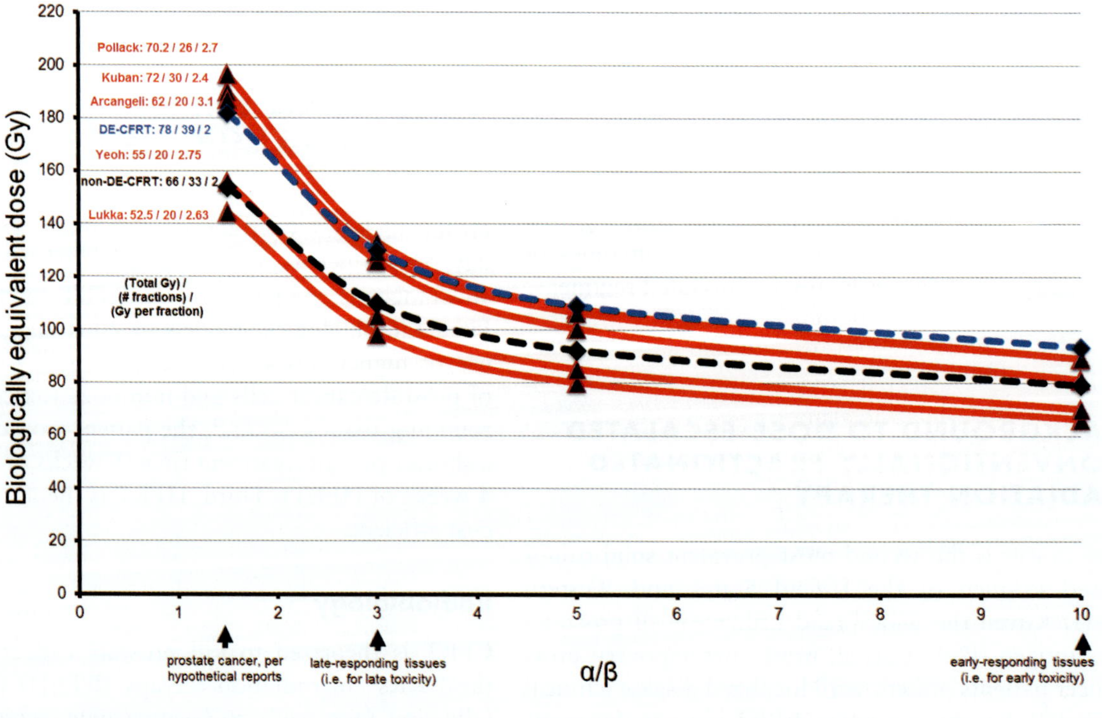

FIGURE 10.1.2.1 Biologically equivalent dose (BED) versus α/β ratios for initial and modern trials of hypofractionated radiation therapy (HFRT) compared to conventionally fractionated radiation therapy (CFRT). A plot of BED curves for HFRT studies included in this chapter (red lines); compared to CFRT, at 2.0 Gy/fraction, to a total dose of 66 in 33 fractions (nondose escalated, dotted black lines), or 78 Gy in 39 fractions (dose escalated, dotted black lines).

Cost Effectiveness

Resource allocation could be improved with HFRT. According to calculations models, wage costs outweigh the cost of machines due to the labor-intensive nature of RT planning and delivery (25–28). Moreover, although treatment planning complexity increases with novel technologies, the planning is only done at the start of EBRT, while cost builds with the delivery of each fraction (29). For example, it is estimated that staffing RT facilities accounts for 50% of their cost (30). Thus, changing to HFRT from DE-CFRT may decrease the number of work hours and overall cost of treating each patient.

■ INITIAL TRIALS COMPARING CFRT AND HFRT

From 1986 to 1993, nonrandomized studies from around the world reported similar outcomes between HFRT and non-DE-CFRT schedules (31–34). Two "initial" HFRT phase III prospective studies (shown in Table 10.1.2.1) were published in 2005 (13) and 2006 (14, 15). Lukka et al. (13) reported that freedom from biochemical failure (FFBF) and acute toxicity were worse in the HFRT arm, and late toxicities were equal. Yeoh et al. (14, 15) similarly compared HFRT to CFRT. Thirty-six of 108 patients developed BF in the HFRT arm, compared to 49 of 109 patients in the CFRT arm. Multivariate analyses revealed that the CFRT schedule was the only statistically significant variable for increased BF and worse GU symptoms at 4 years.

Lukka et al. (13) and Yeoh et al. (14, 15) reached opposite conclusions about HFRT compared to CFRT. These conclusions are likely due to a few factors. First, the trials were designed to compare widely used non-DE-CFRT regimens in their respective countries with no specific assumptions about the α/β ratio before the trial. To highlight this difference, the total dose of the CFRT arms were 66 (13) and 64 Gy (14, 15) [at an α/β ratio of 1.5, the BEDs are 154 (13) and 144 (14, 15)], which is lower than more contemporary conventional doses of 78 to 80 Gy (Figure 10.1.2.1) (4–6). Second, the arms were not designed to be isoeffective. Third, the study by Lukka et al. (13) reported that the percent of positive biopsies at 2 years was equal between the arms, which is in contradiction to the FFBF rates, possibly suggesting that local control was equivalent, but that patients in the HFRT arm had failed distantly.

In addition, the study by Lukka et al. (13) used the American Society for Therapeutic Radiology and Oncology (ASTRO) definition (35) (i.e., three consecutive PSA rises) and other definitions of BF; in contrast, the study by Yeoh et al. (14, 15) used the ASTRO (35) and Phoenix (i.e., nadir + 2 ng/mL) (36, 37) definitions. Yeoh et al. (14, 15) found a significant difference between their FFBF rates with the use of the Phoenix definition, but not with the ASTRO definition. The relationship between ASTRO-defined BF and overall survival (OS) or prostate cancer–specific survival (PCSS) has not been clearly demonstrated (38, 39). The Phoenix definition has since been shown to be a better predictor of distant metastasis, OS, and PCSS (36, 37). Thus, although these initial studies provide valuable insight in comparing HFRT and CFRT, they do not conclusively show that one schedule has improved outcomes or toxicities compared to the other schedule, likely because their methods were so different from modern trials.

■ MODERN TRIALS COMPARING CFRT AND HFRT

Prospective phase III superiority studies (17–22) (also on Table 10.1.2.1) have been published based on the assumption that the α/β ratio for prostate cancer is 1.5 Gy. The hypotheses of the trials were designed to show one of two endpoints: (1) if the HFRT course had a higher BED than the CFRT arm, then HFRT FFBF rates should be improved while having equal toxicity; or (2) if the BED of the HFRT course were isoeffective to a CFRT course, then FFBF rates should be equivalent, and there should be reduced toxicity in the HFRT arm. The modern trials failed to reach either endpoint.

Pollack et al. (20, 21) predicted equivalent acute toxicities between the HFRT (BED at α/β of 3 = 133) and the CFRT (BED at α/β of 3 = 127) with improved tumor control in the HFRT arm. In their 2011 update (21), they reported that 5-year rates and FFBF were not significantly different (both 86%). Radiation therapy oncology group (RTOG) grade ≥2 GU toxicities were statistically higher in the HFRT arm (18.3% vs. 8.3%, $P = .028$). Moreover, men on the HFRT schedule had a significantly higher rate of GI toxicity during weeks 2 through 4. Pollack et al. attributed the higher incidence of toxicities to the shorter course of the HFRT schedule, the inclusion of lymph nodes in the high-risk patients, the use of a modified RTOG toxicity scale, and the mean biological doses to the prostate (including the urethra) being >80 Gy. Unexpectedly, their initial assumption of isoeffectiveness of the trial design appears to be incorrect.

Arcangeli et al. (17–19) hypothesized that the delivery of an isoeffective dose to prostate tumors using HFRT would reduce the incidence of late complications, have a sparing effect on early responding tissues, and produce equal FFBF rates compared to CFRT. The BED difference between the two arms (at an α/β ratio of 1.5) was only 3, yet a statistically significant difference in 5-year FFBFs was noted: 85% versus 79%, respectively. In addition, there was no reported difference in late toxicity at 5 years between the two schedules. To put this

Table 10.1.2.1 Multi-arm phase III studies comparing CFRT and HFRT

Era	Reference	*n*	Risk Groups	Median FU (mo)	Total dose (Gy)	Total Fractions	Gy/ Fraction	BED (Gy), at α/β = 1.5	3	10	FFBF	Other Outcomes	RTOG Late Toxicity Grade ≥2 (%) GU	GI
Initial	Lukka et al. (13)	470	L, I, H	64	66	33	2	154	110	79	5-y ASTRO: 60%	5-y OS: 85% (NS) 2-y positive biopsy rate: 53% (NS)	1.3	1.9
		466			52.5	20	2.63	144	98	66	5-y ASTRO: 53%	5-y OS: 87% (NS) 2-y positive biopsy rate: 51% (NS)	1.3	1.9
	Yeoh et al. (14,15)	109	NR	90	64	32	2	149	107	77	7.5-y Phoenix: 34% ($P < .05$) 7.5-y ASTRO: 44% (NS)	7.5-y OS: 71% (NS)	NR	NR
		108			55	20	2.75	156	105	70	7.5-y Phoenix: 53% ($P < .05$) 7.5-y ASTRO: 44% (NS)	7.5-y OS: 69% (NS)	NR	NR
Modern	Arcangeli et al. (17–19)	85	H	35	80	40	2	187	133	96	5-y Phoenix: 79% ($P = .04$)	5-y DM: 14% (NS) 5-y LF: 11% (NS)	16	17
		83			62	20	3.1	190	126	81	5-y Phoenix: 85% ($P = .04$)	5-y DM: 10% (NS) 5-y LF: 7% (NS)	11	14
	Pollack et al. (20,21)	152	I, H	60	76	38	2	177	127	91	5-y Phoenix: 86% (NS)	5-y LRF/DM: 1.0% (NS)	8.3	5
		151			70.2	26	2.7	197	133	89	5-y Phoenix: 86% (NS)	5-y LRF/DM: 1.3% (NS)	18.3	6.8
	Kuban et al. (22)	102	Mostly L, I	56	75.6	42	1.80	166	121	89	5-y ASTRO: 92% (NS) 5-y Phoenix: 94% (NS)	5-y clinical failure: 0% (NS)	19	6
		102			72	30	2.40	187	130	89	5-y ASTRO: 96% (NS) 5-y Phoenix: 97% (NS)	5-y clinical failure: 0% (NS)	19	14

Abbreviations: ASTRO, American Society of Therapeutic Radiology and Oncology; BED, biologically equivalent dose; CFRT, conventionally fractionated radiotherapy; DM, distant metastasis; L, low risk; LRF, local-regional failure; FFBF, freedom from biochemical failure; FU, follow-up; GI, gastrointestinal; GU, genitourinary; H, high risk; HFRT, hypofractionated radiotherapy; I, intermediate risk; NS, not significant; NR, not reported; OS, overall survival.

Source: Adapted from Ref. (61). Zaorsky NG, Ohri N, Showalter TN, et al. Systematic review of hypofractionated radiation therapy for prostate cancer. *Cancer Treat Rev.* 2013;39:728–736.

in perspective, the dose escalation RCTs (4–8), which showed significant improvements of BF, had BED differences of approximately 20. Arcangeli et al. did not provide a clear reason for this observation, but noted that patients at high risk (in particular, those with Gleason >7 and PSA > 20 ng/mL) were those who had improved BF rates following HFRT. Finally, there was no reported difference in late toxicity at 5 years between the two schedules.

A few factors may have contributed to the lack of difference in observed toxicity rates. The study by Arcangeli et al. included high-risk patients, which may have affected planning target volumes (prostate alone vs. prostate and seminal vesicles) and treatment setup. In addition, there is a possibility of different mechanisms of radiation damage or repair for late rectal and bladder effects with HFRT in the presence of concomitant androgen deprivation therapy. Finally, they used different toxicity grading methods.

The third modern RCT to compare HFRT to CFRT was performed by Kuban et al. (22). The authors hypothesized that the arms would have equivalent acute toxicities and that there would be improved outcomes in the HFRT arm. They randomized 102 men to receive CFRT (BED at α/β of 1.5 = 166) to a dose of 75.6 Gy in 42 fractions and 102 men to receive HFRT (BED at α/β of 1.5 = 187) to a dose of 72 Gy in 30 fractions. The 5-year Phoenix FFBF rates were 92% and 96% (not significant), respectively, and no patient had a clinical failure. GI and GU toxicity rates were similar between the two groups. Thus, they did not prove their hypothesis.

Dose escalation studies (4–8) have helped to determine the standard of care in determining the optimal CFRT schedule. To compare the outcomes and toxicities in the HFRT studies, the rates of FFBF (Figure 10.1.2.2), GU toxicity (Figure 10.1.2.3), and GI toxicity (Figure 10.1.2.4) of phase III HFRT RCTs are benchmarked dose escalations studies of CFRT.

■ LIMITATIONS AND FUTURE DIRECTION

Intertrial Comparisons

There are a number of important caveats to consider when interpreting results of trials that compare HFRT to CFRT. First, the methods of the initial studies differed greatly from the modern studies. Second, all three modern studies were designed as superiority studies; thus, it would be incorrect to infer that the absence of a difference in any study implies equivalence between the arms. Moreover, although dose escalation studies indicated that DE-CFRT was associated with improved FFBF when compared to non-DE-CFRT, all studies of HFRT are inconsistent in their results. Finally, when compared to dose escalation studies, the follow-up of the HFRT studies is not yet as

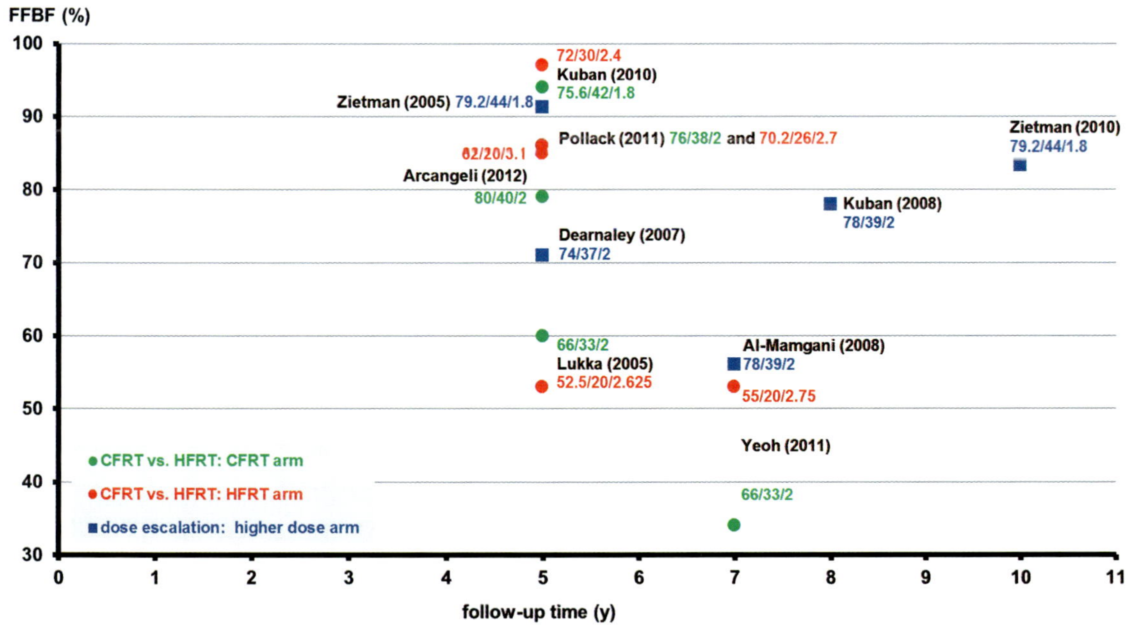

FIGURE 10.1.2.2 Freedom from biochemical failure (FFBF) versus follow-up time of conventionally fractionated radiation therapy (CFRT) versus hypofractionated radiation therapy (HFRT) randomized controlled trials (RCTs) benchmarked to high-dose radiation therapy (RT) arm of escalation RCTs for prostate cancer. The *y*-axis shows the FFBF, and the *x*-axis shows the median follow-up time in years. Individual arms of phase III RCTs comparing CFRT (green circles) and HFRT (red circles) are shown on the plot with first author and year of publication. As a benchmark for these studies, the higher dose arms of dose escalation studies (blue squares) are shown on the plot with first author and year of publication. The individual RT schedule of an arm is shown near each data point: total dose, number of fractions, and Gy/fraction.

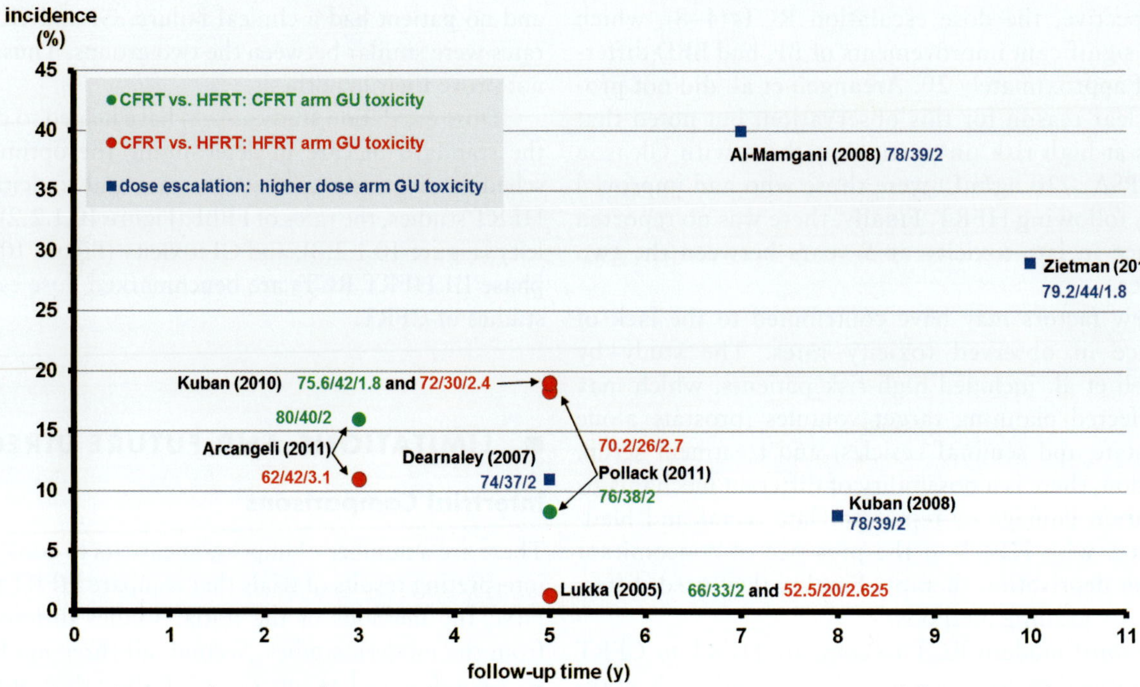

FIGURE 10.1.2.3 Radiation therapy oncology group (RTOG) grade ≥2 genitourinary (GU) toxicity versus follow-up time of conventionally fractionated radiation therapy (CFRT) versus hypofractionated radiation therapy (HFRT) randomized controlled trials (RCTs) benchmarked to high-dose radiation therapy (RT) arm of escalation RCTs for prostate cancer. The *y*-axis shows incidence of late RTOG grade ≥2 toxicity (%), and the *x*-axis shows the follow-up time in years. Individual arms of phase III RCTs comparing CFRT and HFRT are shown on the plot with first author and year of publication. As a benchmark for these studies, the higher dose arms of dose escalation RCTs are shown on the plot with first author and year of publication. Green circles refer to the GU toxicity rates of CFRT arms. Red circles refer to the GU toxicity rates of HFRT arms. Blue squares refer to the GU toxicity rates of the higher dose arm of dose escalation studies. The individual RT schedule of an arm is shown near each data point: total dose, number of fractions, and Gy/fraction.
Source: Adapted from Ref. (61). Zaorsky NG, Ohri N, Showalter TN, et al. Systematic review of hypofractionated radiation therapy for prostate cancer. *Cancer Treat Rev.* 2013;39:728–736.

long, and the significance of the results may change. In addition, a number of factors preclude comparing the results of HFRT trials to the expected outcomes and toxicities of DE-CFRT regimens used today.

Efficacy

With respect to efficacy, HFRT trials had differing planning target margins, treatment techniques, and fractionations schedules, which may all affect outcomes (40). The specific endpoints evaluated in these studies vary. For example, as Yeoh et al. (14, 15) reported, FFBF rates may be significant with the Phoenix definition, but not with the ASTRO definition.

In addition, the study by Yeoh et al. did not report on differing FFBFs among risk groups, and their inclusion criteria were based on the American Joint Committee on Cancer (AJCC). The National Comprehensive Cancer Network (NCCN) model is a superior prognosticator of FFBF to the AJCC and remains the preferred method for risk-based clinical management of prostate cancer with radiotherapy (41); thus, the reported rates of FFBF may have changed if they had used NCCN criteria.

Although Arcangeli et al. (17–19) noted improved FFBF among high-risk patients, no HFRT study has looked at the effect of the optimal fractionation schedule among individual risk groups. Cancer- and patient-specific biomarkers including Ki-67 (42, 43); p53 (44); p21/waf1 (44); P120 (43); Bcl-2, Bax, and the Bcl2/Bax ratio (42, 44–46); and PCNA (43) affect rates of cellular growth and have been shown to predict cancer aggressiveness and recurrence. These biomarkers may contribute to variations in α/β ratios among individual prostate cancer cell lines. Future models will likely combine these markers with traditional pretreatment variables (e.g., PSA, Gleason) to create personalized fractionation schedules and predict outcomes (47).

Toxicity

Late effects from radiation can technically occur decades after therapy (48). Moreover, the RTOG toxicity score does not report on anorectal symptoms such as urgency of defecation and fecal incontinence (49). In addition, assessing quality of life has become an integral component of prostate cancer care. None of the HFRT trials used quality-of-life questionnaires nor did they asses how toxicities affect individual patient subpopulations (e.g., minority communities, men who have sex with men), who make up a large proportion of the prostate

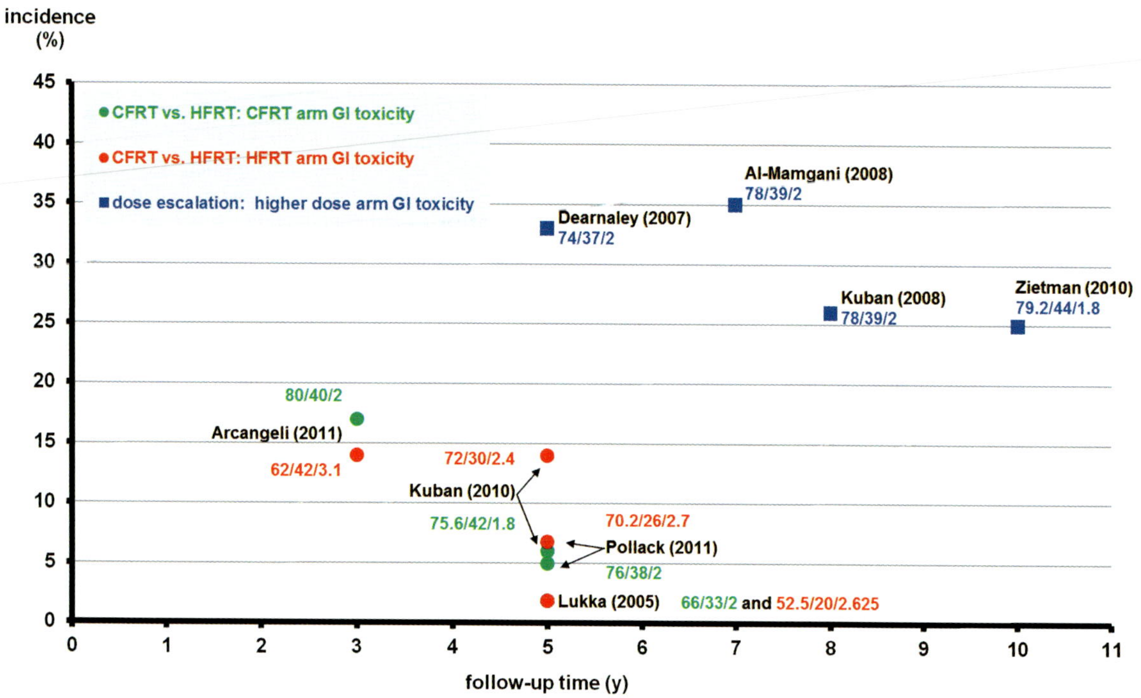

FIGURE 10.1.2.4 Radiation therapy oncology group (RTOG) grade ≥2 gastrointestinal (GI) toxicity versus follow-up time of conventionally fractionated radiation therapy (CFRT) versus hypofractionated radiation therapy (HFRT) randomized controlled trials (RCTs) benchmarked to high-dose radiation therapy (RT) arm of escalation RCTs for prostate cancer. The *y*-axis shows incidence of late RTOG grade ≥2 toxicity (%), and the *x*-axis shows the follow-up time in years. Individual arms of phase III RCTs comparing CFRT and HFRT are shown on the plot with first author and year of publication. As a benchmark for these studies, the higher dose arms of dose escalation RCTs are shown on the plot with first author and year of publication. Green circles refer to the GI toxicity rates of CFRT arms. Red circles refer to the GI toxicity rates of HFRT arms. Blue squares refer to the GI toxicity rates of the higher dose arm of dose escalation studies. The individual RT schedule of an arm is shown near each data point: total dose, number of fractions, and Gy/fraction.
Source: Adapted from Ref. (61). Zaorsky NG, Ohri N, Showalter TN, et al. Systematic review of hypofractionated radiation therapy for prostate cancer. *Cancer Treat Rev.* 2013;39:728–736.

cancer patient demographic and often have specific quality-of-life concerns (50).

Assessing Available Treatment Options

Currently, there are multiple comparative treatment options used for localized disease, and their efficacies vary among risk groups (51). Novel modalities, including stereotactic body radiation therapy (SBRT; a single 3.5–15.0 Gy fraction lasting 1 hour per day, 5 days per week, for about 2 weeks) and hadron therapy (specifically, protons), are gaining popularity as alternatives to DE-CFRT and HFRT schedules. Although neither SBRT (52) nor proton therapy (53) has proven to have improved outcomes of lower toxicities compared to other forms of EBRT, it will be necessary to consider them as possible treatment options alongside HFRT. Comparative effectiveness research will help to define the proper role of RT modalities for specific prostate cancer patients (54).

Evolving Technology

Technology has evolved since the publication of the earliest HFRT studies, and image-guided radiation therapy (IGRT) is now an integral component of SBRT (52,55). To put this in perspective, 72% of the patients in the study by Yeoh et al. (14,15) were treated with two-dimensional radiation therapy; today, the patients could be treated with volumetric-modulated arc therapy and 4D radiofrequency tracking to increase normal organ sparing (56) and decrease intrafractional motion (57). Some retrospective studies show that IGRT improves outcomes with EBRT (58–60), and it is unknown how the use of novel technologies would impact HFRT.

■ CONCLUSIONS

DE-CFRT is an established treatment modality for almost all prostate cancer patients. Determining the optimal fractionation scheme has been one of the goals of radiation oncologists. HFRT is hypothesized to improve tumor control, patient quality of life, and cost. RCTs comparing HFRT and CFRT have been inconsistent in their results. The methods of initial HFRT studies do not compare to modern techniques of DE-CFRT. The modern HFRT studies have rejected their hypotheses of superiority of HFRT. As of 2013, HFRT regimens are still under investigation.

■ REFERENCES

1. Siegel R, Naishadham D, Jemal A. Cancer statistics, 2012. *CA Cancer J Clin*. 2012;62(1):10–29.
2. Hanks GE. External-beam radiation therapy for clinically localized prostate cancer: patterns of care studies in the United States. *NCI Monogr*. 1988;(7):75–84.
3. Zagars GK, von Eschenbach AC, Johnson DE, Oswald MJ. The role of radiation therapy in stages A2 and B adenocarcinoma of the prostate. *Int J Radiat Oncol Biol Phys*. 1988;14(4):701-709.
4. Kuban DA, Tucker SL, Dong L, et al. Long-term results of the M. D. Anderson randomized dose-escalation trial for prostate cancer. *Int J Radiat Oncol Biol Phys*. 2008;70(1):67–74.
5. Al-Mamgani A, van Putten WL, Heemsbergen WD, et al. Update of Dutch multicenter dose-escalation trial of radiotherapy for localized prostate cancer. *Int J Radiat Oncol Biol Phys*. 2008;72(4):980–988.
6. Zietman AL, DeSilvio ML, Slater JD, et al. Comparison of conventional-dose vs high-dose conformal radiation therapy in clinically localized adenocarcinoma of the prostate: a randomized controlled trial. *JAMA*. 2005;294(10):1233–1239.
7. Zietman AL, Bae K, Slater JD, et al. Randomized trial comparing conventional-dose with high-dose conformal radiation therpay in early-stage adenocarcinoma of the prostate: long-term results from Proton Radiation Oncology Group/American College of Radiology 95-09. *J Clin Oncol*. 2010;28(7):1106–1111.
8. Dearnaley DP, Sydes MR, Graham JD, et al. Escalated-dose versus standard-dose conformal radiotherapy in prostate cancer: first results from the MRC RT01 randomised controlled trial. *Lancet Oncol*. 2007;8(6):475–487.
9. Fowler J, Chappell R, Ritter M. Is alpha/beta for prostate tumors really low? *Int J Radiat Oncol Biol Phys*. 2001;50(4):1021–1031.
10. Wang JZ, Li XA. Impact of tumor repopulation on radiotherapy planning. *Int J Radiat Oncol Biol Phys*. 2005;61(1):220–227.
11. Fowler JF, Ritter MA, Chappell RJ, Brenner DJ. What hypofractionated protocols should be tested for prostate cancer? *Int J Radiat Oncol Biol Phys*. 2003;56(4):1093-1104.
12. Brenner DJ, Martinez AA, Edmundson GK, et al. Direct evidence that prostate tumors show high sensitivity to fractionation (low alpha/beta ratio), similar to late-responding normal tissue. *Int J Radiat Oncol Biol Phys*. 2002;52(1):6–13.
13. Lukka H, Hayter C, Julian JA, et al. Randomized trial comparing two fractionation schedules for patients with localized prostate cancer. *J Clin Oncol*. 2005;23(25):6132–6138.
14. Yeoh EE, Holloway RH, Fraser RJ, et al. Hypofractionated versus conventionally fractionated radiation therapy for prostate carcinoma: updated results of a phase III randomized trial. *Int J Radiat Oncol Biol Phys*. 2006;66(4):1072–1083.
15. Yeoh EE, Botten RJ, Butters J, et al. Hypofractionated versus conventionally fractionated radiotherapy for prostate carcinoma: final results of phase III randomized trial. *Int J Radiat Oncol Biol Phys*. 2011;81(5):1271–1278.
16. Miles EF, Lee WR. Hypofractionation for prostate cancer: a critical review. *Semin Radiat Oncol*. 2008;18(1):41–47.
17. Arcangeli G, Saracino B, Gomellini S, et al. A prospective phase III randomized trial of hypofractionation versus conventional fractionation in patients with high-risk prostate cancer. *Int J Radiat Oncol Biol Phys*. 2010;78(1):11–18.
18. Arcangeli G, Fowler J, Gomellini S, et al. Acute and late toxicity in a randomized trial of conventional versus hypofractionated three-dimensional conformal radiotherapy for prostate cancer. *Int J Radiat Oncol Biol Phys*. 2011;79(4):1013–1021.
19. Arcangeli S, Strigari L, Gomellini S, et al. Updated results and patterns of failure in a randomized hypofractionation trial for high-risk prostate cancer. *Int J Radiat Oncol Biol Phys*. 2012;84(5):1172–1178.
20. Pollack A, Hanlon AL, Horwitz EM, et al. Dosimetry and preliminary acute toxicity in the first 100 men treated for prostate cancer on a randomized hypofractionation dose escalation trial. *Int J Radiat Oncol Biol Phys*. 2006;64(2):518–526.
21. Pollack A, Walker G, Buyyounouski M, et al. Five year results of a randomized external beam radiotherapy hypofractionation trial for prostate cancer. *Int J Radiat Oncol Biol Phys*. 2011;81(2):S1.
22. Kuban DA, Nogueras-Gonzalez GM, Hamblin L, et al. Preliminary report of a randomized dose escalation trial for prostate cancer using hypofractionation. *Int J Radiat Oncol Biol Phys*. 2010;78(3):S58–S59.
23. Holmboe ES, Concato J. Treatment decisions for localized prostate cancer: asking men what's important. *J Gen Intern Med*. 2000;15(10):694–701.
24. Sethukavalan P, Cheung P, Tang CI, et al. Patient costs associated with external beam radiotherapy treatment for localized prostate cancer: the benefits of hypofractionated over conventionally fractionated radiotherapy. *Can J Urol*. 2012;19(2):6165–6169.
25. Parthan A, Pruttivarasin N, Taylor D, et al. CyberKnife for prostate cancer: is it cost-effective? ASCO: Genitourinary Cancers Symposium. *J Clin Oncol*. 2011;29(suppl 7):abstr 87.
26. Perez CA, Kobeissi B, Smith BD, et al. Cost accounting in radiation oncology: a computer-based model for reimbursement. *Int J Radiat Oncol Biol Phys*. 1993;25(5):895–906.
27. Lievens Y, van den Bogaert W, Kesteloot K. Activity-based costing: a practical model for cost calculation in radiotherapy. *Int J Radiat Oncol Biol Phys*. 2003;57(2):522–535.
28. Norlund A. Costs of radiotherapy. *Acta Oncol*. 2003;42(5-6):411–415.
29. Van de Werf E, Lievens Y, Verstraete J, et al. Time and motion study of radiotherapy delivery: economic burden of increased quality assurance and IMRT. *Radiother Oncol*. 2009;93(1):137–140.
30. Kesteloot K, Lievens Y, van der Schueren E. Improved management of radiotherapy departments through accurate cost data. *Radiother Oncol*. 2000;55(3):251–262.
31. Duncan W, Warde P, Catton CN, et al. Carcinoma of the prostate: results of radical radiotherapy (1970–1985). *Int J Radiat Oncol Biol Phys*. 1993;26(2):203–210.
32. Read G, Pointon RC. Retrospective study of radiotherapy in early carcinoma of the prostate. *Br J Urol*. 1989;63(2):191–195.
33. Kearsley JH. High-dose radiotherapy for localized prostatic cancer. An analysis of treatment results and early complications. *Med J Aust*. 1986;144(12):624–628.
34. Preston CI, Duncan W, Kerr GR. Radical treatment of prostatic carcinoma by mega voltage X-ray therapy. *Clin Radiol*. 1986;37(5):473–477.
35. Consensus statement: guidelines for PSA following radiation therapy. American Society for Therapeutic Radiology and Oncology Consensus Panel. *Int J Radiat Oncol Biol Phys*. 1997;37(5):1035–1041.
36. Abramowitz MC, Li T, Buyyounouski MK, et al. The Phoenix definition of biochemical failure predicts for overall survival in patients with prostate cancer. *Cancer*. 2008;112(1):55–60.
37. Buyyounouski MK, Hanlon AL, Eisenberg DF, et al. Defining biochemical failure after radiotherapy with and without androgen deprivation for prostate cancer. *Int J Radiat Oncol Biol Phys*. 2005;63(5):1455–1462.
38. Horwitz EM, Vicini FA, Ziaja EL, et al. The correlation between the ASTRO Consensus Panel definition of biochemical failure and clinical outcome for patients with prostate cancer treated with external beam irradiation. American Society of Therapeutic Radiology and Oncology. *Int J Radiat Oncol Biol Phys*. 1998;41(2):267–272.
39. Kupelian PA, Buchsbaum JC, Patel C, et al. Impact of biochemical failure on overall survival after radiation therapy for localized prostate cancer in the PSA era. *Int J Radiat Oncol Biol Phys*. 2002;52(3):704–711.
40. McBride SM, Wong DS, Dombrowski JJ, et al. Hypofractionated stereotactic body radiotherapy in low-risk prostate

adenocarcinoma: preliminary results of a multi-institutional phase 1 feasibility trial. *Cancer.* 2012;118(15):3681–3690.

41. Zaorsky NG, Li T, Devarajan K, et al. Assessment of the American Joint Committee on Cancer staging (sixth and seventh editions) for clinically localized prostate cancer treated with external beam radiotherapy and comparison with the National Comprehensive Cancer Network risk-stratification method. *Cancer.* 2012;118(22):5535–5543.
42. Pollack A, Cowen D, Troncoso P, et al. Molecular markers of outcome after radiotherapy in patients with prostate carcinoma. *Cancer.* 2003;97(7):1630–1638.
43. Bantis A, Giannopoulos A, Gonidi M, et al. Expression of p120, Ki-67 and PCNA as proliferation biomarkers in imprint smears of prostate carcinoma and their prognostic value. *Cytopathology.* 2004;15(1):25–31.
44. Zhou JR, Yu L, Zerbini LF, et al. Progression to androgen-independent LNCaP human prostate tumors: cellular and molecular alterations. *Int J Cancer.* 2004;110(6):800–806.
45. Khor LY, Moughan J, Al-Saleem T, et al. Bcl-2 and Bax expression predict prostate cancer outcome in men treated with androgen deprivation and radiotherapy on radiation therapy oncology group protocol 92-02. *Clin Cancer Res.* 2007;13(12):3585–3590.
46. Pollack A, Cowen D, Troncoso P, et al. Molecular markers of outcome after radiotherapy in patients with pro*state carcinoma: Ki-67, bcl-2, bax, and bcl-x. Cancer.* 2003;97(7):1630–1638.
47. Roach MIII, Waldman F, Pollack A. Predictive models in external beam radiotherapy for clinically localized prostate cancer. *Cancer.* 2009;115(13 suppl):3112–3120.
48. Potters L, Kavanagh B, Galvin JM, et al. American Society for Therapeutic Radiology and Oncology (ASTRO) and American College of Radiology (ACR) practice guideline for the performance of stereotactic body radiation therapy. *Int J Radiat Oncol Biol Phys.* 2010;76(2):326–332.
49. Denham JW, O'Brien PC, Dunstan RH, et al. Is there more than one late radiation proctitis syndrome? *Radiother Oncol.* 1999;51(1):43–53.
50. Kleinmann N, Zaorsky NG, Showalter TN, et al. The effect of ethnicity and sexual preference on prostate-cancer-related quality of life. *Nat Rev Urol.* 2012;9(5):258–265.
51. Grimm P, Billiet I, Bostwick D, et al. Comparative analysis of prostate-specific antigen free survival outcomes for patients with low, intermediate and high risk prostate cancer treatment by radical therapy. Results from the Prostate Cancer Results Study Group. *BJU Int.* 2012;109(suppl 1):22–29.
52. Zaorsky NG, Studenski MT, Dicker AP, et al. Stereotactic body radiation therapy for prostate cancer: is the technology ready to be the standard of care? *Cancer Treat Rev.* 2013;39(3):212–218.
53. Zietman A, Goitein M, Tepper JE. Technology evolution: is it survival of the fittest? *J Clin Oncol.* 2010;28(27):4275–4279.
54. Shen X, Zaorsky NG, Mishra MV, et al. Comparative effectiveness research for prostate cancer radiation therapy: current status and future directions. *Future Oncol.* 2012;8(1):37–54.
55. Button MR, Staffurth JN. Clinical application of image-guided radiotherapy in bladder and prostate cancer. *Clin Oncol (R Coll Radiol).* 2010;22(8):698–706.
56. Zwahlen DR, Lang S, Hrbacek J, et al. The use of photon beams of a flattening filter-free linear accelerator for hypofractionated volumetric modulated arc therapy in localized prostate cancer. *Int J Radiat Oncol Biol Phys.* 2012;83(5):1655–1660.
57. Klayton T, Price R, Buyyounouski MK, et al. Prostate bed motion during intensity-modulated radiotherapy treatment. *Int J Radiat Oncol Biol Phys.* 2012;84(1):130–136.
58. Zelefsky MJ, Kollmeier M, Cox B, et al. Improved clinical outcomes with high-dose image guided radiotherapy compared with non-IGRT for the treatment of clinically localized prostate cancer. *Int J Radiat Oncol Biol Phys.* 2012;84(1):125–129.
59. de Crevoisier R, Tucker SL, Dong L, et al. Increased risk of biochemical and local failure in patients with distended rectum on the planning CT for prostate cancer radiotherapy. *Int J Radiat Oncol Biol Phys.* 2005;62(4):965–973.
60. Heemsbergen WD, Hoogeman MS, Witte MG, et al. Increased risk of biochemical and clinical failure for prostate patients with a large rectum at radiotherapy planning: results from the Dutch trial of 68 GY versus 78 Gy. *Int J Radiat Oncol Biol Phys.* 2007;67(5):1418–1424.
61. Zaorsky NG, Ohri N, Showalter TN, et al. Systematic review of hypofractionated radiation therapy for prostate cancer. *Cancer Treat Rev.* 2013;39:728–736.

Stereotactic Body Radiation Therapy for Localized Prostate Cancer

10.1.3

NICHOLAS G. ZAORSKY

ROBERT B. DEN

■ OVERVIEW

This chapter discusses the use of stereotactic body radiation therapy (SBRT) for the treatment of localized prostate cancer. Since 2001, SBRT has been touted as a superior type of external beam radiation therapy (EBRT) for the treatment of various tumors. SBRT developed from the theory that high doses of radiation from high-dose rate brachytherapy (HDR-BT) implants could be recapitulated from radiation treatment planning and delivery systems. In addition, SBRT has been theorized to be advantageous compared with other radiation therapy (RT) techniques in terms of radiobiology, radiophysics, patient convenience, and resource allocation. In this chapter, we discuss the impetus behind SBRT and the clinical evidence supporting its use for prostate cancer. As of 2013, studies of SBRT provide encouraging results of biochemical control and late toxicity rates. However, they are limited by a number of factors; these include short follow-up, exclusion of intermediate- and high-risk patients, and relatively small number of patients treated.

■ BACKGROUND AND HISTORY OF INCREASING DOSE PER FRACTION

Given the widespread use of prostate-specific antigen testing, most prostate cancer patients present with localized disease (clinical stage T1–T2). Treatment options for localized disease include radical prostatectomy (RP) and RT. RT is delivered as either a BT or an EBRT. Currently, most men who receive EBRT are treated with conventionally fractionated radiation therapy (CFRT; a single 1.8–2.0 Gy fraction lasting 15 minutes per day, 5 days per week, for about 8 weeks) to a total dose of 76 to 80 Gy.

In the mid-1990s, the most commonly used method to deliver CFRT was a four-field technique. At that time, there was no consistent agreement on the optimal schedule or dose used for patient treatment (1). CFRT schedules were typically administered over 6 to 7 weeks with doses of 60 to 70 Gy (2). Dose-escalated CFRT (i.e., using the same dose per fraction, but up to ~80 Gy, for 8–9 weeks) was shown in multiple phase III randomized controlled trials to improve biochemical control rates and became the standard of care EBRT schedule (3–7).

In 2001, hypothesis-generating reports suggested that prostate cancer had a low α/β ratio of ~1.5 Gy (8), implying that those cells were more sensitive to doses delivered in larger fraction size. Given the lower α/β ratio for prostate cancer than bladder and rectal mucosa (where the most late toxicity occurs), reduced morbidity was expected from hypofractionated radiation therapy (HFRT; 2.1–3.5 Gy/fraction, 5 days per week, for about 4 weeks) (9).

Although there has been controversy in calculating the accurate α/β ratio for prostate cancer (10), prospective phase III superiority studies using HFRT (11–19) have been published based on the assumption that the α/β ratio for prostate cancer is 1.5 Gy. The results of these studies have been inconclusive (20). The older studies (11–13) reached opposite conclusions about HFRT compared with CFRT and differed greatly in their methodology from the modern studies. The more modern studies comparing HFRT with CFRT (14–18) have not shown a clear reduction in the incidence of late complications while maintaining biochemical control rates.

There has been interest in increasing fraction size even further than 3.5 Gy/fraction to provide for tumor control, decrease toxicity, and reduce overall treatment time. SBRT (a single 3.5–15.0 Gy fraction lasting 1 hour per day, 5 days per week, for about 2 weeks), also called extreme hypofractionation, was shown to recapitulate HDR-BT plans closely and deliver such doses noninvasively (21). Use of SBRT increased in the 2000s due to the advent of image-guided technologies that improved the accuracy of delivering high doses of radiation. Moreover, SBRT has been theorized to have advantages (1) from a radiobiological perspective; (2) in treatment delivery from a radiophysics perspective; (3) to the patient himself, compared with other treatment modalities; and (4) for resource allocation (22).

■ POTENTIAL BENEFITS OF SBRT

Radiobiology

CFRT has several theoretical advantages of killing prostate cancer cells though the "3 Rs" of RT: (1) reoxygenation, that is, allowing more cells to become oxic, which makes RT more effective; (2) redistribution, that is, allowing for tumor cells to cycle into more radiosensitive phases of the cell cycle; and (3) repair, that is, allowing normal cells to repair sublethal damage.

There is also a possibility of increasing tumor cell death and a minimizing radiation-related toxicity with higher doses per fraction. In general, as the total dose delivered increases, the number of surviving cells decreases. However, the advantages of increasing dose are countered by the toxicity to surrounding normal tissues. An α/β ratio is used to estimate the effects of radiation on tissues and compare various dose and fractionation schemes.

The α/β ratio is generally believed to be >10 Gy for early-responding tissue (e.g., skin, mucosa, and most tumors); and it is believed to be 3 to 5 Gy for late-responding tissue (e.g., connective tissues, muscles), where genitourinary (GU) and gastrointestinal (GI) toxicity occurs. The α/β ratio is used in the calculation of the biologically equivalent dose (BED):

$$\text{BED} = (nd[1 + d/(\alpha/\beta)]),$$

where n is the number of radiation fractions and d is the fraction size.

Dose-escalated CFRT (a single 1.8–2.0 Gy fraction lasting 15 minutes per day, 5 days per week, up to ~80 Gy, for about 8 weeks) has been shown in multiple phase III randomized controlled trials to improve biochemical control over nondose-escalated fractionation schedules, which deliver the same Gy per fraction, but typically to a total dose of ~66 Gy (3–7). Using these two sample schedules, dose-escalated CFRT and nondose-escalated CFRT have BEDs (at an α/β ratio of 1.5 Gy) of 182 versus 154 Gy, respectively and (at an α/β ratio of 3.0 Gy) of 130 versus 110 Gy, respectively.

In 2001, hypothesis-generating reports suggested that prostate cancer cells had a low α/β ratio of ~1.5 Gy, implying that the cells were more sensitive to large fraction doses (8). In addition, calculation models with an α/β ratio of 1.5 Gy showed that a prolonged course of RT (i.e., from CFRT) would be disadvantageous because (1) dose escalation is necessary to offset accelerated cancer cell repopulation (23); and (2) given the lower α/β ratio for prostate cancer than late-responding tissues, there would be potential for therapeutic gain and minimized toxicity to surrounding tissues with larger fraction sizes (9, 24).

Thus, investigators have tried to maintain a high BED (at an α/β ratio of 1.5) to kill prostate cancer cells while minimizing the BED (at α/β ratios of 3–10) for toxicities. The BED curves for α/β ratios of 1.5 to 10 Gy for EBRT and sample SBRT schedules from articles included in this chapter are juxtaposed in Figure 10.1.3.1.

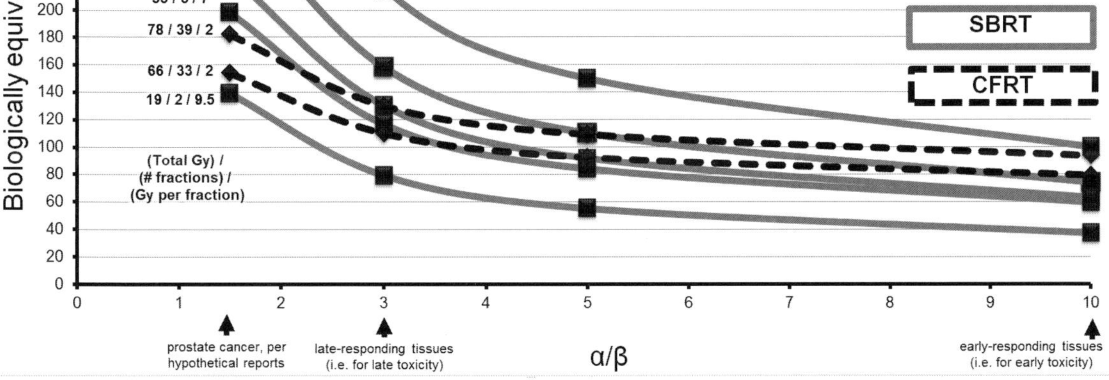

FIGURE 10.1.3.1 Biologically equivalent dose (BED) versus α/β ratios for stereotactic body radiation therapy (SBRT) compared with conventionally fractionated radiation therapy (CFRT). A plot of BED curves for SBRT studies included in this chapter (gray lines); compared to CFRT to a total dose of 66 to 78 Gy in 2.0 Gy/fraction, for 33 to 39 fractions (dashed black lines).

Radiophysics

Since SBRT uses only one to five fractions to deliver the dose, there is little chance for adjustment once treatment has been initiated. Considerable time is spent by radiation oncologists and medical physicists ensure accuracy and precision in dose delivery on the treatment plan (25). Treatment planning is aided by advanced technologies that help to maximize dose to the tumor (minimizing dose to surrounding tissues), detect target movement, and compensate for movement. Two treatment delivering technologies used with SBRT help to achieve these goals: intensity-modulated radiation therapy (IMRT) and image-guided radiation therapy (IGRT).

Currently, IMRT is the standard of care for prostate cancer because it maximizes the dose delivered to the tumor volume and minimizes the dose delivered to the surrounding organs. However, the sharp dose gradients that exist with IMRT plans could result in the volumetric error of missing the tumor because of the movement of the patient on the treatment table and the IGRT is a component of IMRT to ensure accuracy and precision of each fraction.

IGRT detects and corrects random and systematic errors that occur during treatment delivery. Currently, multiple solutions exist for IGRT, including portal imaging using implanted fiducial markers (26), electromagnetic transponders (27), cone beam computed tomography (CT) (28), and CT-on-rails (29). IGRT has shown that the prostate moves daily, and these movements influence dosimetric coverage during RT. Prostate movements occur both interfractionally (i.e., between two RT sessions) (30,31) and intrafractionally (i.e., during one RT session) (32,33). The movements are also both translational (i.e., shifting of the isocenter) and rotational (i.e., around the isocenter). Although translations may be more easily detected and managed using image guidance, rotations are more difficult to detect and could cause significant underdosing (34). It is possible that a shortened treatment course with SBRT would lead to a reduction in intrafraction and interfraction motion compared to CFRT, thus decreasing toxicity, although this hypothesis has not yet been tested in clinical trials.

The two major types of delivery systems of SBRT are gantry-based linear accelerators and the robotic arm-based systems. The conformality of robotic arm-based systems has been shown to be superior to IMRT, although the dose fall-off appears similar in both plans (35), and neither has been proven to be more efficacious than the other. The studies included in this chapter use both gantry-based and robotic arm-based systems.

Patient Perspective

Treatment options for low-risk, localized prostate cancer include CFRT, HFRT, RP, and BT. SBRT has unique advantages for the patient when compared with these options. The 8 weeks of therapy of CFRT is inconvenient to those who live far from treatment centers or have difficulty with travel. This long treatment course is the most frequently patient-cited disadvantage of CFRT (36). Moreover, CFRT has commonly associated early rectal toxicity, and sometimes late rectal, urinary, and sexual toxicities (37). Currently, HFRT is only available in the setting of clinical trials (20). Finally, although studies of both RP (38–44) and BT (41,45–60) (both of which last for a few hours in 1 day) have shown improved biochemical outcomes, these modalities have limitations. RP commonly causes impotence and incontinence, and BT commonly causes irritative and obstructive urinary symptoms (37).

Thus, the shorter treatment course (i.e., 2 weeks) and noninvasive nature of SBRT make it an attractive treatment option to patients with localized prostate cancer. Moreover, in certain regions of the world where RT centers may be difficult to access or are few in number, SBRT could become the standard of care.

Resource Allocation

SBRT has potential to improve resource allocation. Calculation models show that wage costs outweigh the cost of machines in RT; planning and delivery are labor intensive (61–64). Moreover, although treatment planning complexity is increasing with evolving technology, the planning is only done at the beginning of therapy. Cost, however, builds with the delivery of each fraction (65). Staffing RT facilities is estimated to account for 50% of their cost (66). Thus, changing from CFRT to an SBRT schedule may decrease the number of work hours and overall cost of treating each patient.

■ OUTCOMES

Results of efficacy from recent studies with SBRT are listed in Table 10.1.3.1 (67–81). The longest follow-up times currently available are at 5 years. Freedom from biochemical failure (FFBF) rates for low-, intermediate-, and high-risk patients have generally been ≥90% at up to 5 years. Outcomes from both gantry and robotic arm-based systems have been similar: 2-year FFBF rates have been 90% to 100% versus 94% to 100%, respectively.

There are a number of differences among SBRT, RP, and BT studies. Figure 10.1.3.2 shows the FFBF versus time of SBRT studies with the FFBF rates of low-risk patients in published studies of RP (38–44) and BT (41,45–60) studies co-plotted. The mean median follow-up times of SBRT, RP, and BT studies are co-plotted on the inset in Figure 10.1.3.2. First, the follow-up times of SBRT studies

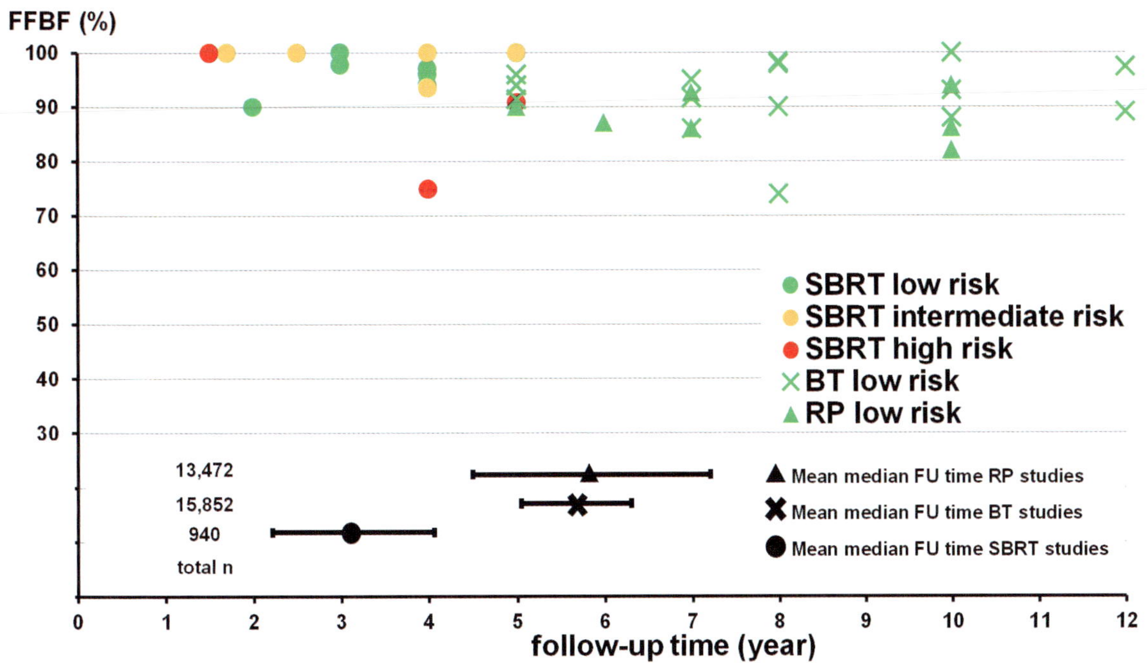

FIGURE 10.1.3.2 Freedom from biochemical failure (FFBF) versus year plot of prostate cancer patients treated with stereotactic body radiation therapy (SBRT), compared with those treated with brachytherapy (BT) and radical prostatectomy (RP). The *y*-axis shows the FFBF rate, and the *x*-axis shows time in years. Among the men treated with SBRT (circles), FFBF rates for low-, intermediate-, and high-risk patients have generally been ≥90% at up to 5 years (67–81). FFBF rates of low-risk patients from trials with BT(Xs) (41, 45–50) and RP (triangles) (38–44) are co-plotted for comparison. The mean median follow-up times (with their respective standard deviations) of SBRT, RP, and BT studies are co-plotted on the inset.

(mean 3.1 years) are significantly shorter than those of studies of RP (5.8 years) or BT (5.6 years). Second, there have been many more patients treated with RP and BT than SBRT (>20,000 vs. <1,000). Third, most of the patients treated in the reported SBRT trials have low-risk disease. It will be necessary to enroll intermediate- and high-risk patients to see whether they have comparable outcomes. Thus, although the biochemical results of SBRT studies appear promising, a number of issues must be addressed before SBRT becomes the standard of care.

TOXICITY

The late GI and GU Radiation Therapy Oncology Group (RTOG) toxicities are summarized in Table 10.1.3.1 and Figure 10.1.3.3. Among the studies analyzed, 57% (95% confidence interval [CI] 43%–71%) of patients had RTOG grade 0 GU toxicity and 63% (95% CI 46%–79%) of patients had RTOG grade 0 GI toxicity. Further, 15% (95% CI 10%–20%) had grade 1 GU toxicity and 9% (95% CI 4%–15%) had grade 2 GU toxicity. Less than 4% of patients had grade 3 to 4 GI or GU toxicity.

In comparison, phase III studies of CFRT have shown RTOG late GU toxicity grade ≥2 in 8% to 40% of patients and GI toxicity grade ≥2 in 9% to 26% of patients (3–7). Phase III studies using HFRT have shown RTOG late GU and GI toxicity grade ≥2 in 1% to 19% and 2% to 14% of patients, respectively (11–19). The results of SBRT studies are very encouraging and highlight the potential of SBRT in the management of certain patients with prostate cancer.

There are a number of important caveats to consider when interpreting the SBRT toxicities. Late effects from radiation can technically occur decades after therapy (25). Moreover, the RTOG toxicity score does not include the evaluation of anorectal symptoms such as urgency of defecation and fecal incontinence (82). When compared with studies that measure quality of life for RP, BT, and CFRT (37, 83), studies with SBRT do not yet integrate more detailed quality-of-life measures. Thus, further patient-reported quality-of-life metrics should be incorporated (e.g., the short-form-36 and expanded prostate cancer index composite). Erectile preservation is defined differently on questionnaires in studies. These questionnaires are often not tailored to homosexual and minority communities, although these are large subpopulations of the prostate cancer patient demographics (84).

Phase III studies of CFRT included low-, intermediate-, and high-risk groups. Subsequently, areas outside of the prostate, including the seminal vesicles, were frequently included in RT planning, and these are not included in SBRT plans of low-risk patients. The CFRT studies did not use advanced forms of IMRT and IGRT available

Table 10.1.3.1 Prospective studies of SBRT for prostate cancer

Reference	Phase	*n*	Risk Groups	RT System	Median Actuarial FU (mo)	Total Dose (Gy)	Total Fractions	Gy/ Fraction	BED (Gy), at α/β = 1.5	BED (Gy), at α/β = 3	FFBF[a]	RTOG Late Toxicity Grade ≥2 (%) GU	RTOG Late Toxicity Grade ≥2 (%) GI
Friedland et al. (67)	N/A	112	L, I, H	RA	48	35	5	7.0	170	89	3 y: 97%	NR	NR
McBride et al. (68)	I	10	L	RA	45	37.5	5	7.5	195	101	3 y: 98%	19.2	12
		34				36.3	5	7.3	182	95			
		1				—							
Fuller et al. (69)	N/A	51	L, I	RA	42	38	4	9.5	250	130	4 y: 98%	24	2
SHARP: Madsen et al. (70)	I/II	40	L	G	41	33.5	5	6.7	156	82	2 y: 90%	20	37.5
Katz et al. (71,72)	I/II	50	L, I, H	RA	40	35	5	7.0	170	89	4 y: 98.5%, 93%, 75%	7.8	4.2
		254				36.3	5	7.3	182	95			
Kang et al. (73)	N/A	5	L, I, H	RA	40	32	4	8.0	179	93	5 y: 100%, 100%, 90.8%	6.8	11
		28				34	4	8.5	201	105			
		11				36	4	9.0	225	117			
Mantz et al. (74)	II	65	L	G	36	40	5	8.0	221	115	3 y: 100%	NR	NR
King et al. (75)	II	16	L	RA	32	36.3	5	7.3	182	95	4 y: 94%	8.7	2
		41		RA		36.3	5	7.3	182	95			
Boike et al. (76)	I	15	L, I	G	30	45	5	9.0	279	144	2.5 y: 100%	31	18
		15				47.5	5	9.5	310	160			
		15				50	5	10.0	343	177			
Bolzicco et al. (77)	N/A	45	L, I	RA	20	35	5	7.0	170	89	20 mo: 100%	2.2	2.2
pHART3: Tang et al. (78) and Quon et al. (79)	I/II	84	L	G	18	35	5	7.0	170	89	18 mo: 100%	13	13
Jabbari et al. (80)	N/A	20	L, I, H	G	18	38	4	9.5	250	130	18 mo: 100%	13	3
		18		G		19	2	9.5	130	70			
Aluwini et al. (81)	I/II	10	L, I	RA	5	38	4	9.5	250	130	NR	37	0

Note: Studies ordered by median actuarial FU time.

[a]Listed as overall FFBF; or for low-, intermediate-, and high-risk groups.

Abbreviations: BED, biological equivalent dose; FFBF, freedom from biochemical failure; FU, follow up; G, Gantry; GI, gastrointestinal; GU, genitourinary; H, high; I, intermediate; L, low; N/A, not applicable NR, not reported; RA, robotic arm; RTOG, Radiation Therapy Oncology Group.

Source: Adapted from Ref. (22). Zaorsky NG, Studenski MT, Dicker AP, et al. Stereotactic body radiation therapy for prostate cancer: is the technology ready to be the standard of care? *Cancer Treat Rev.* 2013;39(3):212–218.

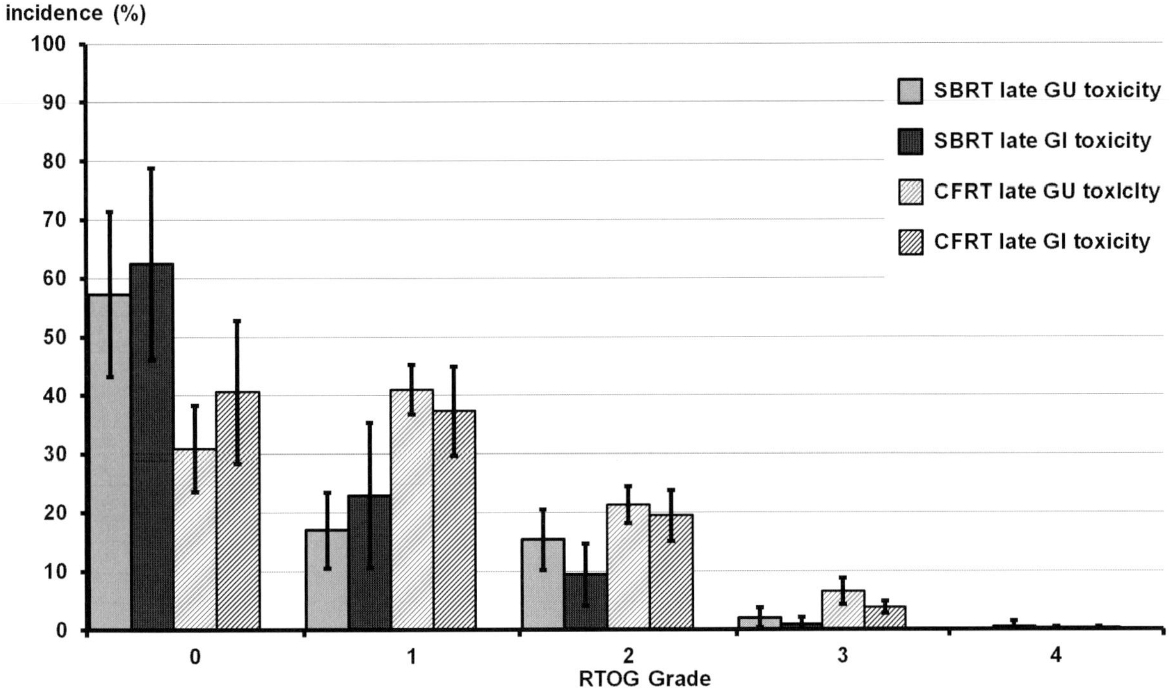

FIGURE 10.1.3.3 Radiation therapy oncology group (RTOG) late grade genitourinary (GU) and gastrointestinal (GI) toxicity from studies of stereotactic body radiation therapy (SBRT) compared with those of conventionally fractionated radiation therapy for prostate cancer. The *y*-axis shows the incidence of toxicity (as a %), and the *x*-axis shows GU (light shade) and GI (dark shade) RTOG late toxicity. Black bars indicate 95% confidence intervals. The toxicity rates of SBRT studies included in the review (67–81) are benchmarked to those of dose escalation studies (3–7), which provide the current standard of care fractionation schedule.

Source: Adapted from Ref. (22). Zaorsky NG, Studenski MT, Dicker AP, et al. Stereotactic body radiation therapy for prostate cancer: is the technology ready to be the standard of care? *Cancer Treat Rev.* 2013;39(3):212–218.

today. Finally, the SBRT studies were all single-institution experiences, and the toxicities might not be representative if conducted in a larger setting with a more diversified patient population. As of 2013, it is currently inappropriate to conclude that toxicities from SBRT studies are noninferior to those of CFRT. Given the number of treatment options available for men with localized prostate cancer, comparative effectiveness research will help to personalize RT for individual prostate cancer patients (85).

■ CONCLUSION

Dose-escalated CFRT is an established treatment modality for almost all prostate cancer patients. Determining the optimal EBRT fractionation scheme has been one of the goals of radiation oncologists. Hypofractionation and extreme hypofractionation (i.e., with SBRT) are two relatively novel types of EBRT fractionation. SBRT is hypothesized to improve tumor control, decrease toxicity, improve patient quality of life, and reduce resource consumption. Phase I/II studies of SBRT have had some encouraging results in terms of biochemical control and treatment toxicity. However, as of 2013, a number of limitations are still present among all of the trials that preclude recommending SBRT monotherapy for prostate cancer outside the setting of a clinical trial.

■ REFERENCES

1. Hanks GE. External-beam radiation therapy for clinically localized prostate cancer: patterns of care studies in the United States. *NCI Monogr.* 1988;(7):75–84.
2. Zagars GK, von Eschenbach AC, Johnson DE, Oswald MJ. The role of radiation therapy in stages A2 and B adenocarcinoma of the prostate. *Int J Radiat Oncol Biol Phys.* 1988;14(4):701–709.
3. Kuban DA, Tucker SL, Dong L, et al. Long-term results of the M. D. Anderson randomized dose-escalation trial for prostate cancer. *Int J Radiat Oncol Biol Phys.* 2008;70(1):67–74.
4. Al-Mamgani A, van Putten WL, Heemsbergen WD, et al. Update of Dutch multicenter dose-escalation trial of radiotherapy for localized prostate cancer. *Int J Radiat Oncol Biol Phys.* 2008;72(4):980–988.
5. Zietman AL, DeSilvio ML, Slater JD, et al. Comparison of conventional-dose vs high-dose conformal radiation therapy in clinically localized adenocarcinoma of the prostate: a randomized controlled trial. *JAMA.* 2005;294(10):1233–1239.
6. Zietman AL, Bae K, Slater JD, et al. Randomized trial comparing conventional-dose with high-dose conformal radiation therpay in early-stage adenocarcinoma of the prostate: long-term results from Proton Radiation Oncology Group/American College of Radiology 95-09. *J Clin Oncol.* 2010;28(7):1106–1111.
7. Dearnaley DP, Sydes MR, Graham JD, et al. Escalated-dose versus standard-dose conformal radiotherapy in prostate cancer: first results from the MRC RT01 randomised controlled trial. *Lancet Oncol.* 2007;8(6):475–487.
8. Fowler J, Chappell R, Ritter M. Is alpha/beta for prostate tumors really low? *Int J Radiat Oncol Biol Phys.* 2001;50(4):1021–1031.
9. Brenner DJ, Martinez AA, Edmundson GK, et al. Direct evidence that prostate tumors show high sensitivity to fractionation (low alpha/beta ratio), similar to late-responding normal tissue. *Int J Radiat Oncol Biol Phys.* 2002;52(1):6–13.

10. Miles EF, Lee WR. Hypofractionation for prostate cancer: a critical review. *Semin Radiat Oncol.* 2008;18(1):41–47.
11. Lukka H, Hayter C, Julian JA, et al. Randomized trial comparing two fractionation schedules for patients with localized prostate cancer. *J Clin Oncol.* 2005;23(25):6132–6138.
12. Yeoh EE, Botten RJ, Butters J, et al. Hypofractionated versus conventionally fractionated radiotherapy for prostate carcinoma: final results of phase III randomized trial. *Int J Radiat Oncol Biol Phys.* 2011;81(5):1271–1278.
13. Yeoh EE, Holloway RH, Fraser RJ, et al. Hypofractionated versus conventionally fractionated radiation therapy for prostate carcinoma: updated results of a phase III randomized trial. *Int J Radiat Oncol Biol Phys.* 2006;66(4):1072–1083.
14. Arcangeli G, Saracino B, Gomellini S, et al. A prospective phase III randomized trial of hypofractionation versus conventional fractionation in patients with high-risk prostate cancer. *Int J Radiat Oncol Biol Phys.* 2010;78(1):11–18.
15. Arcangeli G, Fowler J, Gomellini S, et al. Acute and late toxicity in a randomized trial of conventional versus hypofractionated three-dimensional conformal radiotherapy for prostate cancer. *Int J Radiat Oncol Biol Phys.* 2011;79(4):1013–1021.
16. Arcangeli S, Strigari L, Gomellini S, et al. Updated results and patterns of failure in a randomized hypofractionation trial for high-risk prostate cancer. *Int J Radiat Oncol Biol Phys.* 2012;84(5):1172–1178.
17. Pollack A, Hanlon AL, Horwitz EM, et al. Dosimetry and preliminary acute toxicity in the first 100 men treated for prostate cancer on a randomized hypofractionation dose escalation trial. *Int J Radiat Oncol Biol Phys.* 2006;64(2):518–526.
18. Pollack A, Walker G, Buyyounouski M, et al. Five year results of a randomized external beam radiotherapy hypofractionation trial for prostate cancer. *Int J Radiat Oncol Biol Phys.* 2011;81(2):S1.
19. Kuban DA, Nogueras-Gonzalez GM, Hamblin L, et al. Preliminary report of a randomized dose escalation trial for prostate cancer using hypofractionation. *Int J Radiat Oncol Biol Phys.* 2010;78(3):S58–S59.
20. Zaorsky NG, Ohri N, Showalter TN, et al. Systematic review of hypofractionated radiation therapy for prostate cancer. *Cancer Treat Rev.* 2013;39:728–736.
21. Fuller DB, Naitoh J, Lee C, et al. Virtual HDR CyberKnife treatment for localized prostatic carcinoma: dosimetry comparison with HDR brachytherapy and preliminary clinical observations. *Int J Radiat Oncol Biol Phys.* 2008;70(5):1588–1597.
22. Zaorsky NG, Studenski MT, Dicker AP, et al. Stereotactic body radiation therapy for prostate cancer: is the technology ready to be the standard of care? *Cancer Treat Rev.* 2013;39(3):212–218.
23. Wang JZ, Li XA. Impact of tumor repopulation on radiotherapy planning. *Int J Radiat Oncol Biol Phys.* 2005;61(1):220–227.
24. Fowler JF, Ritter MA, Chappell RJ, Brenner DJ. What hypofractionated protocols should be tested for prostate cancer? *Int J Radiat Oncol Biol Phys.* 2003;56(4):1093–1104.
25. Potters L, Kavanagh B, Galvin JM, et al. American Society for Therapeutic Radiology and Oncology (ASTRO) and American College of Radiology (ACR) practice guideline for the performance of stereotactic body radiation therapy. *Int J Radiat Oncol Biol Phys.* 2010;76(2):326–332.
26. Munoz F, Fiandra C, Franco P, et al. Tracking target position variability using intraprostatic fiducial markers and electronic portal imaging in prostate cancer radiotherapy. *Radiol Med.* 2012;117:1057–1070.
27. Klayton T, Price R, Buyyounouski MK, et al. Prostate bed motion during intensity-modulated radiotherapy treatment. *Int J Radiat Oncol Biol Phys.* 2012;84(1):130–136.
28. Wierzbicki M, Schaly B, Peters T, Barnett R. Automatic image guidance for prostate IMRT using low dose CBCT. *Med Phys.* 2010;37(7):3677–3686.
29. Cavalieri R, Gay HA, Liu J, et al. Total error shift patterns for daily CT on rails image-guided radiotherapy to the prostate bed. *Radiat Oncol.* 2011;6:142.
30. Graf R, Boehmer D, Budach V, Wust P. Interfraction rotation of the prostate as evaluated by kilovoltage X-ray fiducial marker imaging in intensity-modulated radiotherapy of localized prostate cancer. *Med Dosim.* 2012;37:396–400.
31. Owen R, Kron T, Foroudi F, et al. Interfraction prostate rotation determined from in-room computerized tomography images. *Med Dosim.* 2011;36(2):188–194.
32. Li JS, Jin L, Pollack A, et al. Gains from real-time tracking of prostate motion during external beam radiation therapy. *Int J Radiat Oncol Biol Phys.* 2009;75(5):1613–1620.
33. Litzenberg DW, Balter JM, Hadley SW, et al. Prostate intrafraction translation margins for real-time monitoring and correction strategies. *Prostate Cancer.* 2012;2012:130579.
34. Amro H, Hamstra DA, McShan DL, et al. The dosimetric impact of prostate rotations during electromagnetically guided external-beam radiation therapy. *Int J Radiat Oncol Biol Phys.* 2013;85:230–236.
35. Hossain S, Xia P, Chuang C, et al. Simulated real time image guided intrafraction tracking-delivery for hypofractionated prostate IMRT. *Med Phys.* 2008;35(9):4041–4048.
36. Holmboe ES, Concato J. Treatment decisions for localized prostate cancer: asking men what's important. *J Gen Intern Med.* 2000;15(10):694–701.
37. Dandapani SV, Sanda MG. Measuring health-related quality of life consequences from primary treatment for early-stage prostate cancer. *Semin Radiat Oncol.* 2008;18(1):67–72.
38. Bhatta-Dhar N, Reuther AM, Zippe C, Klein EA. No difference in six-year biochemical failure rates with or without pelvic lymph node dissection during radical prostatectomy in low-risk patients with localized prostate cancer. *Urology.* 2004;63(3):528–531.
39. Boorjian SA, Karnes RJ, Rangel LJ, et al. Mayo Clinic validation of the D'amico risk group classification for predicting survival following radical prostatectomy. *J Urol.* 2008;179(4):1354–1360; discussion 1360-1351.
40. Kane CJ, Im R, Amling CL, et al. Outcomes after radical prostatectomy among men who are candidates for active surveillance: results from the SEARCH database. *Urology.* 2010;76(3):695–700.
41. Kupelian PA, Potters L, Khuntia D, et al. Radical prostatectomy, external beam radiotherapy <72 Gy, external beam radiotherapy > or =72 Gy, permanent seed implantation, or combined seeds/external beam radiotherapy for stage T1-T2 prostate cancer. *Int J Radiat Oncol Biol Phys.* 2004;58(1):25–33.
42. Nguyen PL, Chen MH, Catalona WJ, et al. Biochemical recurrence after radical prostatectomy for prevalent versus incident cases of prostate cancer : implications for management. *Cancer.* 2008;113(11):3146–3152.
43. Weight CJ, Reuther AM, Gunn PW, et al. Limited pelvic lymph node dissection does not improve biochemical relapse-free survival at 10 years after radical prostatectomy in patients with low-risk prostate cancer. *Urology.* 2008;71(1):141–145.
44. Menon M, Bhandari M, Gupta N, et al. Biochemical recurrence following robot-assisted radical prostatectomy: analysis of 1384 patients with a median 5-year follow-up. *Eur Urol.* 2010;58(6):838–846.
45. Bittner N, Merrick GS, Galbreath RW, et al. Primary causes of death after permanent prostate brachytherapy. *Int J Radiat Oncol Biol Phys.* 2008;72(2):433–440.
46. Burri RJ, Ho AY, Forsythe K, et al. Young men have equivalent biochemical outcomes compared with older men after treatment with brachytherapy for prostate cancer. *Int J Radiat Oncol Biol Phys.* 2010;77(5):1315–1321.
47. Critz FA, Levinson K. 10-year disease-free survival rates after simultaneous irradiation for prostate cancer with a focus on calculation methodology. *J Urol.* 2004;172(6 pt 1):2232–2238.
48. Hinnen KA, Battermann JJ, van Roermund JG, et al. Long-term biochemical and survival outcome of 921 patients treated with I-125 permanent prostate brachytherapy. *Int J Radiat Oncol Biol Phys.* 2010;76(5):1433–1438.

49. Jabbari S, Weinberg VK, Shinohara K, et al. Equivalent biochemical control and improved prostate-specific antigen nadir after permanent prostate seed implant brachytherapy versus high-dose three-dimensional conformal radiotherapy and high-dose conformal proton beam radiotherapy boost. *Int J Radiat Oncol Biol Phys*. 2010;76(1):36–42.
50. Martin AG, Roy J, Beaulieu L, et al. Permanent prostate implant using high activity seeds and inverse planning with fast simulated annealing algorithm: a 12-year Canadian experience. *Int J Radiat Oncol Biol Phys*. 2007;67(2):334–341.
51. Merrick GS, Butler WM, Wallner KE, et al. Prognostic significance of perineural invasion on biochemical progression-free survival after prostate brachytherapy. *Urology*. 2005;66(5):1048–1053.
52. Merrick GS, Butler WM, Wallner KE, et al. Androgen-deprivation therapy does not impact cause-specific or overall survival after permanent prostate brachytherapy. *Int J Radiat Oncol Biol Phys*. 2006;65(3):669–677.
53. Morris WJ, Keyes M, Palma D, et al. Population-based study of biochemical and survival outcomes after permanent 125I brachytherapy for low- and intermediate-risk prostate cancer. *Urology*. 2009;73(4):860-865; discussion 865–867.
54. Moyad MA, Merrick GS, Butler WM, et al. Statins, especially atorvastatin, may favorably influence clinical presentation and biochemical progression-free survival after brachytherapy for clinically localized prostate cancer. *Urology*. 2005;66(6):1150–1154.
55. Pickles T, Keyes M, Morris WJ. Brachytherapy or conformal external radiotherapy for prostate cancer: a single-institution matched-pair analysis. *Int J Radiat Oncol Biol Phys*. 2010;76(1):43–49.
56. Potters L, Morgenstern C, Calugaru E, et al. 12-year outcomes following permanent prostate brachytherapy in patients with clinically localized prostate cancer. *J Urol*. 2008;179(5 suppl):S20–S24.
57. Stone NN, Stock RG, Cesaretti JA, Unger P. Local control following permanent prostate brachytherapy: effect of high biologically effective dose on biopsy results and oncologic outcomes. *Int J Radiat Oncol Biol Phys*. 2010;76(2):355-360.
58. Taira AV, Merrick GS, Galbreath RW, et al. Natural history of clinically staged low- and intermediate-risk prostate cancer treated with monotherapeutic permanent interstitial brachytherapy. *Int J Radiat Oncol Biol Phys*. 2010;76(2):349–354.
59. Zelefsky MJ, Kuban DA, Levy LB, et al. Multi-institutional analysis of long-term outcome for stages T1-T2 prostate cancer treated with permanent seed implantation. *Int J Radiat Oncol Biol Phys*. 2007;67(2):327–333.
60. Zelefsky MJ, Yamada Y, Cohen GN, et al. Five-year outcome of intraoperative conformal permanent I-125 interstitial implantation for patients with clinically localized prostate cancer. *Int J Radiat Oncol Biol Phys*. 2007;67(1):65–70.
61. Parthan A, Pruttivarasin N, Taylor D, et al. CyberKnife for prostate cancer: is it cost-effective? ASCO: Genitourinary Cancers Symposium. *J Clin Oncol*. 2011;29(suppl 7):abstr 87.
62. Perez CA, Kobeissi B, Smith BD, et al. Cost accounting in radiation oncology: a computer-based model for reimbursement. *Int J Radiat Oncol Biol Phys*. 1993;25(5):895–906.
63. Lievens Y, van den Bogaert W, Kesteloot K. Activity-based costing: a practical model for cost calculation in radiotherapy. *Int J Radiat Oncol Biol Phys*. 2003;57(2):522–535.
64. Norlund A. Costs of radiotherapy. *Acta Oncol*. 2003;42(5-6):411–415.
65. Van de Werf E, Lievens Y, Verstraete J, et al. Time and motion study of radiotherapy delivery: economic burden of increased quality assurance and IMRT. *Radiother Oncol*. 2009;93(1):137–140.
66. Kesteloot K, Lievens Y, van der Schueren E. Improved management of radiotherapy departments through accurate cost data. *Radiother Oncol*. 2000;55(3):251–262.
67. Friedland JL, Freeman DE, Masterson-McGary ME, Spellberg DM. Stereotactic body radiotherapy: an emerging treatment approach for localized prostate cancer. *Technol Cancer Res Treat*. 2009;8(5):387–392.
68. McBride SM, Wong DS, Dombrowski JJ, et al. Hypofractionated stereotactic body radiotherapy in low-risk prostate adenocarcinoma: preliminary results of a multi-institutional phase 1 feasibility trial. *Cancer*. 2012;118(15):3681–3690.
69. Fuller DB, Shirazi R, Naitoh J, Mardirossian G. Virtual HDR SBRT for localized prostate carcinoma: efficacy and quality-of-life assessment. *J Clin Oncol*. 2012;30(suppl 5):abstr 45.
70. Madsen BL, Hsi RA, Pham HT, et al. Stereotactic hypofractionated accurate radiotherapy of the prostate (SHARP), 33.5 Gy in five fractions for localized disease: first clinical trial results. *Int J Radiat Oncol Biol Phys*. 2007;67(4):1099–1105.
71. Katz AJ, Santoro M, Ashley R, et al. Stereotactic body radiotherapy as boost for organ-confined prostate cancer. *Technol Cancer ResTreat*. 2010;9(6):575–582.
72. Katz AJ, Santoro M, DiBlasio F, Ashley R. Stereotactic body radiation therapy for low-, intermediate- and high-risk prostate cancer: disease control and quality of life. *Int J Radiat Oncol Biol Phys*. 2011;81:S100.
73. Kang JK, Cho CK, Choi CW, et al. Image-guided stereotactic body radiation therapy for localized prostate cancer. *Tumori*. 2011;97(1):43–48.
74. Mantz CA, Fernandez E, Zucker I, Harrison S. A phase IItrial of real-time target tracking sbrt for low-risk prostate cancer utilizing the calypso 4D localization system: patient-reported quality of life and toxicity outcomes. *Int J Radiat Oncol Biol Phys*. 2011;81(2):S100.
75. King CR, Brooks JD, Gill H, Presti JC Jr. Long-term outcomes from a prospective trial of stereotactic body radiotherapy for low-risk prostate cancer. *Int J Radiat Oncol Biol Phys*. 2012;82(2):877–882.
76. Boike TP, Lotan Y, Cho LC, et al. Phase I dose-escalation study of stereotactic body radiation therapy for low- and intermediate-risk prostate cancer. *J Clin Oncol*. 2011;29(15):2020-2026.
77. Bolzicco G, Favretto MS, Scremin E, et al. Image-guided stereotactic body radiation therapy for clinically localized prostate cancer: preliminary clinical results. *Technol Cancer Res Treat*. 2010;9(5):473–477.
78. Tang CI, Loblaw DA, Cheung P, et al. Phase I/II study of a five-fraction hypofractionated accelerated radiotherapy treatment for low-risk localised prostate cancer: early results of pHART3. *Clin Oncol (R Coll Radiol)*. 2008;20(10):729–737.
79. Quon H, Cheung P, Cesta A, et al. Phase II study of a five-fraction hypofractionated accelerated radiotherapy treatment for low-risk localized prostate cancer: toxicity results of pHART3. Paper presented at: ASCO 2010 Genitourinary Cancers Symposium; 2010; San Francisco, CA.
80. Jabbari S, Weinberg VK, Kaprealian T, et al. Stereotactic body radiotherapy as monotherapy or post-external beam radiotherapy boost for prostate cancer: technique, early toxicity, and PSA response. *Int J Radiat Oncol Biol Phys*. 2012;82(1):228–234.
81. Aluwini S, van Rooij P, Hoogeman M, et al. CyberKnife stereotactic radiotherapy as monotherapy for low- to intermediate-stage prostate cancer: early experience, feasibility, and tolerance. *J Endourol*. 2010;24(5):865–869.
82. Denham JW, O'Brien PC, Dunstan RH, et al. Is there more than one late radiation proctitis syndrome? *Radiother Oncol*. 1999;51(1):43–53.
83. Sanda MG, Dunn RL, Michalski J, et al. Quality of life and satisfaction with outcome among prostate-cancer survivors. *N Engl J Med*. 2008;358(12):1250–1261.
84. Kleinmann N, Zaorsky NG, Showalter TN, et al. The effect of ethnicity and sexual preference on prostate-cancer-related quality of life. *Nat Rev Urol*. 2012;9(5):258–265.
85. Shen X, Zaorsky NG, Mishra MV, et al. Comparative effectiveness research for prostate cancer radiation therapy: current status and future directions. *Future Oncol*. 2012;8(1):37–54.

Treatment of Low-Risk, Localized Prostate Cancer: Use of Proton Therapy

10.1.4

PHILLIP J. GRAY
AYAL A. AIZER
JASON A. EFSTATHIOU

INTRODUCTION

Although developed more than a half century ago, the use of proton therapy (PT) for the treatment of localized prostate cancer has only recently emerged as a topic of great interest among patients, care providers, and policy makers. Much of this attention has surrounded the increased cost of PT relative to other treatment options in an era of economic austerity and increasing desire for the delivery of cost-conscious care. Despite this, PT has shown itself to be a promising emerging technology with many, at least hypothetical, advantages over other available therapies. This chapter will briefly review the promise of and controversies surrounding the use of PT in the treatment of prostate cancer and the potential role for improved multidisciplinary care in defining its appropriate use.

BASICS OF PROTON THERAPY

Given the length limitations of this chapter, an in-depth review of all of the unique attributes and areas of controversy surrounding PT is impossible, and for more information, the reader is directed to several recent reviews on the topic (1–4). Unlike radiation techniques reliant on high-energy x-rays (photons), PT, as its name suggests, involves the therapeutic delivery of positively charged particles accelerated to relativistic speeds. The unique physical properties of protons allows them to deliver the majority of their tumor-killing energy at an end-of-range maximum known as the Bragg peak, while, unlike x-rays, having little or no penetration beyond the target of interest. This property allows for high doses of radiation to be delivered with high precision while using a minimal number of beams in areas of anatomic complexity such as the pelvis.

Other techniques have also been developed in recent years to overcome the drawbacks of beam penetration and radiation exit dose when photons are used. Chief among these is intensity-modulated radiation therapy (IMRT), which relies on five to nine angled beams to increase dose conformality and "spread out" the spillover effects of exit dose and radiation scatter. Compared with PT, this approach can provide similar radiation dose distributions in regions near the prostate but greatly increases the amount of normal tissue receiving low-to-moderate doses of radiation (5–7) (Figure 10.1.4.1). Furthermore, the use of IMRT greatly increases integral radiation dose to the entire body, theoretically putting the patient at risk for complications such as radiation-induced cancers (8, 9). The relative benefit for PT remains highly theoretical, however, and intense debate continues regarding the relative contributions of these effects on clinical outcomes.

COMPARATIVE EFFECTIVENESS OF PROTON THERAPY

Although strong data exist supporting the safety and efficacy of PT in the treatment of prostate cancer, there is as of yet no level 1 evidence to demonstrate that this approach improves patient outcomes compared to other modern techniques such as IMRT (10). In the absence of randomized data, several recent studies have attempted to quantitate the relative clinical toxicity of PT. Two recent studies that relied on data mined from the linked Surveillance Epidemiology and End Results–Medicare databases identified relatively higher rates of gastrointestinal toxicity in patients treated with PT compared with IMRT (11, 12). These findings, however, were greatly limited by data missing from these databases (such as radiation dose and target volume) and the high potential for misclassification bias inherent in defining toxicity according to billing claims. A third study utilizing a larger claims database identified similar rates of gastrointestinal complications between PT and IMRT with transiently lower rates of genitourinary complications in those receiving PT (13). This study also identified the somewhat higher

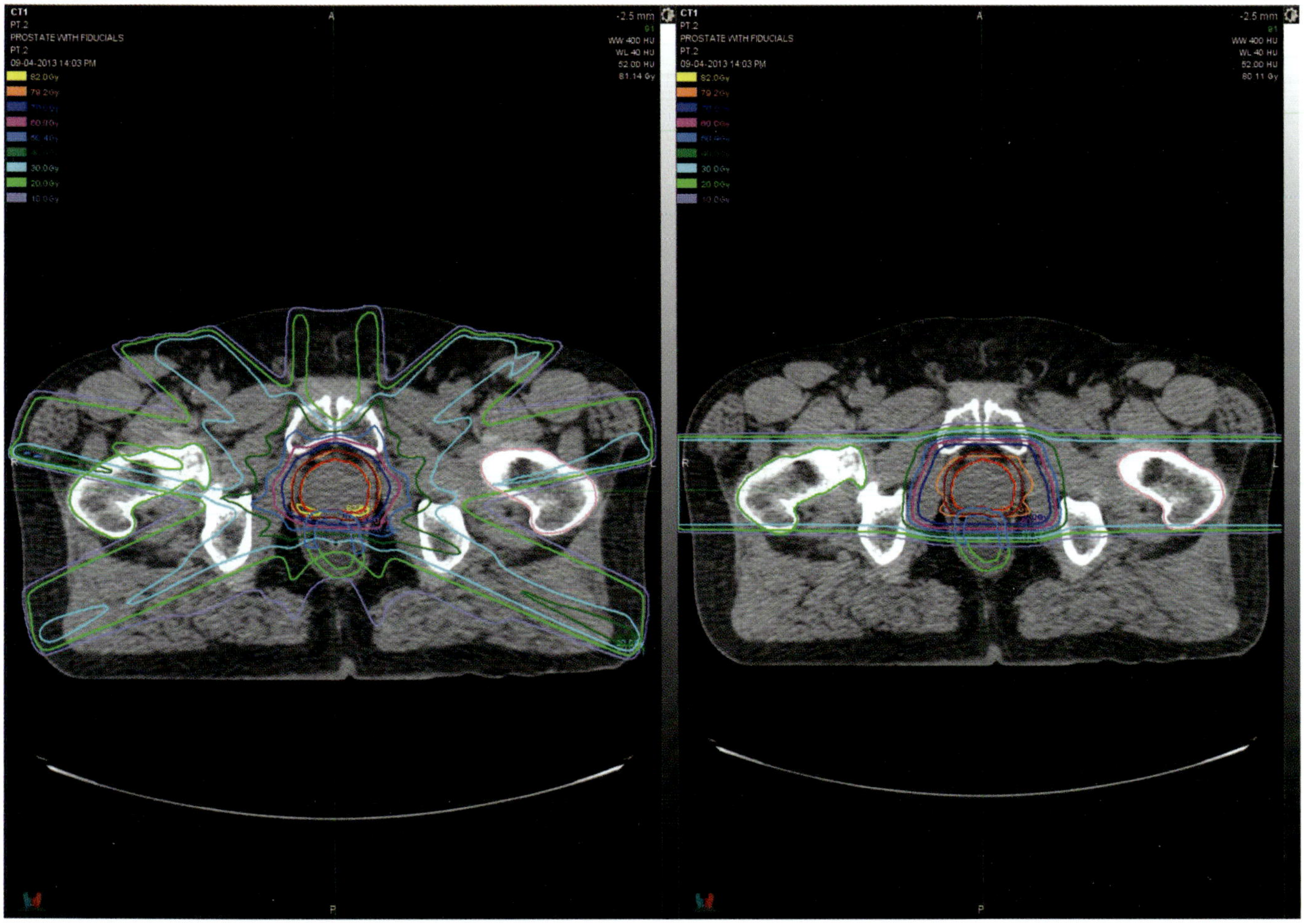

FIGURE 10.1.4.1 Comparison of dose distributions achieved using IMRT (left) and PT (right). Both radiation plans were prescribed to 79.2 Gy (RBE). Prostate is outlined in red, anterior rectum in blue, and posterior rectum in green.

cost of PT relative to IMRT with median Medicare reimbursements of $32,428 and $18,575, respectively.

Only one study to date has analyzed patient-reported outcomes in patients receiving PT and other radiation modalities (14). In this study, patients treated with PT reported minimal acute decrements in gastrointestinal or genitourinary quality of life, whereas those treated with IMRT reported modest but clinically relevant decrements in the first few months following therapy. By 2 years, however, similar quality-of-life decrements were reported by all patients. Given the disagreement and limitations of these and other retrospective studies, strong randomized evidence is needed to define the role of PT in the future of prostate cancer care. The Massachusetts General Hospital and University of Pennsylvania have recently partnered and opened a randomized trial of PT versus IMRT for low- and intermediate-risk prostate cancer patients (15). Other centers are expected to join this effort in the near future. Although cost considerations are ever-changing in an era of advancing technology, the results of this trial will be vital to place PT for prostate cancer in an appropriate context.

■ ROLE FOR MULTIDISCIPLINARY CARE

The management of patients with low-risk prostate cancer (Gleason score of ≤6, pretreatment PSA of <10 ng/mL, and clinical stage of T1c or T2a) is complicated by the relative paucity of data to suggest the superiority of one management modality versus another (16). It is not known whether definitive treatment improves prostate cancer–specific survival when compared to active surveillance, as randomized trials comparing observation to radical prostatectomy employed expectant management approaches consistent with watchful waiting, in which patients were not rigorously screened for progression and/or did not receive definitive therapy at the time of earliest progression (17–19). As an example, the recently published Prostate Cancer Intervention versus Observation Trial, which compared radical prostatectomy to watchful waiting in men with localized prostate cancer, showed that the 12-year prostate cancer–specific survival rate with both expectant management and radical prostatectomy were 97.7% (18). Therefore, the benefit of definitive therapy in patients with low-risk disease remains unknown, especially when compared with approaches such as active surveillance. In addition, no accepted, prospective trials from the United States or Europe have compared radical prostatectomy with radiation therapy—an older trial has been largely discredited due to significant limitations in design (20–22).

Given the multitude of management options available to men with low-risk prostate cancer, such patients often experience difficulty selecting a particular management option. Confounding the matter, physician bias, in which radiation oncologists and urologists recommend the therapeutic modality that they are capable of delivering, complicates the delivery of objective information to patients deciding among management options for prostate cancer (23, 24). As a result of the multitude of therapeutic modalities offered to prostate cancer patients, the lack of a clear "best" treatment option, and the presence of physician bias, multidisciplinary clinics offer an appealing approach to managing patients with prostate cancer. In such clinics, patients are provided the opportunity to meet with urologists, radiation oncologists, and medical oncologists concurrently during a single consultation. Such a model of care has the potential to minimize physician bias and lead to a consensus recommendation from the group (Figure 10.1.4.2).

Disadvantages of multidisciplinary clinics include the fact that fewer patients are likely be seen in a given morning or afternoon (relative to three practitioners seeing patients individually), and such clinics may be difficult to implement in the community setting, where specialists can be separated by great distances. Despite increasing popularity of multidisciplinary clinics, little data exist to support the notion that they provide a tangible benefit to patients or health care systems at large. Jefferson Medical

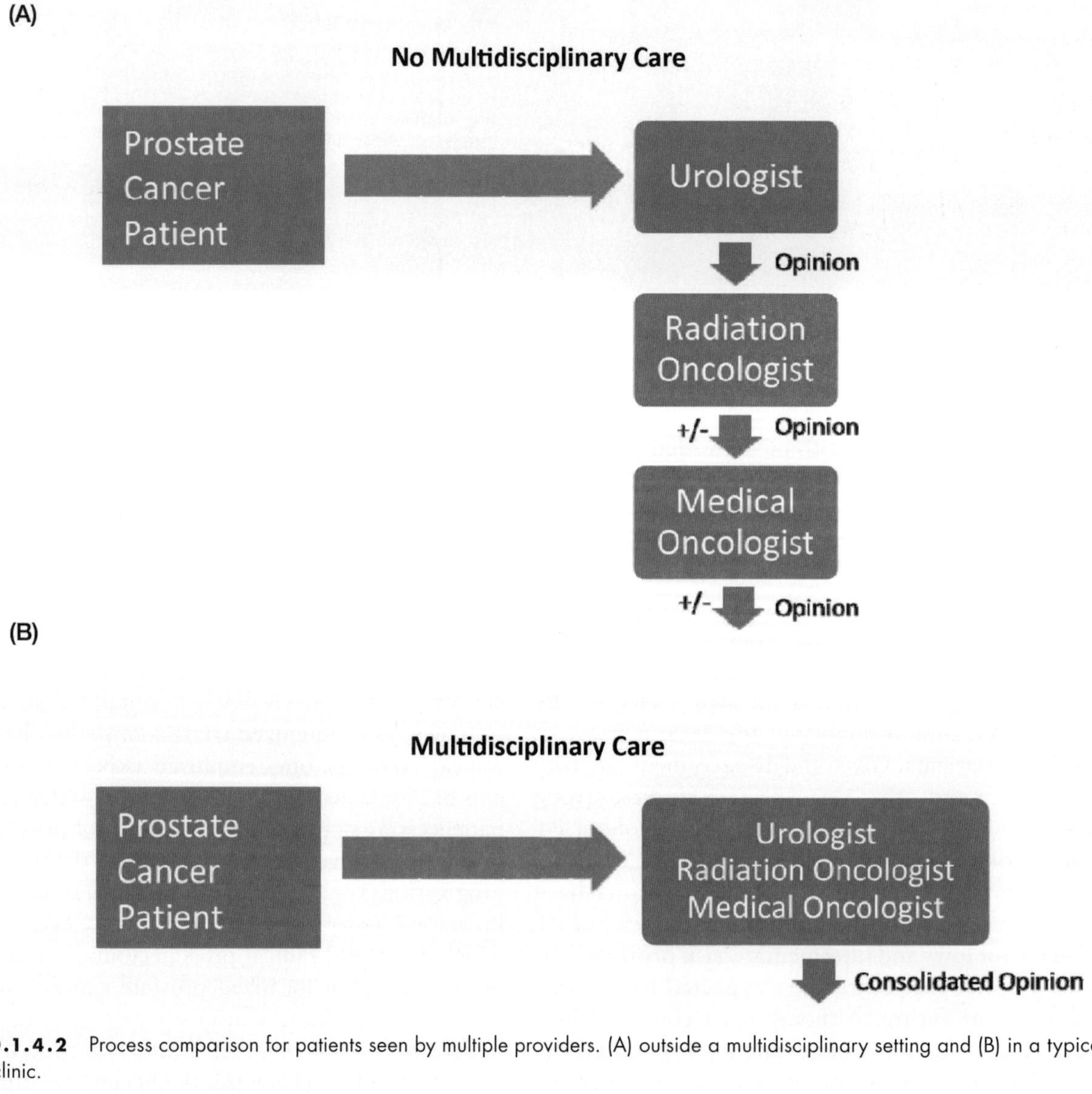

FIGURE 10.1.4.2 Process comparison for patients seen by multiple providers. (A) outside a multidisciplinary setting and (B) in a typical multidisciplinary clinic.

College at Thomas Jefferson University established one of the first multidisciplinary prostate cancer clinics in the United States. Patients have reviewed the clinic very favorably; >90% of patients rated their experience as "good" or "very good" within all measured domains and many patients chose to receive their treatment at this institution after a consultation at the multidisciplinary clinic (25,26). The Center for Prostate Disease Research/Walter Reed Army Medical Center has demonstrated that clinical research can be readily incorporated into the multidisciplinary setting (27). Our group has published on the impact of multidisciplinary models of care on management selection among patients with low-risk prostate cancer. In this study, 701 low-risk prostate cancer patients managed at Massachusetts General Hospital, Brigham and Women's Hospital, and Beth Israel Deaconess Medical Center in the year 2009 were identified (28). Patients were either seen at a multidisciplinary clinic (defined as a setting in which concurrent consultation with at least two of the following specialties were obtained: urology, radiation oncology, medical oncology) or, alternatively, by individual practitioners in sequential settings. It was found that multidisciplinary care doubled the rate of active surveillance as an initial management strategy. Rates of selection of prostatectomy, external beam radiation therapy, and brachytherapy all decreased. After adjustment for pertinent demographic-, clinical-, and provider-related variables, the effect of multidisciplinary care on active surveillance remained significant (odds ratio 2.15, 95% confidence interval 1.13–4.10; $P = .02$). Notably, both the number of physicians and the specialties encountered were associated with selection of active surveillance on univariable analysis, but not multivariable analysis, implying that multidisciplinary care itself, and not merely the number or type of physicians seen, was important to the shared decision making process for selection of active surveillance (28). In summary, this was a key study in demonstrating that multidisciplinary clinics can affect management.

The use of protons versus photons may also be a decision for which multidisciplinary models of care may be helpful, as both protons and photons have their own set of associated benefits, risks, and costs. The input of several physicians in a potentially less biased setting can ultimately help patients to decide the optimal modality of management given their own priorities and goals of care. Further research investigating the role of multidisciplinary clinics on patient selection of protons versus photons (and other new and emerging therapies) may be warranted.

REFERENCES

1. Efstathiou JA, Gray PJ, Zietman AL. Proton beam therapy and localised prostate cancer: current status and controversies. *Br J Cancer*. 2013;108:1225–1230.
2. Gray PJ, Efstathiou JA. Proton beam radiation therapy for prostate cancer—is the hype (and the cost) justified? *Curr Urol Rep.* 2013;14:199–208.
3. Gray PJ, Efstathiou JA. Prostate cancer: proton therapy—revolutionary advance or diminishing returns? *Nat Rev Urol.* 2013;10:128–129.
4. Mouw KW, Trofimov A, Zietman AL, et al. Clinical controversies: proton therapy for prostate cancer. *Semin Radiat Oncol.* 2013;23:109–114.
5. Trofimov A, Nguyen PL, Coen JJ, et al. Radiotherapy treatment of early-stage prostate cancer with IMRT and protons: a treatment planning comparison. *Int J Radiat Oncol Biol Phys.* 2007;69:444–453.
6. Vargas C, Fryer A, Mahajan C, et al. Dose-volume comparison of proton therapy and intensity-modulated radiotherapy for prostate cancer. *Int J Radiat Oncol Biol Phys.* 2008;70:744–751.
7. Zhang X, Dong L, Lee AK, et al. Effect of anatomic motion on proton therapy dose distributions in prostate cancer treatment. *Int J Radiat Oncol Biol Phys.* 2007;67:620–629.
8. Fontenot JD, Lee AK, Newhauser WD. Risk of secondary malignant neoplasms from proton therapy and intensity-modulated x-ray therapy for early-stage prostate cancer. *Int J Radiat Oncol Biol Phys.* 2009;74:616–622.
9. Yoon M, Ahn SH, Kim J, et al. Radiation-induced cancers from modern radiotherapy techniques: intensity-modulated radiotherapy versus proton therapy. *Int J Radiat Oncol Biol Phys.* 2010;77:1477–1485.
10. Zietman AL, Bae K, Slater JD, et al. Randomized trial comparing conventional-dose with high-dose conformal radiation therapy in early-stage adenocarcinoma of the prostate: long-term results from proton radiation oncology group/american college of radiology 95-09. *J Clin Oncol.* 2010;28:1106–1111.
11. Kim S, Shen S, Moore DF, et al. Late gastrointestinal toxicities following radiation therapy for prostate cancer. *Eur Urol.* 2011;60:908–916.
12. Sheets NC, Goldin GH, Meyer AM, et al. Intensity-modulated radiation therapy, proton therapy, or conformal radiation therapy and morbidity and disease control in localized prostate cancer. *JAMA.* 2012;307:1611–1620.
13. Yu JB, Soulos PR, Herrin J, et al. Proton versus intensity-modulated radiotherapy for prostate cancer: patterns of care and early toxicity. *J Natl Cancer Inst.* 2013;105:25–32.
14. Gray PJ, Paly JJ, Yeap BY, et al. Patient-reported outcomes after 3-dimensional conformal, intensity-modulated, or proton beam radiotherapy for localized prostate cancer. *Cancer.* 2013;119:1729–1735.
15. Proton Therapy vs. IMRT for Low or Intermediate Risk Prostate Cancer (PARTIQoL). http://clinicaltrials.gov/ct2/show/NCT01617161.
16. National Comprehensive Cancer Network. NCCN Clinical Practice Guidelines in Oncology. Prostate Cancer. Vol 2012. *www.nccn.org.* Accessed October 1, 2012.
17. Bill-Axelson A, Holmberg L, Ruutu M, et al. Radical prostatectomy versus watchful waiting in early prostate cancer. *N Engl J Med.* 2011;364:1708–1717.
18. Wilt TJ, Brawer MK, Jones KM, et al. Radical prostatectomy versus observation for localized prostate cancer. *N Engl J Med.* 2012;367:203–213.
19. Widmark A. Prospective randomized trial comparing external beam radiotherapy versus watchful waiting in early prostate cancer. Annual Meeting of the American Society of Radiation Oncology; 2011 (Abstract). Miami Beach, Florida, USA.
20. Paulson DF, Lin GH, Hinshaw W, et al. Radical surgery versus radiotherapy for adenocarcinoma of the prostate. *J Urol.* 1982;128:502–504.
21. Hanks GE. More on the Uro-Oncology Research Group report of radical surgery vs. radiotherapy for adenocarcinoma of the prostate. *Int J Radiat Oncol Biol Phys.* 1988;14:1053–1054.

22. Byhardt RW, Greenlaw RH, Jensen R, et al. Re: radical surgery versus radiotherapy for adenocarcinoma of the prostate. *J Urol.* 1983;130:1205–1206.
23. Fowler FJ Jr, McNaughton Collins M, Albertsen PC, et al. Comparison of recommendations by urologists and radiation oncologists for treatment of clinically localized prostate cancer. *JAMA.* 2000;283:3217–3222.
24. Moore MJ, O'Sullivan B, Tannock IF. How expert physicians would wish to be treated if they had genitourinary cancer. *J Clin Oncol.* 1988;6:1736–1745.
25. Gomella LG, Lin J, Hoffman-Censits J, et al. Enhancing prostate cancer care through the multidisciplinary clinic approach: a 15-year experience. *J Oncol Pract.* 2010;6:e5–e10.
26. Valicenti RK, Gomella LG, El-Gabry EA, et al. The multidisciplinary clinic approach to prostate cancer counseling and treatment. *Semin Urol Oncol.* 2000;18:188–191.
27. Brassell SA, Dobi A, Petrovics G, et al. The Center for Prostate Disease Research (CPDR): a multidisciplinary approach to translational research. *Urol Oncol.* 2009;27:562–569.
28. Aizer AA, Paly JJ, Zietman AL, et al. Multidisciplinary care and pursuit of active surveillance in low-risk prostate cancer. *J Clin Oncol.* 2012;30:3071–3076.

10.2 Treatment of Low-Risk, Localized Prostate Cancer: Brachytherapy

PETER GRIMM

■ LDR AND HDR FOR LOW-RISK PROSTATE CANCER

Two forms of brachytherapy are used for low-risk disease, low-dose rate (LDR) that employs permanently placed radioactive seeds and high-dose rate (HDR) that employs temporary placement of radioactive sources. Both methods operate with the same principle, delivering a high-targeted dose to the prostate and suitable margin. Early experience with single seed placement technique using a retropubic technique prevented LDR treatments from consistently achieving high-quality implants. However, in the past 30 years, multiple technologic advances in both LDR and HDR have resulted in consistent high-quality implants and outcomes (1,20, 21, 24). These advances include introduction of preplanned and intraoperatively planned dosimetry, connected seeds, postoperative computed tomography (CT) dosimetry, and improved ultrasound and magnetic resonance imaging (MRI) imagery for planning (1–8, 78).

■ RATIONALE FOR BRACHYTHERAPY IN LOW-RISK DISEASE

The primary rationale of brachytherapy with either HDR or LDR in low-risk disease is the ability to deliver significantly higher dose of radiation than external beam radiation therapy (EBRT) to the prostate and the immediate surrounding margin. There is no dispute that higher radiation dose, with any radiation modality, results in higher prostate cancer control rates (12,15–18). The low-risk prescription dose for modern intensity-modulated radiotherapy (IMRT) and protons is typically 81 Gy, whereas the prescription doses for LDR, for example, are 125 Gy for Pd and 145 Gy for I-125. A typical HDR dose is 38 Gy over two separate treatments. LDR and HDR can achieve significantly high radiobiological doses, which has correlated with improved long-term cancer control cancer control over IMRT treatments (18, 80, 81). LDR and HDR are considered to be radiobiologically similar (13). Although dose inhomogeneity with LDR and HDR brachytherapy is unavoidable because individual radioactive sources are emitting radiation from single sources, the calculated contributed dose from all of the sources to any point in the prostate and surrounding area remains substantially higher than EBRT. Technique, careful planning, and standardization of the prescription dose can insure adequate doses to the prostate and immediate surrounding area.

■ PATIENT SELECTION WITH LOW-RISK DISEASE

Virtually all patients with low-risk disease are candidates for LDR or HDR brachytherapy. Brachytherapy as "monotherapy" can be a confusing term to patients because patients often think it means a single treatment. Although LDR monotherapy means a single outpatient treatment, HDR monotherapy means usually two separate sessions. HDR for low-risk disease is often a multimodality treatment, delivered as a combination of EBRT and a single HDR application.

LDR and HDR are appropriate treatments for low-risk disease because there is a high likelihood of disease being confined to the implant target volume. Partin et al. demonstrated that the risk of lymph node and seminal vesicle risk is low in this group (9), and Davis et al. demonstrated that extracapsular extension (ECE) is within 3 mm from the edge of the gland in 98% of cases. Both LDR and HDR deliver high doses to the prostate and this margin of disease surrounding the prostate (10).

■ TECHNICAL ISSUES

Large glands greater than 60 cc may create a technical challenge due to pubic interference and/or result in large volume of high dose. Pubic arch interference can occur with any size gland (8). Large prostates also require more needles and seeds or more source placement locations to achieve adequate dosimetric coverage. An increase in trauma and swelling can increase the risk of temporary acute urinary retention. Thus, ideally, the prostate should be less than 60 cc at the time of the implant. Ultrasounds, CT scans, and MRIs can be very useful to evaluate this problem preoperatively. In addition, preoperative antiandrogens can help reduce the prostate size to this goal prior to implant.

A previous transurethral resection of the prostate (TURP) does not exclude brachytherapy (79). However, large TURP defects can prevent adequate needle or seed placement. Patients with a history of a small TURP may be good candidates for an implant but should be counseled that their risk of incontinence may be slightly higher than non-TURP patients (79).

■ ONCOLOGIC ISSUES

As noted in the Partin tables, low-risk patients usually have low likelihood of extraprostatic disease beyond the treatment volume (9). Extracapsular disease (ECE) is typically within a short distance of the prostate and easily within a LDR or HDR target volume (10). Surgical studies, however, suggest that the exception to using LDR or HDR monotherapy in low-risk patients may involve patients with a high percentage of positive biopsies (14). Although percentage biopsies has not yet been demonstrated in LDR or HDR monotherapy to have a significant effect on prognosis, we usually perform a pretreatment multiparametric MRI and consider combining EBRT with an implant in these patients.

■ CLINICAL ISSUES

Overall and local tissue tolerance must be considered before selecting brachytherapy and should involve both the urologist and the radiation oncologist. Patients with a life expectancy of <5 years, generally, should not be considered for any treatment in this category. Absolute contraindications are rare but include patient intolerance to anesthesia and severe pubic arch interference. Active inflammatory bowel disease in the rectum should be considered with some caution (25). A retrospective study from Mt. Sinai, however, demonstrated that patients with Crohn's disease or ulcerative colitis did not have elevated rectal toxicity (82).

Relative contraindications are those that the patient or physician may find unacceptable. Severe obstructive voiding symptoms, as defined as persistent International Prostate Symptom Score over 20 despite medications will increase the risk of temporary urinary obstruction or symptoms. Patients with bladder neck contracture or large median lobes can undergo prebrachytherapy transurethral incision of the prostate or TURP 6 to 8 weeks prior to implantation to decrease the risk of obstruction problems (22). Challenging patients, such as those with a history of prior low-dose pelvic radiation therapy, large prostate volume, large median lobe, unusual pelvic anatomy, or poor quality implant as noted at the time of postimplantation dosimetry after initial implant, will likely benefit from a consultation with an experienced radiation oncologist and urologist who are experts in prostate brachytherapy.

■ RESULTS

Biochemical relapse-free survival (BRFS) is the most sensitive endpoint for treatment efficacy as it is the least influenced by confounding factors. Low-risk patients have a very long natural history with or without treatment, making survival, for example, a poor early endpoint for comparative analysis. Long-term, brachytherapy BRFS survival results for low-risk disease are demonstrated in Figure 10.2.1. This figure is updated from a comprehensive comparative study conducted by the Prostate Cancer Results Study Group (19,27–77). Figure 10.2.1 includes all studies to date meeting study criteria for low-risk disease with a minimum median follow-up of 5 years and minimum 100 patients in each study. Long-term BRFS for low-risk disease is expected to be 89% to 98% for LDR and 92% to 94% for HDR at 10 years (19,27–77). Updates are done every six months and can be obtained at www.pctrf.org.

■ TOXICITY

Intraoperative or postoperative morbidity is rare (23). In our experience in Seattle with over 10,000 patients treated in an outpatient ambulatory surgery center, there have been no perioperative infections or deaths. Acute postoperative side effects are common and are primarily Radiation Therapy Oncology Group grade 1 to 2 irritative and obstructive lower urinary symptoms, including increased urinary frequency, urgency, dysuria, and weakening of the urinary stream. The symptoms are at their worst weeks 2 to 6 postoperatively, diminish gradually, and can be bothersome for 2 to 12 months. Short-term (<3 weeks) acute urinary retention occurs in approximately 3% to 10% of patients (23) and is generally associated with large gland size, high pretreatment urinary symptom score, and pretreatment with androgen ablation. Acute retention is treated with short-term self-catheterization or a suprapubic catheterization.

Mild hematuria is to be expected for at least a few days after LDR or HDR. Mild hematospermia or orgasmalgia

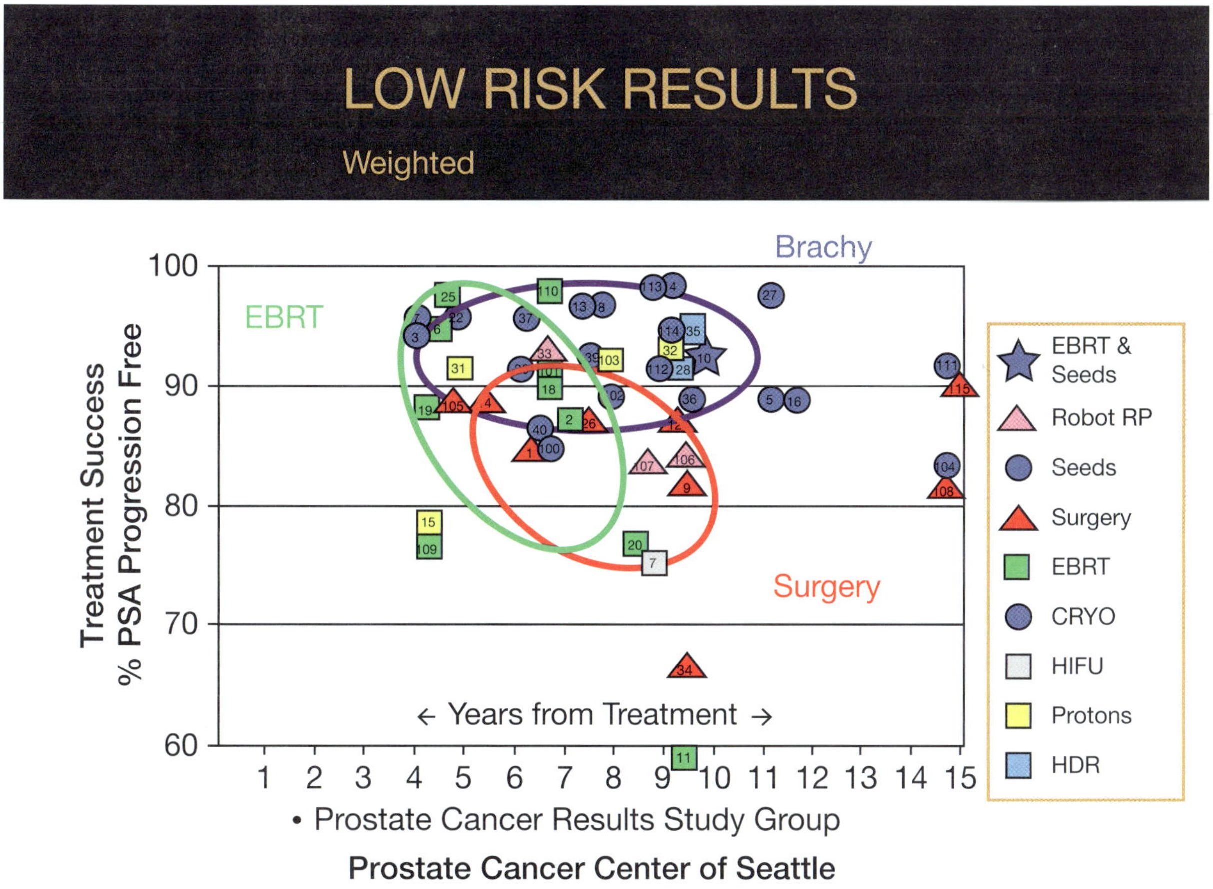

FIGURE 10.2.1 Low-risk results. Numbers within symbols refer to original source references.
Source: Updated from Ref. (19). Grimm P, Billiet I, Bostwick D, et al. Results of the prostate cancer results study group; comparative effectiveness of prostate cancer treatments. *BJU.* 2012;109(suppl 1):22–29. Update 0913.

can occur with first orgasms and generally resolves. Prostatic and seminal vesicle fluid components (~90%) of the ejaculate will usually decrease dramatically but should not be considered contraceptive by the patient.

Chronic or delayed rectal bleeding occurs with a 2% to 3% in modern series but has been reported as high as (84) 10% incidence (83). Postimplant dosimetric rectal volume receiving 100% of the prescribed dose (RV100) correlate to this, and the recommended targeted RV100 goal is less than 1.0 cc. Proctitis may be conservatively managed with dietary changes, steroids, suppositories, and sucralfate enemas. Significant rectal bleeding should be investigated with colonoscopy or flexible sigmoidoscopy. We advise against biopsy or electrocautery of the anterior rectum, due to risk of acquired rectal-urethral fistula or nonhealing rectal ulcer. In Seattle, we also require a colonoscopy within 5 years prior to brachytherapy. Chemical cautery with dilute formalin of the rectal mucosa for rectal bleeding is an effective chemical cautery measure. Late urinary retention due to urethral stricture occurs in approximately 5% of LDR and 8% to 10% of HDR patients (88, 89). This highly correlates with dose (87). This can be corrected in ~90% of patients with dilation or urethotomy (86).

Erectile dysfunction (ED) can occur with all prostate cancer treatments and is highly dependent on pretreatment ability (26, 27). At 3 years post LDR treatment in patients with normal erectile function, approximately 50% will retain this ability and another 30% will have near normal ability with the use of PFDE5 inhibitors (27). In the prospective trial by Talcott and coworkers, significantly higher rates of ED were noted in the surgical patients than brachytherapy-treated patients (27).

■ REFERENCES

1. Grimm PG, Blasko JC, Sylvester JE, et al. Technical improvement in permanent seed implantation: a 2-stage brachytherapy system: description and comparison with current technique. *Brachytherapy.* 2004;3(1):34–40.
2. Holm HH, Juul N, Pedersen JF, Hansen H, Stroyer I. Transperineal I-125 seed implantation in prostatic cancer guided by transrectal ultrasonography. *J Urol.* 1983;130:283–286.
3. Blasko JC, Wallner K, Grimm PD, Ragde H. Prostate specific antigen based disease control following ultrasound guided 125iodine implantation for stage T1/T2 prostatic carcinoma. *J Urol.* 1995;154:1096–1099.
4. Blasko JC, Grimm PD, Ragde H. Brachytherapy and organ preservation in the management of carcinoma of the prostate. *Semin Radiat Oncol.* 1993;3:240–249.

5. Sylvester J, Blasko JC, Grimm P, Ragde H. Interstitial implantation techniques in prostate cancer. *J Surg Oncol.* 1997;66:65-75.
6. Stock RG, Stone NN, Wesson MF, DeWyngaert JK. A modified technique allowing interactive ultrasound-guided three-dimensional transperineal prostate implantation. *Int J Radiat Oncol Biol Phys.* 1995;32:219–225.
7. Wallner K, Chiu-Tsao ST, Roy J, et al. An improved method for computerized tomography-planned transperineal 125iodine prostate implants. *J Urol.* 1991;146:90–95.
8. Grimm PD, Blasko JC, Ragde H. Ultrasound-guided transperineal implantation of iodine-125 and palladium-103 for the treatment of early-stage prostate cancer: technical concepts in planning, operative technique, and evaluation. In: Schellhammer PF, ed. New Techniques in Prostate Surgery. Vol 2. Philadelphia, PA: W.B. Saunders Co; 1994:113–126.
9. Partin AW, Mangold LA, Lamm DM, Walsh PC, Epstein JI, Pearson JD. Contemporary update of prostate cancer staging nomograms (Partin Tables) for the new millennium. *Urology.* 2001;58:843–848.
10. Davis BJ, Pisansky TM, Wilson TM, et al. The radial distance of extraprostatic extension of prostate carcinoma: implications for prostate brachytherapy. *Cancer.* 1999;85:2630–2637.
11. Kupelian P, Kuban D, Thames H, et al. Radical prostatectomy, external beam radiotherapy <72 Gy, external beam radiotherapy ≥72 Gy, permanent seed implantation, or combined seeds/external beam radiotherapy for stage T1-T2 prostate cancer. *Int J Radiat Oncol Biol Phys.* 2004;58(1):25–33.
12. Zelefsky M, Yamada Y, Fuks Z, et al. Long-term results of conformal radiotherapy for prostate cancer: impact of dose escalation in biochemical tumor control and distant metastases-free survival outcomes. *Int J Radiat Oncol Biol Phys.* 2008;71(4):1028–1033.
13. Stock RG, Stone NN. Biologically effective dose values for prostate brachytherapy: effects on PSA failure and post treatment biopsy results. *Int J Radiat Oncol Biol Phys.* 2006;64(2):527–533.
14. D'Amico AV, Whittington R, Malkowicz SB, et al. Clinical utility of the percentage of positive prostate biopsies in defining biochemical outcome after radical prostatectomy for patients with clinically localized prostate cancer [see comments]. *J Clin Oncol.* 2000;18:1164–1172.
15. Zelefsky MJ, Leibel SA, Gaudin PB, et al. Dose escalation with three-dimensional conformal radiation therapy affects the outcome in prostate cancer. *Int J Radiat Oncol Biol Phys.* 1998;41:491–500.
16. Zeitman AL, Bae K, Slater JD, et al. Randomized trial comparing conventional-dose with high-dose conformal radiation therapy in early-stage adenocarcinoma of the prostate: long-term results from proton radiation oncology group/american college of radiology 95-09. *J Clin Oncol.* 2010;28 (7):1106–1111.
17. Kupelian P, Kuban D, Thames H, et al. Improved biochemical relapse-free survival with increased radiation doses in patients with localized prostate cancer: the combined experience of nine institutions in 1994 and 1995. *Int J Radiat Oncol Biol Phys.* 2005;61(2):415–419.
18. Pollock A, Hanlon A, Horwitz EM, Feigenberg S, Uzzo RG, Price RA. Radiation therapy dose escalation for prostate cancer a rationale for IMRT. *World J Urol.* 2003;21:200–208.
19. Grimm P, Billiet I, BostwickD, et al. Results of the prostate cancer results study group; comparative effectiveness of prostate cancer treatments. *BJU.* 2012;109(suppl 1):22–29. Update 0913.
20. Wong J, Grimm P, Sylvester J, et al. First report on the use of a thinner I125 radioactive seed that fits into 20 gauge needles for permanent seed prostate brachytherapy: a report on post-implant dosimetry and acute toxicity. 51st American Society for Radiation Oncology Annual Meeting, abstract; November 1–5, 2009; Chicago, IL.
21. Holm HH, Juul N, Pedersen JF, Hansen H, Stroyer I. Transperineal I-125 seed implantation in prostatic cancer guided by transrectal ultrasonography. *J Urol.* 1983;130:283–286.
22. Stone NN, Ratnow ER, Stock RG. Prior transurethral resection does not increase morbidity following real-time ultrasound-guided prostate seed implantation. *Techn Urol.* 2000;6:123–127.
23. Bottomley D, AshD, Al-Qaisieh, et al. Side effects of permanent I125 prostate seed implants in 667 patients treated in Leeds. *Radiother Oncol.* 2007;82(1):46–49.
24. Deger S, Boehmer D, Roigas J, et al. HDR brachytherapy with conformal radiation therapy for localized PCa. *Eur Urol.* 2005;47:441–448.
25. PaiH, Keyes M, Morris J, Christie J. Toxicity after I-125 prostate brachytherapy in patients with inflammatory bowel disease. *Brachytherapy.* 2013;12:126–1333.
26. Chen RC, Clark JA, Talcott JA. Individualizing QOL outcomes for localized PCA. *J Clin Oncol.* 2009;27(24):3916–3922.
27. Kupelian P, Potters L, Khuntia D, et al. Radical prostatectomy, external beam radiotherapy <72 Gy, external beam radiotherapy ≥72 Gy, permanent seed implantation, or combined seeds/external beam radiotherapy for stage T1-T2 prostate cancer. *Int J Radiat Oncol Biol Phys.* 2004;58:(1):25–33.
28. Thames H, Kuban DA, DeSilvio ML,et al. Increasing external beam dose for T1-T2 prostate cancer: effect on risk groups. *Int J Radiat Oncol Biol Phys.* 2006;65(4):975–981.
29. Martin AG, Roy J, Beaulieu L, et al. Permanent prostate implant using high activity seeds and inverse planning with fast simulated annealing algorithm: a 12-year Canadian experience. *Int J Radiat Oncol Biol Phys.* 2007;67(2):334–341.
30. Potters L, Morgenstern C, Calugaru E, et al. 12-year outcomes following permanent prostate brachytherapy in patients with clinically localized prostate cancer. *J Urol.* 2005;173:1562–1566.
31. Sabolch A, Feng FY, Daignault-Newton S, et al. Gleason patter 5 is greatest risk factor for clinical failure and death from prostate cancer after dose-escalation radiation therapy and hormonal ablation. *Int J Radiat Oncol Bio Phys.* 2011;81(4):e351–e360.
32. Zelefsky M, Yamada Y, Cohen GN, et al. Five-year outcome of intraoperative conformal permanent I-125 interstitial implantation for patients with clinically localized prostate cancer. *Int J Radiat Oncol Biol Phys.* 2007;67(1):65–70.
33. Boorjian S, Karnes RJ, Rangel LJ, Bergstralh EJ, Blute ML. Mayo Clinic validation of the D'Amico risk group classification for predicting survival following radical prostatectomy. *J Urol.* 2008;179:1354–1361.
34. Critz J, Levinson K. 10-year disease free survival rates after simultaneous irradiation for prostate cancer with a focus on calculation and methodology. *J Urol.* 2004;172:2232–2238.
35. Kuban D, Thames HD, Levy LB, et al. Long-term multi-institutional analysis of stage T1-T2 prostate cancer treated with radiotherapy in the PSA era. *Int J Radiat Oncol Biol Phys.* 2003;57(4):915–928.
36. Weight C, Reuther AM, Gunn PW, Zippe CR, Dhar NB, Klein EA. Limited pelvic lymph node dissection does not improve biochemical relapse free survival at 10-years after radical prostatectomy in patients with low risk prostate cancer. *J Urol.* 2008;71(1):141–145.
37. Merrick G, Butler WM, Wallner KE, Galbreath RW, Allen ZA, Adamovich E. Prognostic significance of perineural invasion on biochemical progression-free survival after prostate brachytherapy. *J Urol.* 2005;66(5):1048–1053.
38. Merrick G, Butler WM, Wallner KE, Galbreath RW, Allen ZA, Adamovich E. Androgen deprivation therapy does not impact cause-specific overall survival after permanent prostate brachytherapy. *Int J Radiat Oncol Biol Phys.* 2006;65(3):669–667.
39. Rossi C. Conformal proton beam radiation therapy for prostate cancer: concepts and clinical results. *Commun Oncol.* 2007;4(4):235–240.
40. Stone NN, Stone MM, Rosenstein BS, Unger P, Stock RG. Influence of pretreatment and treatment factors on intermediate to long-term outcome after prostate brachytherapy. *J Urol.* 2011;185:495–500.

41. Zelefsky M, Yamada Y, Fuks Z, et al. Long-term results of conformal radiotherapy for prostate cancer: impact of dose escalation in biochemical tumor control and distant metastases-free survival outcomes. *Int J Radiat Oncol Biol Phys.* 2008;71(4):1028–1033.
42. Pickles T, Keyes M, Morris WJ. Brachytherapy or conformal external radiotherapy for prostate cancer: a single-institutional matched pair analysis. *Int J Radiat Oncol Biol Phys.* 2010;76(1):43–49.
43. Vora SA, Wong WW, Schild SE, et al. Nine year outcomes and toxicity in patients treated with IMRT for localized PCa. *J Urol.* 2013;190(2):521–526.
44. Morris W, Keyes M, Palma D, et al. Population-based study of biochemical and survival outcomes after permanent 125i brachytherapy for low and intermediate-risk prostate cancer. *Urology.* 2009;73(4):860–867.
45. Dickinson P, Malik J, Mandall P, et al. Five year outcomes after I-125 seed brachytherapy for low risk prostate cancer at three cancer centres in UK. *BJUI int.* 2014;1133:748–753.
46. Bhatta-Dhar N, Reuther AM, Zippe C, Klein EA. No difference in 6 year biochemical failure rates with or without pelvic lymph node during radical prostatectomy in low risk patients with prostate cancer. *Urology.* 2004;63(3):528–531.
47. Zietman A, DeSilvio ML, Slater JD, et al. Comparison of conventional dose vs high dose conformal radiation therapy in clinically localized adenocarcinoma of the prostate. *JAMA.* 2005;294(10):1233-1239; Correction: *JAMA.* 2008;299(8):898–900.
48. Nguyen P, Chen MH, Catalona WJ, et al. Biochemical recurrence after radical prostatectomy for prevalent versus incident cases of prostate cancer. *Cancer.* 2008;113(11):3146–3152.
49. Taira A, Merrick GS, Galbreath RW, Wallner KE, Butler WM. Natural history of clinically staged low- and intermediate risk prostate cancer treated with monotherapeutic permanent interstitial brachytherapy. *Int J Radiat Oncol Biol Phys.* 2010;76(2): 349-354. Update Paper: Taira AV, Merrick GS, Butler WM, et al. Long-term outcomes for clinically localized prostate cancer treated with permanent interstitial brachytherapy. *Int J Radiat Oncol Bio Phys.* 2011;79(5):1336–1342.
50. Demanes J, Brandt D, Schour L, Hill DR. Excellent results from high dose rate brachytherapy and external beam for prostate cancer are not improved by androgen deprivation. *Am J Clin Oncol.* 2009;32(4):342–347.
51. Stone N, Stock RG, Cesaretti JA, Unger P. Local control following permanent prostate brachytherapy: effect of high biologically effective dose on biopsy results and oncologic outcomes. *Int J Radiat Oncol Biol Phys.* 2010;76(2):355–360.
52. Jabbari S, Weinberg VK, Shinohara K, et al. Equivalent biochemical control and improved prostate-specific antigen nadir after permanent prostate seed implant brachytherapy versus high-dose three-dimensional conformal radiotherapy and high-dose conformal proton beam radiotherapy boost. *Int J Radiat Oncol Biol Phys.* 2010;76(1):36–42.
53. Zeitman A, Bae K, Slater JD, et al. Randomized trial comparing conventional dose with high dose conformal radiation therapy in early-stage adenocarcinoma of the prostate: long term results from proton radiation oncology group/American College of Radiology 95-09. *J Clin Oncol.* 2010;28(7):1106–1111.
54. Menon M, Bhandari M, Gupta N, et al. Biochemical recurrence following robot-assisted radical prostatectomy: analysis of 1384 patients with a median 5-year follow-up. *Eur Urol.* 2010;58:838–846.
55. Kane CJ, Im R, Amling CL, et al. Outcomes after radical prostatectomy among men who are candidates for active surveillance: results from the SEARCH database urology. *Urology.* 2010;76(3):695–700.
56. Ellis R, Kaminsky DA, Zhou EH, et al. Ten year outcomes: the clinical utility of single photon emission computed tomography/computed tomography capromab pendetide (prostascint) in a cohort diagnosed with localized prostate cancer. *Int J Radiat Oncol Biol Phys.* 2011;81(1):29–34.
57. Hinnen K, Battermann JJ, van Roermund JG, et al. Long term biochemical and survival outcome of 921 patients treated with I-125 permanent prostate brachytherapy. *Int J Radiat Oncol Biol Phys.* 2010;76(5):1433–1438.
58. Zelefsky MJ, Yamada Y, Pei X, et al. Comparison of tumor control and toxicity outcomes of IMRT and brachytherapy for patients with favorable risk PCa. *J Urol.* 2011;77(4):986–990.
59. Burri R, Ho AY, Forsythe K, Cesaretti JA, Stone NN, Stock RG. Young men have equivalent biochemical outcomes compared with older men after treatment with brachytherapy for prostate cancer. *Int J Radiat Oncol Biol Phys.* 2010;77(5):1315–1321.
60. Jabbari S, Weinberg VK, Shinohara K, et al. Equivalent biochemical control and improved prostate-specific antigen nadir after permanent prostate seed implant brachytherapy versus high-dose three-dimensional conformal radiotherapy and high-dose conformal proton beam radiotherapy boost. *Int J Radiat Oncol Biol Phys.* 2010;76(1):36–42.
61. Kupelian P, Kuban D, Thames H, et al. Radical prostatectomy, external beam radiotherapy <72 Gy, external beam radiotherapy ≥72 Gy, permanent seed implantation, or combined seeds/external beam radiotherapy for stage T1-T2 prostate cancer. *Int J Radiat Oncol Biol Phys.* 2004;58:(1):25–33.
62. Kupelian P, Kuban D, Thames H, et al. Radical prostatectomy, external beam radiotherapy <72 Gy, external beam radiotherapy ≥72 Gy, permanent seed implantation, or combined seeds/external beam radiotherapy for stage T1-T2 prostate cancer. *Int J Radiat Oncol Biol Phys.* 2004;58:(1):25–33.
63. Coen J, Zietman AL, Rossi CJ, et al. Comparison of high-dose-rate proton radiotherapy and brachytherapy in localized prostate cancer: a case-matched analysis. *Int J Radiat Oncol Biol Phys.* 2012;81(1):e25–e31.
64. Coen J, Zietman AL, Rossi CJ, et al. Comparison of high-dose-rate proton radiotherapy and brachytherapy in localized prostate cancer: a case-matched analysis. *Int J Radiat Oncol Biol Phys.* 2012;81(1):e25–e31.
65. Sylvester J, Grimm PD, Wong J, Galbreath RW, Merrick G, Blasko JC. Fifteen year biochemical RFS CSS, OS following I-125 prostate brachytherapy in clinically localized prostate cancer. *Int J Radiat Oncol Biol Phys.* 2011;81:376–381.
66. Gonzales S, Herranz-Amo F, Alvarez-González A, et al. RP vs EBRT for localized PCa: long term effect on biochemical control. *Ann Surg Oncol.* 2011;18:2980–2987.
67. Busch J, Stephan C, Herold A, et al. Long-term oncological and continence outcomes after laparoscopic radical prostatectomy: a single-centre experience. *BJU Int.* 2012;110(11):E985–E990.
68. Sooriakumaran P, Haendler L, Nyberg T, et al. Biochemical recurrence after robot-assisted radical prostatectomy in a European single-centre cohort with a minimum follow-up time of 5 years. *Eur Urol.* 2012;62(5):768–774.
69. Mullins J, Han M, Pierorazio PM, Partin AW, Carter HB. Radical prostatectomy outcome in men 65 years old or older with low risk prostate cancer. *J Urol.* 2012;187(5):1620–1625.
70. Michalski AA, Gonzalez J, Ye H, et al. Clinical outcomes of patient treated with 3 D conformal RT (74-79Gy) (3D-CRT) for PCa on RTOG 9406. *Int J Radiat Oncol Biol Phys.* 2012;83(3): 363–370.
71. Spratt DE, Pei X, Yamada J, Kollmeier MA, Cox B, Zelefsky MJ. Long term outcome of high dose intensity modulated radiation therapy (86 Gy) for patients with clinically localized prostate cancer. *Int J Radiat Oncol Biol Phys.* 2013;85(3):686–692.
72. Critz FA, Benton JB, Shrake P, Merlin ML. 25 year disease free survival rates after irradiation of PCa calculated with the PSA definition of recurrences used for RP. *J Urol.* 2013;189(3):878–883.
73. Ding W, Lee J, Chamberlain D, Cunningham J, Yang L, Tay J. Twelve month PSA values and perineural invasion as strong independent variables of long term biochemical outcome after prostate brachytherapy. *Int J Radiat Oncol Biol Phys.* 2012;84 (4):962–967.

74. Vargas C, Swartz D, Vashi A, et al. Long term outcome and prognostic factors in patients treated with intraoperatively planned prostate brachytherapy. *Brachytherapy.* 2013;12(2):120–125.
75. Morris WJ, Keyes M, Spadinger I, et al. Population based 10 year oncologic outcomes after low dose rate brachytherapy for low risk and intermediate risk PCA. *Cancer.* 2013;8:1537–1546.
76. Mullins JK, Feng Z, Trock BJ, Epstein JI, Walsh PC, Loeb S. The impact of RR prostatectomy on cancer control: the 30 year anniversary. *J Urol.* 2012;188(6):22205–22210.
77. Dinkla AM, Pieters BR, Koedooder K, et al. Improved tumour control probability with MRI-based prostate brachytherapy treatment planning. *Acta Oncol.* 2013;52(3):658–665.
78. Stone NN, Ratnow ER, Stock RG. Prior transurethral resection does not increase morbidity following real-time ultrasound-guided prostate seed implantation. *Tech Urol.* 2000;6:123–127
79. Stone NN, Stock RG, Cesaretti JA, Unger P. Local control following permanent prostate brachytherapy: effect of high biologically effective dose on biopsy results and oncologic outcomes. *Int J Radiat Oncol Biol Phys.* 2010;76(2):355–360.
80. Stone NN, Stock RG, Cesaretti JA, Unger P. Local control following permanent prostate brachytherapy: effect of high biologically effective dose on biopsy results and oncologic outcomes. *Int J Radiat Oncol Biol Phys.* 2010;76:355-360.
81. Peters CA, Cesaretti JA, Stone NN, Stock RG. Low-dose rate prostate brachytherapy is well tolerated in patients with a history of inflammatory bowel disease. *Int J Radiat Oncol Biol Phys.* 2006;66(2):424–429.
82. Akimoto T, Katoh H, Kitamoto Y, Tamaki T, Harada K, Shirai K, Nakano T. Rectal bleeding after high-dose-rate brachytherapy combined with hypofractionated external-beam radiotherapy for localized prostate cancer: impact of rectal dose in high-dose-rate brachytherapy on occurrence of grade 2 or worse rectal bleeding. *Int J Radiat Oncol Biol Phys.* 2006;65(2):364–370.
83. Keyes M, Morris J, Pickles T, McKenzie M. Cancer agency prostate brachytherapy experience: indications, procedure, and outcomes. *BCMJ.* 2010;52(2):76–83.
84. Clarke RE, Tenorio LM, Hussey JR, et al. Hyperbaric oxygen treatment of chronic refractory radiation proctitis: a randomized and controlled double-blind crossover trial with long-term follow-up. *Int J Radiat Oncol Biol Phys.* 2008;72(1):134–143.
85. Merrick G, Butler W, Tollenaar B, Galbreath R, Lief J. The dosimetry of prostate brachytherapy-induced urethral strictures. *Int J Radiat Oncol Biol Phys.* 2002;52(2):461–468.
86. Earley JJ, Abdelbaky AM, Cunningham MJ, Chadwick E, Langley SE, Laing RW. Correlation between prostate brachytherapy-related urethral stricture and peri-apical urethral dosimetry: a matched case-control study. *Radiother Oncol.* 2012;104(2):187–191.
87. Hindson BR, Millar JL, Matheson B. Urethral strictures following high-dose-rate brachytherapy for prostate cancer: analysis of risk factors. *Brachytherapy.* 2013;12(1):50–55.
88. Sullivan L, Williams SG, Tai KH, Foroudi F, Cleeve L, Duchesne GM. Urethral stricture following high dose rate brachytherapy for prostate cancer. *Radiother Oncol.* 2009;91(2):232–236.

11.1 Treatment of Low-Risk, Localized Prostate Cancer: General Principles of Ablative and Focal Therapies

JOSHUA A. COHN
AYTEKIN OTO
SCOTT E. EGGENER

■ INTRODUCTION

With an estimated 238,000 incident cases in the United States in 2013, prostate cancer (PC) remains the most common cancer in men (1). Approximately 29,700 men in the U.S. will die from PC in 2013. Consequently, most men die with PC rather than from the disease. In the era of widespread prostate-specific antigen (PSA) testing, most PC is clinically localized at diagnosis (2–4), and nearly half of incident cases are classified as low-risk (5) by D'Amico criteria (i.e., PSA <10 ng/mL, Gleason score ≤6, and clinical T2a or less) (6). Unfortunately, treatment of PC can be associated with significant side effects such as urinary incontinence and erectile dysfunction (7). Therefore, despite disease-specific mortality benefits associated with thoughtfully applied PSA screening and PC treatment (8, 9), overtreatment of the disease—particularly low-risk disease in older men—is a significant concern (10).

In the case of low-risk disease, clinicians and patients are faced with the dilemma of balancing the side effects of treatment against the potential harms of "doing nothing." The decision is made more challenging by the potential for significant understaging of clinical disease by transrectal ultrasound-guided prostate biopsy (11–13). Though traditional therapy for all clinically localized PC has been whole gland treatment with radical prostatectomy or radiotherapy, treatment approaches that aim to limit overtreatment while mitigating the risk of death from disease are garnering increased interest. One approach is active surveillance, which defers treatment until clinical upstaging is found on repeat biopsies performed at regular intervals. Active surveillance has been well studied since the mid-1990s with excellent intermediate-term results (10-year disease-specific mortality of 3%) in appropriately selected patients (14). A recent study estimated that on average active surveillance defers therapy by 6.4 years at a cost of less than 2 months in decreased life expectancy (15). Nonetheless, concerns remain regarding side effects associated with patient anxiety, repeated biopsies, and the possibility of delayed whole-gland therapy. In addition, there is potential loss of the therapeutic window in which a potentially curable cancer becomes incurable (16).

Focal therapy is an alternative to active surveillance or immediate whole gland treatment that aims to provide definitive therapy while limiting side effects by treating only the portion of the prostate burdened with cancer. This chapter will focus on the challenges associated with focal therapy for PC, which include patient selection, identification of lesions, selection of treatment modality, and follow-up after treatment.

■ PATIENT SELECTION

Clinical Stage

It has been argued that patients who are candidates for focal therapy should be similar to those who are enrolled in active surveillance, which in the majority of American series has been limited to those patients with very low-risk disease, defined by Epstein (17) as: clinical stage ≤T2a, PSA <10 ng/mL, Gleason grade ≤6, low PSA density (<0.15), and low volume disease (no more than 2/12 cores positive or involvement of >50% of one core) (14). Nevertheless, active surveillance was associated with a low PC-specific mortality rate in a large Canadian series that included older patients with Gleason pattern 3+4 disease and PSA up to 15 ng/mL (18). It has therefore also been argued that because focal therapy involves active treatment of cancer rather than surveillance, it is reasonable to consider its use in patients with low volume Gleason grade 3+4 disease and potentially applicable to older patients with primary Gleason pattern 4 PC.

After much debate, a recently published 18-physician Consensus Report (19) recommended that appropriately selected intermediate-risk patients should be considered for focal therapy. Specifically, the panel recommended focal therapy be limited to patients with life expectancy >10 years, those with low- to intermediate-risk disease, and clinical stage T2aN0M0 and radiologic stage T2bN0M0 or less. Unsurprisingly, it was difficult for this international panel to reach a consensus on candidate selection: recently completed and ongoing focal therapy trials in the United States and Europe have inclusion criteria varying from PSA<10 to <15 ng/mL and Gleason score ranging from ≤6 to ≤8 (www.clinicaltrials.gov, Table 11.1.1) (20).

Confirmation of Eligibility

Porten and colleagues (21) found that 81 of 377 (21%) men enrolled in active surveillance were upgraded on repeat 12-core transrectal biopsy. Therefore, if a patient is eligible and interested in focal therapy following diagnostic prostate biopsy, a repeat biopsy and/or MRI should be considered to rule out larger volume or higher grade cancers that may represent a greater threat of disease progression and metastases. Detailed localization of the disease has been attempted with transperineal mapping biopsies. Onik and colleagues (22) evaluated 180 patients with unilateral cancer on TRUS-biopsy considering conservative management. Using a brachytherapy grid and ultrasound guidance, a median of 50 cores were taken from each patient at 5 mm intervals. Bilateral disease was identified in 110 patients (61%) and Gleason score was upgraded to 7 or higher in 41 of 120 (34%) patients with Gleason grade 6 cancer on initial biopsy. The findings of Onik et al. underscore the relative rarity of unilateral and unifocal cancer as well as the potential limitations of TRUS-biopsy alone prior to pursuing focal therapy.

MRI in combination with TRUS-biopsy has also been used to evaluate eligibility for focal therapy. Girouin and colleagues (23) compared whole-mount radical prostatectomy pathology with preoperative dynamic contrast-enhanced (DCE) MRI in 46 men. Although DCE imaging performed significantly better than standard T2-weighted MRI, significant nodules (defined as >0.3 cc) were missed in about 20% of cases. The likelihood of a missed nodule decreased with increasing Gleason grade. Improved results have also been obtained with use of endorectal coil MRI (24), though smaller lesions (<0.5 cc) may still be missed. Advanced ultrasonography modalities such as computer-aided ultrasonography (HistoScanning) may also prove useful in determining the location and extent of localized disease (25,26).

Focal therapy may still be considered even if multifocal disease is found on transperineal mapping biopsy or focused prostatic imaging. Bott and colleagues (27) identified 374 tumor foci in 100 radical prostatectomy specimens which included 68 Gleason 6 cancers by preoperative biopsy. The median volume of the index lesion was 0.95 cc (range 0.1–18.2) whereas the median volume of secondary lesions was 0.2 cc (range 0.05–1.7), with only 9 having volume >0.5 cc. Of the 274 secondary lesions, 12 contained cancers of Gleason grade >6, and 4 were responsible for

Table 11.1.1 Summary of ongoing clinical trials in focal therapy for the treatment of localized prostate cancer

Clinical Trial ID	Modality	Phase	Study Site	PSA	GS	*n*	Expected Completion
NCT00295802	HIFU vs. Cryoablation	Phase 2/3	Multi-institutional, United States	<10	≤6	446	07/2012
NCT00770822	HIFU vs. Std Brachytherapy	Phase 2/3	Multi-institutional, United States	<10	≤6	466	07/2013
NCT00774436	Cryoablation	Phase 2	Memorial Sloan-Kettering	<10	≤6	50	10/2013
NCT01094665	Laser ablation	Phase 1/2	University Health Network	<15	not specified	60	12/2013
NCT01377753	Laser ablation	Phase 2	National Cancer Institute	<15	≤3+4	15	04/2014
NCT00877682	Cryoablation	Phase 1	M.D. Anderson	<10	≤3+4	100	04/2014
NCT01354951	Brachytherapy	Phase 2	Multi-institutional, United States	<10	≤3+4	80	05/2014
NCT01194648	HIFU	Phase 2	University College London	<10	≤4+3	272	06/2014
NCT00928603	Cryoablation	Phase 1	Università Vita-Salute San Raffaele	<10	≤6	100	09/2014
NCT01792024	Laser ablation	Phase 2	University of Chicago	<15	≤7	27	05/2015
NCT01310894	PDT vs. Active Surveillance	Phase 3	Multi-institutional, Europe	<10	≤6	400	09/2015
NCT01830166	Brachytherapy	Phase 1	British Columbia Cancer Agency	<10	≤3+4	10	05/2017
NCT01802307	Brachytherapy	Phase 2	University of Maryland	<15	≤3+4	50	03/2018

Abbreviations: PSA, prostate-specific antigen; GS, Gleason score; *n*, expected enrollment; HIFU, high-intensity focused ultrasound; PDT, photodynamic therapy.

extraprostatic extension. Similarly, Noguchi et al. (28) found that 140 of 222 (63%) radical prostatectomy specimens contained either unifocal cancer or cancers with secondary lesions <0.5 cc in volume. Further suggesting the potential use of focal therapy in multifocal disease are several studies documenting that adverse pathology, if present, is likely to be associated with the index lesion (27–31). Nonetheless, the long-term risk associated with untreated secondary lesions is unknown.

■ TREATMENT MODALITIES

Cryotherapy

Cryosurgical ablation induces tissue damage through several mechanisms (32). As the tissue is cooled and ice forms, an osmotic gradient is created between the dehydrated extracellular environment and relatively hypotonic intracellular environment. Water then exits cells, creating a toxic hyperosmolar intracellular environment. In addition, further cooling leads to direct damage to endothelial cells and intracellular freezing, which disrupts intracellular structures. It is thought that cells ultimately die from both direct cell killing related to freeze-rupture as well as by induction of apoptosis.

Nerve-sparing focal cryoablation was first described by Onik and colleagues (33) in 2002 in a cohort of 9 men with unilateral PC by sextant biopsy. In the technique described by Onik et al., a 22-gauge needle was placed transperineally into Denonvillier's fascia and saline injected to separate the rectum from the prostate then a urethral warmer placed. While monitoring the temperature of the contralateral neurovascular bundle (the ipsilateral neurovascular bundle is destroyed with this hemiablation technique), cryoprobes were transperineally placed 1 cm apart within the areas to be destroyed, 5 mm from the edge of the prostate on the side of the tumor, and at the confluence of the seminal vesicles posterior to the urethra. Tissue temperatures of −35°C were achieved using the Argon gas-based system, and two cycles of freezing and thawing were performed. All patients had a negative follow-up biopsy and stable PSA after a mean follow-up of 3 years. Seven out of nine patients remained potent.

Results of four more recent studies (34–37) evaluating cryosurgical hemiablation of the prostate as initial therapy for PC have been similarly encouraging. Inclusion criteria of these generally smaller series (n = 25–77) were varied: mean PSA ranged from 4.9 to 7.2 ng/mL, and two studies were inclusive of Gleason grade ≤7 disease (34, 35), one inclusive of ≤8 disease (37), and one inclusive of ≤10 disease (36). PC was diagnosed in all studies by TRUS-biopsy. By ASTRO or Phoenix criteria, biochemical disease-free survival at follow-up of 15 to 70 months was reported at 73% to 93%. Biopsy-proven recurrences were identified in 4% to 23% of patients, nearly all of which were found in untreated areas. Potency was maintained in 71% to 89% and continence in 96% to 100%.

Onik and colleagues (38) sought to improve on their initial hemiablation experience by focal ablation of lesions after detailed 3D-mapping by transperineal biopsy in a recent study inclusive of men with Gleason grade ≤8 PC. Cryotherapy was directed only at areas of cancer with attempted sparing of both neurovascular bundles, if possible. At mean follow-up of 4.5 years, biochemical disease-free survival was maintained in 94% of patients, with 10% having biopsy-proven recurrences, all of which were in untreated areas. Potency was maintained in 90% of men. In contrast, imaging-based rather than transperineal mapping-dependent focal cryoablation may also be an option for those patients whose lesions are visible on MRI, and results have been encouraging (39).

Complications of cryotherapy are rare but can include urinary retention, erectile dysfunction, and rectourethral fistula. Cryotherapy may be more challenging to administer to patients with anterior cancers or very large prostates. In addition, long-term outcomes are somewhat more challenging to ascertain based on relatively short follow-up in many studies and high rates (up to 92%) of administration of preoperative androgen deprivation therapy (40). Potential to miss significant (i.e., >0.5 cc) secondary lesions is a concern and may be as high as 20% (41).

Results of a Phase II study of the use of focal cryotherapy for low-risk disease are expected and should provide further insight with respect to its applicability in this setting (NCT00774436). A similar study (NCT00877682) in low and intermediate-risk disease is also ongoing and should provide additional efficacy and quality of life data. However, neither study is likely to answer questions regarding the long-term cancer-related outcomes associated with cryotherapy.

High Intensity Focused Ultrasound (HIFU)

High intensity focused ultrasound (HIFU) uses focused ultrasound energy to generate temperatures within tissue of greater than 60°C, resulting in coagulative necrosis. The two most common systems are the Ablatherm® and Sonoblate® 500, both of which function by similar principles. Under general or regional anesthesia, a cooling probe is placed in the rectum, and hundreds of cycles of therapy are delivered to a focused area under ultrasound guidance. Transurethral resection of the prostate is sometimes performed concomitantly. Unfortunately, HIFU may be limited in treatment of anterior lesions and smaller prostates.

Though HIFU has mainly been studied as whole gland therapy, in 1995 Madersbacher and colleagues (42) published the first study investigating the feasibility of focal HIFU therapy as treatment for PC. Only 3 of 10 patients, all of whom had presumed unilateral disease prior to treatment, were found to have had their cancer completely eradicated by HIFU at radical prostatectomy. More recent studies of whole gland ablation, however, have produced more encouraging results.

Poissonnier and colleagues (43) studied 227 men with clinical stage T1–T2 PC treated with whole gland HIFU with the Ablatherm device between 1994 and 2003. Patients underwent a mean of 419 cycles per treatment session. At a mean follow-up of 27 months, 86% had a negative 6-core biopsy; however, 31% had received neoadjuvant hormone deprivation. Five-year disease-free survival was reported at 66%. Forty-three percent of men required retreatment for persistent disease, 13% developed urinary incontinence, and 12% developed urethral stricture. In a similar study, Uchida et al. (44) reported on treatment of 517 patients with T1c-T3N0M0 disease with whole gland HIFU over an 8-year period using the Sonablate 500. Using the Phoenix criteria (PSA nadir + 2 ng/mL) to define biochemical failure, 74%, 79%, 72%, 24%, and 33% of patients with stage T1c, T2a, T2b, T2c, and T3 disease, respectively, remained biochemically disease-free at 5 years. Twenty-nine percent of patients who were potent preoperatively had erectile dysfunction at a median follow-up of 2 years.

There is limited data published on HIFU for partial gland ablation as definitive therapy. We are aware of three studies, each including between 12 and 29 patients (45–47). Negative biopsy rates after therapy were reported in 77% to 89% of patients. Muto et al. (45) reported biochemical disease-free recurrence at two years at 83% in low-risk and 54% in intermediate-risk cancers, whereas El Fegoun et al. (46) reported 90% of men were biochemically free of disease at 5 years.

Reported complications of HIFU include urinary retention (12%–22%), urethral stricture and/or bladder neck contracture (0%–41%), urinary tract infection (0%–48%), incontinence (1%–18%), fistula (0%–1%), and erectile dysfunction (18%–53%) (44). At this time, its use in the United States for focal PC treatment remains largely investigational. There is currently one ongoing nonrandomized study of HIFU for initial treatment of localized PC in the United States comparing HIFU with brachytherapy for initial treatment of low-risk PC and whose results are expected shortly (NCT00295802). A large, multi-institutional study is investigating HIFU as salvage therapy after external beam radiation (NCT00772317). Results of both studies may have implications for the frequency of HIFU treatment in the U.S. going forward.

Photodynamic Therapy

In photodynamic therapy (PDT), light activates a topically or systemically delivered photosensitizer in the presence of oxygen to generate free radicals that damage cells and/or microvasculature and cause tissue necrosis (48). Initially used to treat skin lesions, PDT has subsequently been tested in a number of other cancer sites. Tissue-activated agents can take several days to achieve desired levels in target organs, requiring a delay of several days between administration of the photosensitizer and light treatment. In addition, these agents can accumulate in nontarget tissues, such as the eyes and skin. As such, light-protection may be required for up to 6 weeks. In contrast, vascular-targeted phototherapy (VTP) agents achieve peak concentrations relatively quickly, allowing administration of the drug and light therapy in the same treatment session.

The first clinical trial evaluating PDT in PC was published in 2002 and included men with locally recurrent disease (49). The same group subsequently conducted a study of the tissue-based PDT agent mTHPC (Foscan®) as primary therapy in 6 men with organ-confined Gleason 6 PC. A 652 nm laser was used to activate the mTHPC 2 to 5 days following intravenous administration. The results were discouraging: four patients required repeat treatment for residual cancer at follow-up biopsy, all patients experienced lower urinary tract symptoms for 2 weeks, two men developed urinary retention, and one patient developed gram-negative sepsis.

Since its initial application, studies have aimed to determine optimal dosing of photosensitizing agents and timing to light therapy, which is typically delivered transperineally under MRI or ultrasound template-based guidance. Initially encouraging oncologic outcomes have been achieved with the VTP palladium pheophorbide photosensitizers (WST-09 Tookad® and WST-11 Tookad® Soluble) (48), however optimal therapy and long-term outcomes are still unknown. Additionally, its use in recurrent localized PC following radiotherapy has been associated with rectourethral fistula (50), which raises concerns for this potential complication resulting from initial therapy.

A European randomized clinical trial aiming to compare oncologic and quality of life outcomes associated with Tookad Soluble PDT versus active surveillance is currently recruiting patients (NCT01310894). With an estimated enrollment of 400 men, this phase III study should provide much-needed insight as to the appropriate application and expected outcomes associated with PDT as primary therapy for low-risk PC.

Radiation Therapy

Though almost exclusively used for whole gland therapy, radiotherapy with both intensity-modulated radiation therapy (IMRT) and brachytherapy have also been studied as partial gland therapy. In one such example with IMRT, van Lin et al. (51) irradiated the entire prostate to 70 Gy with a boost dose of 90 Gy to the affected lobe in a feasibility study. Brachytherapy, however, remains a more encouraging option than IMRT for focally delivered therapy. Nguyen and colleagues (52) recently reported outcomes on 318 men (cT1c, Gleason grade ≤7, PSA <15 ng/mL) over 10 years who underwent MRI-guided brachytherapy limited to the peripheral zone. Freedom from PSA failure (defined as nadir + 2 ng/mL and PSA velocity >0.75 ng/mL/yr) was observed in 96% and 90% of men with low-risk disease at 5 and 8 years, respectively, and 73% and 66% at 5 and 8 years, respectively, in men with intermediate-risk disease. Though, based on this study, limited-template brachytherapy appears to be inappropriate for intermediate-risk disease, focal brachytherapy may be promising in low-risk disease. Several clinical trials designed to further investigate the feasibility and outcomes associated with focal brachytherapy as initial management for low-risk PC are in the early stages (NCT01802307, NCT01354951).

Focal Laser Ablation

Lindner and colleagues (53) used laser energy to ablate MRI-visible lesions under real-time monitoring in 12 patients with low-risk PC in a phase I study. Follow-up using a combination of prostate biopsy and MRI revealed no evidence of disease in 50% of patients and no evidence of disease at the site of treatment in 67%. No patients experienced worsening of erectile function or voiding symptoms. In a concurrent study, Lindner et al. (54) confirmed histopathology at radical prostatectomy to be well correlated with ablated volume on MRI after laser therapy in four patients. Most recently, Oto and colleagues (55) published a phase I study in nine patients with Gleason ≤7 disease treated with focal laser ablation. MRI-guided biopsy following treatment revealed no disease in 7 patients and Gleason 6 cancer in 2. There was no significant change in mean erectile function or urinary symptom scores. One additional phase I study in the United States is underway (NCT01377753). Oto and colleagues are currently enrolling patients in a Phase II efficacy study whose results are expected in the year 2015 (NCT01792024).

■ FOLLOW-UP

Laboratory Studies

Whereas PSA is a very reliable marker of recurrent disease following radical prostatectomy, its use in focal therapy is not well defined. Criteria well studied in the radiated population include the ASTRO (3 consecutive rising PSA values following a nadir with backdating to halfway between the nadir and first rise) (56) and Phoenix criteria (nadir + 2 ng/mL) (57). Although these criteria have been applied in direct or modified form in many focal therapy studies to define biochemical recurrence-free survival, neither set of criteria has been validated in this setting. Acknowledging the uncertainty associated with PSA in follow-up after focal therapy, the 2010 Consensus Report (19) recommended PSA be measured every 3 months for the first year and every 6 months thereafter. However, the panel did not provide any direct insight regarding what PSA criteria define treatment failure.

Biopsy

The 2010 Consensus Report, having recommended detailed transperineal biopsy mapping in all patients prior to initiating therapy, stressed that ideal assessment of oncologic outcomes would involve a similar repeat biopsy after therapy. However, the panel recognized the challenges involved and acknowledged that an office-based TRUS-biopsy at 6 to 12 months post therapy was reasonable. Although expert consensus is a helpful guide, at this time decisions regarding rebiopsy will generally have to be an individualized decision based upon clinical suspicion.

Imaging

MRI may obviate the need for invasive follow-up after focal therapy. Rouvière and colleagues (58) lauded the ability of combined T2-weighted and DCE MRI to distinguish between areas of posttreatment fibrosis and tumor after HIFU therapy. In follow-up after cryotherapy, adding MR-spectroscopy imaging to endorectal MRI greatly improved the ability to detect cancer over endorectal MRI or TRUS alone (59). Nevertheless, relying exclusively on imaging has limitations: not all tumors are visible on MRI, T2-weighted imaging alone poorly differentiates ablated areas from tumor, and even with advanced imaging techniques sensitivity to detect recurrent or de novo disease may be suboptimal (60).

■ CONCLUSIONS

At a time when the urologic community is under increasing pressure to balance the risk of PC treatment with treatment-related side effects, investigation of focal therapy holds promise. However, long-term oncologic and functional outcomes are largely unknown. Before any of the existing treatment modalities are deserving of widespread use, further studies will be required to better characterize outcomes with focal therapy in comparison to existing established treatment approaches, including active surveillance.

■ REFERENCES

1. American Cancer Society. *Cancer Facts and Figures 2013*. Atlanta, GA: American Cancer Society; 2013. http://www.cancer.org/research/cancerfactsfigures/cancerfactsfigures/cancer-facts–wfigures-2013. Accessed April 5, 2013.

2. Catalona WJ, Smith DS, Ratliff TL, Basler JW. Detection of organ-confined prostate cancer is increased through prostate-specific antigen-based screening. *JAMA*. 1993;270(8):948–954.
3. Etzioni R, Gulati R, Falcon S, Penson DF. Impact of PSA screening on the incidence of advanced stage prostate cancer in the United States: a surveillance modeling approach. *Med Decis Making*. 2008;28(3):323–331.
4. Jacobsen SJ, Katusic SK, Bergstralh EJ, et al. Incidence of prostate cancer diagnosis in the eras before and after serum prostate-specific antigen testing. *JAMA*. 1995;274(18):1445–1449.
5. Cooperberg MR, Broering JM, Kantoff PW, Carroll PR. Contemporary trends in low risk prostate cancer: risk assessment and treatment. *J Urol*. 2007;178(3 pt 2):S14–S19.
6. D'Amico AV, Whittington R, Malkowicz SB, et al. Biochemical outcome after radical prostatectomy, external beam radiation therapy, or interstitial radiation therapy for clinically localized prostate cancer. *JAMA*. 1998;280(11):969–974.
7. Sanda MG, Dunn RL, Michalski J, et al. Quality of life and satisfaction with outcome among prostate-cancer survivors. *N Engl J Med*. 2008;358(12):1250–1261.
8. Gulati R, Gore JL, Etzioni R. Comparative effectiveness of alternative prostate-specific antigen–based prostate cancer screening strategies: model estimates of potential benefits and harms. *Ann Intern Med*. 2013;158(3):145–153.
9. Holmberg L, Bill-Axelson A, Steineck G, et al. Results from the Scandinavian Prostate Cancer Group Trial Number 4: a randomized controlled trial of radical prostatectomy versus watchful waiting. *J Natl Cancer Inst Monogr*. 2012;2012 (45):230–233.
10. Welch HG, Black WC. Overdiagnosis in cancer. *J Natl Cancer Inst*. 2010;102 (9):605–613.
11. Epstein JI, Walsh PC, Carmichael M, Brendler CB. Pathologic and clinical findings to predict tumor extent of nonpalpable (stage T1c) prostate cancer. *JAMA*. 1994;271(5):368–374.
12. Cookson MS, Fleshner NE, Soloway SM, Fair WR. Correlation between Gleason score of needle biopsy and radical prostatectomy specimen: accuracy and clinical implications. *J Urol*. 1997;157(2):559–562.
13. Steinberg GD, Bales GT, Brendler CB. An analysis of watchful waiting for clinically localized prostate cancer. *J Urol*. 1998;159(5):1431–1436.
14. Klotz L. Active surveillance for low-risk prostate cancer. *F1000 Med Rep*. 2012;4(16):1–7.
15. Xia J, Trock BJ, Cooperberg MR, et al. Prostate cancer mortality following active surveillance versus immediate radical prostatectomy. *Clin Cancer Res*. 2012;18(19):5471–5478.
16. Harlan SR, Cooperberg MR, Elkin EP, et al. Time trends and characteristics of men choosing watchful waiting for initial treatment of localized prostate cancer: results from CaPSURE. *J Urol*. 2003;170(5):1804–1807.
17. Epstein JI. Prognostic significance of tumor volume in radical prostatectomy and needle biopsy specimens. *J Urol*. 2011;186(3):790–797.
18. Klotz L, Zhang L, Lam A, Nam R, Mamedov A, Loblaw A. Clinical results of long-term follow-up of a large, active surveillance cohort with localized prostate cancer. *J Clin Oncol*. 2010;28(1):126–131.
19. De la Rosette J, Ahmed H, Barentsz J, et al. Focal therapy in prostate cancer-report from a consensus panel. *J Endourol*. 2010;24(5):775–780.
20. Borofsky MS, Ito T, Rosenkrantz AB, Taneja SS. Focal therapy for prostate cancer - where are we in 2011? *Ther Adv Urol*. 2011;3(4):183–192.
21. Porten SP, Whitson JM, Cowan JE, et al. Changes in prostate cancer grade on serial biopsy in men undergoing active surveillance. *J Clin Oncol*. 2011;29(20):2795–2800.
22. Onik G, Miessau M, Bostwick DG. Three-dimensional prostate mapping biopsy has a potentially significant impact on prostate cancer management. *J Clin Oncol*. 2009;27(26):4321–4326.
23. Girouin N, Mège-Lechevallier F, Tonina Senes A, et al. Prostate dynamic contrast-enhanced MRI with simple visual diagnostic criteria: is it reasonable? *Eur Radiol*. 2007;17(6):1498–1509.
24. Turkbey B, Mani H, Aras O, et al. Correlation of magnetic resonance imaging tumor volume with histopathology. *J Urol*. 2012;188(4):1157–1163.
25. Braeckman J, Autier P, Soviany C, et al. The accuracy of transrectal ultrasonography supplemented with computer-aided ultrasonography for detecting small prostate cancers. *BJU Int*. 2008;102(11):1560–1565.
26. Turkbey B, Pinto PA, Choyke PL. Imaging techniques for prostate cancer: implications for focal therapy. *Nat Rev Urol*. 2009;6(4):191–203.
27. Bott SRJ, Ahmed HU, Hindley RG, Abdul-Rahman A, Freeman A, Emberton M. The index lesion and focal therapy: an analysis of the pathological characteristics of prostate cancer. *BJU Int*. 2010;106(11):1607–1611.
28. Noguchi M, Stamey TA, McNeal JE, Nolley R. Prognostic factors for multifocal prostate cancer in radical prostatectomy specimens: lack of significance of secondary cancers. *J Urol*. 2003;170 (2, pt 1): 459–463.
29. Arora R, Koch MO, Eble JN, Ulbright TM, Li L, Cheng L. Heterogeneity of Gleason grade in multifocal adenocarcinoma of the prostate. *Cancer*. 2004;100(11):2362–2366.
30. Wise AM, Stamey TA, McNeal JE, Clayton JL. Morphologic and clinical significance of multifocal prostate cancers in radical prostatectomy specimens. *Urology*. 2002;60(2):264–269.
31. Ruijter ET, van de Kaa CA, Schalken JA, Debruyne FM, Ruiter DJ. Histological grade heterogeneity in multifocal prostate cancer. Biological and clinical implications. *J Pathol*. 1996;180 (3):295–299.
32. Levy D, Avallone A, Jones JS. Current state of urological cryosurgery: prostate and kidney. *BJU Int*. 2010;105(5):590–600.
33. Onik G, Narayan P, Vaughan D, Dineen M, Brunelle R. Focal "nerve-sparing" cryosurgery for treatment of primary prostate cancer: a new approach to preserving potency. *Urology*. 2002;60 (1): 109–114.
34. Bahn DK, Silverman P, Lee F Sr, Badalament R, Bahn ED, Rewcastle JC. Focal prostate cryoablation: initial results show cancer control and potency preservation. *J Endourol*. 2006;20 (9): 688–692.
35. Lambert EH, Bolte K, Masson P, Katz AE. Focal cryosurgery: encouraging health outcomes for unifocal prostate cancer. *Urology*. 2007;69(6):1117–1120.
36. Ellis DS, Manny TB Jr, Rewcastle JC. Focal cryosurgery followed by penile rehabilitation as primary treatment for localized prostate cancer: initial results. *Urology*. 2007;70(suppl 6):9–15.
37. Truesdale MD, Cheetham PJ, Hruby GW, et al. An evaluation of patient selection criteria on predicting progression-free survival after primary focal unilateral nerve-sparing cryoablation for prostate cancer: recommendations for follow up. *Cancer J*. 2010;16(5):544–549.
38. Onik G, Vaughan D, Lotenfoe R, Dineen M, Brady J. The "male lumpectomy": focal therapy for prostate cancer using cryoablation results in 48 patients with at least 2-year follow-up. *Urol Oncol*. 2008;26(5):500–505.
39. Gangi A, Tsoumakidou G, Abdelli O, et al. Percutaneous MR-guided cryoablation of prostate cancer: initial experience. *Eur Radiol*. 2012;22(8):1829–1835.
40. Bozzini G, Colin P, Nevoux P, Villers A, Mordon S, Betrouni N. Focal therapy of prostate cancer: energies and procedures. *Urol Oncol*. 2013;31(2):155–167.
41. Rukstalis DB, Goldknopf JL, Crowley EM, Garcia FU. Prostate cryoablation: a scientific rationale for future modifications. *Urology*. 2002;60(2) (suppl 1):19–25.
42. Madersbacher S, Pedevilla M, Vingers L, Susani M, Marberger M. Effect of high-intensity focused ultrasound on human prostate cancer in vivo. *Cancer Res*. 1995;55(15):3346–3351.

43. Poissonnier L, Chapelon J-Y, Rouvière O, et al. Control of prostate cancer by transrectal HIFU in 227 patients. *Eur Urol.* 2007;51(2):381–387.
44. Uchida T, Nakano M, Hongo S, et al. High-intensity focused ultrasound therapy for prostate cancer. *Int J Urol.* 2012;19(3):187–201.
45. Muto S, Yoshii T, Saito K, Kamiyama Y, Ide H, Horie S. Focal therapy with high-intensity-focused ultrasound in the treatment of localized prostate cancer. *Jpn J Clin Oncol.* 2008;38(3):192–199.
46. El Fegoun AB, Barret E, Prapotnich D, et al. Focal therapy with high-intensity focused ultrasound for prostate cancer in the elderly. A feasibility study with 10 years follow-up. *Int Braz J Urol.* 2011;37(2):213–219.
47. Ahmed HU, Freeman A, Kirkham A, et al. Focal therapy for localized prostate cancer: a phase I/II trial. *J Urol.* 2011;185(4):1246–1254.
48. Arumainayagam N, Moore CM, Ahmed HU, Emberton M. Photodynamic therapy for focal ablation of the prostate. *World J Urol.* 2010;28(5):571–576.
49. Nathan TR, Whitelaw DE, Chang SC, et al. Photodynamic therapy for prostate cancer recurrence after radiotherapy: a phase I study. *J Urol.* 2002;168(4, pt 1):1427–1432.
50. Trachtenberg J, Weersink RA, Davidson SRH, et al. Vascular-targeted photodynamic therapy (padoporfin, WST09) for recurrent prostate cancer after failure of external beam radiotherapy: a study of escalating light doses. *BJU Int.* 2008;102(5):556–562.
51. Van Lin ENJT, Fütterer JJ, Heijmink SWTPJ, et al. IMRT boost dose planning on dominant intraprostatic lesions: gold marker-based three-dimensional fusion of CT with dynamic contrast-enhanced and 1H-spectroscopic MRI. *Int J Radiat Oncol Biol Phys.* 2006;65(1):291–303.
52. Nguyen PL, Chen M-H, Zhang Y, et al. Updated results of magnetic resonance imaging guided partial prostate brachytherapy for favorable risk prostate cancer: implications for focal therapy. *J Urol.* 2012;188(4):1151–1156.
53. Lindner U, Weersink RA, Haider MA, et al. Image guided photothermal focal therapy for localized prostate cancer: phase I trial. *J Urol.* 2009;182(4):1371–1377.
54. Lindner U, Lawrentschuk N, Weersink RA, et al. Focal laser ablation for prostate cancer followed by radical prostatectomy: validation of focal therapy and imaging accuracy. *Eur Urol.* 2010;57(6):1111–1114.
55. Oto A, Sethi I, Karczmar G, et al. MR Imaging-guided focal laser ablation for prostate cancer: phase I trial. *Radiology.* 2013;267:932–940.
56. Consensus statement: guidelines for PSA following radiation therapy. American Society for Therapeutic Radiology and Oncology Consensus Panel. *Int J Radiat Oncol Biol Phys.* 1997;37(5):1035–1041.
57. Roach M 3rd, Hanks G, Thames H Jr, et al. Defining biochemical failure following radiotherapy with or without hormonal therapy in men with clinically localized prostate cancer: recommendations of the RTOG-ASTRO Phoenix Consensus Conference. *Int J Radiat Oncol Biol Phys.* 2006;65(4):965–974.
58. Rouvière O, Girouin N, Glas L, et al. Prostate cancer transrectal HIFU ablation: detection of local recurrences using T2-weighted and dynamic contrast-enhanced MRI. *Eur Radiol.* 2010;20(1):48–55.
59. Parivar F, Hricak H, Shinohara K, et al. Detection of locally recurrent prostate cancer after cryosurgery: evaluation by transrectal ultrasound, magnetic resonance imaging, and three-dimensional proton magnetic resonance spectroscopy. *Urology.* 1996;48(4):594–599.
60. De Visschere PJ, De Meerleer GO, Fütterer JJ, Villeirs GM. Role of MRI in follow-up after focal therapy for prostate carcinoma. *Am J Roentgenol.* 2010;194(6):1427–1433.

11.2 *Hyperthermia for Prostate Cancer*

MARK HURWITZ

Hyperthermia is the use of heat for therapeutic purposes. Thermal ablation is the use of high temperatures that result in direct cellular and tissue destruction. In oncology, moderate temperature elevations in the range of 39°F to 45°F can be used to sensitize or complement radiation, chemotherapy, and potentially immunotherapy. Cancer cells may be resistant to radiation due to many factors including phase of the cell cycle, hypoxia, acidification, and nutritional deprivation. These conditions associated with radiation resistance all make cells more susceptible to killing with heat (1–7). For instance, late s-phase is the point in the cell cycle when cells are most resistant to radiation and the point at which hyperthermia has been shown to have maximal effect. In regard to hypoxia, hyperthermia effect may be greatest in poorly oxygenated cells, which, due to poor perfusion, are more easily heatable (8, 9). The subsequent induction of a physiologic response increasing perfusion to dissipate heat leads to tissue oxygenation prior to radiation therapy. Similarly, hyperthermia results in enhanced effect when given in combination with certain chemotherapeutic agents (10). Hyperthermia through production of heat shock proteins is also associated with modulation of the immune system including the potential to generate a tumor specific cellular immune response (11, 12).

In regard to prostate cancer, hyperthermia has been shown to provide potential benefit in a range of early stage clinical trials. The first reported study to assess hyperthermia with radiation included 21 patients with locally advanced disease defined as clinical T2b through T4 or recurrent prostate cancer. Median Gleason score was 7 and median prostate-specific antigen (PSA) was 69 ng/mL. Five to ten noninvasive local-regional hyperthermia treatments were administered in combination with external beam radiation therapy to a median dose of 6840 cGy. In this heterogeneous high-risk group of patients treated in an era predating most systemic therapies now available, disease free and overall survival at 3 years were 25% and 88%, respectively. There was no significant increase in acute or long-term toxicity with addition of hyperthermia to radiation (13).

In another early study of a heterogeneous group of patients, noninvasive regional hyperthermia was administered weekly for a total of five to six treatments over a nearly 8-week course of radiation therapy to 6840 cGy. Fifteen patients with primary T3N0M0 disease and seven with histologically confirmed local recurrence postprostatectomy were treated. Five patients received short-term androgen deprivation. With 6 years of median follow-up overall survival was 95% and 60% for primary and recurrent disease respectively. Notably higher temperatures and measures of thermal dose correlated with improved biochemical control (14).

Another early phase trial assessed both noninvasive and interstitial hyperthermia techniques with external beam radiation. Twelve patients received a single interstitial treatment on a phase I study and 14 received 5 weekly regional hyperthermia treatments on a phase II study. All patients had clinical T3 or T4 disease. Freedom from biochemical relapse was 70% at 36 months overall and 79% for regional and 57% for interstitial approaches (15).

In the largest study to date of hyperthermia for prostate cancer, patients with either clinical T2 tumors with Gleason scores ≥ 7 and/or PSA > 10 ng/mL or clinical T3 or T4 disease received hyperthermia with a noninvasive annular-phased array radiofrequency device in combination with 7400 cGy. Hyperthermia was administered weekly for up to 5 treatments. Androgen deprivation of variable type and duration was used in nearly two thirds of patients. A total of 144 patients were enrolled on this phase II trial. Five year overall survival and biochemical disease-free survival were 87% and 49%, respectively. Hyperthermia was well tolerated (16).

Transrectal and interstitial approaches to prostate hyperthermia have also been assessed in clinical trials. A phase II trial at the Dana-Farber Cancer Institute included 37 patients with clinical T2b–T3a disease treated with 3D conformal radiation to a median dose of 6660 cGy with two transrectal ultrasound hyperthermia treatments administered in the first 4 weeks of radiation therapy. All but the first four patients received short course androgen deprivation. Median Gleason score and PSA were 7 and 13.3 ng/mL, respectively. With median follow-up of 70 months the 7-year overall survival rate was 94%, and 61% of patients remained failure free. There was a statistically significant increase in the absolute rate of disease-free survival at 2 years, which was the primary study endpoint. Disease-free survival at 2 years was 84% for study participants, which compared favorably with a rate of 64% for similar patients on the 4-month androgen suppression arm of Radiation Therapy Oncology Group (RTOG) 92-02 that served as the benchmark historical control group. When Phoenix criteria were used to define biochemical failure, 89% of patients were failure free at 2 years. Hyperthermia was well tolerated with no significant long-term side effects (17).

Another innovate approach to prostate hyperthermia involves the implantation of self-regulating thermoseeds in an analogous manner to prostate brachytherapy. These seeds are heatable in an alternating magnetic field to a predetermined maximum temperature, or Curie point, based on their composition. Promising early results have been reported in 57 patients with T1 through T3 prostate cancer with median PSA of 11.6 ng/mL and the median World Health Organization (WHO) tumor grade 2. A total of 6 hyperthermia treatments were administered with 55°C Curie thermoseeds after implantation in combination with 6840 cGy. With median follow-up of 36 months, 84% remained free of recurrence with median PSA of 0.55 ng/mL 2 years after therapy (18).

Hyperthermia in combination with radiation has shown promise for palliation of symptoms associated with advanced or recurrent prostate cancer. Thirteen patients treated on a phase I–II study with a noninvasive radiofrequency device all experienced clinical and/or radiographic responses and all achieved complete palliation of symptoms (19). In another study of 15 patients with symptomatic prostate cancer, microwave hyperthermia in combination with radiation resulted in moderate to marked improvement in symptoms in 8 patients. Studies of immune markers also indicated stimulation of response and intriguingly a few patients were noted to have resolution of bone scan findings without additional therapy (20).

New approaches to prostate hyperthermia in preclinical or early clinical development include magnetic nanofluids and transurethral strategies including ultrasound and noninvasive high intensity focused ultrasound used to moderately heat larger areas of tissue as opposed to highly focal tissue ablation (21).

While promising results with prostate hyperthermia have been noted in certain circumstances, future studies will benefit from additional focus on inclusion of uniform patient risk groups and treatment protocols. Phase III trials have been done for a wide range of malignancies with survival advantage noted in several studies (22–24). However, to date none have yet been done for prostate cancer. Completion of such trials will help to define the role of hyperthermia for prostate cancer.

■ REFERENCES

1. Dewey WC, Hopwood LE, Sapareto LA, et al. Cellular response to combinations of hyperthermia and radiation. *Radiology.* 1977;123:463–474.
2. Gerweck L. Modification of cell lethality at elevated temperatures. The pH effect. *Radiat Res.* 1977;70:224–235.
3. Gerweck LE, Nygaard TG, Burlett M. Response of cells to hyperthermia under acute and chronic hypoxic conditions. *Cancer Res.* 1979;9:966–972.
4. Hahn GM, Shiu C. Adaptation to low pH modifies thermal and thermochemical responses of mammalian cells. *Int J Hyperthermia.* 1986;2:379–387.
5. Henle KJ, Leeper DB. Combination of hyperthermia (40°, 45° C) with radiation. *Radiology.* 1976;121:451–454.
6. Kim JH, Kim SH, Dutta P, et al. Preferential killing of glucose-depleted HeLa cells by menadione and hyperthermia. *Int J Hyperthermia.* 1992;8:139–146.
7. Westra A, Dewey WC. Variation in sensitivity to heat shock during the cell cycle of Chinese hamster cells in vitro. *Int J Radiat Biol.* 1971;19:467–477.
8. Eddy HA. Alterations in tumor microvasculature during hyperthermia. *Radiology.* 1980;137:515–521.
9. Song CW. Effect of local hyperthermia on blood flow and microenvironment: a review. *Cancer Res.* 1984;44(suppl 10):S4721–S4730.
10. Kano E. Hyperthermia and drugs. In: Overgaard J, ed. *Hyperthermic Oncology.* London, UK: Taylor & Francis; 1985:277–282.
11. Srivastava PK, Maki RG. Stress-induced proteins in immune response to cancer. *Curr Top Microbiol Immunol.* 1991;167:109–123.
12. Udono H, Srivastava PK. Heat shock protein 70-associated peptides elicit specific cancer immunity. *J Exp Med.* 1993;178:1391–1396.
13. Anscher MS, Samulski TV, Dodge R, Prosnitz LR, Dewhirst MW. Combined external beam irradiation and external regional hyperthermia for locally advanced adenocarcinoma of the prostate. *Int J Radiat Oncol Biol Phys.* 1997;37(5):1059–1065.
14. Tilly W, Gellermann J, Graf R, et al. Regional hyperthermia in conjunction with definitive radiotherapy against recurrent or locally advanced prostate cancer T3 pN0 M0. *Strahlenther Onkol.* 2005;181(1):35–41.
15. Van Vulpen M, De Leeuw JR, Van Gellekom MP, et al. A prospective quality of life study in patients with locally advanced prostate cancer, treated with radiotherapy with or without regional or interstitial hyperthermia. *Int J Hyperthermia.* 2003;19(4):402–413.
16. Maluta S, Dall'Oglio S, Romano M, et al. Conformal radiotherapy plus local hyperthermia in patients affected by locally advanced high risk prostate cancer: preliminary results of a prospective phase II study. *Int J Hyperthermia.* 2007;23(5):451–456.
17. Hurwitz MD, Hansen JL, Prokopios-Davos S, et al. Hyperthermia combined with radiation for the treatment of locally advanced prostate cancer: long-term results from Dana-Farber Cancer Institute study 94–153. *Cancer.* 2011;117(3):510–516.
18. Deger S, Taymoorian K, Boehmer D, et al. Thermoradiotherapy using interstitial self-regulating thermoseeds: an intermediate analysis of a phase II trial. *Eur Urol.* 2004;45(5):574–580.
19. Kalapurakal JA, Pierce M, Chen A, Sathiaseelan V. Efficacy of irradiation and external hyperthermia in locally advanced, hormone-refractory or radiation recurrent prostate cancer: a preliminary report. *Int J Radiat Oncol Biol Phys.* 2003;57(3):654–664.

20. Stawarz B, Zielinski H, Szmigielski S, et al. Transrectal hyperthermia as palliative treatment for advanced adenocarcinoma of prostate and studies of cell-mediated immunity. *Urology.* 1993;41:548–553.
21. Johannsen M, Gneveckow U, Taymoorian K, et al. Morbidity and quality of life during thermotherapy using magnetic nanoparticles in locally recurrent prostate cancer: results of a prospective phase I trial. *Int J Hyperthermia.* 2007;23:315–323.
22. van der Zee J, Gonza´lez Gonza´lez D, van Rhoon GC, et al. Comparison of radiotherapy alone with radiotherapy plus hyperthermia in locally advanced pelvic tumours: a prospective, randomised, multicentre trial. Dutch Deep Hyperthermia Group. *Lancet.* 2000;355:1119–1125.
23. Sneed PK, Stauffer PR, McDermott MW, et al. Survival benefit of hyperthermia in a prospective randomized trial of brachytherapy boost _/_ hyperthermia for glioblastoma multiforme. *Int J Radiat Oncol Biol Phys.* 1998;40:287–295.
24. Valdagni R, Amichetti M. Report of long-term follow-up in a randomized trial comparing radiation therapy and radiation therapy plus hyperthermia to metastatic lymph nodes in stage IV head and neck patients. *Int J Radiat OncolBiol Phys.* 1994;28:163–169.

11.3 Ablative Techniques: Vascular Targeted Photodynamic Therapy

ASHLEY G. WINTER

JONATHAN A. COLEMAN

MECHANISM OF ACTION

Photodynamic therapy (PDT) is a nonthermal ablative technology that utilizes activation of a light-sensitive compound to produce reactive oxygen species (ROS) and subsequent tissue destruction. Traditional PDT is predicated on photosensitive agent extravasation from the vasculature and cellular uptake into tissues followed by local laser irradiation. This form of PDT has two fundamental pitfalls: (a) treatment generally requires two separate patient visits, one for drug administration, and a second for light exposure several days later, and (b) long-term photosensitivity requiring avoidance of sunlight by patients due to prolonged drug half-life (1). Vascular-targeted photodynamic therapy (VTP), however, is a distinct form of PDT that affects tissues directly from the vascular compartment; this permits rapid treatment following photosensitizer administration and eliminates the pitfalls of conventional agents. A number of agents can be used to produce the VTP effect, though for recent urologic applications, VTP is considered as reference to several clinical trials using the bacteriochlorophyll derivatives, TOOKAD® (T or WST-09) and TOOKAD Soluble (TS or WST-11). TOOKAD® is a lipophilic agent that binds to plasma lipoproteins following intravenous co-administration with a cremophor solubilizing agent, while TOOKAD-Soluble complexes with serum albumin (2–4). Prior to elimination, circulating photosensitizer is activated by laser illumination in the near-infrared spectrum (NIR) (753 nm), generating both ROS and secondary reactive nitrogen species (RNS) (4, 5). ROS and RNS induce a rapid sequence of vasodilation, followed by vasoconstriction and blood clotting in the tumor feeding arterioles, leading to ischemia and necrosis. Selectivity for malignant over benign tissues was demonstrated by Madar-Balakirski et al., likely due to the immature, rudimentary and disordered structure of tumor vessels (6). TS-VTP also induces a strong immune reaction, with significant neutrophil and lymphocyte recruitment to treated areas (7).

The chronic effects of TS-VTP can be observed on histopathology. On prostate biopsy tissue 6 months following treatment, there is well-demarcated, fibrotic, and hyaline scarring with interspersed regions of atrophic glands, mild inflammation, and coagulative necrosis (8, 9). Unlike radiation or hormonal therapy, VTP does not induce gland-wide changes that are difficult to interpret on histology. TS-VTP generates clearly demarcated regions of hemorrhagic and coagulative necrosis with sharply defined borders and relative sparing of small caliber blood vessels down to 40 microns in size (10). Outside of treated areas, there is observed preservation of benign and cancerous untreated regions; a finding that has important implications in postfocal therapy surveillance (9).

DELIVERY

Techniques for VTP treatment of the prostate have been described as follows: the patient is placed in lithotomy position under general anesthesia followed by sterile preparation of the perineum and genitalia. Using transrectal ultrasound guidance and 2 dimensional template grid, similar to brachytherapy techniques, hollow translucent catheters are then inserted into the prostate via the perineum (8, 11, 12). Conformationally precise catheter placement is achieved with a predetermined, individualized template developed using MRI and treatment planning software to achieve 5 × 5 mm catheter spacing within the gland (13). Cylindrical laser diffusing fibers are then passed into the translucent catheters at the appropriate predetermined depth. The photosensitizer is given as a single intravenous infusion over 10 minutes for WST-11 or 20 minutes for WST-09. Immediately after completion of photosensitizer infusion, illumination of all diffusion fibers at

Source of Funding: The Thompson Foundation.

Conflict of Interest: Jonathan Coleman, MD is a consultant for AngioDynamics.

753 nm is provided for 20 to 25 minutes. Monitoring of light dose near the rectum and urethra is achieved with separate light sensors placed in these locations. Following treatment the catheters and laser fibers are then removed and the procedure terminated, with a total time of approximately 2 hours including anesthesia (8, 11, 12).

■ CLINICAL TRIALS: SAFETY AND EFFICACY

The developmental pathway of VTP treatment with WST-09 and WST-11 into clinical use is perhaps the most robust and well studied of the current ablative therapies. These include rigorous preclinical testing to establish treatment parameters and associated tissue effects, beyond the scope of this review, and a series of well-designed clinical studies, including a phase III trial. A brief overview of the phases of clinical development follows.

Radiorecurrent Prostate Cancer and WST09

The initial clinical studies of VTP in human prostate utilized WST09 in the postradiotherapy setting. The first phase I-dose-escalation study treated 24 men with WST09 at doses of 0.1, 0.25, 0.5, 1, and 2 mg/kg. Patients were evaluated with contrast-MRI at 7 days postprocedure and prostate biopsy 6 months later (8). A second study of WST09-VTP in postradiotherapy patients looked at light dose escalation with fixed drug dosing at 2 mg/kg (12). These studies established several critical parameters for T-VTP administration and monitoring: (a) a 2 mg/kg threshold of TOOKAD® was required to reliably see treatment associated lesions on 1-week MRI (8), (b) a minimum of 23 J/cm^2 light delivery was required to achieve a 6-month negative biopsy (12), (c) biopsy outcomes were heterogeneous even at optimal treatment parameters, (d) intraprostatic-thermal rise was negligible at these treatment parameters, also seen with TS-VTP in preclinical testing (14), and not monitored in further studies (8), and (e) skin phototoxicity was negligible, permitting same-day hospital discharge. Adverse events were reported as minor, the most common being intraoperative hypotension associated with the cremophor solubilizing carrier agent (8). There were two cases of rectourethral fistulae, one self-resolving and one managed with temporary diverting colostomy (12).

Treatment-Naïve Prostate Cancer and WST09

T-VTP was first used in treatment naïve prostate cancer in a single-center dose-escalation study based out of the UK (15). Per-fiber illumination parameters associated with consistent treatment effects were found at an illumination of 200 J/cm (interestingly, a non-maximal laser fluence). Total dosing was escalated to 3,800 J per lobe with additional fibers, and higher doses had a greater likelihood of negative biopsy. Several adverse events (AE) occurred during this trial, including deep venous thrombosis (1 patient), superficial venous thrombosis (2 patients), intraoperative ischemic EKG changes (1 patient), and one patient with both postprocedural myocardial infarction (MI) and cerebrovascular accident (CVA). These AEs were attributed to cremophor, and WST09 use was halted (15).

Treatment-Naïve Prostate Cancer and WST11

The replacement of WST09 with WST11 lead to several exploratory and phase II studies performed in the United States and Europe, the largest to date being the European trial PCM203 (11). In this prospective, open-label trial, 85 men with localized prostate cancer deemed suitable for active surveillance underwent either uni- or bilateral TS-VTP. They were assigned to 4 mg/kg or 6 mg/kg dosing (based on prostate volume), and illumination dose of 200 or 300 J/cm. Follow up was conducted with contrast-MRI at 1 week postprocedure and biopsy 6 months later. AEs were recorded along with quality-of-life (QoL) questionnaires, including International Prostate Symptom Score (IPSS) and International Index of Erectile Function-5 (IIEF-5). Sixty-one of the 83 men who underwent biopsy at 6 months were negative for cancer (74%). Analysis of the subset deemed to have received optimal treatment parameters (4 mg/kg TS, 200 J/cm, and unilateral VTP), revealed 38/46 or 83% had negative prostate biopsy at 6 months. Although 78% of patients had evidence of extraprostatic necrosis on 1-week MRI, none of these were associated with clinical sequelae. Overall, there were 5 serious adverse events related to the treatment: prostatitis (2 patients), hematuria (1 patient), epididymo-orchitis (1 patient), prostatic stricture (1 patient), and 2 serious adverse events related to the drug—ischemic optic neuropathy (1 patient) and inflammatory prostatic cyst (1 patient). An overall worsening of urinary symptoms was reported at 1-month post-VTP (as indicated by an increase of mean IPSS), but this improved to below baseline by 3 months post-VTP. Mean IIEF-5 score decreased modestly from 19.7 at baseline to 15.3 at 6 months, indicating a decline in overall erectile function (11). In addition to the promising efficacy and mild side-effect profile, TS-VTP treatment effects were predictable and well correlated with imaging assessment of tissue treatment volumetric data. A subgroup analysis of patients from PCM203 and an earlier phase II study, PCM201, demonstrated a satisfactory correlation between total energy delivered and volume of necrosis on 1 week MRI (R^2=0.78) (16).

The promising results from the phase 2 program have led to the ongoing phase III trials of WST11. PCM301, a randomized trial comparing TS-VTP to active surveillance, has completed patient accrual with >400 patients at the time of writing and awaits assessment of the primary trial endpoint of treatment efficacy in controlling measures of localized tumor growth and grade progression.

FUTURE STEPS

TS-VTP is capable of generating large or small regions of nonthermal tissue ablation with histologic analysis from animal studies demonstrating an intense inflammatory reaction isolated to treated areas (7). Further understanding of these secondary effects may prove important in further characterizing the mechanism of action and suitability of this treatment for other forms of malignancy. The oncologic benefit from PDT as a class of agents has long been established; in addition to local, acute control of the primary lesion, PDT has been known to confer improved survival over surgery alone (17), and has been shown anecdotally to generate spontaneous involution of metastatic lesions (18). Animal studies have highlighted the systemic antitumor protection conferred by VTP (7). Clinical trials capturing the immunologically mediated benefit of VTP on nonorgan-confined prostate cancer are expected in the near future as we await the results of treatment outcomes from accrued phase III trials in localized low-risk disease.

REFERENCES

1. Windahl T, Andersson SO, Lofgren L. Photodynamic therapy of localised prostatic cancer. *Lancet*. 1990;336(8723):1139.
2. Brun PH, DeGroot JL, Dickson EF, Farahani M, Pottier RH. Determination of the in vivo pharmacokinetics of palladium-bacteriopheophorbide (WST09) in EMT6 tumour-bearing Balb/c mice using graphite furnace atomic absorption spectroscopy. *Photochem Photobiol Sci*. 2004;3(11–12):1006–1010.
3. Weersink RA, Forbes J, Bisland S, et al. Assessment of cutaneous photosensitivity of TOOKAD (WST09) in preclinical animal models and in patients. *Photochem Photobiol*. 2005;81(1):106–113.
4. Ashur I, Goldschmidt R, Pinkas I, et al. Photocatalytic generation of oxygen radicals by the water-soluble bacteriochlorophyll derivative WST11, noncovalently bound to serum albumin. *J Phys Chem A*. 2009;113(28):8027–8037.
5. Coleman J, Scherz A. Focal therapy of localised prostate cancer by vascular targeted photodynamic therapy with WST-11 (TOOKAD® Soluble). *Eur Urol Rev*. 2012;7(2):106–108.
6. Madar-Balakirski N, Tempel-Brami C, Kalchenko V, et al. Permanent occlusion of feeding arteries and draining veins in solid mouse tumors by vascular targeted photodynamic therapy (VTP) with Tookad. *PLoS One*. 2010;5(4):e10282.
7. Preise D, Oren R, Glinert I, et al. Systemic antitumor protection by vascular-targeted photodynamic therapy involves cellular and humoral immunity. *Cancer Immunol Immunother*. 2009;58(1):71–84.
8. Trachtenberg J, Bogaards A, Weersink RA, et al. Vascular targeted photodynamic therapy with palladium-bacteriopheophorbide photosensitizer for recurrent prostate cancer following definitive radiation therapy: assessment of safety and treatment response. *J Urol*. 2007;178(5):1974–1979; discussion 1979.
9. Eymerit-Morin C, Zidane M, Lebdai S, Triau S, Azzouzi AR, Rousselet MC. Histopathology of prostate tissue after vascular-targeted photodynamic therapy for localized prostate cancer. *Virchows Arch*. 2013;463(4):547–552.
10. Kimm S, Gerber, D, Wimmer, D, et al. Histologic characterization and comparison of ablations produced by irreversible electroporation, vascular targeted photodynamic therapy, radiofrequency ablation, and cryotherapy: implications for focal therapy. *J Urol*. 2013;189(4):e579.
11. Azzouzi AR, Barret E, Moore CM, et al. TOOKAD® Soluble Vascular Targeted Photodynamic (VTP) therapy: determination of optimal treatment conditions and assessment of effects in patients with localised prostate cancer. *BJU Int*. 2013;112:766–774.
12. Trachtenberg J, Weersink RA, Davidson SR, et al. Vascular-targeted photodynamic therapy (padoporfin, WST09) for recurrent prostate cancer after failure of external beam radiotherapy: a study of escalating light doses. *BJU Int*. 2008;102(5):556–562.
13. Davidson SR, Weersink RA, Haider MA, et al. Treatment planning and dose analysis for interstitial photodynamic therapy of prostate cancer. *Phys Med Biol*. 2009;54(8):2293–2313.
14. Tarin T, Kimm S, Zhao P, et al. Photothermal effect in vascular targeted photodynamic therapy. *J Urol*. 2012;187(4):e609.
15. Moore CM, Mark Emberton M. *Photodynamic Therapy for Early Prostate Cancer, in Imaging and Focal Therapy of Early Prostate Cancer*. New York, NY: Springer; 2013:283–295.
16. Azzouzi A, Barret E, Villers A, et al. 86 Results of TOOKAD® Soluble Vascular Targeted Photodynamic Therapy (vtP) for low risk loCalized Prostate CanCer (PCM201/PCM203). *Eur Urol Suppl*. 2011;10(2):54.
17. Schreiber S, Gross S, Brandis A, et al. Local photodynamic therapy (PDT) of rat C6 glioma xenografts with Pd-bacteriopheophorbide leads to decreased metastases and increase of animal cure compared with surgery. *Int J Cancer*. 2002;99(2):279–285.
18. Thong PS, Ong KW, Goh NS, et al. Photodynamic-therapy-activated immune response against distant untreated tumours in recurrent angiosarcoma. *Lancet Oncol*. 2007;8(10):950–952.

11.4 Laser Ablative Techniques for Prostate Cancer

ASHLEY G. WINTER

JONATHAN A. COLEMAN

■ MECHANISM OF ACTION

Lasers have been widely utilized in the management of benign prostatic hypertrophy for their safety and precision of energy delivery (1). With these principles in mind, laser ablation of prostate cancer has become an area of interest(2). Several terms in the literature refer to the process of laser-based prostate cancer ablation: focal laser ablation (FLA), laser interstitial photocoagulation, photo-thermal therapy, or laser interstitial tumor therapy (2). FLA has three inherent qualities: (a) it is focal—FLA can be targeted using fiberoptics to create discreet lesions within tissues and organs including those that may be visualized on MRI, (b) it requires real-time MR thermographic imaging in order to create a large enough lesion while avoiding damage to surrounding organs, and (c) it utilizes a thermal based mechanism for tissue ablation(3). The first two topics will be addressed in the "Delivery" section of this chapter, while the third is discussed here. Briefly, when radiant energy (emitted by a surgically placed laser) is absorbed by tissue chromophores, rapid heating occurs along with subsequent tissue damage (2, 4). When heated to temperatures above 60°C, instantaneous tissue coagulation occurs (5–7). At supraphysiologic temperatures below 60°C, longer heating periods are required to cause cellular damage. The intrinsic lytic enzymes of cells heated to these temperatures become denatured and complete histologic effects are not seen until 48 to 72 hours after treatment, when digestion by inflammatory cells occurs (8). FLA generally results in a combination of these two types of thermal effects, with delayed tissue damage occurring at the periphery of lesions (8). For this reason, thermal damage planning and preoperative modeling have become key elements of this therapy (9).

■ DELIVERY

A number of unique systems have been employed in clinical studies to date, but there are unifying features throughout (2, 10–16). Qualifying patients generally have a solitary focus of disease (detected on transrectal ultrasound-guided prostate biopsy [TRUSBx]), and a clearly identifiable corresponding lesion on multiparametric prostate MRI (16). Patients are administered anesthesia and placed in the dorsal lithotomy position. Using a brachytherapy type grid and open-ended obturators, between 1 and 3 lasers are placed transperineally into the target lesion (2). Initial laser placement and subsequent ablation are conducted under image guidance. In several studies, MRI is used in real time (12, 14, 16). Other studies use 3-dimensional (3D) contrast-enhanced ultrasound (CEUS) with an onlay of preoperative MRI images (10, 11). Given the poor resolution of CEUS in delineating and localizing tumors relative to MRI, when using CEUS the ablation zone is intentionally overestimated (11). Using either a 805 nm (Diomed diode laser) (2), 830 nm (Indigo diode laser) (10, 11), or 980 nm (Visualase diode laser) (12, 15), the prostate is heated and the lesion created. Ablation is terminated when a target temperature and affected volume has been created based on either fluoroptic temperature probe feedback (10) or real-time MRI thermometry (15). Between 2880 and 5900 J are delivered to the prostate over 500 to 700 s (11, 13, 17). Following treatment, the lasers are removed and the procedure terminated.

■ CLINICAL TRIALS

The use of FLA in prostate cancer ablation was first reported by Amin et al. in 1993 (18). They performed FLA in one 65-year-old male with a focal recurrence following external beam radiation. Under TRUS and CT guidance, three laser fibers were inserted transperineally through 18-gauge needles. An 805 nm diode laser was activated

Conflict of Interest: Jonathan Coleman, MD is a consultant for AngioDynamics.

at 2W for 500 s, developing a gradually enlarging echogenic zone. Ten days postprocedure, biopsy revealed persistent tumor in the anterior zone, and the procedure was repeated. The patient tolerated the procedure without serious adverse events (18).

Since the initial experience, several small-scale studies have been conducted, none enrolling more than 12 patients (2). In 2009, Linder et al. (11) reported on the treatment of 12 men with biopsy-proven, low-risk prostate cancer with FLA. Patients were between 51 and 62 years old, had clinical stage T1c, and a mean PSA of 5.7 ng/mL. While in lithotomy position under general anesthesia, 1 or 2 Indigo Optima® laser fibers were inserted under real-time guidance of 3D CEUS with MRI based fusion images. MRI was not used in real time. Fluoroptic temperature probes were placed at the expected ablation boundaries to ensure a temperature >55°C. Patients were followed with 7 day posttreatment MRI and CEUS, 3- to 6-month posttreatment biopsy, and serial International Prostate Symptom Score (I-PSS) and International Index of Erectile Function (IIEF-5) assessments (11). Despite an ablated lesion size on average 12 times larger than the tumor, there was only an approximate 53% overlap in pretreatment and posttreatment MRI. In follow-up, six patients had negative biopsies, two patients had disease in the lobe contralateral to FLA, and four had disease on the side of ablation. Poor correlation between image guidance and actual therapy was considered a main barrier to efficacy in these cases. All patients maintained similar IPSS and IIEF-5 scores prior to and following therapy (11). In a follow up study by the same group, four men received FLA one week prior to radical prostatectomy (13). Patients underwent MRI one week following FLA, on the day on their surgery. Correlation between the ablated region on MR-imaging and H&E was considered good, Pearson correlation $r = 0.79$, indicating that post-FLA imaging was a reasonably accurate indicator of localizing histologic effects (13).

In 2010 to 2011, several studies enrolling one to four patients using the Visualase diode laser (980 nm) were reported (12–15). Raz et al. (12) used MRI-guided fiber placement and real-time MR thermometry (Visualase system) to perform FLA in two patients. There were no major adverse events reported and 2-week posttreatment MRI showed no damage to the rectum or neurovascular bundles. Histopathologic posttreatment data was not provided (12). The same team subsequently described a case of robotic MRI-guided FLA in one patient (14).

In the most recent clinical report of FLA, Oto et al. treated nine patients, 52 to 77 years of age, with low- or intermediate-risk prostate cancer (16). Using the Visualase system, the authors performed FLA under real-time MRI imaging and MR thermal imaging. There were no immediate complications, and the procedure was performed under conscious sedation over a 2.5- to 4-hour period. Average urinary and sexual function scores were not significantly changed from baseline at 1, 3, or 6 months postprocedure (16). At 6 month postoperative biopsy, seven patients had no cancer detected, and two patients (22%) had Gleason 3+3 disease. Retrospective review of these patients revealed incomplete coverage of the lesion site by the surgical ablation zone (16). There are currently two additional phase I/II clinical trials of FLA recruiting patients, NCT01377753 and NCT01094665, with no results yet reported.

■ FUTURE STEPS

While promising, FLA is still an exploratory technology for prostate cancer management that takes advantage of advanced MR imaging techniques for therapeutic targeting of discreet tumors within the gland. Larger clinical trials are necessary to validate its treatment outcomes in regard to thermal toxicity relative to increasing volumes of treated tissue that would be needed for larger tumors and cancers located close to critical structures. As discordance between preoperative planning and actual treatment zone appear responsible for most treatment failures, optimization of these technologies is also of critical interest in future development.

■ REFERENCES

1. Issa MM. The evolution of laser therapy in the treatment of benign prostatic hyperplasia. *Rev Urol.* 2005;7(suppl 9):S15.
2. Colin P, Mordon S, Nevoux P, et al. Focal laser ablation of prostate cancer: definition, needs, and future. *Adv Urol.* 2012;2012:589160.
3. Coleman JA, Scardino PT. Targeted prostate cancer ablation: energy options. *Curr Opin Urol.* 2013;23(2):123–128.
4. Mordon S, WassmeR B, Reynaud JP, Zemmouri J, et al. Mathematical modeling of laser lipolysis. *Biomed Eng Online.* 2008;7(1):10.
5. Heisterkamp JR, van Hillegersberg R, IJzermans JN. Critical temperature and heating time for coagulation damage: implications for interstitial laser coagulation (ILC) of tumors. *Lasers Surg Med.* 1999;25(3):257–262.
6. Colin P, Nevoux P, Marqa M, et al. Focal laser interstitial thermotherapy (LITT) at 980 nm for prostate cancer: treatment feasibility in Dunning R3327-AT2 rat prostate tumour. *BJU Int.* 2012;109(3):452–458.
7. Van Nimwegen S, L'Eplattenier HF, Rem AI, van der Lugt JJ, Kirpensteijn J. Nd: YAG surgical laser effects in canine prostate tissue: temperature and damage distribution. *Phys Med Biol.* 2009;54(1):29.
8. Peters RD, Chan E, Trachtenberg J, et al. Magnetic resonance thermometry for predicting thermal damage: an application of interstitial laser coagulation in an in vivo canine prostate model. *Magn Reson Med.* 2000;44(6):873–883.

9. Marqa M-F, Colin P, Nevoux P, Mordon SR, Betrouni N. Focal laser ablation of prostate cancer: numerical simulation of temperature and damage distribution. *Biomed Eng Online*. 2011;10(1):45.
10. Atri M, Gertner MR, Haider MA, Weersink RA, Trachtenberg J. Contrast-enhanced ultrasonography for real-time monitoring of interstitial laser thermal therapy in the focal treatment of prostate cancer. *Can Urol Assoc J*. 2009;3(2):125.
11. Lindner U, Weersink RA, Haider MA, et al. Image guided photothermal focal therapy for localized prostate cancer: phase I trial. *J Urol*. 2009;182(4):1371–1377.
12. Raz O, Haider MA, Davidson SR, et al. Real-time magnetic resonance imaging–guided focal laser therapy in patients with low-risk prostate cancer. *Eur Urol*. 2010;58(1):173–177.
13. Lindner U, Lawrentschuk N, Weersink RA, et al. Focal laser ablation for prostate cancer followed by radical prostatectomy: validation of focal therapy and imaging accuracy. *Eur Urol*. 2010;57(6):1111–1114.
14. Lindner U, Louis AS, Colquhoun AJ, et al. First robotic magnetic resonance-guided laser focal therapy for prostate cancer: a case report and review of the literature. *Int Oncol Soc J*. 2011;1(1):69–77.
15. Woodrum DA, Mynderse LA, Gorny KR, Amrami KK, McNichols RJ, Callstrom MR. 3.0 T MR-guided laser ablation of a prostate cancer recurrence in the postsurgical prostate bed. *J Vasc Int Radiol*. 2011;22(7):929–934.
16. Oto A, Sethi I, Karczmar G, et al. MR imaging-guided focal laser ablation for prostate cancer: phase I trial. *Radiology*. 2013;267(3):932–940.
17. Lindner U, Lawrentschuk N, Weersink RA, et al. Construction and evaluation of an anatomically correct multi-image modality compatible phantom for prostate cancer focal ablation. *J Urol*. 2010;184(1):352–357.
18. Amin Z, Lees W, Bown S. Interstitial laser photocoagulation for the treatment of prostatic cancer. *Br J Radiol*. 1993;66(791):1044–1047.

11.5 Irreversible Electroporation (IRE) Prostate Ablation

ASHLEY G. WINTER

JONATHAN A. COLEMAN

■ MECHANISM OF ACTION

Within the past decade, irreversible electroporation (IRE) has emerged as a new tissue ablation technology. IRE is the application of nonthermal pulsed electrical fields to an organ/tumor of interest, resulting in irreversible cellular damage (1). Pulsed electrical fields cause nanoscale pores to develop on the cellular membrane (1). Specifically, charging of the plasma membrane results in destabilization; aqueous fingers then span the membrane and become lined by phospholipid head groups resulting in hydrophilic pores (2, 3). Following removal of the electrical stimulus, small pores reseal, whereas large pores persist, resulting in cell death (1). The aforementioned phenomenon marks the difference between *reversible* electroporation, commonly used for the introduction of genetic material and chemotherapeutics into cells, and *irreversible* electroporation, discussed in this chapter (4). The downstream pathways by which these critically large pores activate cell death have not been fully elucidated. Histopathologic analysis following IRE has appeared predominantly apoptotic in some studies (5) and mostly necrotic in others (6).

IRE as surgical ablative modality was first proposed by Davalos, Mir, and Rubinsky in 2005 (7). Using mathematical modeling, they demonstrated that it was possible to destroy clinically relevant tissue volumes using surgically placed electrodes. Furthermore, this could be done without detrimental thermal effects (7). Their critical hypothesis was that the nonthermal mechanism of IRE would lead to unique advantages over existing thermal ablative modalities (for instance, cryotherapy) (7). This hypothesis has been confirmed in subsequent animal and clinical studies, with several of the following findings. Lack of heat-sink effect tumoricidal efficacy near large arteries and veins may be dampened when using thermal-based mechanisms; IRE, on the other hand, appears unaltered by this phenomenon (8, 9). With preservation of the "tissue scaffold" by affecting only living cells, IRE leaves behind organ structural elements. This preservation enables rapid regeneration of functional tissues (10), permits nerve re-growth along intact myelin sheaths (11, 12), and preserves patency of vessels (13). Additionally, IRE creates a sharply demarcated region of treatment effect (8), permitting treatment of tumors abutting vital structures. Given its delicate anatomic relationship to erectile, bowel, and bladder function, the prostate may receive unique benefit from IRE-based ablation. This benefit is the impetus for ongoing investigations.

There is mixed evidence regarding whether or not IRE elicits a strong immunologic reaction. Al-Sakere et al saw negligible infiltration of immune cells following IRE ablation in a mouse sarcoma model (14), whereas Onik et al. found a marked reaction in the lymph nodes draining a canine prostate following IRE (15). Use of immune reactivity for systemic anti-tumorigenic potentiation is a target of future IRE research.

■ DELIVERY

IRE ablation of the prostate has yet to be carried out on a large clinical scale, but initial reports detail the procedure (16). Patients are placed in dorsal lithotomy position following induction of general anesthesia. Muscle paralysis is required to reduce the intense muscular contractions elicited by the intensity of the electrical stimulation on the pelvic musculature. In the method described by Onik et al, 18 g IRE electrodes were placed by transperineal template grid technique using biplanar transrectal ultrasound (TRUS) guidance (16). Based on the results of a preprocedural transperineal prostate-mapping biopsy, electrodes were oriented in a four-probe square array, centered on the cancerous lesion (16). Sets of 90 IRE pulses, 70 to 100 microseconds in length, were delivered at 1500 V between two electrodes at a time, and repeated until all paired electrode combinations were utilized. The electrodes are then removed and the procedure terminated.

Conflict of Interest: Jonathan Coleman, MD is a consultant for AngioDynamics.

A Foley catheter is placed preprocedurally and removed between postoperative day 0 and 3. Patients are typically discharged from the hospital on the day of therapy (16).

One consideration to IRE ablation of organs in proximity to the heart is the principle of cardiac synchronization. In the first clinical experience with IRE, four instances of ventricular arrhythmias occurred in a group of eight patients (17). Ventricular dysrhythmias did not occur when pulses were delivered during the refractory phase of the cardiac cycle (17), and IRE systems now incorporate cardiac synchronization (18). Still, occasional supraventricular arrhythmias have been reported when using synchronized devices (17, 19), and caution is advised in patients with known cardiac disease. The only commercially produced IRE system is the NanoKnife (AngioDynamics). The NanoKnife is currently FDA-approved for ablation of soft tissue.

■ IRE EXPERIENCE—PROSTATE

Exploratory Studies—In Vitro and In Vivo

As mentioned previously, the prostate is considered a meaningful target for IRE-based ablations due to the expected potency and continence preservation. Several preclinical studies have explored the treatment parameters associated with IRE of various prostate and prostate cancer models. Rubinsky et al. applied IRE in vitro to prostate cancer cells, finding that sets of 90 pulses, 100 microseconds in duration, at 250 V/cm would completely ablate prostate cancer without collateral thermal damage (20). Neal et al. studied the effect of brachytherapy seeds on IRE field distribution and histologic damage in canine models (21). They found that brachytherapy seeds did not significantly alter ablations or electrical properties, proposing the feasibility of salvage IRE in this setting (21). Using a mouse dorsal skinfold chamber implanted with human prostate cancer cells, Qin et al. measured the effects of IRE in a novel microvascular environment (22). Live tumor patches persisted following treatment, raising concerns that the electrical heterogeneity of tumors must be considered in future clinical applications (22).

Onik et al. performed a trial of IRE in canine prostate using a clinically relevant delivery modality (15). Six male beagles had 18-gauge electrodes placed transperineally into the prostate under TRUS guidance. Each subject underwent prostate hemi-ablation (at varying settings), along with a safety component that involved direct ablation to nearby sensitive structures, either urethra, rectum, or neurovascular bundles (15). At 1 day postablation, lesions were sharply demarcated, grossly hemorrhagic, and contained no viable glandular elements. When subject to direct ablation, both the urethra and rectum appeared unaffected. Despite demonstrating necrotic endothelial cells, the vessels of the neurovascular bundle remained patent and associated nerves appeared unaffected (15). At 2 weeks, hemorrhage had resolved and lesion volume reduced markedly in size (15).

Clinical Trials

The initial clinical experience with prostatic IRE ablation was described by Onik and Rubinsky in 2010 (16). Sixteen patients between the ages of 40 and 78 were treated using the procedure described earlier in this chapter. Seven patients had Gleason 6 disease, six had Gleason pattern 7, and three men had Gleason 8. Preprocedural prostate-specific antigen (PSA) ranged from 2.2 to 7 ng/mL. They were administered 6 sets of 90 IRE pulses, each 70–100 microseconds in length, at 1500 V. Intraoperative TRUS showed immediate mixed echogenicity in the treated areas. All patients had preserved continence. In two patients with bilateral ablations, there was a 6-month delay in return of potency; all other potent patients remained potent immediately following the procedure (16). One patient refused postoperative biopsy, but all other men underwent sampling known cancerous area. There was no residual cancer within any of the ablation zones. One patient had residual cancer on biopsy, but this was beyond the region of treatment effect. Histologic analysis showed no residual viable glandular elements in the treated areas. Interestingly, nerve bundles and vascular structures remained intact (16).

Another early experience with prostate IRE was reported by Dickinson et al. (23). Fifteen men between the ages of 48 and 73 received focal IRE therapy, nine as a primary treatment and six in the salvage setting. Of the six salvage patients, four had primarily been treated with HIFU and two with EBRT. Similar to the Onik series, patients had a range of low-, intermediate-, and high-risk disease (7%, 80%, and 13%, respectively). On multiparametric MRI, mean lesion size was 0.84 cc and mean ablative volume 10 cc. There were no intraoperative complications or serious adverse events. Mean PSA nadir was 3.3 from a preoperative of 5.9 ng/mL. All patients maintained potency and continence. No follow-up biopsy data was reported (23).

While these reports show promising safety and efficacy profiles, systematic, randomized trials are clearly needed. Several future and ongoing studies are registered with the National Institutes of Health. In NCT01790451, 16 men will undergo IRE 1 month prior to prostatectomy. Efficacy will be assessed from serial MRI and prostatectomy specimens. The other, NCT01726894, aims to assess the use of MRI in characterizing the IRE lesions, with an approximate 20 patient accrual. NCT01835977, which is not yet enrolling, is a multi-center trial that will randomize approximately 200 patients with unilateral Gleason 3+3 or Gleason 3+4 disease to either prostate hemi-ablation or whole-gland ablation.

FUTURE STEPS

The clear and immediate next step for the advancement of IRE in prostate cancer therapy is to establish the treatment parameters defining the boundaries of safety and toxicity associated with prostate treatment as a step toward trials of treatment efficacy in the settings of primary therapy or for salvage in previously treated patients. Large, multicenter randomized phase III studies may then be able to help define the benefits that this therapy may provide as a critical new tool in the management of this complex disease.

REFERENCES

1. Golberg A, Yarmush ML. Nonthermal irreversible electroporation: fundamentals, applications, and challenges. *IEEE Trans Biomed Eng.* 2013;60(3):707–714.
2. Böckmann RA, de Groot BL, Kakorin S, Neumann E, Grubmüller H. Kinetics, statistics, and energetics of lipid membrane electroporation studied by molecular dynamics simulations. *Biophys J.* 2008;95(4):1837–1850.
3. Weaver JC.> *Electroporation theory*, in *Animal Cell Electroporation and Electrofusion Protocols.* New York, NY: Springer; 1995:3–28.
4. Gehl J. Electroporation: theory and methods, perspectives for drug delivery, gene therapy and research. *Acta Physiol Scand.* 2003;177(4):437–447.
5. Guo Y, Zhang Y, Klein R, et al. Irreversible electroporation therapy in the liver: longitudinal efficacy studies in a rat model of hepatocellular carcinoma. *Cancer Res.* 2010;70(4):1555–1563.
6. José A, Sobrevals L, Ivorra A, Fillat C. Irreversible electroporation shows efficacy against pancreatic carcinoma without systemic toxicity in mouse models. *Cancer Lett.* 2012;317(1):16–23.
7. Davalos R, Mir L, Rubinsky B. Tissue ablation with irreversible electroporation. *Ann Biomed Eng.* 2005;33(2):223–231.
8. Charpentier KP, Wolf F, Noble L, Winn B, Resnick M, Dupuy DE. Irreversible electroporation of the liver and liver hilum in swine. *HPB (Oxford).* 2011;13(3):168–173.
9. Deodhar A, Monette S, Single GW Jr, et al. Renal tissue ablation with irreversible electroporation: preliminary results in a porcine model. *Urology.* 2011;77(3):754–760.
10. Lu DS, Kee ST, Lee EW. Irreversible electroporation: ready for prime time? *Tech Vasc Interv Radiol.* 2013;16(4):277–286.
11. Li W, Fan Q, Ji Z, Qiu X, Li Z. The effects of irreversible electroporation (IRE) on nerves. *PLoS One.* 2011;6(4):e18831.
12. Schoellnast H, Monette S, Ezell PC, et al. Acute and subacute effects of irreversible electroporation on nerves: experimental study in a pig model. *Radiology.* 2011;260(2):421–427.
13. Cannon R, Ellis S, Hayes D, Narayanan G, Martin RC 2nd. Safety and early efficacy of irreversible electroporation for hepatic tumors in proximity to vital structures. *J Surg Oncol.* 2013;107(5):544–549.
14. Al-Sakere B, Bernat C, Andre F, et al. A study of the immunological response to tumor ablation with irreversible electroporation. *Technol Cancer Res Treat.* 2007;6(4):301–306.
15. Onik G, Mikus P, Rubinsky B. Irreversible electroporation: implications for prostate ablation. *Technol Cancer Res Treat.* 2007;6(4):295–300.
16. Onik G, Rubinsky B. *Irreversible Electroporation: First Patient Experience Focal Therapy of Prostate Cancer*, in *Irreversible Electroporation.* New York, NY: Springer; 2010:235–247.
17. Thomson KR, Cheung W, Ellis SJ, et al. Investigation of the safety of irreversible electroporation in humans. *J Vasc Interv Radiol.* 2011;22(5):611–621.
18. Deodhar A, Dickfeld T, Single GW, et al. Irreversible electroporation near the heart: ventricular arrhythmias can be prevented with ECG synchronization. *AJR Am J Roentgenol.* 2011;196(3):W330–W335.
19. Pech M, Janitzky A, Wendler JJ, et al. Irreversible electroporation of renal cell carcinoma: a first-in-man phase I clinical study. *Cardiovasc Interv Radiol.* 2011;34(1):132–138.
20. Rubinsky J, Onik G, Mikus P, Rubinsky B. Optimal parameters for the destruction of prostate cancer using irreversible electroporation. *J Urol.* 2008;180(6):2668–2674.
21. Neal RE 2nd, Smith RL, Kavnoudias H, et al. The effects of metallic implants on electroporation therapies: feasibility of irreversible electroporation for brachytherapy salvage. *Cardiovasc Intervent Radiol.* 2013;36(6):1638–1645.
22. Qin Z, Jiang J, Long G, Lindgren B, Bischof JC. Irreversible electroporation: an in vivo study with dorsal skin fold chamber. *Ann Biomed Eng.* 2013;41(3):619–629.
23. Dickinson C, Valerio M, Ahmed HU, Freeman A, Allen C, Emberton M. 584 Early clinical experience of focal therapy for localised prostate cancer using irreversible electroporation. *Eur Urol Suppl.* 2013;12(1):e584–e584.

12.1 Quality of Life With Surgery

ALANA M. MURPHY
PATRICK J. SHENOT

■ INTRODUCTION

Radical prostatectomy (RP) offers excellent long-term prostate cancer control (1). Although no consensus has been reached regarding an absolute survival advantage associated with RP versus watchful waiting, a randomized study of 695 Scandinavian men demonstrated a survival benefit with RP even with low-risk cancers if the men were less than 65 years old (2). Recent data extracted from the Cancer of the Prostate Strategic Urological Research Endeavor (CaPSURE) database indicated that RP accounts for the treatment choice in approximately 50% of newly diagnosed clinically localized prostate cancer (3). Although the number of men undergoing prostate cancer screening and subsequent treatment may decrease in the wake of the recent scrutiny of prostate cancer screening, the proportion of newly diagnosed men who elect to undergo a RP will likely remain relatively high. In order to improve patient counseling and postoperative expectations, clinicians who treat men with prostate cancer should be well versed in the potential quality of life (QoL) changes associated with RP.

Assessment of treatment-related morbidity has become an increasingly important topic in clinical research and is a particularly relevant focus as the urologic community is criticized for the treatment of indolent prostate cancer. Historically, studies investigating QoL after RP have lacked validated metrics and baseline functional assessments from which to draw postoperative comparisons. The use of validated QoL metrics is of paramount importance, since urologists have been shown to consistently underestimate impairment in QoL domains after prostate cancer treatment (4, 5). Despite the absence of robust QoL studies, the functional changes after RP are well described in the literature.

■ ERECTILE DYSFUNCTION

Sexual function is the QoL domain most commonly impaired after RP (6, 7). Postoperative sexual function depends on several factors, including age, preoperative erectile function, and degree of nerve sparing. Nerve sparing RP was first described by Walsh and Donker in 1982 (8). Since the importance of neurovascular bundle preservation was recognized, the technique of nerve sparing has been refined and is now the preferred dissection method for potent patients with locally confined prostate cancer. Despite refinement of surgical technique, the reported rates of postoperative potency rates vary largely from 31% to 86% for men with localized disease undergoing bilateral nerve sparing RP (9). The significant discrepancy in postoperative potency rates is due to variable definitions of potency, various metrics for reporting potency and heterogeneous patient populations. While data from high-volume RP centers has reported potency rates of 78% to 86%, data from a community based study reported a potency rate of only 44% (10, 12). Although the majority of men who achieve postoperative erectile function do so in the first 6 months, a smaller number of men may experience improvement in erectile function up to 4 years following RP (13).

Management options for erectile dysfunction (ED) following RP include oral phosphodiesterase-5 (PDE-5) inhibitors, vacuum-assisted erection devices, intraurethral alprostadil, penile injection therapy (prostaglandin E1, papaverine, phentolamine), and insertion of a penile prosthesis. Oral pharmacologic therapy should be the first line treatment, followed by more invasive treatment modalities. Although men prefer noninvasive treatments to address postoperative ED, invasive treatments in the form of injection therapy and penile implants are associated with higher efficacy rates (14).

Penile rehabilitation regimens have been developed to speed the return of erectile function and to reduce the rates of postoperative ED. Treatment regimens are highly variable but typically include either isolated oral pharmacotherapy or a combination of PDE-5 inhibitors, vacuum-assisted devices, intraurethral suppositories, and injection therapy. While earlier regimens employed regular use of PDE-5 inhibitors, more recent data suggests that on-demand dosing may provide similar efficacy. In a randomized, double blind trial of 628 men who underwent bilateral nerve sparing RP, there was no significant difference in sexual function between men who took nightly vardenafil versus men who took vardenafil on demand for 9 months (15). Both treatment groups demonstrated superior erectile function rates compared to a placebo group. Implementation of penile rehabilitation regimens has become widespread. A survey of International Society of Sexual Medicine members indicated that 87% utilized penile rehabilitation, with oral PDE-5 inhibitors being the most common treatment modality (16).

As the most common impairment in QoL following RP, ED should be a primary focus of the preoperative counseling session when patients are considering RP. The physician should provide a realistic expectation of postoperative ED and outline treatment options to facilitate the return of erectile function to allow for informed medical decision making on the part of the patient. Similar to oncologic parameters following RP, a nomogram has been developed as a counseling tool to help physicians provide an individualized prediction of postoperative erectile function based on preoperative characteristics (17).

■ URINARY INCONTINENCE

Postprostatectomy urinary incontinence (PPUI) largely refers to stress urinary incontinence (SUI) due to intrinsic sphincter deficiency, with a minority of men experiencing de novo urgency urinary incontinence (UUI) or mixed urinary incontinence after RP. Regardless of the mechanism of UI, studies have demonstrated that UI following RP has a negative impact on QoL (18, 19). Similar to postoperative potency rates, PPUI rates vary considerably due to the lack of a standard definition of UI and heterogeneous patient populations. A stringent definition of postprostatectomy continence does not even allow for use of a safety pad, which is in line with evidence that any degree of pad usage is associated with significantly greater patient bother than no pad utilization (20). Postprostatectomy continence also improves over time and the rates of PPUI depend on the interval from RP. A number of single surgeon series have reported continence rates in excess of 90%, while other multi-institutional series have reported rates in the range of 66% to 72% (12, 21–23).

Although the majority of men who experience some degree of postoperative UI will not seek treatment, there are available options for motivated patients who are significantly bothered by their PPUI. Studies indicate that between 8% and 20% of men who undergo an RP will ultimately undergo treatment for PPUI (19, 24, 25). Since postprostatectomy continence can significantly improve within the first year following RP, conservative management in the form of pelvic floor muscle training is an appropriate first line therapy. The management of postprostatectomy UUI would mimic overactive bladder guidelines, including behavioral modification followed by antimuscarinic therapy (26).

If bothersome SUI persists, then more invasive treatment modalities are warranted to improve QoL. Urethral bulking agents offer a minimally invasive endoscopic treatment option but success rates have been cited as low as 20% (27). Male slings have gained popularity since 1998, when Schaeffer et al. reported a 75% success rate with a male sling at 16 months (28). Although male slings have been widely adopted as a minimally invasive technique for treating PPUI, the artificial urinary sphincter (AUS) remains the gold standard. In a long-term retrospective series of 124 consecutive men undergoing AUS implantation, 27% of men were able to stop wearing pads and 52% used 1 pad per day (29).

■ ROBOTIC-ASSISTED RADICAL PROSTATECTOMY (RARP) VERSUS RETROPUBIC RADICAL PROSTATECTOMY (RRP)

RARP, first introduced in 2001, has been both widely adopted by urologists and embraced by patients seeking improved perioperative and postoperative outcomes (30). Comparison of functional outcomes after RARP and RRP is hindered by a lack of randomized surgical series or well-designed prospective cohort studies. Despite these limitations, there is convincing evidence that RARP is associated with superior postoperative erectile function compared to RRP. A number of prospective single-institution studies have demonstrated higher potency rates and shorter times to potency following RARP, and one systematic review reported mean potency rates at 12 months of 79% and 92% for RRP and RARP, respectively (31–33). In contrast to the favorable data regarding erectile function after RARP, studies focusing on return of continence have reported more variable outcomes regarding a durable advantage for RARP over RRP. A single institution study from a high volume prostate cancer center demonstrated no significant difference in continence rates at 12 months between RARP and RRP (92% vs. 94%, $P = .34$) (34). However, a recent meta-analysis comparing postoperative continence rates found that men undergoing RARP were more likely to achieve urinary continence at 12 months than men undergoing RRP (OR 1.53, $P = .03$) (35).

CONCLUSION

RP is a mainstay of treatment for localized prostate cancer; however, excellent cancer control may be achieved at the expense of adverse QoL outcomes. A thorough discussion of health related QoL factors, such as postoperative ED and PPUI, should be included in the preoperative treatment planning. In order to facilitate a balanced discussion, physicians offering RP as a treatment modality should be well versed in the potential impact on QoL. Finally, future research studies should continue to focus on QoL parameters following RP using validated instruments and comparing the impact on QoL associated with various prostate cancer treatments.

REFERENCES

1. Boorjian SA, Eastham JA, Graefen M, et al. A critical analysis of the long-term impact of radical prostatectomy on cancer control and function outcomes. *Eur Urol.* 2012;6(4):664–675.
2. Bill-Axelson A, Holmberg L, Ruutu M, et al. Radical prostatectomy versus watchful waiting in early prostate cancer. *N Engl J Med.* 2011;364(18):1708–1717.
3. Cooperberg MR, Broering JM, Carroll PR. Time trends and local variation in primary treatment of localized prostate cancer. *J Clin Oncol.* 2010;28(7):1117–1123.
4. Litwin MS, Lubeck DP, Henning JM, et al. Differences in urologist and patient assessments of health related quality of life in men with prostate cancer: results of the CaPSURE database. *J Urol.* 1998;159(6):1988–1992.
5. Cooperberg MR, Master VA, Carroll PR. Health related quality of life significance of single pad urinary incontinence following radical prostatectomy. *J Urol.* 2003;170 (2, pt 1):512–515.
6. Sanda MG, Dunn RL, Michalski J, et al. Quality of life and satisfaction with outcome among prostate-cancer survivors. *N Engl J Med.* 2008;358(12):1250–1261.
7. Madalinska JB, Essink Bot ML, de Koning HJ, et al. Health-related quality-of-life effects of radical prostatectomy and primary radiotherapy for screen-detected or clinically diagnosed localized prostate cancer. *J Clin Oncol.* 2001;19(6):1619–1628.
8. Walsh PC, Donker PJ. Impotence following radical prostatectomy: insight into etiology and prevention. *J Urol.* 1982;128(3):492–497.
9. Dubbelman YD, Dohle GR, Schroder FH. Sexual function before and after radical retropubic prostatectomy: a systematic review of prognostic indicators for a successful outcome. *Eur Urol.* 2006;50(4):711–718.
10. Kundu SD, Roehl KA, Eggener SE, et al. Potency, continence and complications in 3,477 consecutive radical retropubic prostatectomies. *J Urol.* 2004;172 (6, pt 1):2227–2231.
11. Stanford JL, Feng Z, Hamilton AS, et al. Urinary and sexual function after radical prostatectomy for clinically localized prostate cancer: the Prostate Cancer Outcomes Study. *JAMA.* 2000;283(3):354–360.
12. Walsh PC, Marschke P, Ricker D, et al. Patient-reported urinary continence and sexual function after anatomic radical prostatectomy. *Urology.* 2000;55(1):58–61.
13. Glickman L, Godoy G, Lepor H. Changes in continence and erectile function between 2 and 4 years after radical prostatectomy. *J Urol.* 2009;181(2):731–735.
14. Schover LR, Fouladi RT, Warneke CL, et al: The use of treatments for erectile dysfunction among survivors of prostate carcinoma. *Cancer.* 2002;95(11):2397–2407.
15. Montorsi F, Brock G, Lee J, et al. Effect of nightly versus on-demand vardenafil on recovery of erectile function in men following bilateral nerve-sparing radical prostatectomy. *Eur Urol.* 2008;54(4):924–931.
16. Teloken P, Mesquita G, Montorsi F, et al. Post-radical prostatectomy pharmacological penile rehabilitation: practice patterns among the international society for sexual medicine practitioners. *J Sex Med.* 2009;6(7):2032–2038.
17. Alemozaffar M, Regan MM, Cooperberg MR, et al. Prediction of erectile function following treatment for prostate cancer. *JAMA.* 2011;306(11):1205–1214.
18. Miller DC, Sanda MG, Dunn RL, et al. Long-term outcomes among localized prostate cancer survivors: health-related quality-of-life changes after radical prostatectomy, external radiation, and brachytherapy. *J Clin Oncol.* 2005; 23(12):2772–2780.
19. Penson DF, McLerran D, Feng Z, et al. 5-year urinary and sexual outcomes after radical prostatectomy: results from the Prostate Cancer Outcomes Study. *J Urol.* 2008;179(5 suppl):S40–S44.
20. Wallerstedt A, Carlsson S, Nilsson AE, et al. Pad use and patient reported bother from urinary leakage after radical prostatectomy. *J Urol.* 2012;187(1):196–200.
21. Lepor H, Kaci L, Xue X. Continence following radical retropubic prostatectomy using self-reporting instruments. *J Urol.* 2004;171(3):1212–1215.
22. Kao TC, Cruess DF, Garner D, et al. Multicenter patient self-reporting questionnaire on impotence, incontinence and stricture after radical prostatectomy. *J Urol.* 2000;163(3):858–864.
23. Moul JW, Mooneyhan RM, Kao TC, et al. Preoperative and operative factors to predict incontinence, impotence and stricture after radical prostatectomy. *Prostate Cancer Prostatic Dis.* 1998;1(5):242–249.
24. Begg CB, Riedel ER, Bach PB, et al. Variations in morbidity after radical prostatectomy. *N Engl J Med.* 2002;346:1138.
25. Stanford JL, Feng Z, Hamilton AS, et al. Urinary and sexual function after radical prostatectomy for clinically localized prostate cancer: the Prostate Cancer Outcomes Study. *JAMA* 2000;283(3):354–360.
26. Gormley EA, Lightner DJ, Burgio KL, et al. *Diagnosis and Treatment of Overactive Bladder (non-neurogenic) in Adults: AUA/SUFU Guideline.* http://www.auanet.org/common/pdf/education/clinical-guidance/Overactive-Bladder.pdf. Updated 2012. Accessed December 15, 2013.
27. Westney OL, Bevan-Thomas R, Palmer JL, et al. Transurethral collagen injections for male intrinsic sphincter deficiency: the University of Texas-Houston experience. *J Urol.* 2005;174(3):994–997.
28. Schaeffer AJ, Clemens JQ, Ferrari M, et al. The male bulbourethral sling procedure for post-radical prostatectomy incontinence. *J Urol.* 1998;159(5):1510–1515.
29. Kim SP, Sarmast Z, Daignault S, et al. Long-term durability and functional outcomes among patients with artificial urinary sphincters: a 10-year retrospective review from the University of Michigan. *J Urol.* 2008;179(5):1912–1916.
30. Pasticier G, Rietbergen JB, Guillonneau B, et al. Robotically assisted laparoscopic radical prostatectomy: feasibility study in men. *Eur Urol.* 2001;40(1):70–74.
31. Di Pierro GB, Baumeister P, Stucki P, et al. A prospective trial comparing consecutive series of open retropubic and robot-assisted laparoscopic radical prostatectomy in a centre with a limited caseload. *Eur Urol.* 2011;59(1):1–6.
32. Tewari A, Srivasatava A, Menon M et al. A prospective comparison of radical retropubic and robot-assisted prostatectomy: experience in one institution. *BJU Int.* 2003;92(3):205–210.

33. Coelho RF, Rocco B, Patel MB, et al. Retropubic, laparoscopic, and robot-assisted radical prostatectomy: a critical review of outcomes reported by high-volume centers. *J Endourol.* 2010;24(12):2003–2015.
34. Krambeck AE, DiMarco DS, Rangel LJ, et al. Radical prostatectomy for prostatic adenocarcinoma: a matched comparison of open retropubic and robot-assisted techniques. *BJU Int.* 2009;103(4):448–453.
35. Ficarra V, Novara G, Rosen RC et al. Systematic review and meta-analysis of studies reporting urinary continence recovery after robot-assisted radical prostatectomy. *Eur Urol.* 2012;62(3):405–417.

12.2 Quality of Life With Androgen Deprivation Therapy

ALANA M. MURPHY
PATRICK J. SHENOT

■ INTRODUCTION

Androgen deprivation therapy (ADT) is most commonly utilized as first-line treatment for symptomatic metastatic prostate cancer, as neoadjuvant therapy combined with radiation therapy, and for biochemical relapse after surgery or radiation (1). Historically, approximately 40% of patients diagnosed with prostate cancer will receive ADT within 6 months of diagnosis and nearly 50% of treated prostate cancer patients receive ADT at some point in their disease course (2, 3). These trends have led to increasing numbers of patients treated with ADT for disease management over longer periods of time. ADT is associated with a number of physical side-effects, including hot flashes, decreased libido, fatigue, decreased bone and muscle mass, increased total body fat content, possible harmful metabolic and cardiovascular effects, and cognitive defects. The constellation of these side effects associated with castrate levels of testosterone, termed the "androgen deprivation syndrome," may have profound effects on physical, sexual, and social functioning resulting in a dramatic impact on overall quality of life (QoL) (4).

QoL is a broad term that reflects a patient's overall subjective assessment of emotional and physical well-being. ADT may contribute to psychological distress on the partners of prostate cancer patients. QoL is, for many men, just as important as survival. QoL concerns are often a fundamental factor in prostate cancer treatment decision making.

■ HOT FLASHES

Hot flashes are among the most common and early described side effects of ADT. They are characterized by the sensation of intense warmth and subsequent cooling, flushing of the skin, perspiration, and chills which typically involve the neck and face. Associated symptoms may include anxiety and palpitations. Hot flashes are believed to be caused by peripheral vasodilation resulting from inappropriate stimulation of thermoregulatory centers in the hypothalamus (5). The severity of these symptoms range from mild to pervasive, but may result in a significant effect on daily functioning and QoL (6). The incidence of hot flashes, which approaches 15% in uncastrated men, is reported in 80% in men treated with ADT (7). The significance of hot flashes is not only physical, but may be psychological as well, and may be a significant source of distress in prostate cancer patients.

■ SEXUAL DYSFUNCTION

Castrate levels of testosterone can result in changes in both sexual desire (libido) and erectile function. The overwhelming majority of men under ADT will develop some degree of erectile dysfunction due to the lack of androgens. The Prostate Cancer Outcomes Study found that 80% of the men who were potent before ADT treatment lost their potency after treatment (8). Age greater than 70 and the presence of diabetes mellitus are the two most important predictive factors for ED following ADT (9). Sexual dysfunction can negatively impact the self-esteem, self-perception, and QoL of younger, sexually active men who may also experience ADT-related changes in body fat and muscle distribution (10).

■ CHANGES IN BODY COMPOSITION

ADT may negatively impact on psychosocial well-being by causing feminization, characterized by decreased muscle mass, weight gain, altered fat distribution in a postmenopausal female pattern, and body hair loss. Gynecomastia is strongly associated with negative body image perception (11, 12). Men with gynecomastia may employ coping techniques characterized by disguise and avoidance strategies resulting in social isolation (13, 14).

Diminished testicular volume and the loss of penile length related to ADT can diminish sexual self-esteem (15, 16). Efforts to educate patients and their partners about treatment side effects and coping strategies should be employed in patients undergoing ADT.

SKELETAL MORBIDITY

Bone maintenance is an androgen-mediated processes. Approximately one-third of prostate cancer patients have a pre-existing low bone mineral density (BMD) before starting ADT (17, 18). ADT accelerates bone loss and low BMD is strongly associated with an increased risk of fracture. Once ADT has been initiated, the risk of hip fracture increases progressively from the first year, reaching a relative risk of 4% in those patients who have received ADT for more than 5 years (18). The risk of bone fracture cumulatively increases with the duration of ADT starting from 5% at 5 years after the initiation of ADT and reaching nearly 20% by 10 years after the initiation of ADT (19, 20).

Other factors may account for the high fracture rates in men receiving ADT androgen deprivation including increased fall risk due to metastatic disease and to treatment-related frailty. While the relative contributions of these factors have not been adequately characterized, treatment-related changes in BMD remain after adjustment for known confounders and appear sufficient to explain the increase in fracture risk in men with prostate cancer.

METABOLIC SYNDROME AND CARDIOVASCULAR MORBIDITY

Obesity, insulin resistance, and increased triglycerides are common ADT-related metabolic changes that overlap with features of the metabolic syndrome (21). This syndrome is clearly associated with an increased risk of death as a result of myocardial infarction, even in the absence of recognized known cardiovascular disease or diabetes mellitus (22).

A high frequency of cardiovascular disease has been observed in men treated with ADT. The use of ADT is associated with earlier onset of fatal myocardial infarctions in men aged 65 years or older who are treated for 6 months when compared with men who are not treated with ADT (23). The association between ADT and cardiovascular morbidity is hypothesized to be mediated through changes in lipoproteins, arterial stiffness, and QT interval prolongation (24–26). The decision as to whether or not to initiate ADT in patients with cardiac disease should be weighed against any possible risks.

PSYCHOLOGICAL AND COGNITIVE EFFECTS

ADT has been associated with changes in mood, cognitive function, and self-esteem while also negatively effecting memory and attention (27). Cognitive side effects are apparent almost immediately, as shown in a recent 3-month neoadjuvant trial and appear to be reversible after completing treatment; however, sometimes the effects are only partly reversible at 1 year (28). There is evidence of an increased occurrence of anxiety, depression, diminished body image perception, and sleep disturbances in prostate cancer patients undergoing adjuvant AD (29). The relationship between androgen deprivation and depression is supported by studies in hypogonadal men without prostate cancer. Low testosterone is associated with depression and testosterone replacement appears to reduce depressive symptoms in these patients.

IMPACT ON INTIMACY

Prostate cancer may result in significant relationship distress that is compounded by side effects of ADT. Partners of prostate cancer patients may experience more distress than those affected (30). Couples may utilize conflicting coping methods leading to isolation of either or both partners (31). Some partners may experience less attraction to their partner on ADT and some ADT-treated men may doubt their own attractiveness (32). Clinicians working with men diagnosed with prostate cancer should understand how side effects impact on both partners. Some couples may find it beneficial to seek professional counseling to assist with coping with relationship distress related to prostate cancer and treatment-related side effects.

IMPACT OF ADT ON HEALTH-RELATED QUALITY OF LIFE

Health-related quality of life (HRQoL) is a patient reported outcome measure that uses evaluations of the patient's physical, psychological, and social functioning to measure the patient's overall perception of his disease and its treatment (33). It is now widely accepted that the impact of ADT on HRQoL should be an important part of the clinical decision-making process.

The utilization of ADT has significant HRQoL implications in men with prostate cancer. ADT is associated with numerous declines in objective measures of physical function as well as in the physical function, role-physical, bodily pain, and vitality domains (34). A longitudinal study of subjects in the Cancer of the Prostate Strategic Urologic Research Endeavor (CaPSURE) registry found worse physical well-being in patients receiving ADT. ADT was associated with worse physical well-being compared with local treatment at all time-points, even when corrected for age, comorbid conditions, and clinical presentation (35). A number of studies have demonstrated declines in both general HRQoL and prostate cancer–specific HRQoL associated with the initiation of ADT (36–38). There appears to be no difference in HRQoL outcomes between patients who undergo medical versus surgical castration.

Intermittent androgen deprivation therapy (IADT) may minimize the impact of ADT-related side effects, and, to a certain degree, their impact on patient QoL. IADT also has the potential to reduce the morbidity associated with long-term therapy (39). Several studies have demonstrated improvement in the sexual function domains of HRQoL instruments while off ADT therapy (40–42). In selected patients, IADT appears to be noninferior to continuous ADT, minimizes the impact of ADT-related side effects, and limits potential toxicity. The decision to pursue IADT should depend on a number of factors including patient preference, extent of disease, and the degree of comorbidity associated with ADT.

■ CONCLUSION

The potential benefits of any treatment for prostate cancer, including ADT, must outweigh its risks. This principle is particularly important given the expanded use of this therapy, which is sometimes prescribed for localized, asymptomatic prostate cancer. It is essential that the physician managing ADT possess a comprehensive understanding of the potential adverse effects of ADT and the impact that this treatment has on QoL. A shared decision-making process allows patients to deliberate and express their preferences and views regarding treatment options.

■ REFERENCES

1. Cooperberg MR, Grossfeld GD, Lubeck DP, Carroll PR. National practice patterns and time trends in androgen ablation for localized prostate cancer. *J Natl Cancer Inst.* 2003;95(13):981–995.
2. Shahinian VB, Kuo Y, Gilbert SM. Reimbursement policy and androgen-deprivation therapy for prostate cancer. *N Engl J Med.* 2010;363(19):1822–1832.
3. Meng MV, Grossfeld GD, Sadetsky N, Mehta SS, Lubeck DP, Carroll PR. Contemporary patterns of androgen deprivation therapy use for newly diagnosed prostate cancer. *Urology.* 2002;60(3, suppl 1):7–11.
4. Shahinian VB, Kuo YF, Freeman JL, Goodwin JS. Risk of the "androgen deprivation syndrome" in men receiving androgen deprivation for prostate cancer. *Arch Intern Med.* 2006;166(4):465–471.
5. Shanafelt TD, Barton DL, Adjei AA, Loprinzi CL. Pathophysiology and treatment of hot flashes. *Mayo Clin Proc.* 2002;77(11):1207–1218.
6. Jones JM, Kohli M, Loprinzi CL. Androgen deprivation therapy-associated vasomotor symptoms. *Asian J Androl.* 2012;14(2): 193–197.
7. Spetz A, Zetterlund E, Varenhorst E, Hammar M. Incidence and management of hot flashes in prostate cancer. *J Support Oncol.* 2003;1(4):263–272.
8. Potosky AL, Reeve BB, Clegg LX, et al. Quality of life following localized prostate cancer treated initially with androgen deprivation therapy or no therapy. *J Natl Cancer Inst.* 2002;94(6):430–437.
9. DiBlasio CJ, Malcolm JB, Derweesh IH, et al. Patterns of sexual and erectile dysfunction and response to treatment in patients receiving androgen deprivation therapy for prostate cancer. *BJU Int.* 2008;102(1):39–43.
10. Casey RG, Corcoran NM, Goldenberg SL. Quality of life issues in men undergoing androgen deprivation therapy: a review. *Asian J Androl.* 2012;14(2):226–231.
11. Harrington JM, Jones EG, Badger T. Body image perceptions in men with prostate cancer. *Oncol Nurs Forum.* 2009;36(2):167–172.
12. Harrington JM, Badger TA. Body image and quality of life in men with prostate cancer. *Cancer Nurs.* 2009;32(2):E1-E7.
13. Wassersug RJ, Oliffe JL. The social context for psychological distress from iatrogenic gynecomastia with suggestions for its management. *J Sex Med.* 2009;6(4):989–1000.
14. Navon L, Morag A. Advanced prostate cancer patients' ways of coping with the hormonal therapy's effect on body, sexuality, and spousal ties. *Qual Health Res.* 2003;13(10):1378–1392.
15. Munding MD, Wessells HB, Dalkin BL. Pilot study of changes in stretched penile length 3 months after radical retropubic prostatectomy. *Urology.* 2001;58(4):567–569.
16. Haliloglu A, Baltaci S, Yaman O. Penile length changes in men treated with androgen suppression plus radiation therapy for local or locally advanced prostate cancer. *J Urol.* 2007;177:128–130.
17. Morote J, Martinez E, Trilla E, et al. Osteoporosis during continuous androgen deprivation: influence of the modality and length of treatment. *Eur Urol.* 2003;44(6):661–665.
18. Hussain SA, Weston R, Stephenson RN, et al. Immediate dual energy X-ray absorptiometry reveals a high incidence of osteoporosis in patients with advanced prostate cancer before hormonal manipulation. *BJU Int.* 2003;92(7):690–694.
19. Oefelein MG, Ricchuiti V, Conrad W, et al. Skeletal fracture associated with androgen suppression induced osteoporosis: the clinical incidence and risk factors for patients with prostate cancer. *J Urol.* 2001;166(5):1724–1728.
20. Shahinian VB, Kuo Y, Freeman JL, et al. Risk of fracture after androgen deprivation for prostate cancer. *N Eng J Med.* 2005;352(2):154–164.
21. Saylor PJ, Smith MR. Metabolic complications of androgen deprivation therapy for prostate cancer. *J Urol.* 2009;181(5):1998–2008.
22. Lakka H, Laaksonen DE, Lakka TA, et al. The metabolic syndrome and total and cardiovascular disease mortality in middle-aged men. *JAMA.* 2002;288(21):2709–2716.
23. D'Amico AV, Denham JW, Crook J, et al. Influence of androgen suppression therapy for prostate cancer on the frequency and timing of fatal myocardial infarctions. *J Clin Oncol.* 2007; 25(17):2420–2425.
24. Wirth MP, See WA, McLeod DG, et al. Bicalutamide 150 mg in addition to standard care in patients with localized or locally advanced prostate cancer: results from the second analysis of the early prostate cancer program at median followup of 5.4 years. *J Urol.* 2004;172(5 part 1):1865–1870.
25. Beyer DC, McKeough T, Thomas T. Impact of short course hormonal therapy on overall and cancer specific survival after permanent prostate brachytherapy. *Int J Radiat Oncol Biol Phys.* 2005;61(5):1299–1306.

26. Keating NL, O'Malley AJ, Smith MR. Diabetes and cardiovascular disease during androgen deprivation therapy for prostate cancer. *J Clin Oncol.* 2006;24(27):4448–4456.
27. Kumar RJ, Barqawi A, Crawford ED. Adverse events associated with hormonal therapy for prostate cancer. *Rev Urol.* 2005;7 (suppl 5):S37–S43.
28. Bloomfield DJ, Shilling V, Edginton TA. Longitudinal pilot study to investigate whether hormonal therapy for prostate cancer affects cognition. *J Clin Oncol.* 2004;22(14S):4646.
29. Almeida OP, Waterreus A, Spry N, Flicker L, Martins RN. One year follow-up study of the association between chemical castration, sex hormones, beta-amyloid, memory and depression in men. *Psychoneuroendocrinology.* 2004;29(8):1071–1081.
30. Hagedoorn M, Sanderman R, Bolks HN, Tuinstra J, Coyne JC. Distress in couples coping with cancer: a meta-analysis and critical review of role and gender effects. *Psychol Bull.* 2008;134(1):1–30.
31. Roesch SC, Adams L, Hines A, et al. Coping with prostate cancer: a meta-analytic review. *J Behav Med.* 2005;28(3):281–293.
32. Walker LM, Robinson JW. The unique needs of couples experiencing androgen deprivation therapy for prostate cancer. *J Sex Marital Ther.* 2010;36(2):154–165.
33. Arpinelli F, Bamfi F. The FDA guidance for industry on PROs: the point of view of a pharmaceutical company. *Health Qual Life Outcome.* 2006;4:85.
34. Alibhai S, Breunis H, Timilshina T, et al. Impact of androgen-deprivation therapy on physical function and quality of life in men with nonmetastatic prostate cancer. *J Clin Oncol.* 2010;28 (34):5038–5045.
35. Sadetsky N, Greene K, Cooperberg MR, Hubbard A, Carroll PR, Satariano W. Impact of androgen deprivation on physical well-being in patients with prostate cancer: analysis from the CaPSURE (Cancer of the Prostate Strategic Urologic Research Endeavor) registry. *Cancer.* 2011;117(19):4406–4413.
36. Lubeck DP, Grossfeld GD, Carroll PR. The effect of androgen deprivation therapy on health-related quality of life in men with prostate cancer. *Urology.* 2001;58 (2, suppl 1):94–100.
37. Basaria S, Lieb J, Tang A, et al. Long-term effects of androgen deprivation therapy in prostate cancer patients. *Clin Endocrinol (Oxf).* 2002;56(6):779–786.
38. Dacal, K, Sereika SM, Greenspan SL. Quality of life in prostate cancer patients taking androgen deprivation therapy. *J Am Geriatr Soc.* 2006;54 (1):85–90.
39. Calais da Silva FE, Bono AV, Whelan P, et al. Intermittent androgen deprivation for locally advanced and metastatic prostate cancer: results from a randomised phase 3 study of the South European Uroncological Group. *Eur Urol.* 2009;55(6):1269–1277.
40. Malone S, Perry G, Segal R, Dahrouge S, Crook J. Long-term side effects of intermittent androgen suppression therapy in prostate cancer: results of a phase II study. *BJU Int.* 2005;96(4):514–520.
41. Spry NA, Kristjanson L, Hooton B, et al. Adverse effects to quality of life arising from treatment can recover with intermittent androgen suppression in men with prostate cancer. *Eur J Cancer.* 2006;42:1083–1092.
42. Bruchovsky N, Klotz L, Crook J, Phillips N, Abersbach J, Goldenberg SL. Quality of life, morbidity, and mortality results of a prospective phase II study of intermittent androgen suppression for men with evidence of prostate-specific antigen relapse after radiation therapy for locally advanced prostate cancer. *Clin Genitourin Cancer.* 2008;6(1):46–52.

12.3 Quality of Life With External Beam Radiation Therapy

STEVE K. WILLIAMS
SAMEER CHOPRA
FARHANG RABBANI

■ INTRODUCTION

Since the advent of PSA screening, most patients with newly diagnosed prostate cancer have localized disease and are being diagnosed at a younger age (1). There are various definitive treatment options for localized prostate cancer, including radical prostatectomy, cryotherapy, radiofrequency ablation, high-intensity focused ultrasound, hormone therapy, and radiation therapy. The primary goal of treatment in these patients is to eradicate the cancer without future relapse (i.e., achieving complete cure). Secondary goals include minimizing risks of acute morbidities around the time of treatment and decreasing the number and severity of long-term side effects of the treatment course. External beam radiation therapy (EBRT) represents a reasonable nonoperative option for definitive treatment of localized prostate cancer. EBRT uses gamma beam radiation directed toward the prostate and surrounding tissues, targeting multiple fields of radiation delineated by initial anatomic mapping. Although there is no conclusive evidence that any radiation therapy is superior to the other available treatment options for early prostate cancer in terms of overall survival, it is clear that each of these therapies has a unique impact on quality of life (2,3). A rational management decision for any individual patient requires assessment of the risk-benefit ratio. Accurate knowledge of the possible consequences of treatment, including the risk of lasting morbidity or negative impact on quality of life, is integral to this decision-making process.

A thorough review and understanding of the health-related quality of life (HRQoL) enables the physician and patient to have realistic expectations of outcome and is essential in the decision-making process. HRQoL is a patient-centered variable from the field of health services research that encompasses the wide range of human experience, primarily including intrapersonal and interpersonal responses to illness (4). It involves patients' own perceptions of their health and ability to function in life. HRQoL is measured using standardized questionnaires, which collect patient-centric data and provide an objective assessment and perception of both generic and disease-specific domains. These questionnaires have been used to compare the effects of various treatments on quality of life. Four of the most commonly used HRQoL instruments include: the University of California, Los Angeles Prostate Cancer Index (UCLA PCI); the Expanded Prostate Cancer Index-Composite (EPIC); the European Organization for Research and Treatment of Cancer Core Quality of Life Questionnaire with its prostate cancer–specific module (EORTC QLQ-C30); and the Functional Assessment of Cancer Therapy-Prostate Instrument (FACT-P).

■ EFFECT OF EBRT ON URINARY SYMPTOMS

Patient selection affects the risk of developing genitourinary symptoms. Pretreatment genitourinary complaints, prior transurethral resection of the prostate or of a bladder tumor, and the presence of acute genitourinary toxicity are suggested as contributing to urinary morbidity (5,6). Men undergoing EBRT may experience irritative voiding symptoms that can negatively affect overall urinary function and HRQoL. Acute, short-term adverse urinary HRQoL effects are common during and in the few months after EBRT and can persist long-term in a small but significant proportion of treated patients. Fransson compared HRQoL in 120 men who underwent EBRT with 125 age matched control subjects 4 and 8 years after EBRT (7). Eight years after treatment, 54% of the patients and 31% of the control subjects reported urinary problems. No significant changes were noted in either group between the 4th and 8th year assessments. Long-term treatment type–specific changes in quality of life domains were reported by Sanda et al. (8). Long-term total urinary incontinence and other severe urinary symptoms (indicating a complication of Radiation Therapy Oncology Group grade >2) are rare (9, 10).

ERECTILE DYSFUNCTION FOLLOWING RADIATION THERAPY

The specific etiology of erectile dysfunction (ED) after radiation therapy is unclear but may be multifactorial in nature (11). Similar to patients undergoing RP, patient age, use of androgen-deprivation therapy (ADT), and baseline erectile function were identified as important predictors for post-treatment erectile function. In a recent study, Fransson et al. recently analyzed the 15-year follow-up of patient-reported sexual function and identified disease progression and the use of ADT as risk factors for worse sexual and erectile function (7). Mangar and colleagues examined the impact of different doses (64 or 74 Gy) of 3-dimensional conformal radiation therapy after 3 to 6 months of ADT in 51 men (12). The authors reported that 12 men (23.5%) remained potent, 22 men (43.1%) had reduced potency, and 17 men (33.3%) were impotent at 2 years using the UCLA PCI and the FACT-P questionnaires. Moreover, the authors found a dose-volume effect with respect to mean dose received by the penile bulb and ED, where a D90 >50 Gy is associated with a significant risk of ED. Similarly, another study noted actuarial potency rates of 96%, 75%, 59%, and 53% at 1, 20, 40, and 60 months, respectively, after EBRT (13). Sexual dysfunction after EBRT appears to have a major effect on quality of life reported by patients. In a report of 432 EBRT patients identified using the Surveillance, Epidemiology, and End Results (SEER) database registry, 37% reported that their sexual function was a "medium or big problem" (14).

RECTAL TOXICITY FOLLOWING RADIATION THERAPY

EBRT often results in bowel dysfunction that can affect HRQoL. Assessment of bowel symptoms, including diarrhea, rectal urgency, tenesmus, rectal bleeding, and others is also essential, especially for patients who undergo radiation therapy. Like urinary symptoms, bowel dysfunction may be highly disruptive in some men's lives, and the time-course and severity of specific bowel symptoms may diverge. Established risk factors for acute and late toxicities after EBRT for prostate cancer include advanced age; larger rectal volume; a history of prior abdominal surgery; the concomitant use of androgen deprivation; and preexisting diabetes mellitus, hemorrhoids, or inflammatory bowel disease (15). In addition, a diagnosis of acute rectal toxicity is recognized to be associated with an increased risk of developing late rectal complications (16). Long-term results of 561 patients who were treated with up to 81 Gy IMRT between 1996 and 2001 at the Memorial Sloan-Kettering Cancer Center were reported by Zelefsky et al. (17). The authors reported a 1.6% rate of rectal bleeding and a 0.1% rate of National Cancer Institute Common Toxicity Criteria (NCI-CTC) grade 3 rectal toxicity after 8 years of follow-up when using a fraction size of 1.8 Gy.

SUMMARY

When discussing therapeutic options for prostate cancer, patients should be made aware of the potential effect of various treatments on HRQoL. Complications of external beam radiation can affect urinary, sexual, and bowel function. These effects can have a significant effect on a patient's quality of life. As such, consideration of quality of life as an important factor in clinical decision making for prostate cancer would benefit patients in making more informed treatment choices.

REFERENCES

1. Newcomer LM, Stanford JL, Blumenstein BA, Brawer MK. Temporal trends in rates of prostate cancer: declining incidence of advanced stage disease, 1974 to 1994. *J Urol.* 1997;158(4):1427–1430.
2. Ghavamian R, Williams SK, Hakimi AA. High-risk prostate cancer: the role of radical prostatectomy for local therapy. *Future Oncol.* 2011;7(4):543–550.
3. Klein EA. Radiation therapy versus radical prostatectomy in the PSA era: a urologist's view. *Semin Radiat Oncol.* 1998;8(2):87–94.
4. Hamoen EH, De Rooij M, Witjes JA, Barentsz JO, Rovers MM. Measuring health-related quality of life in men with prostate cancer: a systematic review of the most used questionnaires and their validity. *Urol Oncol.* 2014. [Epub ahead of print].
5. Bittner N, Merrick GS, Wallner KE, Lief JH, Butler WM, Galbreath RW. The impact of acute urinary morbidity on late urinary function after permanent prostate brachytherapy. *Brachytherapy.* 2007;6(4):258–266.
6. Fiorino C, Valdagni R, Rancati T, Sanguineti G. Dose-volume effects for normal tissues in external radiotherapy: pelvis. *Radiother Oncol.* 2009;93(2):153–167.
7. Fransson P, Widmark A. Late side effects unchanged 4–8 years after radiotherapy for prostate carcinoma: a comparison with age-matched controls. *Cancer.* 1999;85(3):678–688.
8. Sanda MG, Dunn RL, Michalski J, et al. Quality of life and satisfaction with outcome among prostate-cancer survivors. *N Engl J Med.* 2008;358(12):1250–1261.
9. Williams SG, Zietman AL. Does radical treatment have a role in the management of low-risk prostate cancer? The place for brachytherapy and external beam radiotherapy. *World J Urol.* 2008;26(5):447–456.
10. Zietman AL, DeSilvio ML, Slater JD, et al. Comparison of conventional-dose vs high-dose conformal radiation therapy in clinically localized adenocarcinoma of the prostate: a randomized controlled trial. *JAMA.* 2005;294(10):1233–1239.

11. Pinkawa M, Gagel B, Piroth MD, et al. Erectile dysfunction after external beam radiotherapy for prostate cancer. *Eur Urol.* 2009;55(1):227–234.
12. Mangar SA, Sydes MR, Tucker HL, et al. Evaluating the relationship between erectile dysfunction and dose received by the penile bulb: using data from a randomised controlled trial of conformal radiotherapy in prostate cancer (MRC RT01, ISRCTN47772397). *Radiother Oncol.* 2006;80(3):355–362.
13. Mantz CA, Nautiyal J, Awan A, et al. Potency preservation following conformal radiotherapy for localized prostate cancer: impact of neoadjuvant androgen blockade, treatment technique, and patient-related factors. *Cancer J Sci Am.* 1999;5(4):230–236.
14. Fowler FJ Jr, Barry MJ, Lu-Yao G, Wasson JH, Bin L. Outcomes of external-beam radiation therapy for prostate cancer: a study of Medicare beneficiaries in three surveillance, epidemiology, and end results areas. *J Clin Oncol.* 1996;14(8):2258–2265.
15. Peeters ST, Lebesque JV, Heemsbergen WD, et al. Localized volume effects for late rectal and anal toxicity after radiotherapy for prostate cancer. *Int J Radiat Oncol Biol Phys.* 2006;64(4):1151–1161.
16. Denham JW, O'Brien PC, Dunstan RH, et al. Is there more than one late radiation proctitis syndrome? *Radiother Oncol.* 1999;51(1):43–53.
17. Zelefsky MJ, Chan H, Hunt M, Yamada Y, Shippy AM, Amols H. Long-term outcome of high dose intensity modulated radiation therapy for patients with clinically localized prostate cancer. *J Urol.* 2006;176(4, pt 1):1415–1419.

12.4 Quality of Life With Brachytherapy for Low-Risk Localized Prostate Cancer

STEVE K. WILLIAMS
FARHANG RABBANI

INTRODUCTION

In the past few years, the health care community has placed more emphasis on patient-reported end points such as health-related quality of life (HRQoL). HRQoL in prostate cancer is an assessment of how an individual's well-being may be affected over time by the disease or its treatment. Various acceptable treatment options exist for clinically localized prostate cancer including radical prostatectomy, external beam radiotherapy, and brachytherapy (1). Consideration of HRQoL after treatment is therefore essential since patients often base therapeutic decisions on the side effect profiles of different treatments. American Urological Association clinical guidelines call for structural and process of care measures to improve the quality of care and facilitate better treatment decisions for patients diagnosed with prostate cancer (2).

HRQoL INSTRUMENTS AND PROSTATE CANCER

HRQoL is a patient-centered variable and is measured using questionnaires which may be self-administered by the patient or by an objective third-party interviewer. HRQoL instruments typically contain questions organized into scales. Each scale measures a different aspect or domain of HRQoL.

Domains can be general, addressing aspects of HRQoL that are common to all patients regardless of their disease process, or disease specific. Disease-specific domains focus on the impact of particular organic dysfunctions associated with the disease that may affect HRQoL. Prostate cancer–specific domains include areas such as bone pain; anxiety regarding cancer recurrence; urinary, sexual, and bowel dysfunction; and distress from these dysfunctions. Four of the most commonly used HRQoL instruments for brachytherapy include the European Organization for Research and Treatment of Cancer Core Quality of Life Questionnaire with its prostate cancer–specific module (EORTC QLQ-C30), the University of California, Los Angeles Prostate Cancer Index (UCLA PCI), the Expanded Prostate Cancer Index-Composite (EPIC), and the Functional Assessment of Cancer Therapy-Prostate Instrument (FACT-P) (3–6).

BRACHYTHERAPY AND GENERAL HRQoL

A number of authors have reported on HRQoL after prostate cancer primary treatment with brachytherapy. Lee et al. prospectively measured HRQoL in 46 men before they underwent brachytherapy and then 1 and 3 months after treatment (7). The authors reported clinically and statistically significant decreases in HRQoL scores 1 month after treatment in the physical well-being, functional well-being, and prostate cancer–specific domains of the FACT-P. It was noted that this negative impact on quality of life (QoL) was gone by the third month when mean scores in these domains had returned to baseline levels, although patients still experienced significant irritative voiding symptoms.

BRACHYTHERAPY AND ITS EFFECT ON URINARY FUNCTION

Several authors have reported on the effect of brachytherapy on the urinary tract. In the Cancer of the Prostate Strategic Urological Research Endeavor (CaPSURE) population, mean urinary function scores were significantly more favorable in brachytherapy patients than in radical prostatectomy patients at all time points, but mean urinary bother scores were found to be almost equivalent between the two groups (8). This discrepancy may exist because patients tend to find irritative/obstructive symptoms more bothersome than incontinence. In a single-center prospective study examining factors predicting severe urinary bother, higher American Urological Association Symptom Index (AUA-SI) score, a measure of irritiative/obstructive symptoms, was an independent risk factor for worse urinary bother (OR 1.23, 95% CI 1.17–1.29) (9). Arterbery et al. evaluated the short-term complications of transperineal radioactive prostate seed implantation, and reported nocturia, frequency, dysuria, and hesitancy lasting 12 to 24 weeks (10). In a follow-up study, Arterbery et al. used the validated European Organization for Research in Cancer Therapy QoL instrument to survey 51 patients 6 months after seed implantation (11). The authors reported that 40% of patients reported some degree of urinary frequency and 17% had dysuria (11). Talcott et al. surveyed 72 men with a median of 5 years of follow-up after brachytherapy from a single institution using a validated HRQoL instrument (12). Forty-four percent of the patients reported urinary leakage of any amount, 13% reported more than a few drops of leakage, and 18% wore a pad for protection (12). Pretreatment factors that may influence the likelihood that a brachytherapy recipient will develop incontinence post-treatment include, but are not limited to, the use of neoadjuvant hormonal therapy and radiotherapy boost, preimplant IPSS >15, and urethral D_{10} dose (13, 14).

■ EFFECT OF BRACHYTHERAPY ON SEXUAL FUNCTION

Several authors have reported on the effect of brachytherapy on sexual domains. Pardo and colleagues evaluated in a prospective study the effect on QoL of localized prostate cancer interventions in 435 patients treated with radical prostatectomy, external-beam radiotherapy, or brachytherapy. QoL was assessed before and after treatment with the Short Form-36 and the EPIC (15). They reported that approximately 50% of brachytherapy subjects who had no problems with their sexual function at baseline reported moderate or severe problems 3 years after treatment. Chipman and the PROST-QA study group evaluated the responsiveness of EPIC for Clinical Practice in 1,201 subjects from a multicenter longitudinal cohort (16). The authors reported a statistically and clinically significant difference between baseline and post-treatment average EPIC-26 sexual function scores at every point measured. With potency defined as having an erection sufficient for intercourse, impotence rates increased from 36% pretreatment to 56% at 2 years post-treatment, with 30% of brachytherapy subjects reporting a moderate-to-severe problem with sexual function at 2 years. These HRQoL changes were associated with distress in the patients' partners as well.

■ BRACHYTHERAPY AND BOWEL FUNCTION

The intimate relationship between the prostate and the rectum results in inevitable exposure of the rectum to radioactive dose during treatment with brachytherapy. Bowel function (or dysfunction) in this context includes rectal urgency, loose stools, crampy pelvic pain, and occasional rectal bleeding. Bowel bother refers to the degree of distress or annoyance caused by any impairments in bowel function. In the previously described PROST-QA study, brachytherapy subjects have statistically and clinically significant deficits in bowel function compared to baseline as measured by EPIC-26 at every assessed time point (13). Even at 2 years post-treatment, 8% of subjects considered their bowel symptoms to be a moderate-to-severe problem. Talcott et al. reported a 14% incidence in rectal urgency and a 6% incidence of rectal bleeding (12). Litwin and colleagues reviewed the CaPSURE database to study bowel function and bother in 1,584 men recently diagnosed with early stage prostate cancer and followed for 2 years after radical prostatectomy, external beam radiation, or brachytherapy (17). Principal outcomes were assessed with the UCLA PCI, a validated instrument that includes these two domains. Compared to patients treated with radical prostatectomy, patients treated with brachytherapy experience significantly greater impairment in bowel function following treatment. Bowel function QoL tends to improve markedly during the first 3 months but does not reach a steady state until at least a year after therapy. By 2 years, patients who have had brachytherapy appear to yield similar bowel function outcomes to external beam radiation therapy, but both are worse than that which occurs after surgery. Bowel bother or distress over bowel dysfunction is somewhat more impaired in men opting for brachytherapy than in those treated surgically. Within 3 months of treatment, patients treated with radical prostatectomy have rebounded and bother remains minimal. For those undergoing brachytherapy, significant gains are seen in the first 3 months but it takes at least a year to reach a steady state. The authors reported that the three tumor variables of PSA, Gleason score, and clinical stage did not consistently predict bowel outcomes, however, comorbidity was strongly associated with both bowel outcomes.

■ SUMMARY

When discussing therapeutic options for prostate cancer, patients should be made aware of the potential effect of various treatments on HRQoL. Complications of brachytherapy can affect urinary, sexual, and bowel function and are most pronounced in the first several years after implantation. These effects can have a significant effect on a patient's QoL. By including QoL as an important factor in clinical decision making for prostate cancer, we can help our patients make more informed treatment choices.

REFERENCES

1. Barry MJ, Albertsen PC, Bagshaw MA, et al. Outcomes for men with clinically nonmetastatic prostate carcinoma managed with radical prostactectomy, external beam radiotherapy, or expectant management: a retrospective analysis. *Cancer.* 2001;91(12):2302–2314.
2. Thompson I, Thrasher JB, Aus G, et al. Guideline for the management of clinically localized prostate cancer: 2007 update. J Urol. 2007;177(6):2106–2131.
3. Ware J Jr, Kosinski M, Keller SD. A 12-Item Short-Form Health Survey: construction of scales and preliminary tests of reliability and validity. *Med Care.* 1996;34(3):220–233.
4. Wei JT, Dunn RL, Litwin MS, Sandler HM, Sanda MG. Development and validation of the expanded prostate cancer index composite (EPIC) for comprehensive assessment of health-related quality of life in men with prostate cancer. *Urology.* 2000;56(6):899–905.
5. Litwin MS, Hays RD, Fink A, Ganz PA, Leake B, Brook RH. The UCLA Prostate Cancer Index: development, reliability, and validity of a health-related quality of life measure. *Med Care.* 1998;36(7):1002–1012.
6. Aaronson NK, Ahmedzai S, Bergman B, et al. The European Organization for Research and Treatment of Cancer QLQ-C30: a quality-of-life instrument for use in international clinical trials in oncology. *J Natl Cancer Inst.* 1993;85(5):365–376.
7. Lee WR, McQuellon RP, Harris-Henderson K, Case LD, McCullough DL. A preliminary analysis of health-related quality of life in the first year after permanent source interstitial brachytherapy (PIB) for clinically localized prostate cancer. *Int J Radiat Oncol Biol Phys.* 2000;46(1):77–81.
8. Downs TM, Sadetsky N, Pasta DJ, et al. Health related quality of life patterns in patients treated with interstitial prostate brachytherapy for localized prostate cancer–data from CaPSURE. *J Urol.* 2003;170(5):1822–1827.
9. Gore JL, Gollapudi K, Bergman J, Kwan L, Krupski TL, Litwin MS. Correlates of bother following treatment for clinically localized prostate cancer. *J Urol.* 2010;184(4):1309–1315.
10. Arterbery VE, Wallner K, Roy J, Fuks Z. Short-term morbidity from CT-planned transperineal I-125 prostate implants. *Int J Radiat Oncol Biol Phys.* 1993;25(4):661–667.
11. Arterbery VE, Frazier A, Dalmia P, Siefer J, Lutz M, Porter A. Quality of life after permanent prostate implant. *Semin Surg Oncol.* 1997;13(6):461–464.
12. Talcott JA, Clark JA, Stark PC, Mitchell SP. Long-term treatment related complications of brachytherapy for early prostate cancer: a survey of patients previously treated. *J Urol.* 2001;166(2):494–499.
13. Sanda MG, Dunn RL, Michalski J, et al. Quality of life and satisfaction with outcome among prostate-cancer survivors. *N Engl J Med.* 2008;358(12):1250–1261.
14. McElveen TL, Waterman FM, Kim H, Dicker AP. Factors predicting for urinary incontinence after prostate brachytherapy. *Int J Radiat Oncol Biol Phys.* 2004;59(5):1395–1404.
15. Pardo Y, Guedea F, Aguilo F, et al. Quality-of-life impact of primary treatments for localized prostate cancer in patients without hormonal treatment. *J Clin Oncol.* 2010;28(31):4687–4696.
16. Chipman JJ, Sanda MG, Dunn RL, et al. Measuring and predicting prostate cancer related quality of life changes using EPIC for clinical practice. *J Urol.*. 2014;191:638–645.
17. Litwin MS, Sadetsky N, Pasta DJ, Lubeck DP. Bowel function and bother after treatment for early stage prostate cancer: a longitudinal quality of life analysis from CaPSURE. *J Urol.* 2004;172(2):515–519.

13 Role for Comparative Effectiveness Research in Treatment Decision Making

RYAN T. JONES

MARK V. MISHRA

TIMOTHY N. SHOWALTER

Determining optimal management of prostate cancer (PC) continues to be a major focus of health policy debate. Given the widespread use of prostate-specific antigen (PSA) screening, the vast majority of PC cases are now diagnosed with localized disease. Although multiple treatment options exist for such patients—ranging from observation with active surveillance (AS) or watchful waiting, to definitive treatment with surgery, brachytherapy, external beam therapy, or cryotherapy—little comparative outcomes data exist to help guide patient and clinician treatment decisions today.

Although a randomized controlled clinical trial would provide the most robust method for comparing the relative effectiveness and harms of the different treatment strategies, efforts to do so have often failed due to difficulties with patient accrual and lengthy follow-up times necessary to achieve clinically relevant endpoints for PC.

Recent emphasis has been placed on high-quality comparative effectiveness research (CER) to aid patients, health care provides, payers, and policy makers with timely and relevant information of the relative harms and benefits of the different PC treatment strategies.

In this chapter, we will briefly define the scope and potential of CER and discuss its relevance to PC. We will highlight gaps in current evidence and address how CER can be used to complement existing data. We will further review the tools available for performing CER and discuss relative merit and limitation of each strategy.

■ COMPARATIVE EFFECTIVENESS RESEARCH: BACKGROUND

CER aims to provide clinicians, patients, payers, and policy makers with reliable, relevant, and high-quality evidence to make informed decisions regarding the prevention, diagnosis, treatment, monitoring, or improvement of health care (1). Simply put, the intent of CER is to provide clinicians and patients with the necessary resources to make individualized, educated decisions based on evidence regarding the benefits and harms of the various treatment options. As described by Sox (2) in his analysis of the 2009 Institute of Medicine (IOM) definition of CER, CER incorporates several core aims: (1) generation of primary research; (2) systematic review of previously completed research; (3) head-to-head comparison of available methods; and (4) a focus on guiding clinicians and patients to select and effectively apply the available evidence to make informed decisions. Each portion of this dynamic process qualifies as CER, and the range of methodologies and topics is broad. The robust integration of all these steps is necessary for the formation of reliable, relatable recommendations and decision-making support, which is the overarching aim of CER.

Attention to CER and patient-centered outcomes research has increased immensely over the past several years, related in part to recent steps to reform the U.S. health care system. The American Recovery and Reinvestment Act of 2009 instituted $1.1 billion in funding for CER, using a broad basis for funding qualification (3). Recognizing needs for standards in CER methodology and for a large-scale funding policy, the U.S. Department of Health and Human Services (DHHS) and the Patient Protection and Affordable Care Act of 2010 established the nonprofit Patient-Centered Outcomes Research Institute (PCORI) to guide, contract, and disseminate CER research (4). Given its mission and its governmental support, PCORI is emerging as a leading organization for CER in the United States, with the ability to provide leadership and structure to CER efforts by setting guidelines for methodology and decisions regarding funding priorities. As of May 7, 2013, PCORI had dispersed $129.3 million to fund CER (5).

The DHHS definition of CER states that "the purpose of [CER] is to provide information that helps clinicians and patients choose which option best fits an individual patient's needs and preference" (6). At a glance, definitions such as this may suggest that CER is hardly different from traditional evidence-based medicine; however, there are some important distinctions between these two concepts, and CER methodologies include some approaches that may be new to researchers and physicians who are accustomed to the traditional evidence-based medicine paradigm. Rather than mutually exclusive research paradigms, CER and evidence-based medicine should be viewed as synergistic, with each one's strengths ideally providing the ability to address the other's weaknesses. Evidence-based medicine emphasizes rigorous scientific data generated ideally from "gold-standard" randomized controlled trials (RCTs), an investigational approach highly valued for its ability to control for both known and unknown confounding variables to effectively compare different treatment approaches in the strictest way feasible. However, RCTs often suffer in real-world generalizability and feasibility because of several well-recognized limitations, including use of strict exclusion criteria that often limit the external validity of data from RCTs (specifically, comorbidities and potential patient nonadherence to treatment protocol), experimental setting (academic institutions vs. community-based practices), ethical considerations, lengthy study duration, and cost (7–9). Figure 13.1 contains a Venn diagram that compares and contrasts various aspects of RCTs and CER.

One powerful example of a limitation of RCTs is that of the Southwest Oncology Group (SWOG) 8794 trial comparing adjuvant radiation therapy (RT) versus observation after radical prostatectomy (RP) for patients with PC with adverse pathological features. This trial was designed based on strong preliminary evidence that suggested a potential therapeutic benefit for adjuvant RT for patients with adverse pathological features in the prostatectomy specimen. Although the results of the SWOG 8794 trial demonstrated improved overall survival and distant metastasis-free survival with adjuvant RT compared with observation (10), the results have had limited impact on clinical practice (11). In the interval between the design of SWOG 8794 in the late 1980s and the publication of trial results in 2006, the clinical arrival and widespread adoption of PSA blood testing rendered the design of SWOG 8794 only partially relevant to clinical practice. During this period, PSA provided clinicians the ability to closely monitor patients, with potential to identify recurrence prior to clinical relapse, and transformed the nature of postprostatectomy surveillance and management for PC. Given this change, adoption of the adjuvant RT strategy after the trial published was small, with less than 20% of eligible patients undergoing such treatment (11). Currently, there is much controversy regarding the relative merits of adjuvant RT versus close observation with PSA testing and selective use of early salvage RT (12–14), and contemporary decisions regarding management decisions cannot be wholly informed by the SWOG 8794 data because the standard arm (observation) no longer reflects the current alternative to adjuvant RT (serial PSA testing with early salvage RT for a rising PSA). In this case, the utility of the RCT results was impaired by the long time interval required to conduct the clinical trial and unanticipated changes in diagnostic tools used in this disease. CER methods offer opportunities to rapidly fill evidence gaps in situations like this, provided necessary tools such as high-quality databases are available.

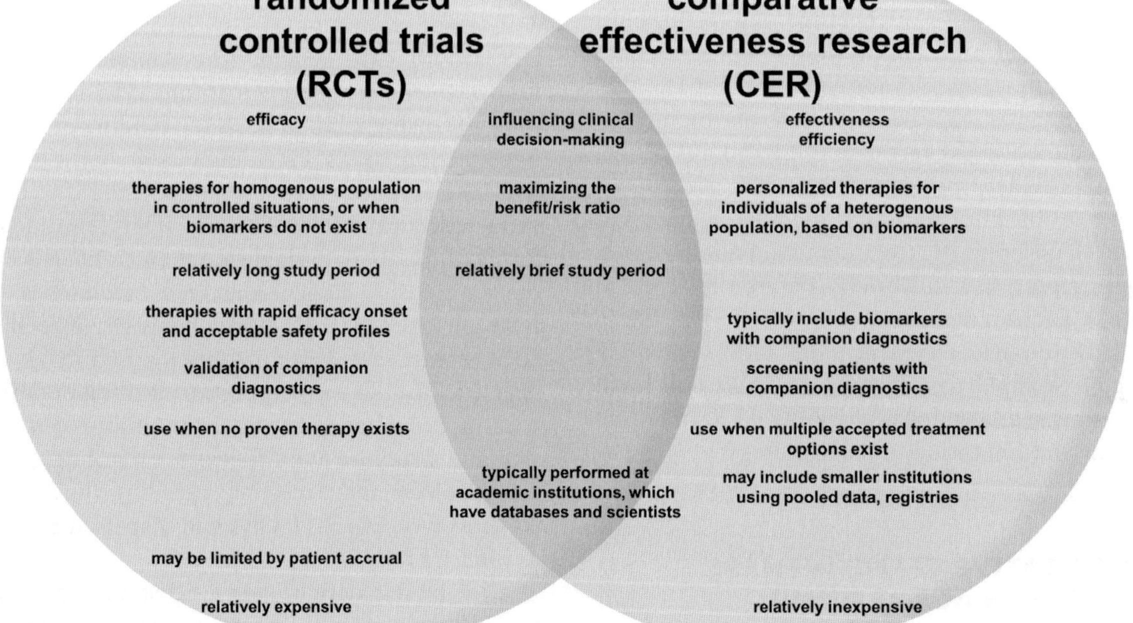

NICHOLAS G. ZAORSKY, M.D.

FIGURE 13.1 A Venn diagram that compares and contrasts various aspects of RCTs and CER.

In contrast to the traditional model for evidence-based medicine, the CER model embraces the use of many study types, including RCTs, pragmatic or practical trials, adaptive studies, and observational data such as retrospective and prospective cohort and case-control studies (15). Pragmatic trials use far fewer exclusion criteria than RCTs and compare treatment effectiveness in usual care conditions (16). Observational studies allow the incorporation of larger sample sizes, permitting the study of interventions across subgroups. The rationale for such allowances is that including comorbidities, larger sample sizes, and natural population variation can assist in obtaining information that is generalizable to real-world scenarios, subgroups, and individuals. For example, CER may help answer which intervention is best for a middle-aged African American male being treated at a community hospital when the only available RCT data include elderly predominately white individuals at academic centers. Furthermore, CER studies using observational data can provide the ability to evaluate new clinical questions when an RCT is not feasible or while awaiting the maturation and publication of RCT results. Adaptive trials allow investigators to incorporate external evidence as the study progresses, such as adding new interventions and dropping less effective ones, thereby maintaining clinical relevance throughout the study duration (17, 18). In essence, CER and traditional evidence-based medicine differ in the same way "effectiveness" differs from "efficacy," the same way pragmatic randomized control trials differ from standard RCTs. In each comparison, the former is focused on a therapy's function in the real world, whereas the latter is focused on function in the ideal setting (19).

There are some important challenges and limitations of CER using observational data that should be considered carefully. CER using observational data is especially prone to methodological and statistical biases that make the results unreliable and thus should be interpreted with great rigor (9). Several authors have expressed concern over the use of CER data to influence clinical intervention given the potential for misinterpretation and rapid dissemination by policy makers and the media (20, 21). There are a variety of methods that CER investigators apply to control for confounding variables and enhance the strength of evidence of observational studies (15, 18).

Observational studies are inherently limited by the fact that decisions made in real-world practice are rarely random. To control for confounding variables and enhance the quality of evidence obtained from observational studies, CER investigators use statistical techniques such as regression models, propensity score methods, and instrumental variable (IV) analysis (22–25). Multivariable regression models allow one to estimate the magnitude of association of an outcome with one variable while holding other covariates constant (15). Propensity score analysis is another strategy to adjust for nonrandom allocation of an intervention in an observational cohort study (26, 27). This method involves first estimating the likelihood ("propensity score") of assignment to the intervention based on measured covariates for each subject and then evaluating the effect of the intervention on the measured outcome after adjusting for propensity score through either propensity score matching or a regression model that includes propensity score. The propensity score may have a value between 0 and 1 and represent the likelihood that a subject would receive an intervention based on the subject's characteristics. Although this is a useful tool, propensity score analysis has limitations, including the ability to adjust only for those potential confounders that exist in the data as measured variables (15).

An IV analysis is an alternative statistical approach that is designed to adjust for both measured and unmeasured confounders (28). This approach is dependent on the identification of an IV, which requires a strong association with assignment of the intervention to subjects and no direct association with the outcome. An example of an IV used in the literature is health service area for the use of androgen deprivation therapy (ADT) alone for localized PC, since variations in clinical practice are observed among areas, but health service area does not independently influence survival outcomes from PC (23). Essentially, an IV analysis involves using the IV itself to mimic the randomization process of a RCT through a two-step analytical process that involves first estimating the probability of assignment to an intervention based on a two-step analytic process that incorporates the IV in predictions of the probabilities of assignment to the intervention and of a subject experiencing the relevant outcome (15). Although all these analytic techniques do have limitations, they serve an important role in the adjustment for potential confounders on CER studies using observational cohorts.

■ IMPORTANCE OF COMPARATIVE EFFECTIVENESS RESEARCH IN ONCOLOGY

CER in oncology has exploded in the last few years, with 103 CER-related studies in oncology funded by the National Cancer Institute's (NCI) Division of Cancer Control and Population Science between 2009 and 2011 (29). The rise in cancer CER has stemmed in part from the emergence of new technologies and drugs, with tremendous associated increases in health care expenditures in oncology (30). One can also not ignore the contributing factor of concerns over the projected increase in cancer diagnoses and long-term cancer survivors to the boost in cancer CER (31). There are a burgeoning number of sources of observational data for cancer CER, such as clinical registries, electronic medical records, and claims databases (18). There has been a tremendous recent emphasis on CER in oncology, including a special issue of the *Journal of Clinical Oncology* in 2012 devoted to the subject (29, 30).

CER investigations in oncology are limited by a variety of challenges, given the extensive complexity of oncological pathology, treatment, and outcomes data. As stated by Shen et al. (8) and Hood and Friend (32), the barriers to cancer CER include choice of an appropriate comparator, control of confounding variables, lack of oncology-specific large-scale data on clinical characteristics and outcomes, lack of large biomarker databases, and the challenge of generating research rapidly enough to keep pace with treatment innovation. As with other CER, cancer CER researchers must pay special attention to methodological rigor in their analyses and data reporting to eliminate confounding variables and maximize real-world relevance. A recent review of 37 published reports relating to breast cancer genetics speaks to the fact that oncological studies vary widely in design (33). Focus must remain on effectively using available resources and generating quality, reliable evidence to inform decision making by patients, clinicians, and policy makers. Glasgow et al. have provided important perspective on future oncology CER directions by evaluating the current body of federally funded cancer CER and by identifying the knowledge gaps and research areas that are in need of methodological improvements. They emphasize, in particular, a need for CER that is designed to help translate discovery and innovation into clinical practice by providing actionable and relevant evidence regarding cancer-related health interventions (29).

Observational studies are an appealing approach for cancer CER due to their rapid turn around, generalizability to real-world clinical situations, and the ability, through large datasets that include individuals who may be underrepresented in RCTs, to explore outcomes of individual subgroups or populations (34). The ability to rapidly evaluate research questions using observational cohorts in existing databases provides the opportunity to obtain evidence while awaiting for results of RCTs, which often require a significant delay before study maturation. Commonly used databases for oncology CER include insurance claims databases, in-house prospective and electronic clinical registries, and the National Cancer Institute's Surveillance, Epidemiology, and End Results (SEER) database (see Table 13.1). In-house registries allow for customization of specific patient and treatment details but are limited in sample size and thus strained in their ability to evaluate effectiveness of interventions. Conversely, the SEER database is composed of 17 population-based registries in the United States that account for 26% of the U.S. population. SEER contains information regarding patient demographics, tumor characteristics, treatment modality, and mortality outcomes but is limited with regard to other clinical outcomes. Previous studies on the reliability of SEER mortality data have shown agreement to medical records of 87% to 92% (35, 36).

The use of evidence obtained from observational research is a potential source of controversy in oncology. A recent exchange among CER and RCT researchers regarding an observational cohort study that compared complications after breast brachytherapy (BBT) and whole breast irradiation (WBI) offers valuable insights into the potential tensions between the paradigms of CER and RCTs (20, 25, 37). Published in late 2012, Presley et al. performed a Medicare database CER study to investigate the national patterns of use in the United States and acute complications of BBT compared with WBI after breast conserving surgery for early-stage invasive breast cancer. By using IV analysis to adjust for potential confounders, the authors reported that BBT had a 16.8% higher (35.2% vs. 18.4%) overall complication rate compared with WBI (25). Cuttino et al. challenged the claim in a commentary, entitled "When retrospective CER hinders science and patient-centered care," citing several RCTs that showed no difference between the complication rates after BBT and WBI and generally discrediting the CER methods used by Presley et al. (20). Cuttino et al., who are BBT specialists and lead investigators for an RCT comparing BBT with WBI, express frustration over CER using claims data when clinical trials are being conducted (20). The authors' rebuttal (38) to the Cuttino et al. commentary presents a compelling review of the limitations of existing RCT-based data for BBT and highlights the value of CER. As Presley et al. point out, the randomized trials cited by Cuttino et al. used either a different form of brachytherapy or used mainly 3D conformal radiation for the partial breast irradiation group as opposed to brachytherapy, confounding the complication rates (38). As a complete set, this *Journal of Clinical Oncology* CER research paper (25), commentary (20), and rebuttal (38) are recommended to the reader as an insightful overview of the limitations and strengths of RCTs and of observational CER, as well as an indicator of the need to expand opportunities for clinical trialists to receive additional training in CER to better understand its role in evidence generation. In addition, the reaction to this study raised a methodological point worthy of mention: Malin (39) pointed out that the complication list used for administrative claims coding in the paper by Presley et al. included the International Classification of Disease code 785.59, "Other shock without mention of trauma," a complication that would very unlikely occur from partial or whole-breast irradiation. As Malin suggests, this is likely not a relevant complication and should not have been included in this investigation. This serves as a reminder that CER investigators must be careful to include only outcomes that may be related to the interventions to be evaluated; otherwise, associations may be inappropriately found and false conclusions drawn (39).

A challenge pertinent to CER in the United States is the decision of whether to include cost. The Affordable Care Act explicitly forbids PCORI from funding research that produces cost-effectiveness results in the form of cost per quality-adjusted life year (QALY) threshold or similar

Table 13.1 Examples of data sources for observational comparative effectiveness research

Source	Advantages	Disadvantages
CISNET	Provides results from statistical modeling analyses of cancer prevention, screening, and treatment alternatives	Available data limited to areas that have been analyzed to date by CISNET
Cancer Research Network	Provides a wealth of patient, tumor, laboratory, cost, and outcomes information Large sample size of over 11 million enrollees Significant data on racial minorities	Limited to data from 14 health maintenance organizations Data kept at the local sites vs. one central database, limiting accessibility
CDC Behavioral Risk Factor Surveillance System	Provides information on health-related risk behaviors, chronic health conditions, and use of preventive services	Risk of volunteer bias—data only garnered from telephone surveys
In-house registries	Customizable data output for specific clinical questions or cohorts	Limited sample size
Linked insurance registry databases	Provides detail of case and treatment Data for younger and older patients, as opposed to Medicare databases	Limited availability
Medicare claims	Technical details of treatment Can link to physician and health care market databases and sometimes to state registries	Data limited to Medicare beneficiaries Limited details of cancer diagnoses and outcomes No RT dosimetric data Requires time-consuming computer programming to perform analysis
Medical records	Detailed information of clinical case, including treatment and outcomes	Level of detail varies by record system Exceedingly difficult to analyze if not in electronic form
National Patient Advocate Foundation CER Database	Lists CER studies funded by the National Institutes of Health (NIH) and Agency for Healthcare Research and Quality	Requires significant work on behalf of the reader to reach meaningful conclusions
SEER Database	Reports clinical details of cancer, patient demographics, and basics of treatment modality	Data limited to 17 regions of the United States Lack of specific treatment information, e.g., dose of radiation therapy, chemotherapy use Lack of data on treatment and outcomes following recurrence
SEER–Medicare database	More specific technical details of treatment compared to SEER Clinical details of cancer Reports on mortality Can link to physician and health care market databases	Data limited to 17 regions of the United States, and patients older than 65 years Limited details on clinical outcomes No information about local control No direct information about patient complications No RT dosimetric data Requires time-consuming computer programming to perform analysis
SEER–MHOS	Provides information from a 95-item questionnaire that includes information on tumor site, race, ethnicity, and patient health care preferences (before and after treatment)	Data limited to 17 regions of the United States Data limited to Medicare beneficiaries who completed at least one survey Data only for years 1998–2007

Abbreviations: BRFSS, behavioral risk factor surveillance system; CDC, Centers for Disease Control and Prevention; CER, comparative effectiveness research; CISNET, Cancer Intervention and Surveillance Modeling Network; CRN, Cancer Research Network; HRQOL, health-related quality of life; MHOS, Medicare Health Outcomes Survey; RT, radiation therapy; SEER, Surveillance, Epidemiology, and End Results.

measures (40,41). However, the rising costs of health care, and cancer care in particular, is a major concern in the United States (42). Smith and Hillner reported that annual costs for cancer care are projected to rise to over $170 billion by 2020, largely due to increased costs of new therapies and more extensive health interventions (42). Given this explosion of costs associated with innovations in cancer care, there is a need for CER that contributes to knowledge regarding the costs and cost-effectiveness of cancer interventions (29,40,43–45). For example, Zhang et al. reported that for oncology patients, a simple discussion of end-of-life wishes alone may result in as much as a 35% reduction in health care spending in the last week of life (46). Organizations other than PCORI, such as the NCI and the Agency for Healthcare Research and Quality (AHRQ), do support including cost-effectiveness and resource analyses in CER (29). Of the 103 NCI-funded CER studies in oncology between 2009 and 2011, 35% included economical modeling (29). Many experts believe that the federal guidelines for cost examination in CER will change as policy makers aim toward both raising the quality of care and limiting health care spending (8, 40).

CER and the related concept of patient-centered outcomes research are particularly compelling in oncology, where individualizing care based on biomarkers, "-omics" information, and patient preferences has gained significant traction and clinical application (29). The constellation of recent advances in personalized medicine, genomics, and CER provides opportunities for CER to accelerate development in these other fields and opportunities for innovation through intersections among these fields (47, 48). CER methods, including systematic reviews, observational cohort studies, and decision analysis models, are essential tools for moving genomic tests and discoveries into clinical practice, including the broad implementation of discoveries beyond the point of "bench to bedside," since these methods can demonstrate effectiveness for individuals, for subgroups, or at the policy level (49, 50). From a development perspective, personalized medicine approaches that use biomarkers to guide therapy decisions suffer from a lack of data on clinical utility, and CER offers methods to rapidly provide evidence when databases exist (48, 51). Furthermore, oncology treatment decisions can be strongly affected by patient characteristics, such as age or comorbidities, and CER provides the potential to evaluate treatment effectiveness within subgroups. For PC in particular, evaluation of the effectiveness of ADT in elderly patients and/or patients with pre-existing cardiac disease is an example of the potential for CER to provide helpful subgroup-level data that is not otherwise available from RCTs (52). Given the complex decisions in oncology, where individual characteristics as varied as patient preference, age, comorbidities, and performance status, as well as biomarkers and genomic profiles, can influence choices and outcomes, CER is particularly a compelling approach to evaluate the effectiveness of interventions in subgroups, strata, or individuals in real-world settings.

■ IMPORTANCE OF COMPARATIVE EFFECTIVENESS RESEARCH IN PROSTATE CANCER

In 2009, the IOM listed treatments for localized PC in the highest quartile of its top 100 national priorities for CER (1). Given the significant public health burden of the disease coupled with the lack of informative RCTs, the need for informative PC CER is tremendous. Currently, it is estimated that one in six men in the United States will develop PC (53). The American Cancer Society estimates that PC will account for 28% of cancer diagnoses among men in 2013 (53) and will account for $16.4 billion in annual direct health care costs by 2020 (54).

Prostate CER is capable of adding valuable insight into the investigation of treatment modalities and outcomes otherwise not feasible with RCTs. The limitations for the generalizability and feasibility of PC RCTs are similar to the general limitations described previously: difficulties with patient accrual which limits statistical power, vast array of comparators, cost, and lengthy duration of follow-up time necessary to achieve clinically significant endpoints (7–9).

For example, the Prostate Cancer Intervention Versus Observation Trial (PIVOT) (55) randomized men with localized PC to prostatectomy versus watchful waiting. The primary endpoint of the study was overall survival with a target accrual of 2,000 patients. Difficulties with patient recruitment caused the trial to close after enrolling 741 patients. With a median follow-up of 8 years, investigators found no significant difference in all-cause mortality between the two treatment arms. However, the validity of the results has been questioned due to concerns of the statistical power of the study. In this instance, prostate CER investigators have used databases to provide supplementary evidence. Lu-Yao et al. (23) performed a SEER database analysis that confirmed the results of the PIVOT trial, and the similar results of another small-sample RCT (56), providing additional evidence that suggests equivalent survival with watchful waiting and surgery in men older than 75 years. Similarly, an RCT aimed at comparing RP versus prostate brachytherapy closed early due to difficulties with patient accrual (57).

The demands upon RCTs are tremendous for PC treatment comparisons, since there is a wide variety of treatment options, which include active observation, ADT, RP, and multiple forms of RT, including intensity-modulated RT (IMRT), brachytherapy, and proton radiation therapy (PRT). A comprehensive RCT designed to evaluate all treatment options for PC would be prohibitively large and costly. Moreover, patient and physician bias about PC treatment would make such a trial difficult to complete. An RCT aimed at comparing surgical prostatectomy versus interstitial radiation intervention closed after enrolling only 56 patients over a 2-year time period in 31 centers in North America (58).

Furthermore, comparisons among treatment options can be considered on multiple levels, since some treatment options, such as PRT and IMRT, are much more costly than RP or AS (59, 60). Yu et al. used a Medicare database analysis to compare the patterns of use, cost, and early toxicity of PRT and IMRT for PC (59). Despite the PRT sample including far younger, healthier men, 12-month toxicity rates were shown to be equivalent among PRT (N = 553) and IMRT (N = 27,094). This finding is particularly important given the nearly double cost to Medicare when using PRT as opposed to IMRT: $32,428 versus $18,575, respectively (59).

Time is also an important consideration for the utility of RCTs for PC. As shown with the SWOG 8794 trial, the relatively low fatality of PC means the RCT follow-up time to reach significant outcomes can take so long that the data may have limited external validity with respect to contemporary practice by the time the trial is published (10). Given these constraints on the feasibility of RCTs, CER can enhance our understanding of available treatment options for PC and help patients, physicians, and policy makers make informed decisions.

The wide array of treatment options with generally equivalent outcomes presents a challenge for PC CER. When health care decisions include multiple options that have similar benefits and harms, or when the clinical evidence is uncertain, the choices are considered "preference-sensitive." PC treatment decisions are a classic example of this, with major implications for prostate CER. Decision analysis models in the CER literature typically evaluate interventions in the average patient, using group-level utilities (61–65). However, individual patients may have preferences that differ dramatically from their peers, with subsequent changes in utilities associated with possible health states following an intervention. Cowen et al. compared decision analytic outcomes using group-level versus individual-level utilities and found that group-level utilities misrepresented individual patients' preferences in 25% to 48% of cases (66). This concept is relevant to interpretation of the medical literature. For example, in the comparison of AS versus active treatment for low-risk PC published in *JAMA* by Hayes et al., the benefit of AS for longer quality-adjusted life expectancy was sensitive to patients' preferences for surveillance versus treatment (62). So, group-level CER may not directly predict nor inform individual patient decisions. There is an existing literature on patient choices and preferences (67–69), and it is important to incorporate such considerations in the design and evaluation of PC CER.

Decision analysis modeling is a useful tool for PC CER, because it synthesizes evidence from a range of sources to compare outcomes of interventions. A decision model incorporates the probabilities of outcomes over time based on the use of interventions. Values, or utilities, are associated with each health outcome, and the output may be expressed as QALYs. Decision analysis models are well suited to evaluating interventions associated with a complex range of outcomes and probabilities. Because development of decision analysis models often involves performing sensitivity analysis of the model inputs, they are particularly well suited to evaluating how individual patient characteristics influence the outcomes of the model (15).

Decision analysis models are also useful tools for evaluating choices for subgroups or individuals, since inputs and probabilities can be adjusted or subjected to sensitivity analyses. Sommers et al. demonstrated that incorporating individualized preferences for PC treatment in decision analysis modeling is feasible and that the preferred treatment depends both on individual clinical factors and patient preferences (70). Decision analysis models can incorporate a range of individual clinical risk factors and patient preferences—essentially any baseline personal characteristics—to inform patient decisions (71). Since the use of individual patient preferences for PC treatments in decision analysis models has been shown to alter outcomes in 30% to 50% of instances (66, 70), and since incorporating individuals' heterogeneity has been shown to improve value over the use of group-level decision-making approaches (72), the authors recommend that these approaches be utilized in PC CER. In a very real sense, the ability to offer personalized cancer care in preference-sensitive decisions is dependent on measuring patients' preferences for cancer treatments and outcomes (73). In addition to explicit assessment of patient preferences to estimate individual utilities for PC CER, the concept of individualization can be extended to include other baseline personal attributes of patients, such as age, comorbid illnesses, tumor genotype (72), or even biomarkers of patient longevity (74). In this fashion, individualized CER methods have the potential to place patients and clinicians at the center of CER to incorporate key baseline attributes and preferences that influence informed health care decisions (72, 75).

■ COMPARATIVE EFFECTIVENESS RESEARCH IN LOW-RISK PROSTATE CANCER

Low-risk PC is defined as PSA <10 mg/mL, Gleason score of ≤6, and a tumor either nonpalpable or only palpable and confined to less than half of one lobe of the prostate, equivalent to clinical stage T1c or T2a (76). The potential impact of low-risk PC CER is comparable with that of prostate CER in general, as 85% of PC is confined within the prostate at diagnosis (77). A brief review of current prostate CER is presented here.

To highlight the current gaps in our knowledge and available evidence, we must first define our target population. The age of the low-risk PC population has recently shifted toward younger age at diagnosis. Although men older than 65 years previously constituted the majority of newly diagnosed PC (78), recent data suggest that men older than 65 years now make up less than half of the new diagnoses (79), likely due to earlier detection of PC from PSA screening. This shift in the mean age of diagnoses raises two important points. First, as our detection ability improves, the proportion of men with early-stage PC is likely to increase. Second, as we move forward with investigations of outcomes for PC treatment modalities, we must use caution to avoid the lead-time bias that earlier detection places on our analyses.

In the absence of RCT data, observational studies have provided a useful framework for comparing outcomes of the different PC treatment options for men with localized PC. For men of all age groups, comparing RT and RP, historical data suggested RT yielded inferior outcomes compared with RP (80, 81), whereas modern studies using higher radiation doses have shown similar outcomes to surgery (82–84). On subgroup analysis, RP appears to be of greatest benefit for men younger than 65 years, with an 11.2% reduction in PC-specific mortality at 12 years of follow-up when compared to watchful waiting (56).

For men older than 65 years, multiple observational studies have shown a survival advantage for surgery compared to RT and observation (85, 86), whereas available randomized evidence suggests that treatment (particularly surgery) and watchful waiting are equivalent in terms of cancer-specific and overall survival (56). From a quality-of-life and cost perspective, observation appears to be more effective and less expensive compared to treatment for men in this age group, granting two additional months to quality-adjusted life expectancy at 65 and 75 years of age and saving patients $12,000 to $15,000 in medical expenses (87).

Unfortunately, despite conservative management being a reasonable alternative for many of these men, a population-based analysis by Cooperberg et al. suggests that less than 10% of eligible men choose conservative management over aggressive treatments (88). Further, despite this relative lack of data favoring treatment over observation for low-risk disease (88), there is a wide variation of patterns of PC care across the United States on a regional level, suggesting that physicians' biases influence the decision-making process. The large discrepancy here between data and actual practice suggests a failure of research to inform decision making of patients and clinicians. By fostering an enhanced understanding of treatment alternatives and outcomes in real-world settings, PC CER may give physicians and patients more accessible tools to help make patient-centered decisions, thus alleviating some of these biases dominating the current decision-making process.

Systematic reviews provide for an additional CER research tool that can be used to methodically review data from published studies to fill gaps in knowledge or identify areas requiring further investigation. A systematic review was recently performed for the AHRQ to help determine the comparative effectiveness and harm associated between and within the different PC treatment strategies (89). After reviewing all available RCTs and observational studies, the panel was only able to identify three RCTs that directly compared the effectiveness between treatment modalities. Two RCTs compared RP with watchful waiting and demonstrated an improvement in all-cause and PC-specific mortality with RP (56, 90). The third RCT compared RP with EBRT among 106 patients with localized PC and showed decreased rates of progression and distant metastasis following RP. However, the generalizability of data from the three RCTs to current practice is limited as the majority of men included in such trials were diagnosed prior to PSA screening. After reviewing available data on adverse events treatment, the panel found that (a) erectile dysfunction was common across all PC treatment modalities; (b) urinary dysfunction was more common following RP; (c) hematuria and urethral strictures were more commonly associated with RT; and (d) bowel complication were rare following RP compared to RT (89). The panel also concluded that assessment of data from observational studies was limited due to varying definitions of adverse events in the literature and overlapping effectiveness estimates between different treatment modalities (89).

Observational cohort CER studies have potential value for PC, since RCT data are limited and require significant lengths of time for data to mature, and can provide useful data regarding the effectiveness of new therapeutic technologies. Hu et al. compared outcomes after minimally invasive RP (MIRP), with and without robotic assistance, with those after open retropubic RP using the SEER-Medicare linked database. They observed a rapid increase in MIRP utilization from 2003 to 2006, with mixed results for outcomes: MIRP was associated with shorter hospital stay and fewer perioperative complications, but with similar rates of additional cancer therapies delivered and higher rates of urinary complications and erectile dysfunction (91). A recent series of studies using the SEER-Medicare database have evaluated the comparative effectiveness of RT techniques, with the purpose of evaluating more expensive, more conformal techniques of IMRT and PRT compared to conformal RT. The results suggested slightly lower rates of gastrointestinal (GI) complications after IMRT compared to conformal RT (92–94) for men receiving definitive RT, but no benefit for IMRT for men receiving radiation after a prostatectomy (95). Another series of SEER-Medicare analyses also demonstrated a surprisingly higher rate of GI complications after PRT compared with IMRT (92, 94). Although these SEER-Medicare studies suffer from limitations arising from the methodology and database itself (15, 96, 97), they serve an important role in helping to fill gaps in evidence regarding PC treatment comparisons. It should be noted that the validity of such data has been questioned given previous research that has clearly demonstrated limitations of the billing claims data for identifying chronic complications following PC treatment (98). Moreover, the use of billing claims data to investigate RT toxicity is further limited due to lack of relevant dosimetric data.

Decision analysis models provide an additional PC research tool to help guide patient-treatment decisions in the absence of robust prospective comparative data (99). Decision analysis modeling provides for another power

CER methodology, and its utility to aid in patient and clinician decision making has been extensively reviewed. A typical decision analysis model includes a pictorial decision tree that displays alternative treatment options and associated outcomes that may occur with different treatment strategies. A decision analysis model is then created to account for the probability of an outcome occurring (obtained from the published literature) and the expected value of each outcome. The expected result of different treatment strategies is then presented, in terms of the outcome of clinical interest, which may vary from expected survival probability or years lived, QALYs, cost, and other clinical parameters of interest. Uncertainty in the different probabilities incorporated into the model can, however, limit the validity of the model. To account for any uncertainty in the probability values incorporated into the model, sensitivity analyses can be performed to assess the differing outcomes based on a range of probability values.

Multiple decision analyses have been performed to help aid the decision-making process for patients with localized PC. Hayes et al. performed a decision analysis to compare the quality-of-life benefits of watchful waiting or AS with definitive treatment (RP, EBRT, or brachytherapy) for a 65- or 75-year-old male with low-risk PC (100). On the basis of this analysis, investigators determined that AS was associated with the highest quality-adjusted life expectancy (11.07 QALYs), followed by brachytherapy (10.57 QALYs), IMRT (10.51 QALYs), and then RP (10.23 QALYs) (100). Konski et al. recently performed a decision analysis to compare the cost and quality-of-life benefit of IMRT versus 3D-CRT for a 70-year-old male with localized PC (101). On the basis of this analysis, investigators found that IMRT was associated with 6.27 QALYs compared to 5.62 QALYs with 3D-CRT. The incremental cost-effectiveness of IMRT was $40,101/QALYs, which meets current willingness-to-pay thresholds in the United States (101). However, the validity of decision analysis modeling is dependent on the quality of published data. Thus, as high-quality comparative data between PC treatments becomes available over the next few years, there will likely be a greater role for PC decision analysis modeling.

■ CONCLUSIONS

CER continues to build the evidence basis for PC decision making. As we have argued, PC presents unique needs and challenges for CER. Given the significant public health burden of PC, the tremendous health care costs associated with treatments, and the relative lack of informative RCTs, PC has been identified as a priority for CER. However, to fill evidence gaps and provide much-needed insights into effectiveness of treatments within subgroups, and based on individual characteristics, CER investigators will require improved data sources and methodologies. Ideally, future CER databases will include technical details regarding treatment, such as radiation doses and techniques, biomarkers and/or linked tissue repositories, clinical outcomes, and patient-reported outcomes. Although the intersection of CER and personalized medicine creates opportunities for accelerating progress toward patient-centered decision making, challenges remain regarding integration of genomics, epigenetics, and proteomics into a CER framework.

CER should be viewed as complementary to the traditional evidence-based medicine paradigm, which prioritizes RCTs. The protracted natural history of PC leads to a long period of maturation for clinical trial results and also makes it likely that secular trends or other diagnostic or therapeutic advances (e.g., PSA blood test) will render irrelevant or uninterpretable results of even the best-conducted RCTs. Therefore, it is critical that investigators embrace CER as a way to obtain rapid, relevant, real-world data to inform PC decisions, even while maintaining emphasis on RCTs and basic and translational science methods. Although current CER methods were reviewed in this chapter, it is expected that CER and patient-centered outcomes research will evolve continually to address the challenges and opportunities of genomics, personalized medicine, and future medical advances.

■ REFERENCES

1. Institute of Medicine of the National Academies. *Initial National Priorities for Comparative Effectiveness Research.* Washington, DC: Institute of Medicine of the National Academies; 2009.
2. Sox HC. Defining comparative effectiveness research: the importance of getting it right. *Med Care.* 2010;48:S7–S8.
3. Department of Health and Human Services. *Text of the Recovery Act Related to Comparative Effectiveness Funding: the American Recovery and Reinvestment Act.* Washington, DC: US Department of Health and Human Services; 2009. http://www.hhs.gov/recovery/programs/cer/recoveryacttext.html.
4. Clancy C, Collins FS. Patient-Centered Outcomes Research Institute: the inter-section of science and health care. *Sci Transl Med.* 2010;2:37cm18.
5. *Patient-Centered Outcomes Research Institute.* Vol. 2013. http://www.pcori.org. Updated 2013.
6. Department of Health and Human Services. *Report to the President and Congress; 6-30-2009.* Vol 2013. http://www.hhs.gov/recovery/programs/cer/execsummary.html. Updated 2009.
7. Haynes B. Can it work? Does it work? Is it worth it? The testing of healthcare interventions is evolving. *BMJ.* 1999;319:652–653.
8. Shen X, Zaorsky NG, Mishra MV, et al. Comparative effectiveness research for prostate cancer radiation therapy: current status and future directions. *Future Oncol.* 2012;8:37–54.
9. Giordano SH, Kuo YF, Duan Z, et al. Limits of observational data in determining outcomes from cancer therapy. *Cancer.* 2008;112:2456–2466.
10. Thompson IM, Tangen CM, Klein EA. Is there a standard of care for pathologic stage T3 prostate cancer? *J Clin Oncol.* 2009;27:2898–2899.
11. Hoffman KE, Nguyen PL, Chen MH, et al. Recommendations for post-prostatectomy radiation therapy in the United States

before and after the presentation of randomized trial. *J Urol.* 2011;185:116–120.
12. Nielsen ME, Trock BJ, Walsh PC. Salvage or adjuvant radiation therapy: counseling patients on the benefits. *J Natl Compr Canc Netw.* 2010;8:228–237.
13. Showalter TN, Ohri N, Teti KG, et al. Physician beliefs and practices for adjuvant and salvage radiation therapy after prostatectomy. *Int J Radiat Oncol Biol Phys.* 2012;82:e233–e238.
14. Mishra MV, Champ CE, Den RB, et al. Postprostatectomy radiation therapy: an evidence-based review. *Future Oncol.* 2011;7:1429–1440.
15. Armstrong K. Methods in comparative effectiveness research. *J Clin Oncol.* 2012;30:4208–4214.
16. Zwarenstein M, Treweek S, Gagnier JJ, et al. Improving the reporting of pragmatic trials: an extension of the CONSORT statement. *BMJ.* 2008;337:a2390.
17. Luce BR, Kramer JM, Goodman SN, et al. Rethinking randomized clinical trials for comparative effectiveness research: the need for transformational change. *Ann Intern Med.* 2009;151:206–209.
18. Bekelman JE, Shah A, Hahn SM. Implications of comparative effectiveness research for radiation oncology. *Pract Radiat Oncol.* 2011;1:72–80.
19. Tunis SR, Stryer DB, Clancy CM. Practical clinical trials: increasing the value of clinical research for decision making in clinical and health policy. *JAMA.* 2003;290:1624–1632.
20. Cuttino LW, Khan A, Wazer DE, et al. When retrospective comparative effectiveness research hinders science and patient-centered care. *J Clin Oncol.* 2013;311:2226–2227.
21. Alemayehu D, Cappelleri JC. Revisiting issues, drawbacks and opportunities with observational studies in comparative effectiveness research. *J Eval Clin Pract.* 2013;19:579–583.
22. McClellan M, McNeil BJ, Newhouse JP. Does more intensive treatment of acute myocardial infarction in the elderly reduce mortality? *JAMA.* 1994;272:859–866.
23. Lu-Yao GL, Albertsen PC, Moore DF, et al. Survival following androgen deprivation therapy among men with localized prostate cancer. *JAMA.* 2008;300:173–181.
24. Earle CC, Tsai JS, Gelber RD, et al. Effectiveness of chemotherapy for advanced lung cancer in the elderly: instrumental variable and propensity analysis. *J Clin Oncol.* 2001;19:1064–1070.
25. Presley CJ, Soulos PR, Herrin J, et al. Patterns of use and short-term complications of breast brachytherapy in the national medicare population from 2008-2009. *J Clin Oncol.* 2012;30:4302–4397.
26. D'Agostino RB Jr. Propensity score methods for bias reduction in the comparison of a treatment to a non-randomized control group. *Stat Med.* 1998;17:2265–2281.
27. Seeger JD, Kurth T, Walker AM. Use of propensity score technique to account for exposure-related covariates: an example and lesson. *Med Care.* 2007;45:S143–S148.
28. Angrist JD, Imbens GW, Rubin DB. Identification of causal effects using instrumental variables. *J Am Stat Assoc.* 1996;91: 444–455.
29. Glasgow RE, Doria-Rose VP, Khoury MJ, et al. Comparative effectiveness research in cancer: what has been funded and what knowledge gaps remain? *J Natl Cancer Inst.* 2013;105:766–773.
30. Lyman GH, Levine M. Comparative effectiveness research in oncology: an overview. *J Clin Oncol.* 2012;30:4181–4184.
31. Parry C, Kent EE, Mariotto AB, et al. Cancer survivors: a booming population. *Cancer Epidemiol Biomarkers Prev.* 2011;20:1996–2005.
32. Hood L, Friend SH. Predictive, personalized, preventive, participatory (P4) cancer medicine. *Nat Rev Clin Oncol.* 2011;8:184–187.
33. Kuderer NM, Culakova E, Huang M, et al. Quality appraisal of clinical validation studies for multigene prediction assays of chemotherapy response in early-stage breast cancer. 2011 ASCO Annual Meeting. *J Clin Oncol.* 2011;29:abstr 2082.
34. Hershman DL, Wright JD. Comparative effectiveness research in oncology data: observational data. *J Clin Oncol.* 2012;30:4215–4222.
35. Albertsen PC, Walters S, Hanley JA. A comparison of cause of death determination in men previously diagnosed with prostate cancer who died in 1985 or 1995. *J Urol.* 2000;163:519–523.
36. Penson DF, Albertsen PC, Nelson PS, et al. Determining cause of death in prostate cancer: are death certificates valid? *J Natl Cancer Inst.* 2001;93:1822–1823.
37. Presley CJ, Soulos PR, Herrin J, et al. Reply to L.W. Cuttino et al. *J Clin Oncol.* 2013;31:2227–2228.
38. Presley CJ, Soulos PR, Herrin J, et al. Reply to L.W. Cuttino et al. *J Clin Oncol.* 2013;31:2227–2229.
39. Malin JL. When hope hindes science and patient-centered care. *J Clin Oncol.* 2012;30:4283–4284.
40. Garber AM, Sox HC. The role of costs in comparative effectiveness research. *Health Aff (Millwood).* 2010;29:1805–1811.
41. United States Congress. Public Law 111-148, 124 STAT. 741. In: Congress US, ed. Washington, DC; 2010.
42. Smith TJ, Hillner BE. Bending the cost curve in cancer care. *N Engl J Med.* 2011;364:2060–2065.
43. Pearson SD. Cost, coverage, and comparative effectiveness research: the critical issues for oncology. *J Clin Oncol.* 2012;30:4275–4281.
44. Konski A. Cost, quality, and value in healthcare: a new paradigm. *Oncology (Willston Park).* 2010;24:542–543.
45. McClellan M, Benner J. *Comparative Effectiveness Research: Will It Bend the Health Care Cost Curve and Improve Quality? Strategies to Improve Comparative Effectiveness Research Methods and Data Infrastructure.* Washington, DC: Engelberg Center for Health Care Reform at Brookings; 2009:P7–P14.
46. Zhang B, Wright AA, Huskamp HA, et al. Health care costs in the last week of life: associations with end-of-life conversations. *Arch Intern Med.* 2009;169:480–488.
47. Mendelsohn J. Personalizing oncology: perspectives and prospects. *J Clin Oncol.* 2013;31:1904–1911.
48. Garber AM, Tunis SR. Does comparative-effectiveness research threaten personalized medicine. *N Engl J Med.* 2009;360:1925–1927.
49. Khoury MJ, Clauser SB, Freedman AN, et al. Population sciences, translational research, and the opportunities and challenges for genomic to reduce the burden of cancer in the 21st century. *Biomarkers Prev.* 2011;20:2105–2114.
50. Khoury MJ, Gwinn ML, Ioannidis JPA. The emergence of translational epidemiology: from scientific discovery to population health impact. *Am J Epidemiol.* 2010;172:517–524.
51. Goddard KAB, Knaus WA, Whitlock E, et al. Building the evidence base for decision making in cancer genomic medicine using comparative effectiveness research. *Genet Med.* 2012;14:633–642.
52. Greenfield S, Kaplan SH. Building useful evidence: changing the clinical research paradigm to account for comparative effectiveness research. *J Comp Eff Res.* 2012;1:263–270.
53. Siegel R, Naishadham D, Jemal A. Cancer Statistics, 2013. *CA Cancer J Clin.* 2013;63:11–30.
54. Mariotto AB, Yabroff KR, Shao Y, et al. Projections of the cost of cancer care in the United States: 2010-2020. *J Natl Cancer Inst.* 2011;103:1–12.
55. Wilt TJ, Brawer MK, Jones KM, et al. Radical prostatectomy versus observation for localized prostate cancer. *N Engl J Med.* 2012;367:203–213.
56. Bill-Axelson A, Holmberg L, Filen F, et al. Radical prostatectomy versus watchful waiting in localized prostate cancer: the Scandinavian prostate cancer group-4 randomized trial. *J Natl Cancer Inst.* 2008;100:1144–1154.
57. Crook JM, Gomez-Iturriaga A, Wallace K, et al. Comparison of health-related quality of life 5 years after SPIRIT: Surgical Prostatectomy Versus Interstitial Radiation Intervention Trial. *J Clin Oncol.* 2011;29:362–368.
58. Wallace K, Fleshner N, Jewett M, et al. Impact of a multi-disciplinary patient education session on accrual to a difficult clinical trial: the Toronto experience with the

surgicalprostatectomyversusinterstitialradiationinterventiontrial. *J Clin Oncol.* 2006;24:4158–4162.
59. Yu JB, Soulos PR, Herrin J, et al. Proton versus intensity-modulated radiotherapy for prostate cancer: patterns of care and early toxicity. *J Natl Cancer Inst.* 2013;105:25–32.
60. Cooperberg MR, Ramakrishna NR, Duff SB, et al. Primarty treatments for clinically localised prostate cancer: a comprehensive lifetime cost-utility analysis. *BJU Int.* 2012;111: 437–450.
61. Elliott SP, Wilt TJ, Kuntz KM. Projecting the clinical benefits of adjuvant radiotherapy versus observation and selective salvage radiotherapy after radical prostatectomy: a decision analysis. *Prostate Cancer Prostatic Dis.* 2011;14:270–277.
62. Hayes JH, Ollendorf DA, Pearson SD, et al. Active surveillance compared with initial treatment for men with low-risk prostate cancer: a decision analysis. *JAMA.* 2010;304:2373–2380.
63. Konski A, Speier W, Hanlon AL, et al. Is proton beam therapy cost effective in the treatment of adenocarcinoma of the prostate? *J Clin Oncol.* 2007;25:3603–3608.
64. Konski A, Watkins-Bruner D, Feigenberg S, et al. Using decision analysis to determine the cost-effectiveness of intensity-modulated radiation therapy in the treatment of intermediate risk porostate cancer. *Int J Radiat Oncol Biol Phys.* 2006;66:408–415.
65. Showalter TN, Foley KA, Jutkowitz E, et al. Costs of early adjuvant radiation therapy after radical prostatectomy: a decision analysis. *Ann Oncol.* 2012;23:701–706.
66. Cowen ME, Miles BJ, Cahill DF, et al. The danger of applying group-level utilities in decision analyses of the treatment of localized prostate cancer in individual patients. *Med Decis Making.* 1998;18:3776–3380.
67. Holmboe ES, Concato J. Treatment decisions for localized prostate cancer: asking men what's important. *J Gen Intern Med.* 2000;15:694–701.
68. Pignone MP, Howard K, Brenner AT, et al. Comparing 3 techniques for eliciting patient values for decision making about prostate-specific antigen screening. *JAMA Intern Med.* 2013;173: 362-368.
69. Llewellyn-Thomas HA, Crump RT. Decision support for patients: values clarification and preference elicitation. *Med Care Res Rev.* 2012;70:50S–79S.
70. Sommers BD, Beard CJ, D'Amico AV, et al. Decision analysis using individual patient preferences to determine optimal treatment for localized prostate cancer. *Cancer.* 2007;110:2210–2217.
71. Vickers AJ, Kattan MW, Sargent DJ. Method for evaluating prediction models that apply the results of randomized trials to individual patients. *Trials.* 2007;8:14.
72. Basu A, Meltzer D. Value of information on preference heterogeneity and individualized care. *Med Decis Making.* 2007;27:112–127.
73. Blinman P, King M, Norman R, et al. Preferences for cancer treatments: an overview of methods and applications in oncology. *Ann Oncol.* 2012;23:1104–1110.
74. Mishra MV, Showalter TN, Dicker AP. Biomarkers of aging and radiation therapy to the elderly: future of the field. *Semin Radiat Oncol.* 2012;22:334–338.
75. Basu A. Individualization at the heart of comparative effectiveness research: the time for i-CER has come. *Med Decis Making.* 2009;29:NP9–NP11.
76. D'Amico AV, Whittington R, Malcowicz SB, et al. A multivariate analysis of clinical and pathological factors that predict for prostate specific antigen failure after radical prostatectomy for prostate cancer. *J Urol.* 1995;154:131–138.
77. Cooperberg MR, Broering JM, Kantoff PW, et al. Contemporary trends in low-risk prostate cancer: risk assessment and treatment. *J Urol.* 2007;178:S14–S19.
78. Cooperberg MR, Broering JM, Litwin MS, et al. Review: the contemporary management of prostate cancer in the United States: lessons from the Cancer of the Prostate Strategic Urologic Research Endeavor (CapSURE), a national disease registry. *J Urol.* 2004;171:1393–1401.
79. Glass AS, Cowan JE, Fuldeore MJ, et al. Patient demographics, quality of life, and disease features of men with newly diagnosed prostate cancer: trends in the PSA era. *Urology.* 2013;82:60–66.
80. Paulson DF, Lin GH, Hinshaw W, et al. Radical surgery versus radiotherapy for adenocarcinoma of the prostate. *J Urol.* 1982;128:502–504.
81. Akakura K, Suzuki H, Ichikawa T, et al. A randomized trial comparing radical prostatectomy plus endocrine therapy versus external beam radiotherapy plus endocrine therapy for locally advanced prostate cancer: results at median follow-up of 102 months. *Jpn J Clin Oncol.* 2006;36:789–793.
82. D'Amico AV, Whittington R, Malkowicz SB, et al. Biochemical outcome after radical prostatectomy, external beam radiation therapy, or interstitial radiation therapy for clinically localized prostate cancer. *JAMA.* 1998;280:969–974.
83. Kupelian PA, Potters L, Khuntia D, et al. Radical prostatectomy, external beam radiotherapy <72 Gy, external beam radiotherapy > or =72 Gy, permanent seed implantation, or combined seeds. external beam radiotherapy for stage T1-T2 prostate cancer. *Int J Radiat Oncol Biol Phys.* 2004;58:25–33.
84. Tward JD, Lee CM, Pappas LM, et al. Survival of men with clinically localized prostate cancer treated with prostatectomy, brachytherapy, or no definitive treatment. *Cancer.* 2006;107:2392–2400.
85. Tewari A, Raman JD, Chang P, et al. Long-term survival probability in men with clinically localized prostate cancer treated either conservatively or with definitive treatment (radiotherapy or radical prostatectomy). *Urology.* 2006;68:1268–1274.
86. Wong YN, Mitra N, Hudes G, et al. Survival associated with treatment vs observation of localized prostate cancer in elderly men. *JAMA.* 2006;296:2683–2693.
87. Hayes JH, Ollendorf DA, Pearson SD, et al. Observation versus initial treatment for men with localized, low-risk prostate cancer: a cost-effectiveness analysis. *Ann Intern Med.* 2013;158:853–860.
88. Cooperberg MR, Broering JM, Carroll PR. Time trends and local variation in primary treatment of localized prostate cancer. *J Clin Oncol.* 2010;28:1117–1123.
89. Wilt TJ, MacDonald R, Rutks I, et al. Systematic review: comparative effectiveness and harms of treatments for clinically localized prostate cancer. *Ann Intern Med.* 2008;148:435–448.
90. Iversen P, Madsen PO, Corle DK. Radical prostatectomy versus expectant treatment for early carcinoma of the prostate. Twenty-three year follow-up of a prospective randomized study. *Scand J Urol Nephrol Suppl.* 1995;172:65–72.
91. Hu JC, Gu X, Lipsitz SR, et al. Comparative effectiveness of minimally invasive vs open radical prostatectomy. *JAMA.* 2009;302:1557–1564.
92. Kim S, Shen S, Moore DF, et al. Late gastrointestinal toxicities following radiation therapy for prostate cancer. *Eur Urol.* 2011;60:908–916.
93. Bekelman JE, Mitra N, Efstathiou JA, et al. Outcomes after intensity-modulated versus conformal radiotherapy in older men with nonmetastatic prostate cancer. *Int J Radiat Oncol Biol Phys.* 2011;81:e325–e334.
94. Sheets NC, Goldein GH, Meyer A-M, et al. Intensity-modulated radiation therapy, proton therapy, or conformal radiation therapy and morbidity and disease control in localized prostate cancer. *JAMA.* 2012;307:1611–1620.
95. Goldin GH, Sheets NC, Meyer AM, et al. Comparative effectiveness of intensity-modulated radiotherapy and conventional conformal radiotherapy in the treatment of prostate cancer after radical prostatectomy. *JAMA Intern Med.* 2013;173: 1136–1143.
96. Virnig B, Warren JL, Cooper GS, et al. Studying radiation therapy using SEER-Medicare-linked data. *Med Care.* 2002;40:IV-49-IV-54.
97. Warren JL, Klabunde CN, Schrag D, et al. Overview of the SEER-Medicare data: content, research applications, and generalizability to the United States elderly population. *Med Care.* 2002;40:IV-3-IV-18.

98. Potosky AL, Warren JL, Riedel ER, et al. Measuring complications of cancer treatment using the SEER-Medicare data. *Med Care*. 2002;40:IV-62-IV-68.
99. Aleem IS, Jalal H, Sheikh AA, et al. Clinical decision analysis: incorporating the evidence with patient preferences. *Patient Prefer Adherence*. 2009;3:21–24.
100. Hayes JH, Ollendorf DA, Pearson SD, et al. Active surveillance compared with initial treatment for men with low-risk prostate cancer: a decision analysis. *JAMA*. 2010;304:2373–2380.
101. Konski A, Watkins-Bruner D, Feigenberg S, et al. Using decision analysis to determine the cost-effectiveness of intensity-modulated radiation therapy in the treatment of intermediate risk prostate cancer. *Int J Radiat Oncol Biol Phys*. 2006;66:408–415.

14 Defining Treatment Failure for Localized Prostate Cancer: PSA and Beyond

NICHOLAS G. ZAORSKY

ROBERT B. DEN

JIANQING LIN

OVERVIEW

This chapter discusses dilemmas faced by physicians who manage a patient with a rising prostate-specific antigen (PSA) value after focal therapy for localized disease. Although primary treatment with radiation or surgery is largely successful at controlling localized disease, about one of three men develop biochemical recurrence (BR), or a rise in PSA to a defined threshold. Presumably, BR will lead to overt progression in men over subsequent years. In this chapter, we focus on the factors that a physician considers when counseling and recommending treatment to a patient with a rising PSA, including various PSA-based definitions of BR; presumed source of PSA (i.e., local disease, distant disease, or residual benign prostate); and the emerging technologies that may help detect treatment failure.

Rising PSA After Focal Therapy: Background

The incidence of prostate cancer rose since the introduction of PSA screening. Consequently, about 80% of men diagnosed in the United States present with localized (i.e., T1–T2, confined to the prostate capsule) disease (2). For men with localized prostate cancer, treatment with external beam radiation therapy (EBRT) or radical prostatectomy (RP) is largely successful at controlling disease (3). However, approximately one third of men develop BR or a rise serum level of PSA to a defined level (4). In the United States, an estimated 20,000 to 35,000 men per year experience BR after RP (5).

Presumably, BR will lead to distant metastasis (DM) and prostate cancer–specific mortality (PCSM) over subsequent years. Management of patients with BR is complex and controversial for a number of reasons: (a) a number of BR definitions exist; (b) a transient PSA rise after RT (i.e., a PSA "bounce") is difficult to differentiate from treatment failure; (c) even after confirmed BR, a further dilemma is the determination of the source of PSA (i.e., local vs. systemic disease vs. benign prostatic tissue); and (d) not all men with BR develop clinical relapse, so it is difficult to correlate BR with DM and PCSM.

PSA AS A MARKER OF TREATMENT SUCCESS

PSA is a soluble 34-kD glycoprotein secreted by the epithelium of the prostate gland and detected in the peripheral blood. PSA is a part of the ejaculate, and its purpose is to liquefy semen in the seminal coagulum and allow sperm to swim freely. PSA is also secreted into the blood, almost exclusively by the prostate gland, and has a reference range of ≤4 ng/mL. PSA remains in the prostate cells after they become malignant; therefore, it is a biomarker used in both the initial detection and subsequent posttreatment monitoring for prostate cancer. PSA production is regulated by the androgen receptor (AR), the main proliferative signal for prostate cancer growth. PSA values are typically measured every 3 to 6 months after RP or RT for the initial 1 to 2 years after therapy; they are checked yearly thereafter. A sample plot of fall in PSA post-RP versus post-RT is shown in Figure 14.1.

Post-RP

Serum PSA should reach undetectable levels by conventional assays in 4 to 6 weeks in the majority of men undergoing RP since that the half-life of PSA is 2.5 to 3 days (6). Despite this short half-life, studies have shown that 65% to 83% of men will have PSA levels that remain stable up to 10 years following RP (7–9). Thus, a low, stable, detectable PSA after RP may reflect presence of benign prostatic tissue, but a rise in PSA may signal cancer recurrence.

RP patients who experience BR have an 88% 10-year OS rate; in contrast, men treated with RP who do not have BR have a 93% 10-year OS rate (10). For men who have BR, the reported median time to clinical progression is 8 years; and DM to PCSM is 5 years. Thus, it is estimated

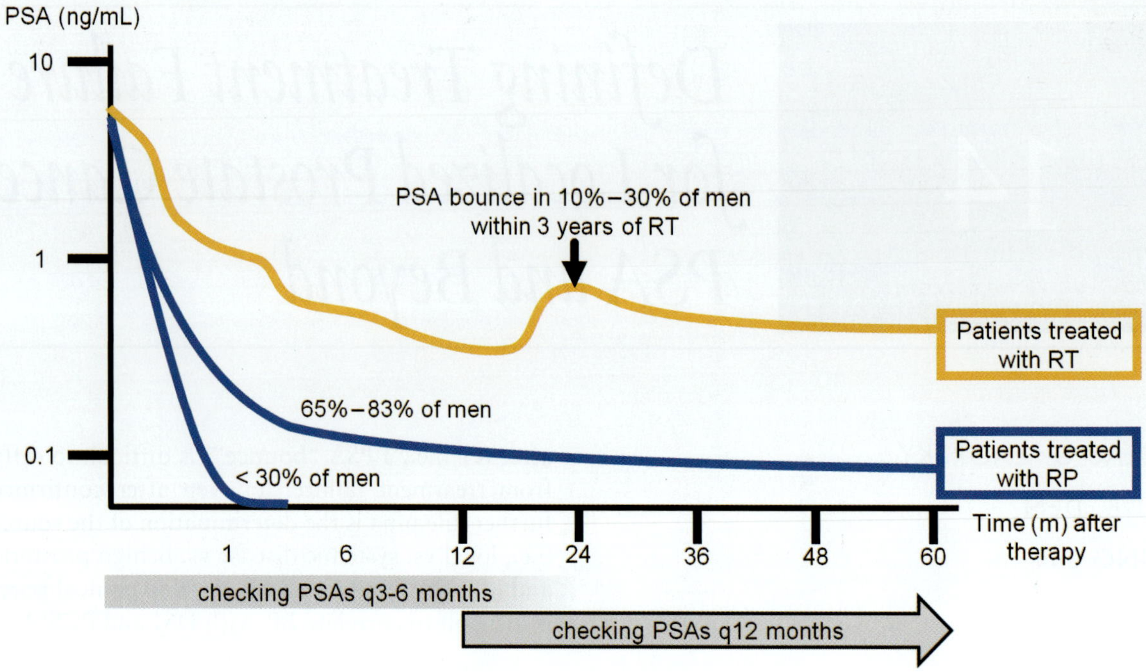

FIGURE 14.1 Typical plots of prostate-specific antigen (PSA) plotted versus time after radical prostatectomy (RP) or radiation therapy (RT). After RP, the majority (65%–83%) of men will have PSA levels that remain stable up to 10 years, and a minority will have undetectable levels. In contrast, RT typically induces a slow and inconsistent decrease in PSA to levels that are typically still detectable. Moreover, 10% to 30% of post-RT patients exhibit a PSA bounce (i.e., a temporary elevation in PSA without disease recurrence) within 3 years after RT, and these bounces may take up to 18 months to normalize. This figure is a descriptive approximation, created by Nicholas G. Zaorsky, MD.

that the time from BR until PCSM is 13 years (11). Although recent studies have demonstrated a median survival of up to 16 years after BR, a subset of men with aggressive prostate cancer die much sooner (12).

Post-RT

Compared to the post-RP setting, it is more difficult to define treatment success and failure based on PSA values alone following RT. RT typically induces a slow and inconsistent decrease in PSA to levels that are typically still detectable. Moreover, 10% to 30% of patients exhibit a PSA bounce (i.e., a temporary elevation in PSA without disease recurrence) within 3 years after RT, and these bounces may take up to 18 months to normalize (13–15). PSA bounces are likely due to radiation and bacterial prostatitis (16).

Five-year BR rates post-RT have been estimated to be 28% to 39% using the ASTRO definition (i.e., three consecutive rises in PSA) and 24% to 32% using the Phoenix definition (i.e., nadir +2 ng/mL) (17, 18). OS remains high at 5 years in men who have experienced BR versus those who have not; moreover, patient's age at failure, pre-RT PSA, PSA nadir, time from RT to failure, time to nadir, Gleason score (GS), T-stage, and rate of rise, both from the nadir and from the beginning of the rise, are not significantly associated with an increased risk of death (19).

The Phoenix definition has since been shown to be a better predictor of DM, PCSM, and OS (20, 21). For men with a rising PSA, the 10-year DM-free survival is estimated to be 90%, while those with stable PSA have a rate of 97% (22). BR has been used as an outcome measure in multiple studies; however, because of variable definitions (18), the difficulty with comparing BR across treatments (23), and post-RT BR not directly translating to mortality, PCSM has been the preferred metric for treatment efficacy after RT. For patients treated with RP, EBRT and androgen deprivation therapy (ADT), and EBRT alone, the 10-year PCSM rates have been estimated to be 8%, 8%, and 12%, respectively (24).

■ PSA AS A MARKER OF PROSTATE CANCER RECURRENCE

A rising PSA after RT or RP may signify existence of benign tissue, local recurrence (LR), or metastatic recurrence. It is important to differentiate among these possibilities to tailor treatment accordingly. The definition of BR varies, and important factors in its definition include the absolute PSA level, PSA kinetics, nomograms, imaging studies, and biopsy of the prostatic bed (summarized in Table 14.1). Although a number of guidelines for trending PSA post-therapy have been published, future markers of failure

Table 14.1 PSA trajectory after RT or RP, and definitions of BR

	Post-RP	Post-RT
PSA trajectory	• PSA should reach undetectable levels in 4 wk (6) • 65%–83% of men have elevated PSA up to 10 y post-RP (7–9)	• PSA falls slowly and unevenly • 10%–30% of men have PSA bounces in 3 y post-RT (13–15) • Bounces take up to 18 m to normalize (13–15) • ADT use confounds the true PSA value
Absolute PSA value cutoffs	• 0.2 ng/mL (25, 26)	• 3 consecutive PSA rises (ASTRO) (34)
	• 2 sequential PSA values ≥ 0.2 ng/mL (27)	• PSAn + 2 ng/mL (Phoenix) (20, 21)
	• ≥ 0.4 ng/mL + subsequent elevated level (25)	
	• ≥ 0.5 ng/mL is "secure evidence of PSA failure" (30)	
PSA kinetics	• time to BR ≤ 2 y predicts DM (12, 31) • PSA-DT of <3 m have highest risk of recurrence (31, 37) • PSA ≥ 0.4 ng/mL + subsequent elevated level predicts for DM, salvage therapy, PSA-DT (25)	• PSA-DT < 3 m predicts PCSS (41) • IBR < 18 m predicts PCSS (44)
Nomograms	• Post-RP specific (12, 31, 37, 45)	• Post-RT specific (46)

Abbreviations: ASTRO, American Society for Radiation Oncology; BR, biochemical recurrence; DM, diabetes mellitus type 2; DT, doubling time; IBR, interval to biochemical recurrence; PCSS, prostate cancer specific survival; PSA, prostate-specific antigen; PSAn, PSA nadir; RP, radical prostatectomy; RT, radiation therapy

will likely use more sensitive and specific PSA tests and employ other modalities alongside the PSA.

The Absolute PSA Level Post-RP

Often, serial evaluation of PSAs can help evaluate the clinical significance of a detectable PSA. For example, a man with a detectable and low PSA level of 0.06 ng/mL after therapy may have a persistently detectable PSA (i.e., 0.06 ng/mL on every visit) without significant change for many years. Such a patient is unlikely to progress and suffer PCSM. Thus, a detectable PSA alone may not mandate salvage intervention. In contrast, a patient with a detectable and serially rising PSA of 0.6 ng/mL (i.e., from 0.6 to 1.2 ng/mL and then to 1.8 ng/mL) is more indicative of residual prostate cancer and may benefit from salvage intervention.

Several studies have evaluated specific PSA cutoffs to define BR after RP at 0.2 ng/mL (25, 26). Friedland et al. (26) demonstrated a risk of post-RP PSA progression of 86% and 100% at 1 and 3 years, respectively. European Association of Urology (EAU) guidelines define BR with both a post-RP PSA cutoff of 0.2 ng/mL, and two sequential PSA values ≥ 0.2 ng/mL (27). These cutoffs are based on studies showing that only half of men with a detectable PSA in the 0.2 to 0.29 ng/mL range had a subsequent PSA progression and could be defined as having BR. A higher PSA level (i.e., ≥ 0.4 ng/mL) correlated with a 79% risk of PSA progression (28). The PSA Working Group defined BR with a PSA cutoff ≥ 0.4 ng/mL with a subsequent elevated level (29). A retrospective evaluation of BR criteria showed that PSA cutoff ≥ 0.4 ng/mL had the highest correlation with the risk of clinical progression (25). Finally, the 1997 ASTRO consensus panel concluded that a PSA ≥ 0.5 ng/mL is "secure evidence of PSA failure" (30).

The Absolute PSA Level Post-RT

After RT, elevated PSA is associated with a poorer prognosis (e.g., risk of DM) (31); however, correlating an absolute PSA value to clinical outcomes is more difficult. Further, a serum PSA level above 1 ng/mL indicates a higher risk of failure of localized salvage therapy (32). The definition of BR based on an absolute PSA value post-RT is controversial because PSA levels may remain at detectable levels. A PSA bounce is common in the first 2 years following RT (14, 15). Notably, the median time to PSA nadir is 18 months (33); and, the concurrent use of ADT either prior to or along with RT complicates the interpretation of the PSA value. Therefore, using an absolute value for PSA to define BR is not recommended.

In 1997, the American Society for Therapeutic Radiology and Oncology (ASTRO) consensus provided an early common definition of three consecutive PSA rises for treatment relapse following RT (34). Since the ASTRO criteria did not specify a PSA cutoff, a man whose post-RT PSA rose from a nadir of 0.03 ng/mL to 0.04, 0.05, and 0.06 ng/mL on subsequent evaluations could be classified as having BR. Moreover, the relationship between ASTRO-defined BR and PCSM or OS has not been clearly demonstrated (35, 36). The ASTRO definition incorporates backdating the date of failure to the point midway between the post-RT PSA nadir and the first rise. Backdating results in an artificial flattening of Kaplan-Meier curves, and therefore falsely reports more favorable BR rates when follow-up is short.

The PSA nadir + 2 ng/mL (PSAn; Phoenix) definition was introduced in 2005, and it has been shown to reduce the artifacts of the ASTRO definition. The Phoenix definition is a more significant predictor of DM, PCSM, and OS after controlling for other covariates (20, 21). Moreover, it has no apparent length of follow-up bias, requires a shorter time to diagnosis (21), provides a BR risk estimate that remains proportional over time with or without ADT (21), and is associated with fewer misclassifications when neoadjuvant and adjuvant ADT is used (13). Thus, the Phoenix definition is preferred in patients treated with RT alone or RT and ADT, though the ASTRO definition is sometimes used in patients treated with RT alone.

PSA Kinetics Post-RP

The main purpose of following PSA after treatment is to predict clinically meaningful outcomes. Although positive surgical margins are associated with an increased likelihood of BR, there is no current standard interpretation of PSA kinetics after RP or RT. A short time period from RP to BR and shorter PSA doubling time (PSA-DT) have been shown to correlate with the site of recurrence as DM (31). In contrast, a longer time to BR (e.g., > 2 years) is associated with localized recurrence (11, 12). Generally, a shorter PSA-DT indicates a rapidly growing tumor and a higher risk of DM and PCSM (37). Patients with PSA-DT of < 3 months represent a minority (10–15%) of men with BR but have the highest risk of systemic recurrence (37).

PSA Kinetics Post-RT

The use of post-RT PSAn and PSA-DT are recommended to define BR. Although, for PSAn, it is unclear whether a PSAn during a patient's lifetime (38), at 12 months (39), or at 24 months (40) is most prognostic. Similar to the post-RP setting, systemic recurrences are associated with higher PSAn and shorter PSA-DT. Patients with a PSA-DT < 3 months have the greatest risk of PCSM, with a median survival of 6 years (41). However, patients with a PSA-DT < 3 months represent a small high-risk subgroup (42); moreover, a rapid DT may be miscalculated (43). A novel measurement of PSA kinetics is the interval to BR (IBR), which uses the Phoenix definition to define BR after RT. An IBR cutoff of 18 months predicts PCSM following RT without ADT (44).

Multivariable Prediction Tools Post-RP and Post-RT

Multivariable prediction tools such as nomograms integrate clinicopathologic and biochemical risk factors including PSA-DT, IBR, and GS to predict clinical progression after RP (12, 31, 37, 45) and RT (46). Notably, parameters that amplify the risk of DM and PCSM in these systems include PSA-DT ≤ 3 months, IBR ≤ 3 years, and GS ≥ 7 (12).

Advanced Methods for PSA Detection

In less than 40% of men, PSA levels are undetectable after RP (i.e., < 0.01 ng/mL, by current standards). NADiA ProsVue is an FDA-cleared in vitro diagnostic assay that uses a reporter monoclonal antibody against PSA, attached to a synthetic double-stranded DNA label. The limit of quantitation of NADiA ProsVue is 0.65 pg/mL, significantly lower than the most sensitive commercially available PSA assays. Three samples may be collected from patients between 6 weeks and 10 months post-RP, and the three samples are tested in a single ProsVue run to calculate the PSA velocity (47).

The characteristics of PSA that are commonly seen and those that define BR are reviewed in Table 14.1. PSA values differ in the post-RP and post-RT settings; thus, the definitions of BR vary and the following factors are often considered: the absolute PSA level, time to recurrence, PSA kinetics, nomograms, imaging, and re-biopsy of the prostatic bed. Currently, there is no consensual BR definition after cryotherapy, high-intensity-focused ultrasound, or brachytherapy (48). When diagnosing BR, a clinician must discern if the PSA is produced from local or systemic disease, as these will drive treatment recommendations.

■ SALVAGE THERAPY RISK ASSESSMENT

Current Methods: PSA and Nomograms

The initial step in management of BR in post-RP or post-RT patients is determination of the region of recurrence. Recurrence sites include (a) locoregional; (b) distant; or (c) a combination of the two. Typically, if LR is suspected, then the patient would likely benefit from additional local therapy. Patients with distant recurrence alone may benefit from systemic therapy.

Notably, local control is important if prostate cancer recurrence is suspected to be both local and systemic. The results of two phase III trials have demonstrated a survival benefit with the addition of RT to ADT (49, 50) without impacting quality of life (51). Increased OS and DM-free survival were seen in men who had RP and adjuvant RT (52). Finally, a post hoc analysis of South Western

Oncology Group 8894 showed that men with metastatic prostate cancer who had a prior RP had a better response to systemic treatment and improved OS (53).

In any case, the benefit of a therapy always comes with a risk, be it PCSM or treatment toxicity. Currently no single marker can clearly delineate local from systemic disease. Moreover, for continuous variables (e.g., initial PSA, time of BR after initial therapy), overlapping timeframes have been published. Various individual factors are considered in differentiating local and systemic recurrence (Table 14.2). Common factors considered include initial disease risk status (54–56), T-stage (57,58), imaging at time of BR (59), GS at time of BR (12,54–56,60), PSA value at time of BR (61–63), IBR (12,31,64,65), PSA-DT (12,37,57,58,63,66), and PSA velocity (67,68). Moreover, life expectancy tables (69) and clinical progression nomograms (12,31,37,45,46) may be combined in computer programs to help determine benefits and risks of treatment. Current research focuses on advanced imaging techniques to help differentiate local from systemic recurrence.

Future Direction: Advanced Imaging

Currently, there is no uniformly accepted imaging modality that can distinguish local from systemic recurrence. Traditional imaging to evaluate BR involves a radionuclide skeletal scintigraphy (bone scan), transrectal ultrasound and biopsy, CT scan, or MRI (70–73). These techniques may detect macroscopic disease, but they have poor sensitivity for microscopic (i.e., low volume) disease or when PSA is < 10 ng/mL. The NCCN (71) has no clear recommendations for imaging in BR after RP. The NCCN recommends a biopsy and bone scan for certain men who are candidates for local therapy in BR after EBRT; that is, those with T1–T2, NX/0 disease, life expectancy > 10 years, and PSA < 10 ng/mL.

A bone scan is probably the most common study requested in the setting of a rising PSA level after RP, and it is most useful in patients with a rapidly rising PSA (70). Unfortunately, probability of a positive bone scan is < 5% unless PSA is > 40 ng/mL, which is well above the threshold where salvage therapy is considered. MRI seems to be the most sensitive technique for detecting LR after RP, particularly in patients with a PSA < 1 ng/mL; however, the accuracy of MRI after RT has not been fully investigated. Both MRI and CT may be used to plan salvage EBRT target volumes, though CT is otherwise not recommended. A TRUS-guided biopsy is typically not recommended because of poor sensitivity. A number of other imaging modalities are under investigation (Table 14.3).

Multiparametric MRI (48,70,74–76)

The role of endorectal MRI is limited in evaluation of patients with BR because of the low signal intensity of T2-weighted images in radiated tissue. Magnetic resonance spectroscopy (MRS) measures elevation in choline or decrease in citrate in prostate cancer tissue. MRS is limited by poor spatial

Table 14.2 Factors suggesting locoregional or distant disease in BR post-RP or post-RT

	Scenario	Favoring Locoregional Recurrence	Favoring Distant Recurrence	Reference
Initial disease risk status	Either	Low	High	(54–56)
T-stage before initial treatment	Post-RT	T1-2	T3-4	(57,58)
Imaging at BR (CT, MRI, choline PET)	Either	Local relapse	Metastases, lymphadenopathy	(59)
Biopsy GS at time of BR	Post-RT	≤ 6	≥ 7	(56)
	Post-RP	≤ 6	≥ 7	(12)
	Post-RP	≤ 7	≥ 8	(60)
	Post-RT	≤ 8	≥ 9	(54,55)
PSA level at time of BR (ng/mL)	Post-RT	< 10	≥ 10	(61)
	Either	≤ 5	> 5	(63)
	Post-RT	< 4	≥ 4	(62)
IBR (months)	Post-RP	> 36	≤ 36	(12)
	Post-RP	> 24	≤ 46	(31)
	Post-RT	> 18	≤ 18	(64,65)
PSA-DT (months)	Post-RP	> 9	< 3	(57)
	Post-RP	> 3	< 3	(66)
	Either	> 10	≤10	(63)
	Post-RT	> 8	≤ 8	(58)
	Either	> 3	≤ 3	(12,37)
PSA velocity (ng/mL/y)	Either	< 2	≥ 2	(67,68)

Abbreviations: BR, biochemical recurrence; CT, computerized tomography; DT, doubling time; GS, Gleason score; IBR, interval to biochemical recurrence; MRI, magnetic resonance imaging; PSA, prostate-specific antigen; PSAn, PSA nadir; RP, radical prostatectomy; RT, radiation therapy.

■ **Table 14.3** Current and future imaging modalities that may detect the source of BR

Modality	Sensitivity (%)	Specificity (%)	Comments (References)
			Current modalities
Skeletal scintigraphy (bone scan)	depends on PSA		Recommended if: PSA-DT <6 m, or PSA velocity > 0.5 ng/mL, or if absolute PSA > 10 ng/mL (70)
TRUS + biopsy	75–76	66–67	Not routinely performed or recommended (70, 71) Detects local, not distant recurrence (70)
Abdomen/pelvis CT	36	N/A	Not routinely performed; may be used for defining salvage RT target volumes (70, 72)
MRI	> 95	N/A	Most sensitive technique for detecting local recurrence compared to other current modalities (if endorectal coil used) (70) May be used for defining salvage EBRT target volumes (73)
MRI + subtypes			(48, 70, 74–76)
MRS	56–89	78	
DCE	84–88	89–100	Compared to T2-weighted MRI alone: sensitivity 84%–88% vs. 48%–61%; specificity, 89%–100% vs. 52%–82%
DW	62	97	Compared to T2-weighted MRI: sensitivity, 62% vs. 25%, specificity, 97% vs. 92%
LTNP	N/A	N/A	Disturbed nodal architecture visible on MRI
SPECT			(48, 70, 75, 78–80)
^{111}In-capromab pendetide (ProstaScint)	75–86	47–86	MAb targeting the intracellular domain of PSMA More sensitive than anatomic imaging at low PSA levels No correlation between response to salvage RT post-RP
^{111}In or ^{177}Lu -J591	98	N/A	MAb targeting the extracellular domain of PSMA
PET			(48, 70, 75, 78–80)
^{18}F-FDG	50–80	72–100	Unsuccessful in practice
^{11}C-choline	38–85	50–90	Use not recommended for PSA < 1 ng/mL, as MRI has higher sensitivity in detecting LR Sensitivity is dependent on cancer-specific variables (e.g., high-risk features)
^{18}F-choline	47–92	N/A	Has metabolism similar to ^{11}C-choline; has the benefit of longer half-life, but is limited by urinary excretion
^{18}F-NaF	81–89	91–93	Compared to ^{18}F-FDG PET-CT, more accurate in the detection of osseous metastases

Abbreviations: BR, biochemical recurrence; DCE, dynamic contrast enhanced; DW, diffusion weighted; ^{18}F-FDG, 18-fluorodeoxyglucose; ^{18}F-DHT, ^{18}F-dihydrotestosterone; CT, computerized tomography; LTNP, lymphotropic nanoparticle; MAb, monoclonal antibody; MRI, magnetic resonance imaging; MRS, magnetic resonance spectroscopy; PSMA, prostate-specific membrane antigen; PET-CT, positron emission tomography- computerized tomography; PSA-DT, prostate-specific antigen doubling time; RP, radical prostatectomy; RT, radiation therapy; SPECT, single-photon emission computed tomography; TRUS, transrectal ultrasound.

Source: Parts of this table are adapted from Ref. (1). Zaorsky NG, Raj GV, Trabulsi EJ, et al. The dilemma of a rising PSA after local therapy: what are our options? *Semin Oncol.* 2013;40(3):322–336.

resolution and high sensitivity to field inhomogeneities induced by surgical clips; and, the best diagnostic criteria are still unclear since normal citrate is in theory undetectable after RP, thus making the classic choline-to-citrate ratio inaccurate (48). Dynamic contrast-enhanced (DCE) MRI shows favorable contrast between poorly vascularized post-RT fibrosis and hypervascular cancer recurrence, and it has a better correlation with biopsy results than those from T2-weighted MRI. Diffusion-weighted (DW) MRI quantifies the water motion in an indirect manner and indirectly measures the degree of cellular crowding. Finally, in lymphotropic nanoparticle (LTNP) MRI, LN-avid supraparamagnetic iron oxide nanoparticles are distributed among the nodal architecture. In 26 men who were candidates for salvage RT post-RP, LTNP MRI was well tolerated, and six patients who were previously believed to be node negative tested lymph node positive (77).

Radio-Labeled Imaging With SPECT and PET (48, 70, 75, 78–80)

Radioimmunoscintigraphy uses radiolabeled monoclonal antibodies specific for prostate cancer epitomes, which are then detected with single-photon emission computerized tomography (SPECT). ProstaScint™ (^{111}In-capromab pendetide) is a murine IgG monoclonal antibody to the intracellular epitope of prostate-specific membrane antigen (PSMA). It has unfortunately shown no correlation between response and salvage RT in a post-RP setting and no clinical utility in detecting local recurrence. J591, labeled with ^{111}In or ^{177}Lu, is the monoclonal antibody targeting the extracellular domain of PSMA, and it has provided improved imaging of bony metastases and prostatic fossa.

Positron emission tomography-computerized tomography (PET-CT) imaging is advantageous in that it can detect LR and DM, but it is less sensitive than MRI in patients with PSA < 1 ng/mL. It is also limited by low spatial resolution and the tracer used. For example, ^{18}F-FDG PET has been unsuccessful in practice.

Recently, investigational PET tracers have shown more promising results. Although sensitivity of ^{11}C-choline may be as high as 85%, it is dependent on PSA levels, PSA-DT, and high-risk features. ^{18}F-choline has cellular metabolism similar to that of ^{11}C-choline, and has the benefit of a longer half-life (110 minutes vs. 20 minutes), which allows the radionuclide to be used in centers without a cyclotron.

^{18}F-NaF, first approved in 1972, was eclipsed by ^{99}Tc-labeled phosphate bone scans, but has made resurgence in 2000. Among men with BR after RP or EBRT, ^{18}F-NaF PET-CT is more useful than ^{18}F-FDG PET-CT in the detection of osseous metastases. The disadvantages of ^{18}F-NaF include its accumulation in benign bone abnormalities (e.g., degenerative joint disease and uncomplicated bone cysts, which are not seen on ^{99m}Tc-MDP scans) and detection of cancers other those of the prostate. The intracellular processes targeted by novel radiotracers are illustrated in Figure 14.2.

CONCLUSION

PSA screening has resulted in an increase in the overall incidence of prostate cancer diagnosis. While many men can be treated with surgery or radiation, a number of patients experience a rising PSA after primary therapy. Currently, a rise in PSA to a predetermined threshold signifies BR. A general assumption is that BR will lead to overt progression in patients over subsequent years. Clinicians face a number of dilemmas when encountering a rising PSA, including how to define BR, if the BR comes from localized or systemic disease, the treatment modality that would work best for an individual patient, and the timing of therapy. A number of studies have been published to help guide clinicians through these problems, and more clinical trials are currently ongoing. The future of detecting recurrent prostate cancer will likely use more sensitive PSA assays and advanced imaging.

REFERENCES

1. Zaorsky NG, Raj GV, Trabulsi EJ, et al. The dilemma of a rising PSA after local therapy: what are our options? *Semin Oncol.* 2013;40(3):322–336.
2. Siegel R, Ward E, Brawley O, Jemal A. Cancer statistics, 2011: the impact of eliminating socioeconomic and racial disparities on premature cancer deaths. *CA Cancer J Clin.* 2011;61(4):212–236.
3. Grimm P, Billiet I, Bostwick D, et al. Comparative analysis of prostate-specific antigen free survival outcomes for patients with low, intermediate and high risk prostate cancer treatment by radical therapy. Results from the Prostate Cancer Results Study Group. *BJU Int.* 2012;109(suppl 1):22–29.

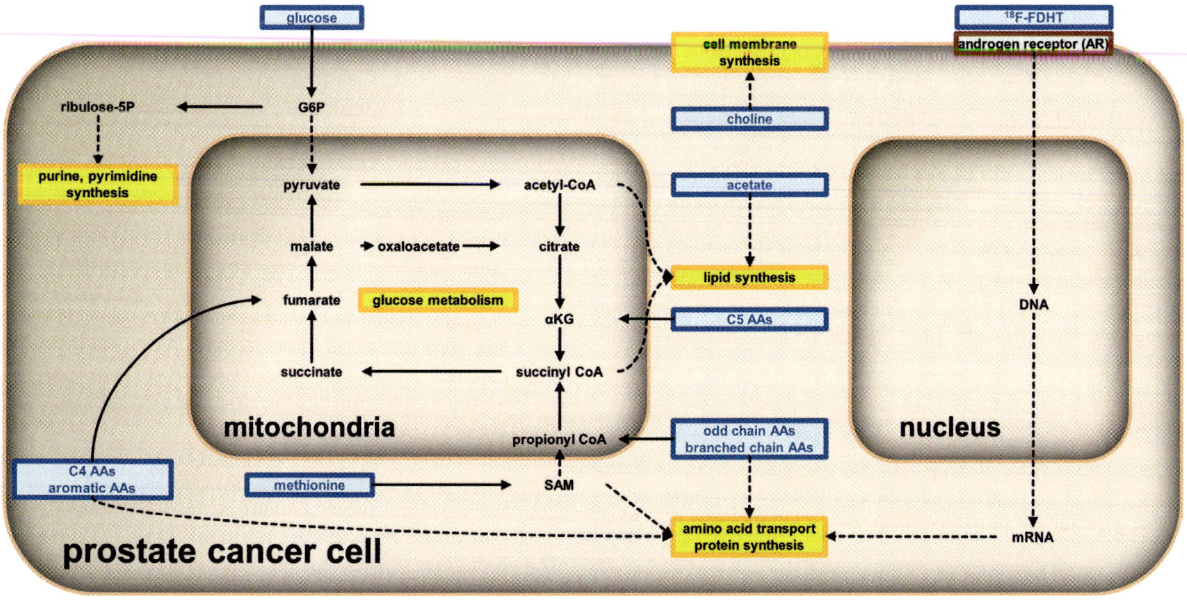

FIGURE 14.2 Prostate cancer cell biochemical pathways targeted by novel radiotracers.
Source: Adapted from Ref. (81). Zaorsky NG, Yamoah K, Thakur M, et al. A paradigm shift from anatomic to functional and molecular imaging in the detection of recurrent prostate cancer. *Future Oncol.* 2014;10(3):457–474. Illustration created by Nicholas G. Zaorsky, MD.

4. Djavan B, Moul JW, Zlotta A, et al. PSA progression following radical prostatectomy and radiation therapy: new standards in the new Millennium. *Eur Urol*. 2003;43(1):12–27.
5. Bianco FJ Jr, Scardino PT, Eastham JA. Radical prostatectomy: long-term cancer control and recovery of sexual and urinary function ("trifecta"). *Urology*. 2005;66(suppl 5):83–94.
6. Partin AW, Oesterling JE. The clinical usefulness of prostate specific antigen: update 1994. *J Urol*. 1994;152(5, pt 1):1358–1368.
7. Liu L, Coker AL, Du XL, et al. Long-term survival after radical prostatectomy compared to other treatments in older men with local/regional prostate cancer. *J Surg Oncol*. 2008;97(7):583–591.
8. Gretzer MB, Trock BJ, Han M, Walsh PC. A critical analysis of the interpretation of biochemical failure in surgically treated patients using the American Society for Therapeutic Radiation and Oncology criteria. *J Urol*. 2002;168(4 pt 1):1419–1422.
9. Roehl KA, Han M, Ramos CG, et al. Cancer progression and survival rates following anatomical radical retropubic prostatectomy in 3,478 consecutive patients: long-term results. *J Urol*. 2004;172(3):910–914.
10. Jhaveri FM, Zippe CD, Klein EA, Kupelian PA. Biochemical failure does not predict overall survival after radical prostatectomy for localized prostate cancer: 10-year results. *Urology*. 1999;54(5):884–890.
11. Pound CR, Partin AW, Eisenberger MA, et al. Natural history of progression after PSA elevation following radical prostatectomy. *JAMA*. 1999;281(17):1591–1597.
12. Freedland SJ, Humphreys EB, Mangold LA, et al. Risk of prostate cancer-specific mortality following biochemical recurrence after radical prostatectomy. *JAMA*. 2005;294(4):433–439.
13. Zietman AL, Christodouleas JP, Shipley WU. PSA bounces after neoadjuvant androgen deprivation and external beam radiation: impact on definitions of failure. *Int J Radiat Oncol Biol Phys*. 2005;62(3):714–718.
14. Hanlon AL, Pinover WH, Horwitz EM, Hanks GE. Patterns and fate of PSA bouncing following 3D-CRT. *Int J Radiat Oncol Biol Phys*. 2001;50(4):845–849.
15. Rosser CJ, Kuban DA, Levy LB, et al. Prostate specific antigen bounce phenomenon after external beam radiation for clinically localized prostate cancer. *J Urol*. 2002;168(5):2001–2005.
16. Critz FA, Williams WH, Benton JB, et al. Prostate specific antigen bounce after radioactive seed implantation followed by external beam radiation for prostate cancer. *J Urol*. 2000;163(4):1085–1089.
17. Beckendorf V, Guerif S, Le Prise E, et al. 70 Gy versus 80 Gy in localized prostate cancer: 5-year results of GETUG 06 randomized trial. *Int J Radiat Oncol Biol Phys*. 2011;80(4):1056–1063.
18. Roach M 3rd, Hanks G, Thames H Jr, et al. Defining biochemical failure following radiotherapy with or without hormonal therapy in men with clinically localized prostate cancer: recommendations of the RTOG-ASTRO Phoenix Consensus Conference. *Int J Radiat Oncol Biol Phys*. 2006;65(4):965–974.
19. Sandler HM, Dunn RL, McLaughlin PW, et al. Overall survival after prostate-specific-antigen-detected recurrence following conformal radiation therapy. *Int J Radiat Oncol Biol Phys*. 2000; 48(3):629–633.
20. Abramowitz MC, Li T, Buyyounouski MK, et al. The Phoenix definition of biochemical failure predicts for overall survival in patients with prostate cancer. *Cancer*. 2008;112(1):55–60.
21. Buyyounouski MK, Hanlon AL, Eisenberg DF, et al. Defining biochemical failure after radiotherapy with and without androgen deprivation for prostate cancer. *Int J Radiat Oncol Biol Phys*. 2005;63(5):1455–1462.
22. Zelefsky MJ, Ben-Porat L, Chan HM, et al. Evaluation of postradiotherapy PSA patterns and correlation with 10-year disease free survival outcomes for prostate cancer. *Int J Radiat Oncol Biol Phys*. 2006;66(2):382–388.
23. Nielsen ME, Makarov DV, Humphreys E, et al. Is it possible to compare PSA recurrence-free survival after surgery and radiotherapy using revised ASTRO criterion–"nadir + 2"? *Urology*. 2008;72(2):389–393; discussion 394–385.
24. Boorjian SA, Karnes RJ, Viterbo R, et al. Long-term survival after radical prostatectomy versus external-beam radiotherapy for patients with high-risk prostate cancer. *Cancer*. 2011;117(13):2883–2891.
25. Stephenson AJ, Kattan MW, Eastham JA, et al. Defining biochemical recurrence of prostate cancer after radical prostatectomy: a proposal for a standardized definition. *J Clin Oncol*. 2006;24(24):3973–3978.
26. Freedland SJ, Sutter ME, Dorey F, Aronson WJ. Defining the ideal cutpoint for determining PSA recurrence after radical prostatectomy. Prostate-specific antigen. *Urology*. 2003;61(2):365–369.
27. Aus G, Abbou CC, Bolla M, et al. EAU guidelines on prostate cancer. *Eur Urol*. 2005;48(4):546–551.
28. Amling CL, Bergstralh EJ, Blute ML, et al. Defining prostate specific antigen progression after radical prostatectomy: what is the most appropriate cut point? *J Urol*. 2001;165(4):1146–1151.
29. Scher HI, Eisenberger M, D'Amico AV, et al. Eligibility and outcomes reporting guidelines for clinical trials for patients in the state of a rising prostate-specific antigen: recommendations from the Prostate-Specific Antigen Working Group. *J Clin Oncol*. 2004;22(3):537–556.
30. Cox J, Gallagher M, Hammond E, et al. Consensus statements on radiation therapy of prostate cancer: guidelines for prostate re-biopsy after radiation and for radiation therapy with rising prostate-specific antigen levels and radical prostatectomy. American Society for Therapeutic Radiology and Oncology Consensus Panel. *J Clin Oncol*. 1999;17(4):1155.
31. Pound CR, Partin AW, Eisenberger MA, et al. Natural history of progression after PSA elevation following radical prostatectomy. *JAMA*. 1999;281(17):1591–1597.
32. Stephenson AJ, Shariat SF, Zelefsky MJ, et al. Salvage radiotherapy for recurrent prostate cancer after radical prostatectomy. *JAMA*. 2004;291(11):1325–1332.
33. Zagars GK. Prostate-specific antigen as a prognostic factor for prostate-cancer treated by external beam radiotherapy. *Int J Radiat Oncol Biol Phys*. 1992;23(1):47–53.
34. Consensus statement: guidelines for PSA following radiation therapy. American Society for Therapeutic Radiology and Oncology Consensus Panel. *Int J Radiat Oncol Biol Phys*. 1997;37(5):1035–1041.
35. Horwitz EM, Vicini FA, Ziaja EL, et al. The correlation between the ASTRO Consensus Panel definition of biochemical failure and clinical outcome for patients with prostate cancer treated with external beam irradiation. American Society of Therapeutic Radiology and Oncology. *Int J Radiat Oncol Biol Phys*. 1998;41(2):267–272.
36. Kupelian PA, Buchsbaum JC, Patel C, et al. Impact of biochemical failure on overall survival after radiation therapy for localized prostate cancer in the PSA era. *Int J Radiat Oncol Biol Phys*. 2002;52(3):704–711.
37. D'Amico AV, Chen MH, Roehl KA, Catalona WJ. Identifying patients at risk for significant versus clinically insignificant postoperative prostate-specific antigen failure. *J Clin Oncol*. 2005;23(22):4975–4979.
38. Ray ME, Thames HD, Levy LB, et al. PSA nadir predicts biochemical and distant failures after external beam radiotherapy for prostate cancer: a multi-institutional analysis. *Int J Radiat Oncol Biol Phys*. 2006;64(4):1140–1150.
39. Alcantara P, Hanlon A, Buyyounouski MK, et al. Prostate-specific antigen nadir within 12 months of prostate cancer radiotherapy predicts metastasis and death. *Cancer*. 2007;109(1):41–47.

40. Zelefsky MJ, Shi W, Yamada Y, et al. Postradiotherapy 2-year prostate-specific antigen nadir as a predictor of long-term prostate cancer mortality. *Int J Radiat Oncol Biol Phys.* 2009;75(5):1350–1356.
41. D'Amico AV, Moul JW, Carroll PR, et al. Surrogate end point for prostate cancer-specific mortality after radical prostatectomy or radiation therapy. *J Natl Cancer Inst.* 2003;95(18):1376–1383.
42. Valicenti RK, DeSilvio M, Hanks GE, et al. Posttreatment prostatic-specific antigen doubling time as a surrogate endpoint for prostate cancer-specific survival: an analysis of Radiation Therapy Oncology Group Protocol 92-02. *Int J Radiat Oncol Biol Phys.* 2006;66(4):1064–1071.
43. Arlen PM, Bianco F, Dahut WL, et al. Prostate Specific Antigen Working Group guidelines on prostate specific antigen doubling time. *J Urol.* 2008;179(6):2181–2185; discussion 2185–2186.
44. Buyyounouski MK, Pickles T, Kestin LL, et al. Validating the interval to biochemical failure for the identification of potentially lethal prostate cancer. *J Clin Oncol.* 2012;30(15):1857–1863.
45. Kattan MW. Nomograms are superior to staging and risk grouping systems for identifying high-risk patients: preoperative application in prostate cancer. *Curr Opin Urol.* 2003;13(2):111–116.
46. Kattan MW, Zelefsky MJ, Kupelian PA, et al. Pretreatment nomogram that predicts 5-year probability of metastasis following three-dimensional conformal radiation therapy for localized prostate cancer. *J Clin Oncol.* 2003;21(24):4568–4571.
47. McDermed JE, Sanders R, Fait S, et al. Nucleic acid detection immunoassay for prostate-specific antigen based on immuno-PCR methodology. *Clin Chem.* 2012;58(4):732–740.
48. Rouviere O, Vitry T, Lyonnet D. Imaging of prostate cancer local recurrences: why and how? *Eur Radiol.* 2010;20(5):1254–1266.
49. Widmark A, Klepp O, Solberg A, et al. Endocrine treatment, with or without radiotherapy, in locally advanced prostate cancer (SPCG-7/SFUO-3): an open randomised phase III trial. *Lancet.* 2009;373(9660):301–308.
50. Warde PR, Mason MD, Sydes MR, et al. Intergroup randomized phase III study of androgen deprivation therapy (ADT) plus radiation therapy (RT) in locally advanced prostate cancer (CaP) (NCIC-CTG, SWOG, MRC-UK, INT: T94-0110; NCT00002633). *J Clin Oncol.* 2010;28:18s.
51. Fransson P, Lund JA, Damber JE, et al. Quality of life in patients with locally advanced prostate cancer given endocrine treatment with or without radiotherapy: 4-year follow-up of SPCG-7/SFUO-3, an open-label, randomised, phase III trial. *Lancet Oncol.* 2009;10(4):370–380.
52. Thompson IM, Tangen CM, Paradelo J, et al. Adjuvant radiotherapy for pathological T3N0M0 prostate cancer significantly reduces risk of metastases and improves survival: long-term followup of a randomized clinical trial. *J Urol.* 2009;181(3):956–962.
53. Thompson IM, Tangen C, Basler J, Crawford ED. Impact of previous local treatment for prostate cancer on subsequent metastatic disease. *J Urol.* 2002;168(3):1008–1012.
54. Chin JL, Pautler SE, Mouraviev V, et al. Results of salvage cryoablation of the prostate after radiation: identifying predictors of treatment failure and complications. *J Urol.* 2001;165(6, pt 1):1937–1941; discussion 1941–1932.
55. Izawa JI, Madsen LT, Scott SM, et al. Salvage cryotherapy for recurrent prostate cancer after radiotherapy: variables affecting patient outcome. *J Clin Oncol.* 2002;20(11):2664–2671.
56. Cheng L, Sebo TJ, Slezak J, et al. Predictors of survival for prostate carcinoma patients treated with salvage radical prostatectomy after radiation therapy. *Cancer.* 1998;83(10):2164–2171.
57. Freedland SJ, Humphreys EB, Mangold LA, et al. Death in patients with recurrent prostate cancer after radical prostatectomy: prostate-specific antigen doubling time subgroups and their associated contributions to all-cause mortality. *J Clin Oncol.* 2007;25(13):1765–1771.
58. Zagars GK, Pollack A. Kinetics of serum prostate-specific antigen after external beam radiation for clinically localized prostate cancer. *Radiother Oncol.* 1997;44(3):213–221.
59. Gleave ME, Coupland D, Drachenberg D, et al. Ability of serum prostate-specific antigen levels to predict normal bone scans in patients with newly diagnosed prostate cancer. *Urology.* 1996;47(5):708–712.
60. Allen GW, Howard AR, Jarrard DF, Ritter MA. Management of prostate cancer recurrences after radiation therapy-brachytherapy as a salvage option. *Cancer.* 2007;110(7):1405–1416.
61. Beyer DC. Permanent brachytherapy as salvage treatment for recurrent prostate cancer. *Urology.* 1999;54(5):880–883.
62. Ng CK, Moussa M, Downey DB, Chin JL. Salvage cryoablation of the prostate: followup and analysis of predictive factors for outcome. *J Urol.* 2007;178(4, pt 1):1253–1257; discussion 1257.
63. Choueiri TK, Dreicer R, Paciorek A, et al. A model that predicts the probability of positive imaging in prostate cancer cases with biochemical failure after initial definitive local therapy. *J Urol.* 2008;179(3):906–910; discussion 910.
64. Buyyounouski MK, Pickles T, Kestin LL, et al. Validating the interval to biochemical failure for the identification of potentially lethal prostate cancer. *J Clin Oncol.* 2012;30(15):1857–1863.
65. Buyyounouski MK, Hanlon AL, Horwitz EM, Pollack A. Interval to biochemical failure highly prognostic for distant metastasis and prostate cancer-specific mortality after radiotherapy. *Int J Radiat Oncol Biol Phys.* 2008;70(1):59–66.
66. Perlmutter MA, Lepor H. Prostate-specific antigen doubling time is a reliable predictor of imageable metastases in men with biochemical recurrence after radical retropubic prostatectomy. *Urology.* 2008;71(3):501–505.
67. D'Amico AV, Chen MH, Roehl KA, Catalona WJ. Preoperative PSA velocity and the risk of death from prostate cancer after radical prostatectomy. *N Engl J Med.* 2004;351(2):125–135.
68. Lee AK, D'Amico AV. Utility of prostate-specific antigen kinetics in addition to clinical factors in the selection of patients for salvage local therapy. *J Clin Oncol.* 2005;23(32):8192–8197.
69. Cowen ME, Halasyamani LK, Kattan MW. Predicting life expectancy in men with clinically localized prostate cancer. *J Urol.* 2006;175(1):99–103.
70. Beresford MJ, Gillatt D, Benson RJ, Ajithkumar T. A systematic review of the role of imaging before salvage radiotherapy for post-prostatectomy biochemical recurrence. *Clin Oncol (R Coll Radiol).* 2010;22(1):46–55.
71. Mohler JL, Armstrong A, Bahnson RR, et al. NCCN Guideline: Prostate Cancer. *Version* 2.2013. http://www.nccn.org/professionals/physician_gls/pdf/prostate.pdf. Updated 2013. Accessed April, 2013.
72. Kane CJ, Amling CL, Johnstone PA, et al. Limited value of bone scintigraphy and computed tomography in assessing biochemical failure after radical prostatectomy. *Urology.* 2003;61(3):607–611.
73. Miralbell R, Vees H, Lozano J, et al. Endorectal MRI assessment of local relapse after surgery for prostate cancer: a model to define treatment field guidelines for adjuvant radiotherapy in patients at high risk for local failure. *Int J Radiat Oncol Biol Phys.* 2007;67(2):356–361.
74. Futterer JJ. Imaging of recurrent prostate cancer. *Radiol Clin North Am.* 2012;50(6):1075–1083.
75. Alfarone A, Panebianco V, Schillaci O, et al. Comparative analysis of multiparametric magnetic resonance and PET-CT in the management of local recurrence after radical prostatectomy for prostate cancer. *Crit Rev Oncol Hematol.* 2012;84(1):109–121.
76. Seitz M, Shukla-Dave A, Bjartell A, et al. Functional magnetic resonance imaging in prostate cancer. *Eur Urol.* 2009;55(4):801–814.
77. Ross RW, Zietman AL, Xie W, et al. Lymphotropic nanoparticle-enhanced magnetic resonance imaging (LNMRI) identifies occult

lymph node metastases in prostate cancer patients prior to salvage radiation therapy. *Clin Imaging.* 2009;33(4):301–305.

78. Beer AJ, Eiber M, Souvatzoglou M, et al. Radionuclide and hybrid imaging of recurrent prostate cancer. *Lancet Oncol.* 2011;12(2):181–191.
79. Bouchelouche K, Tagawa ST, Goldsmith SJ, et al. PET/CT imaging and radioimmunotherapy of prostate cancer. *Semi Nucl Med.* 2011;41(1):29–44.
80. Picchio M, Giovannini E, Crivellaro C, et al. Clinical evidence on PET/CT for radiation therapy planning in prostate cancer. *Radiother Oncol.* 2010;96(3):347–350.
81. Zaorsky NG, Yamoah K, Thakur M, et al. A paradigm shift from anatomic to functional and molecular imaging in the detection of recurrent prostate cancer. *Future Oncol.* 2014;10(3):457–474.

15 Prognosis After Biochemical Failure and Surrogate Endpoints for Prostate Cancer–Specific Mortality

PETER ORIO

NATHAN BITTNER

■ BACKGROUND

The National Comprehensive Cancer Network (NCCN) classifies low-risk prostate cancer according to the following definition: clinical stage T1–T2a, Gleason score ≤ 6, and/or PSA < 10 ng/mL (1). Excellent clinical outcomes have been reported with radical prostatectomy, external beam radiation therapy (EBRT), and brachytherapy in the context of low-risk, organ-confined prostate cancer (2–4). In the subset of low-risk patients who develop biochemical recurrence of disease (BCR) after definitive local therapy, it is often difficult to predict whether BCR will ultimately lead to symptomatic disease and/or prostate cancer–related mortality. When salvage therapies are being considered, surrogate endpoints for prostate cancer–specific mortality (PCSM) may be useful in selecting out the patients who are most likely to benefit from aggressive treatment. In addition, surrogates of PCSM could shorten the long interval of follow-up needed to complete clinical trials with survival as an endpoint. Currently, the FDA-preferred standard for approval of new therapies for metastatic castrate resistant prostate cancer (mCRPC) continues to be overall survival (5). This highlights the importance of surrogates for survival when studying treatment approaches for men with organ confined prostate cancer, as survival can be measured in decades after initial BCR.

■ SURVIVAL AFTER PSA RECURRENCE AFTER DEFINITIVE TREATMENTS OF LOW RISK PROSTATE CANCER

PSA screening is associated with a lead-time of between 5 and 11 years (6). The fact that biochemical recurrences are demonstrated after treatments for low-risk prostate cancer speaks to the heterogeneity of the disease process itself and the need to follow outcomes in the pre- and post-PSA era (7, 8). In the PSA era, biochemical recurrence is demonstrated much sooner than clinical local recurrence or metastatic disease (9). Although biochemical recurrence is associated with prostate cancer–specific mortality, as one often will not occur without the other, it is not predictive because relatively few men will actually die of the disease itself (10, 11). Despite reassurance that many men will "die with" rather than "die from" prostate cancer, this offers little solace to a man faced with a BCR. The varied natural history of biochemically recurrent prostate cancer lends itself to the use of surrogates to help guide additional therapies and predict for men who are at risk of dying from the disease.

The impact of a BCR in the U.S. veteran population has been reported (10). The caveat of this study is that the Veterans Affairs population has a twofold higher burden of comorbidities (12) and patients who received radiation rather than radical prostatectomy were older, had more comorbidities, higher Gleason scores, more extensive cancer, and higher pretreatment PSA values. Among men undergoing a prostatectomy, the biochemical recurrence rates (greater than 0.4 ng/mL) were 34%, 37%, and 37% and PCSM was 3%, 11%, and 21% at 5, 10, and 15 years, respectively. In patients receiving radiation therapy, the biochemical recurrence rates (nadir plus 2 ng/mL) were 35%, 46%, and 48% and PCSM was 11%, 20%, and 42% at 5, 10, and 15 years, respectively. This is in stark contrast to a reported 0% and 1% mortality at 15 years in men without a biochemical recurrence undergoing surgery or radiation, respectively.

Clinicians and patients benefit from an understanding of the natural history of prostate cancer after biochemical failure following definitive therapy. Pound and colleagues (9) reported the natural history of PSA recurrences in a large radical prostatectomy cohort with organ-confined disease not exposed to hormonal therapy or salvage radiation. The actuarial metastatic free survival of the 1997 patient cohort was 82% at 15 years after surgery. Fifteen percent of men had biochemically recurrent disease and of these men 34% developed metastatic disease. The median time from PSA failure to metastatic disease was 8 years and the median time to death after metastatic disease was 5 years. This underscores the long natural history of prostate cancer after PSA failure. Although the majority of men with a PSA recurrence did not die of their disease, the median time to death was 13 years in patients who developed a PSA recurrence and ultimately developed metastatic disease. Additionally, Johns Hopkins reported outcomes of 3,096 men who underwent a prostatectomy from pioneering urologic surgeon Dr. Patrick Walsh (13). Although the generalizability from a single surgeon is reduced, the outcomes are still of interest. Among patients with a BCR, the median time to PSA recurrence was 2 years, the median time from PSA recurrence to metastasis was 3 years and from metastatic disease to death was 7 years.

Nomograms have been created to predict 15 year PCSM. The most important prognostic factors include Gleason grade 4 and 5, seminal vesicle involvement, and surgical year. Surgical year underscores the importance of comparing outcomes in the pre-PSA and PSA era. By Gleason score the 15 year PCSM ranges as follows: (3+3) 0.2% to 1.2%; (3+4) 4.2% to 6.5%; (4+3) 6.6% to 11%; and (8–10) 26% to 37% (14). In men with a documented BCR, the median time from RP to death was 14 years. Again this emphasizes the long natural history of BCR in patients treated for organ-confined prostate cancer and need for surrogates to shorten the duration of clinical trials with survival as an endpoint.

■ WHAT MAKES A GOOD SURROGATE?

For a surrogate to be clinically useful in predicting PCSM, several criteria need to be fulfilled. Not only must the surrogate statistically predict PCSM, it must do so in a time frame that would allow for a meaningful shortening of a clinical trial using the surrogate (15–17). The surrogate would also need to satisfy the Prentice criteria for surrogacy (18), which state that the surrogate must be prognostic for PSCM and also be independent of the treatment received. In this regard, the surrogate can predict for PCSM, without influence from the treatment arm into which a man may have been randomized.

■ PSA KINETICS AS A PREDICTOR OF PCSM AFTER DEFINITIVE LOCAL THERAPY

Although BCR is observed in the treated low-risk population, the likelihood of prostate cancer–related death is relatively small. Arvold and colleagues estimate the 12-year cumulative incidence of PCSM to be less than 1% in the low-risk stratum of patients treated with either prostatectomy or brachytherapy (11). This observation is likely attributable to the generally long natural history of isolated BCR. Freedland et al. report a median interval in excess of 16 years from PSA recurrence to prostate cancer death in patients who fail biochemically after prostatectomy (19). Even so, this interval is known to be highly variable, with some deaths being reported as early as 1 year after BCR (19, 20). This highlights the valuable role a surrogate endpoint may play in the appropriate selection of biochemically relapsed patients for additional therapy or potentially protocol enrollment.

Absolute PSA values have not proven to be a reliable predictor of PCSM and can be problematic because of the varying definitions of biochemical failure used for different treatment modalities (21–23). PSA kinetics on the other hand have routinely been shown to predict for clinical outcome after BCR in the setting of both surgery and radiation therapy. Makarov and colleagues demonstrated that a PSA doubling time (PSADT) < 3 months was predictive of PCSM in men who developed metastatic prostate cancer after undergoing radical prostatectomy (24). In other studies, postprostatectomy PSADT has also been shown to correlate with probability of developing distant metastatic disease (9). D'Amico et al. showed a similar trend in the population of patients who received definitive EBRT, where a posttreatment PSADT of < 6 months was shown to be associated with a significantly shorter survival in patients experiencing biochemical failure (25). In a much larger cohort of patients where 5,918 received radical prostatectomy and 2,751 received definitive radiation for local or locally advanced, nonmetastatic prostate cancer, D'Amico demonstrated that a PSADT of < 3 months was significantly associated with time to prostate cancer–specific mortality.

Assessment of a PSADT < 3 months as a surrogate for PCSM met the Prentice criteria for surrogacy as it was prognostic of survival and independent of the treatment received in terms of prostatectomy or radiation (26). A retrospective analysis of the TROG 96.01 trial has shown findings consistent with those observed by D'Amico (27). This study evaluated a group of 802 patients with locally advanced prostate cancer who developed BCR after definitive EBRT with or without neoadjuvant androgen deprivation therapy (ADT) and demonstrated that PSADT < 4 months as well as time to biochemical failure of less than 1 year were predictive of a poor clinical outcome. More recently, D'Amico analyzed the pooled data from two randomized controlled studies, including the TROG 96.01 data and the Dana Farber Cancer Institute experience, which showed a statistical and clinically significant reduction in PCSM that favored 6 months of ADT over radiation alone in the intermediate-risk population. Two surrogates for PSCM emerged, both satisfying the Prentice criteria for surrogacy: the PSA end and PSA nadir values of > 0.5 ng/mL. This led the authors to conclude that after radiation and 6 months of ADT, patients with a PSA end value exceeding 0.5 ng/mL should be considered for long-term ADT and those with a PSA nadir of >0.5 ng/mL should be considered for inclusion in randomized trials investigating drugs that have shown promise in the treatment of mCRPC (28).

In addition to being predictive of PCSM after local therapy, PSA kinetics have also been shown to correlate with PCSM in the subgroup of patients who are salvaged with AST after experiencing a postoperative or postradiation BCR. Rodrigues et al. examined a population of patients treated with either prostatectomy or EBRT and subsequently salvaged with AST for BCR (29). They found that a pre-AST PSADT ≤ 6 months was associated with an increased risk of PCSM. Other studies have demonstrated that the rate of PSA decline after initiation of AST is also predictive of PCSM. One such study evaluated a group 585 men who were initiated on AST for rising PSA after either surgery or radiation therapy and found that the time to undetectable PSA was significantly associated with PCSM (30).

PSADT is perhaps the most extensively studied surrogate endpoint for PCSM, but other descriptors of PSA kinetics continue to emerge for this purpose. One such parameter is the interval to biochemical failure (IBF) after local therapy. A shorter IBF has consistently been shown to portend a greater incidence of distant metastasis and PCSM. Large prostatectomy series have demonstrated that a time from surgery to biochemical recurrence of ≤ 3 years was significantly associated with higher risk of PCSM (19). Similarly, IBF has been shown to be a reliable predictor of clinical failure and death in patients treated with EBRT. Buyyounouski and colleagues reported that an IBF of < 18 months was independently predictive for distant metastasis and PCSM after definitive EBRT (31). An IBF of < 18 months has also been associated with a higher risk of distant metastasis, PCSM, and overall mortality in patients receiving salvage radiation therapy following prostatectomy (32).

Although the association between PSA kinetics and treatment outcome is readily apparent from the aforementioned data, the clinical utility of this information has not been clearly formulated to date. This is at least partially related to the variability in both the timing and the methodology used to calculate PSA trajectory. For example, there are several different approaches to the calculation of PSADT alone (33, 34). At the present, it seems reasonable to calculate PSADT using a validated metric and to use the information judiciously as a means of identifying those patients who may benefit from intensified salvage therapy or a clinical trial.

■ PATHOLOGIC FEATURES AS A PREDICTIVE TOOL FOR PROSTATE CANCER–SPECIFIC MORTALITY

In addition to PSA kinetics, pathologic features have been used to predict clinical outcome in patients treated for localized prostate cancer. Eggener and colleagues examined a database of 11,521 patients and identified seminal vesicle involvement and primary/secondary Gleason score of 4–5 as the prime pathologic determinants of PCSM after radical prostatectomy (14). The University of California, San Francisco, Cancer of the Prostate Risk Assessment Postsurgical (CAPRA-S) score was developed to use a composite of various pathologic features (PSA, surgical margins, seminal vesicle invasion, Gleason score, extracapsular extension, and lymph node involvement) to predict recurrence and mortality after prostatectomy (35). Recently, the CAPRA-S score was validated externally on a large, multi-institutional, external database (36). Unfortunately, scoring systems such as CAPRA-S are not generalizable to the population of patients who choose nonsurgical treatment modalities. Seminal vesicle biopsies are not routinely performed and the standard 12-core transrectal ultrasound (TRUS)–guided prostate biopsy is known to underestimate Gleason score in a significant proportion of cases, making these scoring systems appropriate only for patients who have undergone surgical staging (37).

■ CONCLUSIONS

Even in the low-risk stratum of prostate cancer patients, treatment is generally recommended because noncurative approaches appear to be associated with an increased risk of PCSM (38). Treatment outcomes with low-risk, organ-confined prostate cancer are excellent, though there is a nontrivial risk of BCR after therapy (2–4). The likelihood that BCR will translate into a prostate cancer–related death is small in the low-risk population, but PSA kinetics can be used as a surrogate endpoint (Table 15.1) to select patients who might benefit from aggressive salvage therapy (11, 24–32).

Table 15.1 Surrogate endpoints for prostate cancer-related mortality and morbidity

Surrogate Endpoint	Clinical Context	Predicted Outcome	Cut-Point
PSADT	Metastatic disease after prostatectomy(24)	PCSM	< 3 months
	Post-prostatectomy with BCR(9)	Metastatic disease	N/A
	Post-radiation therapy with BCR(25)	Mortality	< 6 months
	Post-radiation therapy with BCR(27)	PCSM	< 4 months
	Post-radiation therapy or post-prostatectomy with BCR(26)	PCSM	< 3 months
	Post-radiation therapy or post-prostatectomy with BCR, prior to starting ADT(29)	PCSM	≤ 6 months
IBF	Post-prostatectomy with BCR(19)	PCSM	≤ 3 years
	Post-radiation therapy with BCR(31)	PCSM & DM	< 18 months
	Following salvage radiation post-prostatectomy(32)	PCSM, DM, & Mortality	< 18 months
PSA nadir	Post-radiation therapy with 6 months of ADT(28)	PCSM	> 0.5 ng/mL
SVI or 1°/2° GS 4-5	Post-prostatectomy final pathology (only applicable to surgical staged patients)(14)	PCSM	N/A

Abbreviations: PSADT-prostate-specific antigen doubling time; IBF-interval to biochemical failure; DM-distant metastasis; SVI-seminal vesicle involvement; GS-Gleason score.

REFERENCES

1. http://www.nccn.org/professionals/
2. Kane C, Im R, Amling C, et al. Outcomes after radical prostatectomy among men who are candidates for active surveillance: results from the SEARCH database. *Urology.* 2010;76:695–700.
3. Sylvester J, Grimm P, Wong J, Galbreath RW, Merrick G, Blasko JC. Fifteen-year biochemical relapse-free survival, cause-specific survival, and overall survival following I(125) prostate brachytherapy in clinically localized prostate cancer: Seattle experience. *Int J Radiat Oncol Biol Phys.* 2011;81:376–381.
4. Spratt D, Pei X, Yamada J, Kollmeier MA, Cox B, Zelefsky MJ. Long-term survival and toxicity in patient treated with high-dose intensity modulated radiation therapy for localized prostate cancer. *Int J Radiat Oncol Biol Phys.* 2013;85:686–692.
5. Gomella LG, Sartor AO. The current role and limitations of surrogate endpoints in advanced prostate cancer. *Urol Oncol.* 2014;32:28.e1–28.e9.
6. Draisma G, Etzioni R, Tsodikov A, et al. Lead time and overdiagnosis in prostate specific antigen screening: importance of methods and context. *J Natl Cancer Inst.* 2009;101:374–383.
7. Han M, Partin AW, Piantadosi S, Epstein JI, Walsh PC. Era specific biochemical recurrence-free survival following radical prostatectomy for clinically localized prostate cancer. *J Urol.* 2001;166:416–419.
8. Kupelian PA, Buchsbaum JC, Elshaikh MA, Reddy CA, Klein EA. Improvement in relapse-free survival throughout the PSA era in patients with localized prostate cancer treated with definitive radiotherapy: year of treatment an independent predictor of outcome. *Int J Radiat Oncol Biol Phys.* 2003;57:629–634.
9. Pound C, Partin A, Eisenberger M, Chan DW, Pearson JD, Walsh PC. Natural history of progression after PSA elevation following radical prostatectomy. *JAMA.* 1999;281:1591–1597.
10. Uchio EM, Aslan M, Wells CK, Calderone J, Concato J. Impact of biochemical recurrence in prostate cancer among US veterans. *Arch Intern Med.* 2010;170:1390–1393.

11. Arvold N, Chen M, Moul J, et al. Risk of death from prostate cancer after radical prostatectomy or brachytherapy in men with low or intermediate risk disease. *J Urol.* 2011;186:91–96.
12. Rogers WH, Kazis LE, Miller DR, et al. Comparing the health status of VA and non-VA ambulatory patients: the veterans' health and medical outcomes studies. *J Ambul Care Manage.* 2004;27:249–262.
13. Makarov D, Humphreys E, Mangold L, et al. The natural history of men treated with deferred androgen deprivation therapy in whom metastatic prostate cancer developed following radical prostatectomy. *J Urol.* 2008;179:156–161.
14. Eggener SE, Scardino PT, Walsh PC, et al. Predicting 15 year prostate cancer–specific mortality after radical prostatectomy. *J Urol.* 2011;185:869–875.
15. Fleming TR. Surrogate markers in AIDS and cancer trials. *Stat Med.* 1994;13:1423–1435.
16. O'Shaughnessy JA, Wittes RE, Burke G, et al. Commentary concerning demonstrations of safety and efficacy of investigational anticancer agents in clinical trials. *J Clin Oncol.* 1991;9:2225–2223.
17. Schellhammer P, Cockett A, Boccon-Gibod L, et al. Assessment of endpoints for clinical trials for localized prostate cancer. *Urology.* 1997;49(suppl 4A):27–38.
18. Prentice RL. Surrogate endpoints in clinical trials: definitions and operational criteria. *Stat Med.* 1989;8:431.
19. Freedland S, Humphreys E, Mangold L, et al. Risk of prostate cancer–specific mortality following biochemical recurrence of disease after radical prostatectomy. *JAMA.* 2005;294:433–439.
20. Freedland S, Moul J. Prostate specific antigen recurrence after definitive therapy. *J Urol.* 2007;177:1985–1991.
21. Amling C, Berstrahl E, Blute M, Slezak JM, Zincke H. Defining prostate specific antigen progression after radical prostatectomy: What is the most appropriate cut point? *J Urol.* 2001;165:1146–1151.
22. Freedland S, Sutter M, Dorey F, Aronson WJ. Defining the ideal cutpoint for determining PSA recurrence after radical prostatectomy. *Urology.* 2003;61:365–369.
23. Horwitz E, Thames H, Kuban D, et al. Definitions of biochemical failure that best predict clinical failure in patients with prostate cancer treated with external beam radiation alone: a multi-institutional pooled analysis. *J Urol.* 2005;173:797–802.
24. Makarov D, Humphreys E, Mangold L, et al. The natural history of men treated with deferred androgen deprivation therapy in whom metastatic prostate cancer developed following radical prostatectomy. *J Urol.* 2008;179:156–161.
25. D'Amico A, Kantoff P, Loffredo M, Renshaw AA, Loffredo B, Chen MH. Predictors of mortality after prostate-specific antigen failure. *Int J Radiat Oncol Biol Phys.* 2006;65:656–660.
26. D'Amico AV, Moul JW, Carroll PR, Sun L, Lubeck D, Chen MH. Surrogate end point for prostate cancer–specific mortality after radical prostatectomy of radiation therapy. *J Natl Cancer Inst.* 2003;95:1376–1383.
27. Steigler A, Denham J, Lamb D, et al. Risk stratification after biochemical failure following curative treatment of locally advanced prostate cancer: data from the TROG 96.01 trial. *Prostate Cancer.* 2012;2012:814724.
28. D'Amico AV, Chen MH, De Castro M, et al. Surrogate endpoints for prostate cancer–specific mortality after radiotherapy and androgen suppression therapy in men with localized or locally advanced prostate cancer: an analysis of two randomized trials. *Lancet Oncol.* 2012;13:189–195.
29. Rodrigues N, Chen M, Catalona W, Roehl KA, Richie JP, D'Amico AV. Predictors of mortality after androgen-deprivation therapy in patients with rapidly rising prostate-specific antigen levels after local therapy for prostate cancer. *Cancer.* 2006;107:514–520.
30. D'Amico A, McLeod D, Carroll P, Cullen J, Chen MH. Time to an undetectable prostate-specific antigen (PSA) after androgen suppression therapy for postoperative or postradiation PSA recurrence and prostate cancer–specific mortality. *Cancer.* 2007;109:1290–1295.
31. Buyyounouski M, Hanlon A, Horwitz E, Pollack A. Interval to biochemical failure highly prognostic for distant metastasis and prostate cancer–specific mortality after radiotherapy. *Int J Radiat Oncol Biol Phys.* 2008;70:59–66.
32. Johnson S, Jackson W, Li D, et al. The interval to biochemical failure is prognostic for metastasis, prostate cancer–specific mortality, and overall mortality after salvage radiation therapy for prostate cancer. *Int J Radiat Oncol Biol Phys.* 2013;86:554–561.
33. Ponholzer A, Popper N, Breitenecker F, et al. Proposal for a standardized PSA doubling-time calculation. *Anticancer Res.* 2010;30:1633–1636.
34. http://nomograms.mskcc.org/Prostate/PsaDoublingTime.aspx
35. Cooperberg M, Hilton J, Carroll P. The CAPRA-S score: a straightforward tool for improved prediction of outcomes after radical prostatectomy. *Cancer.* 2011;117:5039–5046.
36. Punnen S, Freedland S, Presti J, et al. Multi-institutional validation of the CAPRA-S score to predict disease recurrence and mortality after radical prostatectomy. *Eur Urol.* 2014;65:1171–1177.
37. Corcoran N, Hong M, Casey R, et al. Upgrade in Gleason score between prostate biopsy and pathology following radical prostatectomy significantly impacts upon the risk of biochemical recurrence. *BJU Int.* 2011;108:E202–E210.
38. Ayal A, Chen M, Hattangadi J, D'Amico AV. Initial management of prostate-specific antigen-detected, low-risk prostate cancer and risk of death from prostate cancer. *BJU* Int. 2014;113(1):43–50.PETER ORIO

Treatment for High-Risk, Localized, and Locally Advanced Disease

III

16 Treatment of High-Risk Prostate Cancer: The Role of Low-Dose Rate (LDR) and High-Dose Rate (HDR) Brachytherapy

THOMAS J. PUGH

■ INTRODUCTION

Contemporary options for the initial treatment of high-risk localized prostate cancer (as defined by any of the following features: clinical state T2c–T4, Gleason score ≥ 8, or PSA ≥ 20) include radiation therapy with long-term androgen deprivation therapy (ADT) or prostatectomy with pelvic lymph node dissection followed by adjuvant radiation with or without ADT contingent upon postsurgical pathologic findings and postoperative biochemical testing. The two major categories of radiation therapy for prostate cancer are external beam radiation therapy (EBRT), where radiation beams generated by a machine outside the body are directed toward the cancer cells, and brachytherapy, with the placement of radioactive material inside the body near the cancer cells. The goal of radiation therapy is to deliver a cancer-sterilizing radiation dose to the treatment target, which may include the prostate, seminal vesicles, and/or pelvic lymph nodes, while limiting dose to surrounding normal tissue including bladder, bowel, erectile tissue, and the femoral heads. Minimizing dose to surrounding normal tissue is critical as the risk of toxicity from radiation therapy is a direct consequence of the amount of inadvertent radiation dose delivered to these tissues. With brachytherapy, a radioactive source is implanted directly into the prostate gland to administer a high dose of radiation directly to the prostate while minimizing radiation to normal tissues. Observational series suggest brachytherapy may have an important role in combination with EBRT and ADT for the management of select patients with high-risk prostate cancer. There is abundant evidence that higher radiation doses are required to optimize local cancer control and improve cancer-free survival in men with localized prostate cancer (1–3). Brachytherapy allows a higher dose of radiation to be given to the target area while minimizing radiation exposure to the surrounding normal tissues. Compared with EBRT, brachytherapy has the advantage of delivering high doses of radiation directly to intraprostatic and periprostatic tissue, without having to traverse normal structures to reach the prostatic target. Furthermore, prostate brachytherapy is a more convenient treatment option for patients compared with EBRT (i.e., the procedure can be completed in perhaps a single outpatient visit). The comparative disadvantages of brachytherapy include the inherent dependence on practitioner skill level, short-term prostate edema related to multiple needles placed into the prostate for delivery of radiation sources, application of spinal or general anesthesia, and the concern that the sharp dose gradient provided by brachytherapy may undertreat cancer spread beyond the planned treatment area (4). Due to concerns for the latter, brachytherapy is often combined with EBRT in men with high risk of extra-prostatic spread (5, 6). Prostate brachytherapy can be delivered through permanent, low-dose rate (LDR) radiation seeds or a temporary high-dose rate (HDR) radiation source. This article will review the indications, techniques, and outcomes from LDR and HDR prostate brachytherapy for high-risk prostate cancer.

■ PATIENT SELECTION FOR BRACHYTHERAPY

The selection of brachytherapy for a patient with high-risk localized prostate cancer is based on technical feasibility, the absence of coexistent urinary conditions, and the ability of the implanted radiation to encompass areas of known disease.

Prostate Size

A large prostate gland (generally defined as a transrectal ultrasound volume greater than 60 cc) is a relative contraindication to brachytherapy due to the consistent finding that a larger prostate confers a greater risk of postprocedure urinary retention (7–14). Furthermore, a large prostate gland may prevent proper radiation source placement as a consequence of pelvic bone interference. Subsequently, the target might receive suboptimal radiation dose along the periphery and excessive dose to central structures such as the urethra. In the setting of high-risk prostate cancer, the therapeutic advantages of using ADT with radiation neoadjuvantly, concurrently, and adjuvantly with radiation therapy also allow for a period of cytoreduction prior to radiation treatment (15, 16). Neoadjuvant ADT is a successful strategy for reducing prostate volume, typically resulting in an approximate 30% reduction in prostate size (17–19).

Baseline Lower Urinary Tract Symptoms (LUTS)

Higher levels of urinary morbidity after brachytherapy may be manifested by an increase in prostate-related symptoms or the development of acute urinary retention. The International Prostate Symptom Score (IPSS) was originally developed for evaluation of LUTS associated with benign prostatic hypertrophy (20). Scores greater than 15 out of 35 are associated with a greater risk of acute urinary retention (21–23). Other objective measurements of urinary function, such as peak urine flow rate, have also shown value for patient selection (14).

Other Considerations

Other relative contraindications for prostate brachytherapy include a history of prior rectal surgery, pelvic radiation therapy, prior prostate surgery including transurethral resection, unacceptable risk from anesthesia application, or inflammatory bowel disease.

■ LDR

LDR brachytherapy is currently indicated for men with high-risk prostate cancer when used in combination with EBRT and ADT (24), where supplemental EBRT is delivered to a total dose of 40 to 50 Gy over approximately 5 to 6 weeks. Observational studies suggest that a strategy such as this, oftentimes referred to as "trimodality" therapy, is well tolerated and effective treatment strategy for high-risk prostate cancer (25–28). Stone et al. published excellent results using trimodality therapy with the combination of 9 months ADT, 45 Gy EBRT, and an LDR brachytherapy boost (28). Biochemical freedom from failure at 5 years was significantly related to the biologic effective dose (76%, 84%, and 88% for doses <200, 200 to 220, and >220 Gy, respectively). In men with Gleason 8 to 10 cancers, there was a trend toward improved 5-year overall survival based on dose (87%, 89%, and 95%, respectively). While these results are excellent, it should be noted that no consistent advantage has been demonstrated from trimodality therapy over ADT+EBRT or surgical alternatives. Although EBRT is generally performed 0 to 8 weeks before brachytherapy, recent reports have demonstrated the viability of initial brachytherapy implant followed by EBRT. No studies have investigated the sequencing or time interval between brachytherapy and EBRT.

Two generally accepted philosophies have emerged with respect to LDR prostate brachytherapy treatment planning. In the first method, intraoperative or real-time treatment planning, all procedures are carried out in the operating room on the day of the procedure. These procedures include setting up the patient, determining the prostate volume, planning treatment, and implanting the patient with preordered radioactive sources. In the second method, preplanning, the prostate implant process is broken up into two separate stages. In the first stage, the patient undergoes an ultrasound simulation, often referred to as a volume study. The simulation consists of setting up the patient in an identical position to positioning at the time of the procedure, determining the prostate volume and cranial to caudal length, evaluating for pelvic bone interference, and deciding whether the patient is a candidate for prostate brachytherapy. Upon completion of the simulation, the patient is discharged home and returns for the procedure at a later date, typically within 2 to 4 weeks. During this period, a treatment plan is generated and seeds are ordered based on the treatment plan needle loading pattern. Quality assurance is performed on the seeds, which are stranded, placed into needles, and sterilized. In the second stage of the preplanning method, patients are set up in the operating room in an identical position to that in their simulation and implanted based on the treatment plan. The relative advantages and disadvantages of each approach have been the subject of extensive debate (29–32). Proponents of the preplanning technique cite cost-effectiveness as a result of all treatment planning and quality assurance being performed outside the operating room. Commonly cited advantages of intraoperative treatment planning over preoperative planning include improved accuracy of prostate volume studies, elimination of the need for a preplan volume study, and the ability to adjust to unanticipated operative findings. Proponents of the intraoperative approach suggest that these advantages result in improved consistency and quality, as assessed by postimplant dosimetry (33). Although real-time dosimetry provides immediate feedback to connect the planned distribution with the final result, imaging at present is not adequate for seed-based real-time dosimetry (34). Furthermore, needle-based dosimetry does not correlate well enough to replace CT-based postplan dosimetry (35). Hybrid approaches in which the treatments are planned on the basis of preoperative imaging with brachytherapy treatment planning software on hand in the operating room in case variation from the predefined treatment plan is necessary (intraoperative optimization) are also an option for LDR brachytherapy delivery (36).

Regardless of the timing for treatment planning, the parameters required to achieve a high-quality implant are similar. Preplan parameters vary considerably but as a general guideline, >99% of the prostate should receive the prescription dose. There are currently three LDR brachytherapy sources routinely used for permanent prostate brachytherapy: I-125, Pd-103, and Cs-131. The half-lives and dosimetry profiles of each isotope are disparate. As a result, the recommended prescription doses for use in combination therapy with EBRT are different for each isotope (I-125 110 Gy, Pd-103 100 Gy, and Cs-131 85 Gy). There is no evidence that one source allows for better outcomes over another (37–43). The planning target volume (PTV) represents an expansion of the prostate. This expansion is generally on the order of 3 to 5 mm. No margin is recommended at the prostate-rectal interface. The prescription dose should cover more than 95% of the PTV. CT-based postplan evaluation is usually performed either immediately after the procedure or within 2 to 6 weeks following the procedure.

The advantage of early (day 0) dosimetry is the provision of immediate feedback which might allow for prompt remediation action if the resultant assessment is suboptimal. However, post-procedural edema and risk of subsequent seed migration may ultimately result in less favorable dosimetry (44,45). Prostate edema typically resolves by 4 weeks postprocedure (45), potentially providing a more accurate representation of dose delivery with longer half-life isotopes, such as I-125. Dose to the rectum and urethra should also be systematically calculated and reported as part of the postplan quality assurance process. Several dosimetry quantifiers have been described for organs at risk (46). For the rectum, the RV100 (volume of rectum receiving the prescription dose) is commonly used and should be less than 1 cc.

■ HDR

HDR brachytherapy is a validated means to escalate radiation dose in men with high-risk prostate cancer (47). Comparatively, HDR may have several advantages over LDR brachytherapy for prostate cancer such as: (a) The overall treatment time is drastically reduced with HDR brachytherapy, thereby eliminating uncertainties created by edema and other prostate volume changes following the procedure. (b) HDR treatment planning allows for three-dimensional reconstruction and optimization of the amount of time/dose delivered by the brachytherapy source (Ir-192) in multiple positions within each brachytherapy needle. The ability to control dose inhomogeneity may be valuable toward increasing tumor dose while minimizing dose delivery to organs at risk. (c) A prevailing hypotheses supports the use of higher dose delivery over time for prostate cancer. HDR treatment is usually completed in about 6 to 8 minutes, with a dose rate of about 100 Gy/hr. This dose rate is similar to that delivered with conventional EBRT and about 1,000 times higher than that for LDR brachytherapy. The relatively high biologic dose delivered in a short period of time may increase prostate cancer cell kill relative to normal tissue injury as modeled by differences in radiation response between tissue these types (48,49). (d) A single HDR radiation source is capable of delivering treatment to multiple patients, whereas LDR brachytherapy requires radioactive sources to be purchased for each individual patient. Therefore, HDR brachytherapy may be a more cost-effective method. (e) Patient-specific radiation safety recommendations are not required for HDR, as patients are not radioactive following the procedure, as is the case with LDR brachytherapy. Conversely, administration of HDR brachytherapy often necessitates hospital admission and monitoring between fractions or multiple procedures to complete the prescribed course of therapy.

The feasibility of combining HDR brachytherapy with EBRT for high-risk prostate cancer was evaluated in a multicenter study conducted by the radiation therapy oncology group (RTOG 0321) (50). Men with high-risk prostate cancer were treated with EBRT (45 Gy over 25 fractions) plus HDR brachytherapy boost (19 Gy in two fractions). At a median follow-up of 2.5 years, 125 patients were evaluable. The rate of late grade 3 or greater gastrointestinal or genitourinary adverse events was 2.6% at 18 months. The combination of HDR and EBRT has been compared with EBRT alone in two small randomized trials. Sathya et al. reported the results of 104 patients with clinical stage T2 and T3 prostate cancer without evidence of metastatic disease. Participants were randomly assigned to EBRT (66 Gy in 33 fractions over 6.5 weeks) vs. EBRT (40 Gy in 20 fractions over 4 weeks) with a 35 Gy HDR boost delivered over 48 hours (6). The median follow-up was 8.2 years. In the HDR boost plus EBRT arm, 17 patients (29%) experienced biochemical or clinical failure compared with 33 patients (61%) in the EBRT only arm (P = .0024). Eighty-seven patients (84%) had a postradiation biopsy; 10 (24%) of 42 in the HDR boost plus EBRT arm had a positive biopsy compared with 23 (51%) of

45 in the EBRT arm (odds ratio, 0.30; *P* = .015). Overall survival was over 90% for both treatment regimens. Hoskin et al. randomized 220 men with prostate cancer and a PSA < 50 ng/mL to receive either EBRT alone (55 Gy in 20 fractions over 4 weeks) or EBRT (35.75 Gy in 13 fractions over 2.5 weeks) followed by an HDR boost of 17 Gy in two fractions over 24 hours (51,52). With a median follow-up of 30 months, a significant improvement in actuarial biochemical relapse-free survival was seen in favor of the combined EBRT plus brachytherapy schedule (*P* = .03). A lower incidence of acute rectal discharge was seen in the EBRT plus brachytherapy group (*P* = .025) and other acute and late toxicities were equivalent. Patients randomized to HDR brachytherapy had a significantly better FACT-P score at 12 weeks (*P* = .02). The interpretation of these trials is complicated by the variable dose and fractionation schedules used with EBRT and HDR brachytherapy, as well as the small size and short follow-up of these trials.

Despite the inconclusive application of the randomized data toward current management of high-risk prostate cancer, multiple prospective series have validated HDR brachytherapy boost as a robust, safe, and reproducible method of dose escalation for prostate cancer. Kestin et al. reported a dose-response relationship for HDR brachytherapy boost combined with 46 Gy EBRT (53). The best results were seen for two fractions of 10.5 Gy, especially in men with larger tumor volumes. Demanes et al. reported 10-year biochemical control of 62% for men with high-risk prostate cancer using EBRT 36 Gy in 20 fractions plus two HDR implants providing two fractions each of 5.5 to 6 Gy (total HDR boost 22 to 24 Gy) (54). Recent publications suggest a 5-year biochemical control advantage of EBRT and HDR brachytherapy compared with intensity-modulated radiotherapy for high-risk prostate cancer (93% vs. 71%) (55). On multivariate analysis, the use of a HDR brachytherapy boost was an independent predictor of PSA relapse-free survival (*P* = .0012).

Since high-risk patients are well represented in HDR brachytherapy series, the use of ADT is often considered. Galalae et al. reported on 611 patients treated at three institutions, of whom 177 received a short course of neoadjuvant and concurrent ADT (56). The 5-year biochemical control was 69% for high-risk disease. In univariate and multivariate analyses, the use of ADT did not affect outcome. Martinez et al. expanded this series in 1260 patients with intermediate or high-risk prostate cancer (57). Forty-three percent of all patients received ADT for 3 to 6 months. The 8-year biochemical control was 85% with ADT and 81% without ADT. However, distant metastases were seen more frequently in men who received neoadjuvant ADT 16.6% versus 7.3%. A short course of ADT was also associated with an increased risk of cancer-related mortality. While many HDR series include a proportion of patients who received trimodality therapy, the benefit of ADT to EBRT plus HDR for high-risk prostate cancer has not been clearly demonstrated. Given an established survival advantage with the combination of ADT and EBRT, ADT will continue to play a role in the management of high-risk prostate cancer despite a lack of evidence specifically addressing the trimodality therapy. Randomized trials will be needed to define value and/or optimal duration of ADT in trimodality therapy.

■ SUMMARY

For men with high-risk prostate cancer, EBRT plus prostate brachytherapy is a viable and highly effective means of intraprostatic dose escalation. As an extrapolation from randomized trials of EBRT+ADT, strong consideration should be given toward inclusion of ADT in combination treatments. HDR/LDR prostate brachytherapy will likely continue to be important tools for optimal dose delivery.

■ REFERENCES

1. Kuban DA, Tucker SL, Dong L, et al. Long-term results of the M. D. Anderson randomized dose-escalation trial for prostate cancer. *Int J Radiat Oncol Biol Phys*. 2008;70:67–74.
2. Zelefsky MJ, Leibel SA, Gaudin PB, et al. Dose escalation with three-dimensional conformal radiation therapy affects the outcome in prostate cancer. *Int J Radiat Oncol Biol Phys*. 1998;41:491–500.
3. Zietman AL, Bae K, Slater JD, et al. Randomized trial comparing conventional-dose with high-dose conformal radiation therapy in early-stage adenocarcinoma of the prostate: long-term results from proton radiation oncology group/american college of radiology 95-09. *J Clin Oncol*. 2010;28:1106–1111.
4. D'Amico AV, Whittington R, Malkowicz SB, et al. Biochemical outcome after radical prostatectomy, external beam radiation therapy, or interstitial radiation therapy for clinically localized prostate cancer. *JAMA*. 1998;280:969–974.
5. Fang FM, Wang YM, Wang CJ, Huang HY, Chiang PH. Comparison of the outcome and morbidity for localized or locally advanced prostate cancer treated by high-dose-rate brachytherapy plus external beam radiotherapy (EBRT) versus EBRT alone. *Jpn J Clin Oncol*. 2008;38:474–479.
6. Sathya JR, Davis IR, Julian JA, et al. Randomized trial comparing iridium implant plus external-beam radiation therapy with external-beam radiation therapy alone in node-negative locally advanced cancer of the prostate. *J Clin Oncol*. 2005;23:1192–1199.
7. Crook J, McLean M, Catton C, Yeung I, Tsihlias J, Pintilie M. Factors influencing risk of acute urinary retention after TRUS-guided permanent prostate seed implantation. *Int J Radiat Oncol Biol Phys*. 2002;52:453–460.
8. Henderson A, Ismail AK, Cunningham M, et al. Toxicity and early biochemical outcomes from 125iodine prostate brachytherapy in the UK. A prospective study. *Clin Oncol (R Coll Radiol)*. 2004;16:95–104.
9. Kelly K, Swindell R, Routledge J, Burns M, Logue JP, Wylie JP. Prediction of urinary symptoms after 125iodine prostate brachytherapy. *Clin Oncol (R Coll Radiol)*. 2006;18:326–332.
10. Keyes M, Miller S, Moravan V, et al. Urinary symptom flare in 712 125I prostate brachytherapy patients: long-term follow-up. *Int J Radiat Oncol Biol Phys*. 2009;75:649–655.

11. Lee N, Wuu CS, Brody R, et al. Factors predicting for postimplantation urinary retention after permanent prostate brachytherapy. *Int J Radiat Oncol Biol Phys*. 2000;48:1457–1460.
12. Locke J, Ellis W, Wallner K, Cavanagh W, Blasko J. Risk factors for acute urinary retention requiring temporary intermittent catheterization after prostate brachytherapy: a prospective study. *Int J Radiat Oncol Biol Phys*. 2002;52:712–719.
13. Mabjeesh NJ, Chen J, Stenger A, Matzkin H. Preimplant predictive factors of urinary retention after iodine 125 prostate brachytherapy. *Urology*. 2007;70:548–553.
14. Martens C, Pond G, Webster D, McLean M, Gillan C, Crook J. Relationship of the International Prostate Symptom score with urinary flow studies, and catheterization rates following 125I prostate brachytherapy. *Brachytherapy*. 2006;5:9–13.
15. Hanks GE, Pajak TF, Porter A, et al. Phase III trial of long-term adjuvant androgen deprivation after neoadjuvant hormonal cytoreduction and radiotherapy in locally advanced carcinoma of the prostate: the Radiation Therapy Oncology Group Protocol 92-02. *J Clin Oncol*. 2003;21:3972–3978.
16. Bolla M, Collette L, Blank L, et al. Long-term results with immediate androgen suppression and external irradiation in patients with locally advanced prostate cancer (an EORTC study): a phase III randomised trial. *Lancet*. 2002;360:103–106.
17. Ebara S, Manabe D, Kobayashi Y, et al. The efficacy of neoadjuvant androgen deprivation therapy as a prostate volume reduction before brachytherapy for clinically localized prostate cancer. *Acta Med Okayama*. 2007;61:335–340.
18. Kucway R, Vicini F, Huang R, Stromberg J, Gonzalez J, Martinez A. Prostate volume reduction with androgen deprivation therapy before interstitial brachytherapy. *J Urol*. 2002;167:2443–2447.
19. Petit JH, Gluck C, Kiger WS 3rd, et al. Bicalutamide alone prior to brachytherapy achieves cytoreduction that is similar to luteinizing hormone-releasing hormone analogues with less patient-reported morbidity. *Urol Oncol*. 2008;26:372–377.
20. Barry MJ, Fowler FJ Jr, O'Leary MP, et al. The American Urological Association symptom index for benign prostatic hyperplasia. The Measurement Committee of the American Urological Association. *J Urol*. 1992;148:1549–1557; discussion 1564.
21. Terk MD, Stock RG, Stone NN. Identification of patients at increased risk for prolonged urinary retention following radioactive seed implantation of the prostate. *J Urol*. 1998;160:1379–1382.
22. Merrick GS, Butler WM, Lief JH, Dorsey AT. Temporal resolution of urinary morbidity following prostate brachytherapy. *Int J Radiat Oncol Biol Phys*. 2000;47:121–128.
23. Bucci J, Morris WJ, Keyes M, Spadinger I, Sidhu S, Moravan V. Predictive factors of urinary retention following prostate brachytherapy. *Int J Radiat Oncol Biol Phys*. 2002;53:91–98.
24. Davis BJ, Horwitz EM, Lee WR, et al. American Brachytherapy Society consensus guidelines for transrectal ultrasound-guided permanent prostate brachytherapy. *Brachytherapy*. 2012;11:6–19.
25. Grimm P, Billiet I, Bostwick D, et al. Comparative analysis of prostate-specific antigen free survival outcomes for patients with low, intermediate and high risk prostate cancer treatment by radical therapy. Results from the Prostate Cancer Results Study Group. *BJU Int*. 2012;109 suppl 1:22–29.
26. Khaksar SJ, Langley SE, Lovell D, Laing RW. Interstitial low dose rate brachytherapy for prostate cancer–a focus on intermediate- and high-risk disease. *Clin Oncol (R Coll Radiol)*. 2006;18:513–518.
27. Koontz BF, Chino J, Lee WR, et al. Morbidity and prostate-specific antigen control of external beam radiation therapy plus low-dose-rate brachytherapy boost for low, intermediate, and high-risk prostate cancer. *Brachytherapy*. 2009;8:191–196.
28. Stone NN, Potters L, Davis BJ, et al. Multicenter analysis of effect of high biologic effective dose on biochemical failure and survival outcomes in patients with Gleason score 7-10 prostate cancer treated with permanent prostate brachytherapy. *Int J Radiat Oncol Biol Phys*. 2009;73:341–346.
29. Blasko JC. Low-dose-rate brachytherapy for prostate cancer: preplanning vs. intraoperative planning-preplanning is best. *Brachytherapy*. 2006;5:139–142; discussion 145.
30. Ishiyama H, Nakamura R, Satoh T, et al. Differences between intraoperative ultrasound-based dosimetry and postoperative computed tomography-based dosimetry for permanent interstitial prostate brachytherapy. *Brachytherapy*. 2010;9:219–223.
31. Stone NN, Hong S, Lo Y-C, Howard V, Stock RG. Comparison of intraoperative dosimetric implant representation with post-implant dosimetry in patients receiving prostate brachytherapy. *Brachytherapy*. 2003;2:17–25.
32. Zelefsky MJ, Zaider M. Low-dose-rate brachytherapy for prostate cancer: preplanning vs. intraoperative planning-intraoperative planning is best. *Brachytherapy*. 2006;5:143–144; discussion 146.
33. Zelefsky MJ, Yamada Y, Marion C, et al. Improved conformality and decreased toxicity with intraoperative computer-optimized transperineal ultrasound-guided prostate brachytherapy. *Int J Radiat Oncol Biol Phys*. 2003;55:956–963.
34. Han BH, Wallner K, Merrick G, Butler W, Sutlief S, Sylvester J. Prostate brachytherapy seed identification on post-implant TRUS images. *Med Phys*. 2003;30:898–900.
35. Nag S, Shi P, Liu B, Gupta N, Bahnson RR, Wang JZ. Comparison of real-time intraoperative ultrasound-based dosimetry with post-operative computed tomography-based dosimetry for prostate brachytherapy. *Int J Radiat Oncol Biol Phys*. 2008;70:311–317.
36. Kudchadker RJ, Pugh TJ, Swanson DA, Bruno TL, Bolukbasi Y, Frank SJ. Preoperative treatment planning with intraoperative optimization can achieve consistent high-quality implants in prostate brachytherapy. *Med Dosim*. 2012;37:387–390.
37. Bice WS, Prestidge BR, Kurtzman SM, et al. Recommendations for permanent prostate brachytherapy with (131)Cs: a consensus report from the Cesium Advisory Group. *Brachytherapy*. 2008;7:290–296.
38. Gelblum DY, Potters L, Ashley R, Waldbaum R, Wang XH, Leibel S. Urinary morbidity following ultrasound-guided transperineal prostate seed implantation. *Int J Radiat Oncol Biol Phys*. 1999;45:59–67.
39. Herstein A, Wallner K, Merrick G, et al. I-125 versus Pd-103 for low-risk prostate cancer: long-term morbidity outcomes from a prospective randomized multicenter controlled trial. *Cancer J*. 2005;11:385–389.
40. Niehaus A, Merrick GS, Butler WM, et al. The influence of isotope and prostate volume on urinary morbidity after prostate brachytherapy. *Int J Radiat Oncol Biol Phys*. 2006;64:136–143.
41. Peschel RE, Colberg JW, Chen Z, Nath R, Wilson LD. Iodine 125 versus palladium 103 implants for prostate cancer: clinical outcomes and complications. *Cancer J*. 2004;10:170–174.
42. Sahgal A, Jabbari S, Chen J, et al. Comparison of dosimetric and biologic effective dose parameters for prostate and urethra using 131 Cs and 125 I for prostate permanent implant brachytherapy. *Int J Radiat Oncol Biol Phys*. 2008;72:247–254.
43. Wallner K, Merrick G, True L, Sutlief S, Cavanagh W, Butler W. 125I versus 103Pd for low-risk prostate cancer: preliminary PSA outcomes from a prospective randomized multicenter trial. *Int J Radiat Oncol Biol Phys*. 2003;57:1297–1303.
44. McLaughlin P, Narayana V, Pan C, et al. Comparison of day 0 and day 14 dosimetry for permanent prostate implants using stranded seeds. *Int J Radiat Oncol Biol Phys*. 2006;64:144–150.
45. Taussky D, Austen L, Toi A, et al. Sequential evaluation of prostate edema after permanent seed prostate brachytherapy using CT-MRI fusion. *Int J Radiat Oncol Biol Phys*. 2005;62:974–980.
46. Crook JM, Potters L, Stock RG, Zelefsky MJ. Critical organ dosimetry in permanent seed prostate brachytherapy: defining the organs at risk. *Brachytherapy*. 2005;4:186–194.
47. Yamada Y, Rogers L, Demanes DJ, et al. American Brachytherapy Society consensus guidelines for high-dose-rate prostate brachytherapy. *Brachytherapy*. 2012;11:20–32.

48. Brenner DJ, Martinez AA, Edmundson GK, Mitchell C, Thames HD, Armour EP. Direct evidence that prostate tumors show high sensitivity to fractionation (low alpha/beta ratio), similar to late-responding normal tissue. *Int J Radiat Oncol Biol Phys.* 2002;52:6–13.
49. Leborgne F, Fowler J, Leborgne JH, Mezzera J. Later outcomes and alpha/beta estimate from hypofractionated conformal three-dimensional radiotherapy versus standard fractionation for localized prostate cancer. *Int J Radiat Oncol Biol Phys.* 2012;82:1200–1207.
50. Hsu IC, Bae K, Shinohara K, et al. Phase II trial of combined high-dose-rate brachytherapy and external beam radiotherapy for adenocarcinoma of the prostate: preliminary results of RTOG 0321. *Int J Radiat Oncol Biol Phys.* 2010;78:751–758.
51. Hoskin PJ, Motohashi K, Bownes P, Bryant L, Ostler P. High dose rate brachytherapy in combination with external beam radiotherapy in the radical treatment of prostate cancer: initial results of a randomised phase three trial. *Radiother Oncol.* 2007;84:114–120.
52. Hoskin PJ, Rojas AM, Bownes PJ, Lowe GJ, Ostler PJ, Bryant L. Randomised trial of external beam radiotherapy alone or combined with high-dose-rate brachytherapy boost for localised prostate cancer. *Radiother Oncol.* 2012;103:217–222.
53. Kestin LL, Goldstein NS, Vicini FA, et al. Pathologic evidence of dose-response and dose-volume relationships for prostate cancer treated with combined external beam radiotherapy and high-dose-rate brachytherapy. *Int J Radiat Oncol Biol Phys.* 2002;54:107–118.
54. Demanes DJ, Rodriguez RR, Schour L, Brandt D, Altieri G. High-dose-rate intensity-modulated brachytherapy with external beam radiotherapy for prostate cancer: California endocurietherapy's 10-year results. *Int J Radiat Oncol Biol Phys.* 2005;61:1306–1316.
55. Deutsch I, Zelefsky MJ, Zhang Z, et al. Comparison of PSA relapse-free survival in patients treated with ultra-high-dose IMRT versus combination HDR brachytherapy and IMRT. *Brachytherapy.* 2010;9:313–318.
56. Galalae RM, Martinez A, Mate T, et al. Long-term outcome by risk factors using conformal high-dose-rate brachytherapy (HDR-BT) boost with or without neoadjuvant androgen suppression for localized prostate cancer. *Int J Radiat Oncol Biol Phys.* 2004;58:1048–1055.
57. Martinez AA, Demanes DJ, Galalae R, et al. Lack of benefit from a short course of androgen deprivation for unfavorable prostate cancer patients treated with an accelerated hypofractionated regime. *Int J Radiat Oncol Biol Phys.* 2005;62:1322–1331.

Treatment of Disseminated Disease

IV

17 *Salvage Therapy for Rising PSA*

JUDD W. MOUL

■ INTRODUCTION

Despite the recent major controversy regarding prostate-specific antigen (PSA) screening for prostate cancer early detection, serum PSA is a sensitive and specific marker for prostate tissue and is the hallmark test for monitoring men after treatment. Monitoring PSA after treatment of localized prostate cancer typically leads to the identification of men with a PSA-only (biochemical) recurrence prior to the development of symptoms or signs of locally recurrent or metastatic disease, and no radiological evidence of recurrent disease may be identifiable even with detailed evaluation. This has been a hot topic since the early to mid-1990s. As a result, intense interest has been focused on workup and treatment, with attention on both survival and the impact of therapy on quality of life.

From a multidisciplinary standpoint, PSA-only recurrence is one of the topics and disease states that stimulate discussion and collaboration between urologic surgeons, radiation oncologists, and medical oncologists. Many a multi-D tumor board has dealt with this issue in many variations. In this chapter, I will intersperse case discussions to further emphasize key teaching points.

■ DEFINITION OF BIOCHEMICAL PROGRESSION

The definition of PSA-only recurrence depends on the initial treatment modality. For radical prostatectomy (RP) patients, all prostate tissue is supposed to be removed during a successful radical prostatectomy. Postoperatively, detectable serum PSA using standard immunoassays is indicative of residual prostatic tissue, which presumably represents loco-regional or systemic cancer or possibly benign residual tissue only (1). Whether such disease is locally confined to the pelvis or represents systemic metastases is an important distinction with significant implications for patient management. If the serum PSA never falls to undetectable levels or is rising rapidly, systemic disease is more likely than residual disease in the prostate or prostatic bed (2, 3). In contrast, if the PSA gradually rises after remaining undetectable for 2 or more years, an isolated local recurrence in the prostatic bed or prostate is more likely (3, 4). The most widely accepted criterion for patients who have undergone radical prostatectomy is that of the American Urological Association (AUA) (5). According to AUA guidelines, a biochemical recurrence is defined as a serum PSA $\geq$ 0.2 ng/mL, which is confirmed by a second determination with a PSA $\geq$ 0.2 ng/mL.

For radiation therapy (RT), the definition of biochemical failure is more complicated than following radical prostatectomy. Some normal prostatic glandular tissue remains and serum PSA levels are unlikely to fall to undetectable levels following a course of RT. The interpretation of serum PSA levels is also complicated by the use of androgen deprivation therapy (ADT) in some patients with intermediate-or high-risk disease. The decline in serum PSA following RT is gradual and the mean time for the PSA to reach its nadir is 18 months or longer (6). The rate of decline in the serum PSA does not appear to correlate with the risk of subsequent disease relapse. The nadir of the serum PSA concentration (i.e., the lowest level to which it drops) is a strong indicator of treatment success following RT (7–11). Although lower nadir values are associated with improved outcomes, no absolute level can distinguish treatment success from treatment failure (6).

To standardize serum PSA testing for outcome assessment following RT, a 1996 American Society for Radiation Oncology (ASTRO) consensus panel defined biochemical recurrence following definitive RT as occurring after three consecutive PSA rises following a nadir (12). The date of biochemical failure was halfway between the nadir and the date of first rise or any rise great enough to provoke the initiation of therapy. A second consensus conference was held by ASTRO in 2005 to address issues that had been identified in the 1996 definition of PSA failure (13). PSA failure was defined in the revised Phoenix criteria as follows: A PSA rise by 2 ng/mL or more above the nadir PSA is considered the standard definition for biochemical failure after external beam RT, regardless of whether a patient receives ADT. The date of failure is defined by the date when the

PSA goes to nadir +2 ng/mL. Serum PSA levels typically fall after RT and can then rise ("bounce") transiently, at a median of 12 to 18 months after treatment(14). This PSA bounce can occur in the absence of recurrent disease and does not necessarily signify a treatment failure or constitute an indication for therapeutic intervention. The PSA bounce phenomenon has been observed after low-dose rate (LDR) brachytherapy(15), high-dose rate (HDR) brachytherapy(16), and external beam RT(17,18). The frequency with which such PSA bounces are observed varies, depending on the definition used(15,17). The most extensive data on the PSA bounce phenomenon come from a consecutive series of 820 patients treated with LDR brachytherapy(19). The incidence of PSA bounce decreased with an increasing threshold to define a PSA bounce (30%, 20%, 13%, and 10%, respectively, using definitions of 0.2, 0.4, 0.6, and 0.8 ng/mL). Regardless of the definition used, PSA bounces occurred significantly earlier when compared with a biochemical failure, as defined by a PSA rise >2 ng/mL above nadir (15–17 vs. 34 months). The clinical implications of a PSA bounce are uncertain. Although some studies have shown an improved prognosis in patients who experience a PSA bounce(19–22), other studies have reported in a worse prognosis in this setting(23,24). There are no definitive methods to distinguish a PSA bounce from recurrent cancer. If an increase in the serum PSA is observed, the patient should be given reassurance, and the PSA can be repeated in 3 to 6 months. If the serum PSA continues to increase, a repeat biopsy can be considered, although the interpretation of a prostate biopsy performed following RT is difficult.

Definition of PSA Only Recurrence Case Scenarios

A 56-year-old white male had a radical prostatectomy 2 years ago and had pT3a pN0 Gleason 3 + 4 = 7 disease and 12% tumor volume. He had one isolated 3-mm posterior-lateral positive surgical margin. His initial postoperative PSA level was <0.1 ng/mL at 3 months postop. He has regained full urinary control and has erections sufficient for intercourse with the use of a low-dose PDE-5 inhibitor. He was lost to follow up and now his PSA is 0.3 ng/mL. What should be done?

a. Immediate salvage radiation to the prostate bed
b. Close observation with PSA levels every 3 months
c. Complete androgen blockade
d. ProstaScint scan, CT scan, and bone scan.

Answer: b: This patient may have a PSA-only recurrence, but his PSA of 0.3 could also represent residual benign tissue in the prostate bed area especially since he had Gleason 3 + 4 = 7 and one isolated positive margin. There is no harm in following him closely and instituting salvage EBRT when his PSA goes to about 0.5 ng/mL. Complete hormonal therapy would be overtreatment at this time and the full metastatic workup would be a waste of resources considering the very low PSA. The key teaching point is that despite the AUA definition of PSA recurrence after surgery being 0.2 ng/mL, this is not always the proper threshold to institute therapy and there is no harm in waiting a bit to get more data points and a better track record on what the PSA levels will do with further close follow-up. Finally, this patient already demonstrated lack of compliance in getting lost to follow up for a while so we do need to emphasize to him the importance of follow-up especially now that his PSA is 0.3 ng/mL. Had his pathologic stage or Gleason sum been more unfavorable, salvage EBRT at 0.3 ng/mL may be appropriate but in this case, there is still uncertainty about the cause of the PSA rise and holding off on further treatment is most prudent.

A 72-year-old African American male received 7,500 cGy of EBRT approximately 3.5 years ago for cT2a, Gleason 3 + 4 = 7 prostate cancer. He had 4/12 cores involved and his prediagnosis PSA level was 8.7 ng/mL. His prostate volume was 44 cc. He did not receive neoadjuvant or adjuvant ADT. His PSA nadir was 0.3 ng/mL occurring 15 months after completion of the radiation. He is now referred to the multi-D clinic by his PCP because his PSA has risen to 1.7 ng/mL. His current digital rectal examination (DRE) reveals a flat postradiation gland with no nodules. Calculation of PSA-DT is approximately 15 months based on 6 values since the nadir. What is the best management?

a. Schedule for prostate biopsy
b. Intermittent hormonal therapy (IHT)
c. Schedule ProstaScint, bone, and CT scans
d. Reassurance and observation

Answer: d: This patient has NOT experienced a PSA recurrence based on ASTRO II (Phoenix) definition. Based on a PSA nadir of 0.3, he would need to rise to >2.3 ng/mL to be considered recurrent. Furthermore, his DRE is not suspicious for recurrence. Furthermore, his PSA-DT is 15 months, which is not a sign of danger. Workup and treatment would be ill-advised at this point and be considered overtreatment that is likely to do more harm than good. However, he does need follow-up every 6 months with DRE and PSA and may require future evaluation and treatment if and when the clinical scenario changes.

■ PROGNOSIS AFTER BIOCHEMICAL FAILURE

The natural history of prostate cancer following a PSA relapse does not necessarily predict the progression to metastases or death(25–27). This is illustrated by a series of 1,973 men treated with radical prostatectomy at

Johns Hopkins between 1981 and 2010 who developed a biochemical recurrence (PSA ≥0.2 ng/mL) following radical prostatectomy (27). Of these, 642 were observed without further treatment; and within this group, 450 had sufficient data for the calculation of PSA doubling time (PSA-DT). With a median follow-up of 8 years, 134 patients (30%) had developed metastases, and the median metastasis-free survival was 10.0 years. Multivariate analysis found that independent factors associated with the development of metastases were the PSA-DT (<3.0 vs. 3.0–8.9 vs. 9.0–14.9 vs. ≥ 15.0 months) and the Gleason score from the radical prostatectomy specimen (≤6 vs. 7 vs. 8–10). Data from an earlier analysis of 321 men at this institution were used to construct tables (the Pound tables) to predict the likelihood of being free of metastases following a biochemical failure after radical prostatectomy (4). A similar table to estimate the 10- and 15-year risk of prostate cancer–related death in men with a rising PSA after radical prostatectomy based on 379 such men was published in 2005 (25). Similar models have been developed to predict the future risk of clinical relapse and death in individual patients initially treated with RT, based on pretreatment variables, radiation dose, and the results of serial posttreatment serum PSA levels (28).

Several parameters (e.g., PSA-doubling time, Gleason score, PSA response to salvage ADT) have been studied to distinguish men who are likely to develop clinically significant disease following either radical prostatectomy or RT from those who have more indolent disease (25,27). This information can be an important factor in determining whether and when to initiate further treatment. The same features that predict biochemical failure after initial treatment for prostate cancer provide insight into the likely natural history of the disease following biochemical recurrence (29). These include the clinical features at original presentation (tumor [T] stage, PSA level, PSA velocity, biopsy Gleason score) as well as pathologic findings at the time of prostatectomy for men who have undergone surgery (T stage, nodal and margin status, and Gleason score). As such, these features can aid in treatment decisions in men with a rising PSA after local treatment.

Multiple studies indicate that a long PSA-DT predicts both clinical metastasis-free survival and prostate cancer–specific mortality in men with a rising serum PSA after radical prostatectomy (30–36). The PSA-DT is less well studied after external beam RT and has not been validated after brachytherapy (21). The prognostic significance of PSA-DT is illustrated by the largest series, which studied the outcomes in 8,669 men with clinically localized or locally advanced nonmetastatic prostate cancer (33). Of these men, 5,918 initially were treated surgically and 2,751 were managed with RT. Men with a PSA-DT of <3 months had a 20-fold increased risk of dying of prostate cancer compared with those with a PSA-DT of ≥3 months. A later analysis found that the use of the Gleason score in conjunction with PSA-DT provided a better estimate of prostate cancer–specific mortality in men with a rising PSA following RT (30). For men with a PSA-DT < 3 months, prostate cancer–specific mortality rates 5 years after biochemical failure were 35% and 75% with Gleason scores of ≤7 and ≥8, respectively. For men with PSA-DT ≥ 3 months, the 5-year prostate cancer–specific mortality rates for Gleason score ≤ 7 and ≥ 8 disease were 4% and 15%, respectively. These data support the view that men who have a short PSA-DT and a Gleason score ≥ 8 disease are at particularly high risk of dying from prostate cancer and are unlikely to achieve long-term disease control from local-only salvage therapies. However, the number of men with a PSA-DT < 3 months was relatively small. Among those who have a biochemical recurrence with a somewhat longer PSA-DT, prostate cancer is still a major cause of mortality. In one study of men with a rising PSA following prostatectomy and a PSA-DT < 15 months, prostate cancer accounted for approximately 90% of all deaths by 15 years after biochemical recurrence (31). Caution should be exercised when an ultrasensitive PSA assay is used to calculate the PSA-DT. The studies that demonstrated the importance of PSA-DT were based on calculations when level of detectability of the serum PSA was ≥0.2 ng/mL. Ultrasensitive PSA assays have a lower limit of detection of 0.01 ng/mL or less, and doubling times using such an assay for the first detection of PSA following treatment correlate poorly with the older methodology (37).

Prognosis After Biochemical Failure Case Scenario

A 61-year-old white male physician/surgeon presented with high-risk prostate cancer Gleason 3 + 4 = 7 (4 cores) and 4 + 4 = 8 (1 core) (overall) in 5/12 cores and a PSA of 11.2 ng/mL. He had T2a N0 M0 disease preop based on a negative metastatic workup (CT and bone scan) that were noted in a progress note in the medical records. Patient came to my center for an open radical prostatectomy with pelvic lymphadenectomy. Surgery was uneventful and revealed pT3a pN0 Mx Gleason 4 + 4 = 8 with 20% cancer volume. He had one 3-mm isolated positive surgical margin and three areas of extracapsular extension but no seminal vesicle invasion. He was told that postoperative adjuvant external beam radiation would likely be needed and this would be addressed at his 3-month follow-up visit. At 6 weeks postop, he called to say that he took a PSA at his own hospital lab and it returned at 5.75 ng/mL. We suggested that this PSA may be a lab error, but repeat PSAs returned at 6.38 and 6.91 ng/mL. What is the next most appropriate step?

a. Reassurance and follow further PSAs
b. Repeat the metastatic workup
c. Start immediate hormonal therapy
d. Refer to radiation oncology to start salvage EBRT

ANSWER: b: A PSA that never falls to undetectable after RP is indicative of residual disease and a very high level, such as in this case, indicates systemic disease. In this case, the patient admitted that he never actually had the bone scan that was scheduled by his local urologist. He was a physician and surgeon and had emergency clinical responsibilities that precluded going to the bone scan appointment. We relied on the progress note stating that the metastatic workup was completed and assumed the bone scan was negative, but did not push for the official report. After surgery, the PSA continued to rise to approximately 10 ng/mL and a repeat metastatic workup with a Sodium-Flouride (F-18) PET bone scan revealed approximately 10 scattered bone metastases. He then started complete androgen blockade and was enrolled in a clinical trial of systemic chemotherapy as well. Referral to a radiation oncologist for salvage radiation when the PSA level was very high would be ill advised in the setting of systemic disease. Certainly, had we questioned the patient further and found out that he did not have a preop bone scan, we may have insisted on a bone scan preop. On the other hand, with the disease characteristics at hand preop, his statistical risk for bone metastases was about 10% and we might not have insisted on the bone scan especially since he did have a negative CT scan preop. This is a real case illustrating the pitfalls we all can face in real-world clinical multi-D practice.

■ DIAGNOSTIC WORKUP FOR PSA RECURRENCE

Patients who have been treated with potentially curative definitive therapy (radical prostatectomy, external beam RT, brachytherapy) are at risk for loco-regional recurrence or distant metastases. Additional local therapy may result in prolonged disease-free survival if the recurrent disease is localized. Unfortunately, the frequency with which unsuspected metastases are detected using imaging studies is very low for men with an early PSA-only progression if the patient has not had prior ADT. Bone scan historically has been the most sensitive imaging procedure for the diagnosis of bone metastases. However, unsuspected bone metastases are only rarely detected in patients undergoing an initial evaluation for an elevated PSA (38–40). The limited yield from routine bone scan is illustrated by a series of 93 men who were evaluated for a PSA-only recurrence after radical prostatectomy (38). The lowest serum PSA that was associated with a positive bone scan in the absence of adjuvant ADT was 46 ng/mL. On multivariate analysis, only the absolute value of the serum PSA and a rapid rise of serum PSA were predictive of a positive bone scan. Based on a logistic regression model, the likelihood of a positive bone scan was less than 5% unless the serum PSA was >40 to 45 ng/mL. In contemporary practice, the serum PSA is monitored after initial treatment and a diagnosis of biochemical recurrence is typically made when the PSA is relatively low (often <1 ng/mL). Thus, bone scans are probably unnecessary unless there are symptoms referable to bone. Our practice is to recommend a bone scan as a part of the initial evaluation for an elevated PSA only for men with a serum PSA ≥ 10 ng/mL (≥5 ng/mL if prior ADT was administered) or a rapid PSA-DT (<3 months) or in whom the rate of PSA rise is >2 ng/mL per month. Men who have a positive or equivocal bone scan are usually evaluated by targeted plain radiographs or with an MRI if radiographic findings are inconclusive.

MRI of the axial skeleton is an alternative to a bone scan to screen high-risk men for the presence of bone metastases. A potential advantage of MRI compared with bone scan was seen in a series of 66 consecutive men with high-risk tumors who underwent MRI of the axial skeleton in addition to a standard sequential workup starting with a bone scan (41). The definition of high-risk disease included newly diagnosed prostate cancer with a biopsy Gleason score ≥ 8 and a PSA ≥ 20 ng/mL (n = 26), a rapidly rising PSA within 3 years of radical prostatectomy (n = 12), or a rapidly rising PSA in men receiving ADT (n = 28). Axial skeleton MRI was more sensitive than any other approach in the 41 men ultimately found to have bone metastases. Screening MRI identified metastases in 7 of 23 men considered negative (30%) and 8 of 17 (46%) considered equivocal by other strategies. As a consequence of the MRI findings, the initial treatment plan was modified in 15 of 66 patients (22%). Five of twenty-six men (19%) scheduled for prostatectomy or RT were instead referred for systemic treatment because of the finding of metastatic disease.

The sensitivity of abdominopelvic CT for detection of low-volume recurrent disease is limited (39, 42). This was illustrated by a study in 86 men who had undergone prostatectomy, in which CT was informative in only 12 (14%) (39). The mean PSA value was significantly higher in those with a positive scan (27.4 vs. 4.9 ng/mL) as was the mean PSA velocity (1.8 vs. 0.7 ng/mL per month). Only eight scans (9%) provided new information to the clinician. Thus, the sensitivity of CT appears to be limited in the setting of PSA-only recurrence unless the PSA value is relatively high. We do not recommend CT unless the serum PSA level is >10 ng/mL or the rate of PSA rise is >20 ng/mL per year.

MRI of the prostate and pelvis with or without an endorectal coil has been suggested as another method of evaluating local recurrences in men with a PSA-only recurrence (43–46). This technique has been used primarily to determine the presence of seminal vesicle involvement or extraprostatic extension in men who are believed to have clinically localized prostate cancer. In men with biochemical recurrence following initial RT, endorectal coil MRI has been used to identify seminal vesicle invasion or extraprostatic extension in those who are being considered for salvage prostatectomy, since the presence of these features (particularly seminal vesicle invasion) identifies men who are unlikely to achieve long-term disease control. There are only limited data on the accuracy of endorectal coil MRI in men with previously irradiated prostate glands (44–46). The largest series included 45 consecutive men who underwent salvage radical prostatectomy for biopsy-proven locally recurrent prostate cancer over a 6-year period, all of whom underwent endorectal coil MRI prior to surgery (44). All scans were read independently by two experienced radiologists. There was significant variation between readers, with sensitivity for seminal vesicle involvement of 38% and 62%, respectively. Further research is needed to establish whether this test is useful to localize prostate cancer recurrences. For men undergoing salvage RT after radical prostatectomy, MRI may complement the treatment planning process by delineating the prostatic bed or localizing a small focus of locally recurrent disease. A number of institutions are rigorously exploring the use of MRI for treatment planning in this setting.

The role of fluorodeoxyglucose (FDG)-PET scanning in men with suspected recurrent prostate cancer is controversial. Some early reports concluded that PET is of limited utility overall, particularly for men with a low serum PSA or PSA velocity (47,48). In contrast, others suggest that PET is useful in imaging local recurrences (49), osseous metastases (50,51), or nodal and soft tissue lesions (48,50,52). FDG is excreted by the kidneys and accumulates in the bladder. This creates a major problem when the goal is to image the prostatic bed and pelvis. The introduction of newer iterative image reconstruction has reduced but not eliminated this problem (49). As an example, in a contemporary series of 91 men with a rising PSA after prostatectomy for early stage disease, PET identified recurrent lesions in the prostatic bed (n = 5, all true-positives), bones (n = 22, 20 true-positives, 2 false-positives), lymph nodes (n = 7, 6 true-positives, 6 false-positive), and one unsuspected liver metastasis (53). Only two patients had an isolated local recurrence or metastatic disease that was shown by other imaging modalities. However, of the 19 men who were thought to have evidence of a local recurrence by virtue of a positive biopsy of the prostatic bed or a drop in the PSA after local radiation treatment, PET was positive in only three. Early studies suggest that 18-fluorine-labeled choline or 11-carbon-labeled acetate may be better tracers for use in recurrent prostate cancer (54–59). PET scanning with either tracer is considered investigational in men with a PSA-only recurrence. Sodium fluoride PET-bone scan is being evaluated for potential utility prior to salvage therapy (60,61). A current demonstration database is underway with Medicare patients with results pending as of mid-2014.

The ProstaScint scan is a radiolabeled monoclonal antibody imaging study that detects prostate-specific membrane antigen (PSMA). ProstaScint lacks sufficient sensitivity and specificity to have a routine role in men with prostate cancer. NCCN guidelines do not recommend ProstaScint as an imaging option for men with known prostate cancer and a rising PSA after definitive treatment (62).

Prostate biopsy may provide useful information to aid in the early diagnosis of a local recurrence in men with a rising PSA following RT (63). However, there are important caveats to its use. The histologic regression of tumor cells after RT may be prolonged; a positive result less than 2 years after treatment does not correlate well with disease progression. An ASTRO consensus panel recommended that routine prostate biopsy for evaluation of PSA recurrence after RT not be performed unless salvage prostatectomy or another local salvage procedure was being considered (64). In this setting, TRUS-guided biopsy is indicated for histologic confirmation of a suspected isolated local recurrence prior to salvage therapy. In such cases, biopsy should be performed at least 18 months after completion of RT. In the setting of prior prostatectomy, the value of TRUS biopsy for men with a rising serum PSA after radical prostatectomy is controversial and rarely indicated. The largest retrospective experience with biopsy in this setting consists of 114 patients who underwent 156 TRUS biopsies at the University of California San Francisco (65). In this series, 61 men (54%) had biopsy-confirmed local recurrence, two-thirds of which were at the anastomotic site. In one-third of cases more than one biopsy was required.

■ THERAPY—SALVAGE RADIATION THERAPY

Management options for men with a PSA-only recurrence after radical prostatectomy include external beam RT to the prostatic bed with or without treatment of the pelvic lymph nodes (salvage RT), ADT, a combination of salvage RT plus ADT, or observation. Most of the available data regarding these approaches have come from observational series. Long-term results of randomized clinical trials will be required to define the optimal approach.

For men with a recurrence following radical prostatectomy, salvage external beam RT can provide long-term disease control if the recurrence is encompassed within the treatment field and a sufficient radiation dose can be delivered to eradicate the residual/recurrent cancer. The success of salvage RT depends on dose and treatment volume (i.e., prostate bed with or without pelvis), in addition to the localization of all malignant cells to the treatment field.

The initial retrospective studies that attempted to define patients who would benefit from salvage RT relied on biochemical relapse-free survival (bRFS), rather than cancer-specific survival or the development of metastatic disease. Numerous studies have analyzed the factors associated with biochemical relapse following salvage RT (66–70). Factors associated with an improved bRFS included a positive surgical margin at prostatectomy, a low PSA level at recurrence, and a long recurrence-free interval following initial surgery. In contrast, a short (e.g., <6 months) PSA-DT, Gleason score ≥ 8, a history of lymph node or seminal vesicle involvement at original diagnosis, and a persistent elevation of PSA following RT were all associated with poorer bRFS in those managed with salvage RT. Although these studies have been used to define patients who were more likely to benefit from salvage RT, these analyses were retrospective and did not include a control group that was managed with observation rather than active intervention. Thus, the factors identified in these studies may have been prognostic for the development of biochemical relapse and not predictive of improved cancer-specific survival in response to treatment with salvage RT (71).

With regard to survival, three large retrospective single-institution series provide conflicting data on whether or not salvage RT as a single modality can prolong survival. In a series of 2,657 men treated at the Mayo Clinic who had a biochemical recurrence following radical prostatectomy, 856 (32%) received salvage RT (72). On multivariate analysis, salvage RT significantly reduced the incidence of subsequent local recurrence (hazard ratio [HR] 0.13, 95% confidence interval [CI] 0.06–0.28). However, salvage RT did not significantly decrease mortality compared with those not receiving salvage RT following biochemical recurrence (5- and 10-year survival rates, 92% vs. 91% and 70% vs. 69%, respectively). A study from Johns Hopkins analyzed 635 patients who had either a biochemical or local recurrence following radical prostatectomy (71). At recurrence, patients were managed with observation, salvage RT alone, or salvage RT in combination with hormonal therapy in 63%, 25%, and 12% of cases, respectively. Cancer-specific survival was significantly prolonged in patients who received RT, with or without hormonal therapy, compared with observation (96% and 96% vs. 88% at 5 years, and 82% and 86% vs. 62% at 10 years). Finally, RT appeared to prolong survival in both groups in a series of 4,036 men who underwent radical prostatectomy at Duke between 1988 and 2008, irrespective of whether the PSA-DT was short or long (73). This cohort included 519 men who had a biochemical recurrence and were fully evaluable. Salvage RT was given, either alone or as part of a combined approach that included ADT, in 219 of these patients (37%). At a median follow-up of 11.3 years, multivariate analysis demonstrated a significant decrease in all-cause mortality both in those with a PSA-DT less than 6 months and in those with a PSA-DT greater than or equal to 6 months (adjusted hazard ratios 0.53 and 0.52, respectively). Despite the limitations inherent in these retrospective studies, these results provide good evidence that salvage RT shortly after biochemical relapse can alter the natural history of prostate cancer.

Careful surveillance and early salvage RT following surgery (e.g., before PSA rises above 0.4–0.5 ng/mL) may be an appropriate alternative to immediate adjuvant RT for patients with high-risk primary prostate cancer managed with surgery. Immediate, postoperative adjuvant RT and early salvage RT are being compared in the RADICALS trial sponsored by the Medical Research Council in the United Kingdom (NCT00541047) (74).

As far as dose and treatment volume, there are no randomized trials that study the optimal radiation dose in salvage RT. In 1999, ASTRO guidelines recommended that the dose should be at least 64 Gy for salvage RT (75). More recently, a number of retrospective series report better outcomes when doses above 65 Gy are used (76–78). Whether RT should be limited to the prostate bed or should include pelvic irradiation is controversial. In our practice, we recommend small-field RT for two reasons. Two randomized trials (EORTC 2291 and SWOG 8794) that demonstrated a treatment benefit from early postprostatectomy RT compared with observation following radical prostatectomy used small field RT (79, 80). The role of more extensive pelvic irradiation was assessed in two trials in men whose prostate cancer was managed with definitive RT. In that setting, two large randomized trials (RTOG 9413 and GETUG-01) failed to show an improvement in survival among men who were assigned to treatment with prostate plus pelvic lymph node RT compared with treatment limited to the prostate (81, 82). However, these trials used RT for primary therapy of prostate cancer rather than in the salvage setting. The effect of elective pelvic irradiation in men with a rising PSA following surgery is being addressed in an ongoing multicenter trial (RTOG 0534, NCT00567580), although only in the context of men who are receiving ADT (74). That trial does not include an arm with RT to the pelvic lymph nodes without ADT.

With regard to side effects and toxicity, salvage RT after a previous radical prostatectomy is generally well tolerated (83, 84). In a multi-institution database study of 959 men who received postoperative RT (81% as salvage and 19% as adjuvant therapy), the 5-year rates of late grade 3 genitourinary and gastrointestinal side effects were 1 and 0.4%, respectively (83).

The addition of ADT to definitive RT benefits men with high-risk clinically localized prostate cancer as well as those with locally advanced disease. Two large randomized trials being conducted by the Radiation Therapy

Oncology Group (RTOG) eventually should provide important information about the role of hormonal therapy in conjunction with RT in the management of patients with a rising serum PSA. RTOG 9601 (NCT00002874) and RTOG 0534 (NCT00567580) both include patients with persistent elevation of PSA after radical prostatectomy as well as those with a rising PSA after radical prostatectomy. In RTOG 9601, there was a statistically significant improvement in freedom from PSA progression when adjuvant bicalutamide was added to RT compared with RT alone (57% vs. 40%) and a statistically significant decrease in the incidence of metastatic disease (7% vs. 13%). The actuarial overall survival rates at 7 years were 91% and 86%, respectively, which did not reach statistical significance. However, there were too few deaths to permit a statistical comparison of overall survival. In addition, the trial used bicalutamide monotherapy, not a GnRH agonist, an approach that is unconventional in the United States. In RTOG 0534, patients were randomly assigned to RT alone to the prostate bed, RT to the prostate bed combined with neoadjuvant and concurrent ADT, or RT to the prostate bed and pelvic lymph nodes with neoadjuvant and concurrent ADT (74). The trial did not include an arm with RT to the pelvic lymph nodes without ADT. RTOG 0534 is awaiting maturation. Given the available preliminary data from RTOG 9601 and from observational series, it is reasonable to recommend short-term ADT (4–6 months) with salvage RT for men with very unfavorable risk factors at the time of radical prostatectomy (e.g., PSA > 20 ng/mL, Gleason score ≥ 8).

■ THERAPY—SALVAGE RADICAL PROSTATECTOMY

Salvage prostatectomy provides disease control for 10 years or more in many patients. In the pre-PSA era, surgery was not widely used because of concerns about operative morbidity and frequent development of disseminated metastases. More contemporary experience, utilizing better patient selection criteria and improved operative techniques, has made radical prostatectomy an important option for appropriately selected patients. Most of the literature is based on open radical prostatectomy. However, salvage laparoscopic robotic prostatectomy has been described in carefully selected patients (85, 86). The key is not the type of surgery (open or robotic) but the experience of the surgeon. In the setting of salvage RP, very highly experienced surgeons are even more critical than with primary radical prostatectomy,

If salvage RP is being considered, a transrectal ultrasound (TRUS) biopsy is indicated for histologic confirmation of a suspected local recurrence. Cystoscopic examination is helpful to rule out bladder neck involvement.

Results from retrospective series in the PSA-era provide some insight into the ability of radical prostatectomy to control disease (87, 88). As an example, one series included 138 men who underwent salvage radical prostatectomy at the Mayo Clinic since PSA monitoring became routine; at a median follow-up of 92 months, the 5-year failure-free survival rate was 63% (87). Similar results were seen in a series from Memorial Sloan-Kettering, where the 5-year recurrence-free survival rate was 54% (88). In general, men with disease confined to the prostate have better outcomes than those with either extraprostatic extension or seminal vesicle invasion (89, 90). The status of the surgical margins is also a strong predictor of both disease-specific and disease-free survival (91). The reported long-term outcomes following salvage radical prostatectomy are consistently better in men with low serum PSA levels (87, 90, 92, 93). As an example, in a report of 100 consecutive men undergoing salvage prostatectomy after initial RT, 5-year progression-free survival rates stratified by preoperative PSA level were as follows (92): <4 ng/mL—86%; 4 to 10 ng/mL—55%; >10 ng/mL—28%. Whether these results reflect an effect of treatment is uncertain. Men with a low serum PSA may have more indolent disease, and these men might have had a high likelihood of remaining free of clinical disease progression without surgical intervention.

With regard to complications, older series of patients treated with salvage prostatectomy reported major complications in one-third to one-half of all men (94–96). These included rectal injury, bladder neck contractures, hemorrhage, ureteral injury, vesicorectal or vesicoperineal fistulas, venous thromboembolism, and chronic urinary incontinence. These series included many patients who had undergone staging pelvic lymph node dissection and/or open radioactive seed implantation. The degree of fibrosis after modern conformal external beam RT or transperineal brachytherapy is much less, permitting the majority of men to undergo a salvage operation that is similar to the standard nonsalvage prostatectomy (97). In three large contemporary series, the rate of early perioperative complications ranged from 13% to 27% (87, 89, 92). However, late rates of urinary incontinence (30%–50%) and anastomotic stricture (17%–32%) do not appear to have improved substantially despite better patient selection, less pelvic fibrosis, and better surgical technique (92, 98). These rates are substantially higher than those observed after radical prostatectomy as initial therapy. This may reflect the persistence of radiation-induced sphincter dysfunction. When the assessment is based on patient-reported data, even higher rates of incontinence have been reported (97). The incidence of incontinence may also be biased by the use of an artificial urinary sphincter in some patients. Erectile dysfunction was previously thought to be an inevitable consequence of salvage prostatectomy. However, nerve preservation is sometimes feasible, and some men with good preoperative erectile function may recover potency after bilateral nerve-sparing salvage prostatectomy (99). In one retrospective series, 45% of men who were potent preoperatively maintained potency (97), and men were more likely to recover erectile function if they had bilateral preservation of the neurovascular bundles (99).

With regard to neoadjuvant ADT, there are no randomized trials that address the role of adjuvant or neoadjuvant ADT in men undergoing salvage prostatectomy. Small retrospective series have reported on the use of perioperative ADT in this setting, but these reports do not provide reliable information on the efficacy of these approaches (91, 96, 100).

■ THERAPY—CRYOTHERAPY

The use of cryotherapy as salvage treatment following local recurrence after RT remains controversial. On one hand, prostate cryotherapy is FDA approved and is reimbursed by Medicare and virtually all private insurance plans and is a reasonable option for well-selected men treated by very experienced surgeons. On the other hand, there is no level I evidence for its use and there are still some who consider it less effective than salvage radical prostatectomy. There are no prospective studies that directly compare cryosurgery versus prostatectomy as salvage therapy for men with a local recurrence of prostate cancer. The relative effectiveness and safety of cryotherapy compared with salvage prostatectomy are uncertain.

A retrospective study compared 42 men treated with salvage prostatectomy at the Mayo Clinic to 56 patients treated by salvage cryotherapy at M. D. Anderson Cancer Center. Patients were matched for pretreatment PSA and biopsy Gleason score (101). Biochemical progression occurred more frequently in patients treated with salvage cryotherapy than with radical prostatectomy (5-year bRFS 66% vs. 42%, based upon a criterion of two increases in serum PSA above nadir). At a median follow-up of 8 years, there was no difference in disease-specific survival (96% vs. 98%). Although salvage prostatectomy appeared to be more effective, the choice of therapy needs to be individualized, and cryotherapy is appropriate for older patients and those with significant comorbidity.

Cryotherapy can freeze and destroy tissue beyond the confines of the prostate gland, and this may be an advantage compared with radical prostatectomy for selected cases. Thus, we suggest cryotherapy rather than salvage radical prostatectomy for men with a rising PSA if they have clinical stage T3 disease, either prior to initial RT or at the time of disease recurrence. Guidelines from the AUA support cryotherapy as an option in this setting (102).

■ THERAPY—BRACHYTHERAPY AFTER RT

Another option that has been used for men with a biochemical recurrence following initial external beam RT is brachytherapy. Brachytherapy is typically given by a LDR methodology using iodine-125 (I-125) or palladium-103 (Pd-103) (103–107), but can also be given using a HDR technique (108). There are no randomized trials comparing brachytherapy with other forms of salvage therapy. In the largest series, 49 men with biopsy-proven local recurrence after EBRT underwent salvage LDR brachytherapy (104). At 64 months average follow-up, the bRFS rates at 3 and 5 years were 48% and 34%, respectively. Men whose PSA nadir was <0.5 ng/mL after salvage brachytherapy (47% of the cohort) fared better than those who failed to do so (5-year bRFS 56% vs. 15%, respectively). In series of 30 men treated with LDR brachytherapy and followed for a median of 46 months, bRFS was approximately 50% at both 5 and 10 years among men who underwent the procedure at a time when their PSA was <10 ng/mL (105). Although urinary incontinence was reported infrequent, two men developed rectal ulcers and one required a colostomy. In the largest series using HDR brachytherapy, 21 men were treated for recurrent prostate cancer after external beam RT (108). At a median follow-up of 19 months, 13 had achieved a PSA nadir of ≤0.1 ng/mL. There were two biochemical failures, both of which occurred in the setting of distant metastases.

Although these limited results suggest that salvage brachytherapy has promise, further study is required, and brachytherapy should not be considered a standard approach for men with a local recurrence after external beam RT.

■ THERAPY—SYSTEMIC THERAPIES

Systemic treatment may be indicated for some men with PSA recurrence when clinical and pathologic factors suggest that disseminated disease is highly probable and hence salvage local therapy is not indicated. In others cases, comorbidity and advanced age preclude aggressive local therapy. Systemic therapy is generally patterned after approaches taken in men with advanced prostate cancer. Typically such treatment utilizes ADT as the initial therapy. Patients who eventually relapse after treatment with ADT are managed following the same treatment algorithm that is used for patients with overt metastatic disease.

ADT with either a gonadotropin releasing hormone (GnRH) agonist or antagonist or with orchiectomy is the standard initial treatment for men with advanced or metastatic prostate cancer. ADT effectively palliates symptoms in 80% to 90% of men and may prolong survival.

Such treatment is clearly beneficial but not curative. The majority of men progress to androgen independence within 2 to 5 years, and require additional therapy. In men with a PSA-only recurrence after initial treatment, overt metastatic disease may not become evident for many years. No randomized trials have assessed the role of ADT in this setting, and it is unclear how applicable the data from men with more advanced disease is to this group.

ADT causes side effects that can significantly lower the quality of life. These adverse effects are particularly important in otherwise asymptomatic men whose only manifestation of disease is a rising serum PSA. The potential development of hot flashes, loss of libido, decreased muscle mass, mild anemia, and osteoporosis are significant concerns that need to be considered in deciding whether or not to treat immediately. Furthermore, concerns about ADT-induced diabetes mellitus, cardiac disease, and metabolic syndrome add credence to the use of a risk-stratified approach.

Key questions concerning the use of ADT include whether treatment should be initiated as soon as a rising PSA is detected or can be delayed, whether ADT should use monotherapy (a GnRH agonist, GnRH antagonist, or orchiectomy) or combined androgen blockade (a GnRH agonist or orchiectomy plus an antiandrogen), and the role of intermittent androgen deprivation (IAD). There are very few randomized trials that address these issues in this population. The optimal timing of ADT for men with a PSA-only recurrence is controversial. Proponents of early treatment argue that this approach can delay disease progression and may prolong survival. Others contend that treatment is best deferred until clinical metastases or symptoms develop since there is no consistent evidence for a significant survival benefit with ADT in this setting, and treatment is associated with adverse effects. In randomized trials in patients with advanced prostate cancer, early initiation of therapy has been associated with a decrease in prostate cancer mortality but no improvement in overall survival (109).

Observational data from studies in patients with a biochemical recurrence provide only weak evidence in support of early intervention. In an analysis of 1,352 men with a rising PSA (>0.2 ng/mL) as the only evidence of recurrent disease after radical prostatectomy, hormone therapy was administered to 355, while the remainder were observed without therapy until the development of overt metastases (110). In the entire cohort, 103 (8%) developed metastases. In patients with a Gleason score > 7 or a PSA-DT ≤12 months, initiation of ADT significantly delayed the appearance of clinical metastases. Two ongoing multicenter phase III trials are examining the role of early ADT in patients with a rising serum PSA (74). A Canadian trial (NCT00439751) is comparing early versus delayed treatment with goserelin in patients who have a recurrence following radical radiotherapy. An Australian study (NCT00110162) is evaluating hormonal therapy in patients with a biochemical recurrence or asymptomatic metastatic disease. In the absence of more definitive data, we favor early intervention, especially in younger men with high-grade disease (e.g., Gleason score 8–10), a serum PSA-DT < 10 to 12 months, or clear evidence of high-risk features on the initial prostatectomy specimen (grossly positive margins, seminal vesicle invasion, high tumor volume [>30%]), or a combination of these features.

ADT can be accomplished by preventing androgen production (orchiectomy, GnRH agonists, GnRH antagonists) or by androgen receptor blockade with antiandrogens; these methods can be used alone or in combination. The combination of a GnRH agonist or orchiectomy plus an antiandrogen is commonly referred to as complete androgen blockade, since it removes the influence of both testicular and adrenal androgens. There are no randomized trials comparing GnRH agonists or orchiectomy alone versus complete androgen blockade in men with a PSA-only recurrence. Current ASCO guidelines support a consideration of complete androgen blockade for treatment in this setting (109), but this remains very controversial.

One of the major disadvantages of ADT are side effects such as sexual dysfunction and loss of bone and muscle mass. Periodically reversing the effects of ADT, which is presumably associated with fewer side effects, can be achieved using intermittent compared with continuous androgen deprivation. IAD refers to cyclic administration of ADT with induction treatment until maximal response, usually defined by serum PSA criteria. Then, temporary withdrawal of ADT and later reinitiation based on predefined threshold levels of serum PSA, which vary from 2.5 to 20 ng/mL, or on serum testosterone levels rising out of the castrate range (typically >20–50 ng/mL).

Men managed with IAD can be expected to be off therapy approximately 35% to 50% of the time. Time off treatment in the first cycle ranges from 6 to 15 months, and may be longer for men with less advanced disease such as PSA-only progression compared with those with overt metastatic disease. The off-treatment period is generally associated with an improvement in the sense of well-being and recovery of libido and potency in men who report normal or near-normal sexual function before the start of therapy.

The most extensive data on IAD in patients with a rising serum PSA come from an international phase III trial (111). In this trial, 1,386 men with a rising PSA following radical prostatectomy were randomly assigned to either intermittent or continuous androgen deprivation. Patients assigned to IAD were treated for 8 months; treatment was then restarted when the serum PSA reached >10 ng/mL of treatment. The primary endpoint of the trial was overall survival. The statistical design of the trial was based on the demonstration of noninferiority, with noninferiority defined by a true difference in overall survival of less than 8% points, which corresponded to a hazard ratio < 1.25. At a median follow-up of 6.9 years, overall survival with IAD met the study criterion for noninferiority compared with continuous androgen deprivation (median 8.8 vs. 9.1 years, HR 1.02, 95% CI 0.86–1.21). Men treated with IAD had more disease or treatment-related deaths but fewer deaths unrelated to prostate cancer compared with continuous ADT (120 vs. 94 and 148 vs. 162 deaths, respectively). Analyses of quality of life suggested that there were modest benefits, but the results may have been limited by the timing of quality-of-life assessments. Differences in functional domain did not show a statistically significant benefit for IAD. Specific symptoms that did show a statistically significant benefit included hot flashes, desire for sexual activity, and urinary symptoms. Among the patients treated with IAD, serum testosterone levels returned to pretreatment levels in only 35% within 2 years after initial cycle of treatment, and only 29% of men who were potent at baseline had a return of potency. These results suggest that there is a potential benefit for IAD compared with continuous ADT in terms of quality of life. Furthermore, overall survival does not appear to be inferior. However, additional data from randomized trials are required to further assess the long-term value of this approach. We offer IAD only to well-informed patients, carefully explaining and documenting that long-term outcomes (including the potential for harm) are incompletely characterized. Despite this, IAD has become a very popular strategy for ADT in PSA recurrence as a way to combat the growing concerns of side-effects with ADT.

Antiandrogen monotherapy has several advantages compared with other forms of hormone therapy, including ease of administration, a favorable toxicity profile, and better quality of life. However, the efficacy of antiandrogen monotherapy is controversial. A meta-analysis of eight trials comparing flutamide or bicalutamide monotherapy versus orchiectomy, DES, or a GnRH agonist in men with advanced prostate cancer suggested that overall survival with antiandrogen monotherapy was inferior to other treatments (112). Despite the concerns about efficacy, antiandrogen monotherapy may be a reasonable option for carefully selected men with well-differentiated tumors and a PSA-only recurrence who wish to minimize side effects during therapy. ASCO guidelines suggest that monotherapy with a nonsteroidal antiandrogen be discussed with individuals as an alternative, but do not specifically recommend this strategy (109).

Antiandrogens plus 5-alpha reductase inhibition can also be considered and some have called this peripheral androgen blockade (PAD). The 5-alpha reductase inhibitors block the intraprostatic conversion of testosterone to dihydrotestosterone ([DHT], the most potent androgen acting on the prostate), while the nonsteroidal antiandrogen blocks the cytoplasmic DHT receptor. Since testosterone conversion is blocked selectively within the prostate, serum testosterone levels are maintained during treatment. As a result, most men retain their pretreatment libido, potency, muscle mass, and erythropoietic capacity. These observations provide the rationale for treatment with the combination of finasteride and flutamide. Uncontrolled studies have suggested that the combination of finasteride plus flutamide may be useful in this setting (113–117). In the largest of these, 101 men with a rising PSA after definitive local therapy were treated with finasteride (5 mg daily) and flutamide (250 mg three times daily) (118). With a median follow-up of 10 years, 96% of patients had a greater than 80% decline in serum PSA. Toxicity was described as mild, with 18 patients stopping treatment for toxicity. A nonrandomized single center trial in 56 men with a biochemical recurrence compared with flutamide plus finasteride versus low-dose flutamide alone (119). With median follow-ups of 54 and 43.5 months, respectively, men on the combined low-dose therapy had lower PSA levels and lower rates of progression. A randomized phase III trial in men with early progression following local therapy will be required to validate this approach. Bicalutamide is also used with a 5-alpha reductase inhibitor in this setting. Smith et al. recently (2013) reported a phase II trial of enzalutamide 160 mg, orally, once daily in 67 men who were previously hormone-naïve (120). Approximately 60% of this cohort did not have metastases (i.e., PSA recurrence). The median PSA was 18.2 ng/mL in the overall group. There was a 92% PSA response (> 90% decline with a value < 4 ng/mL at 6 months). Among PSA-only recurrence patients, half dropped PSA to < 0.1 ng/mL. As with prior generation oral antiandrogens, gynecomastia occurred in 36%, fatigue in 34%, nipple pain in 19%, and hot flashes in 18%. However, published studies specifically in PSA-only recurrence are lacking. With the emergence of more potent oral hormonal agents (enzalutamide, abiraterone acetate), there will undoubtedly be future trials assessing these agents in the PSA-only recurrence setting. However, as of mid-2014, the use of these newer agents for biochemical progression would be considered investigational/experimental.

Cytotoxic chemotherapy is generally reserved for men with castrate-resistant disease and is investigational for the initial systemic therapy of patients with a rising serum PSA (121–123). Chemotherapy may have a role in the management of patients with a rising PSA who have progressed on ADT but remain free of overt metastases. Several studies have shown that chemotherapy is active as the initial therapy in men with a rising PSA after local therapy, used either alone or in combination with ADT (13–15). However, additional studies will be required to determine whether chemotherapy has a role in this setting.

■ REFERENCES

1. Ravery V. The significance of recurrent PSA after radical prostatectomy: benign versus malignant sources. *Semin Urol Oncol.* 1999;17:127.
2. Pound CR, Partin AW, Epstein JI, Walsh PC. Prostate-specific antigen after anatomic radical retropubic prostatectomy. Patterns of recurrence and cancer control. *Urol Clin North Am.* 1997;24:395.
3. Partin AW, Pearson JD, Landis PK, et al. Evaluation of serum prostate-specific antigen velocity after radical prostatectomy to distinguish local recurrence from distant metastases. *Urology.* 1994;43:649.
4. Pound CR, Partin AW, Eisenberger MA, et al. Natural history of progression after PSA elevation following radical prostatectomy. *JAMA.* 1999;281:1591.
5. Cookson MS, Aus G, Burnett AL, et al. Variation in the definition of biochemical recurrence in patients treated for localized prostate cancer: the American Urological Association Prostate Guidelines for Localized Prostate Cancer Update Panel report and recommendations for a standard in the reporting of surgical outcomes. *J Urol.* 2007;177:540.
6. Crook JM, Choan E, Perry GA, et al. Serum prostate-specific antigen profile following radiotherapy for prostate cancer: implications for patterns of failure and definition of cure. *Urology.* 1998;51:566.
7. Critz FA, Levinson AK, Williams WH, et al. The PSA nadir that indicates potential cure after radiotherapy for prostate cancer. *Urology.* 1997;49:322.
8. Hanlon AL, Diratzouian H, Hanks GE. Posttreatment prostate-specific antigen nadir highly predictive of distant failure and death from prostate cancer. *Int J Radiat Oncol Biol Phys.* 2002;53:297.
9. Perez CA, Michalski JM, Lockett MA. Chemical disease-free survival in localized carcinoma of prostate treated with external beam irradiation: comparison of American Society of Therapeutic Radiology and Oncology Consensus or 1 ng/mL as endpoint. *Int J Radiat Oncol Biol Phys.* 2001;49:1287.
10. Yock TI, Zietman AL, Shipley WU, et al. Long-term durability of PSA failure-free survival after radiotherapy for localized prostate cancer. *Int J Radiat Oncol Biol Phys.* 2002;54:420.
11. Ray ME, Thames HD, Levy LB, et al. PSA nadir predicts biochemical and distant failures after external beam radiotherapy for prostate cancer: a multi-institutional analysis. *Int J Radiat Oncol Biol Phys.* 2006;64:1140.
12. Consensus statement: guidelines for PSA following radiation therapy. American Society for Therapeutic Radiology and Oncology Consensus Panel. *Int J Radiat Oncol Biol Phys.* 1997;37:1035.
13. Roach M 3rd, Hanks G, Thames H Jr, et al. Defining biochemical failure following radiotherapy with or without hormonal therapy in men with clinically localized prostate cancer: recommendations of the RTOG-ASTRO Phoenix Consensus Conference. *Int J Radiat Oncol Biol Phys.* 2006;65:965.
14. Satoh T, Ishiyama H, Matsumoto K, et al. Prostate-specific antigen 'bounce' after permanent 125I-implant brachytherapy in Japanese men: a multi-institutional pooled analysis. *BJU Int.* 2009;103:1064.
15. Caloglu M, Ciezki J. Prostate-specific antigen bounce after prostate brachytherapy: review of a confusing phenomenon. *Urology.* 2009;74:1183.
16. Bachand F, Martin AG, Beaulieu L, et al. An eight-year experience of HDR brachytherapy boost for localized prostate cancer: biopsy and PSA outcome. *Int J Radiat Oncol Biol Phys.* 2009;73:679.
17. Pickles T, British Columbia Cancer Agency Prostate Cohort Outcomes Initiative. Prostate-specific antigen (PSA) bounce and other fluctuations: which biochemical relapse definition is least prone to PSA false callsŒ An analysis of 2030 men treated for prostate cancer with external beam or brachytherapy with or without adjuvant androgen deprivation therapy. *Int J Radiat Oncol Biol Phys.* 2006;64:1355.
18. Horwitz EM, Levy LB, Thames HD, et al. Biochemical and clinical significance of the posttreatment prostate-specific antigen bounce for prostate cancer patients treated with external beam radiation therapy alone: a multiinstitutional pooled analysis. *Cancer.* 2006;107:1496.
19. Caloglu M, Ciezki JP, Reddy CA, et al. PSA bounce and biochemical failure after brachytherapy for prostate cancer: a study of 820 patients with a minimum of 3 years of follow-up. *Int J Radiat Oncol Biol Phys.* 2011;80:735.
20. Hinnen KA, Monninkhof EM, Battermann JJ, et al. Prostate specific antigen bounce is related to overall survival in prostate brachytherapy. *Int J Radiat Oncol Biol Phys.* 2012;82:883.
21. Ciezki JP, Reddy CA, Garcia J, et al. PSA kinetics after prostate brachytherapy: PSA bounce phenomenon and its implications for PSA doubling time. *Int J Radiat Oncol Biol Phys.* 2006;64:512.
22. Patel C, Elshaikh MA, Angermeier K, et al. PSA bounce predicts early success in patients with permanent iodine-125 prostate implant. *Urology.* 2004;63:110.
23. Stock RG, Stone NN, Cesaretti JA. Prostate-specific antigen bounce after prostate seed implantation for localized prostate cancer: descriptions and implications. *Int J Radiat Oncol Biol Phys.* 2003;56:448.
24. Merrick GS, Butler WM, Wallner KE, et al. Prostate-specific antigen spikes after permanent prostate brachytherapy. *Int J Radiat Oncol Biol Phys.* 2002;54:450.
25. Freedland SJ, Humphreys EB, Mangold LA, et al. Risk of prostate cancer-specific mortality following biochemical recurrence after radical prostatectomy. *JAMA.* 2005;294:433.
26. Kupelian PA, Buchsbaum JC, Patel C, et al. Impact of biochemical failure on overall survival after radiation therapy for localized prostate cancer in the PSA era. *Int J Radiat Oncol Biol Phys.* 2002;52:704.
27. Antonarakis ES, Feng Z, Trock BJ, et al. The natural history of metastatic progression in men with prostate-specific antigen recurrence after radical prostatectomy: long-term follow-up. *BJU Int.* 2012;109:32.
28. D'Amico AV, Renshaw AA, Sussman B, Chen MH. Pretreatment PSA velocity and risk of death from prostate cancer following external beam radiation therapy. *JAMA.* 2005;294:440.
29. Lee AK, D'Amico AV. Utility of prostate-specific antigen kinetics in addition to clinical factors in the selection of patients for salvage local therapy. *J Clin Oncol.* 2005;23:8192.
30. Zhou P, Chen MH, McLeod D, et al. Predictors of prostate cancer-specific mortality after radical prostatectomy or radiation therapy. *J Clin Oncol.* 2005;23:6992.
31. Freedland SJ, Humphreys EB, Mangold LA, et al. Death in patients with recurrent prostate cancer after radical prostatectomy: prostate-specific antigen doubling time subgroups and their associated contributions to all-cause mortality. *J Clin Oncol.* 2007;25:1765.
32. Ward JF, Zincke H, Bergstralh EJ, et al. Prostate specific antigen doubling time subsequent to radical prostatectomy as a prognosticator of outcome following salvage radiotherapy. *J Urol.* 2004;172:2244.
33. D'Amico AV, Moul JW, Carroll PR, et al. Surrogate end point for prostate cancer-specific mortality after radical prostatectomy or radiation therapy. *J Natl Cancer Inst.* 2003;95:1376.
34. Zelefsky MJ, Ben-Porat L, Scher HI, et al. Outcome predictors for the increasing PSA state after definitive external-beam radiotherapy for prostate cancer. *J Clin Oncol.* 2005;23:826.
35. Albertsen PC, Hanley JA, Penson DF, Fine J. Validation of increasing prostate specific antigen as a predictor of prostate cancer death after treatment of localized prostate cancer with surgery or radiation. *J Urol.* 2004;171:2221.
36. Lee AK, Levy LB, Cheung R, Kuban D. Prostate-specific antigen doubling time predicts clinical outcome and survival in prostate cancer patients treated with combined radiation and hormone therapy. *Int J Radiat Oncol Biol Phys.* 2005;63:456.
37. Teeter AE, Presti JC Jr, Aronson WJ, et al. Does early prostate-specific antigen doubling time (ePSADT) after radical

prostatectomy, calculated using PSA values from the first detectable until the first recurrence value, correlate with standard PSADTŒ A report from the Shared Equal Access Regional Cancer Hospital Database Group. *BJU Int.* 2009;104:1604.
38. Cher ML, Bianco FJ Jr, Lam JS, et al. Limited role of radionuclide bone scintigraphy in patients with prostate specific antigen elevations after radical prostatectomy. *J Urol.* 1998;160:1387.
39. Kane CJ, Amling CL, Johnstone PA, et al. Limited value of bone scintigraphy and computed tomography in assessing biochemical failure after radical prostatectomy. *Urology.* 2003;61:607.
40. Dotan ZA, Bianco FJ Jr, Rabbani F, et al. Pattern of prostate-specific antigen (PSA) failure dictates the probability of a positive bone scan in patients with an increasing PSA after radical prostatectomy. *J Clin Oncol.* 2005;23:1962.
41. Lecouvet FE, Geukens D, Stainier A, et al. Magnetic resonance imaging of the axial skeleton for detecting bone metastases in patients with high-risk prostate cancer: diagnostic and cost-effectiveness and comparison with current detection strategies. *J Clin Oncol.* 2007;25:3281.
42. Krämer S, Görich J, Gottfried HW, et al. Sensitivity of computed tomography in detecting local recurrence of prostatic carcinoma following radical prostatectomy. *Br J Radiol.* 1997;70:995.
43. Silverman JM, Krebs TL. MR imaging evaluation with a transrectal surface coil of local recurrence of prostatic cancer in men who have undergone radical prostatectomy. *AJR Am J Roentgenol.* 1997;168:379.
44. Sala E, Eberhardt SC, Akin O, et al. Endorectal MR imaging before salvage prostatectomy: tumor localization and staging. *Radiology.* 2006;238:176.
45. Huch Böni RA, Meyenberger C, Pok Lundquist J, et al. Value of endorectal coil versus body coil MRI for diagnosis of recurrent pelvic malignancies. *Abdom Imaging.* 1996;21:345.
46. Sella T, Schwartz LH, Swindle PW, et al. Suspected local recurrence after radical prostatectomy: endorectal coil MR imaging. *Radiology.* 2004;231:379.
47. Hofer C, Laubenbacher C, Block T, et al. Fluorine-18-fluorodeoxyglucose positron emission tomography is useless for the detection of local recurrence after radical prostatectomy. *Eur Urol.* 1999;36:31.
48. Seltzer MA, Barbaric Z, Belldegrun A, et al. Comparison of helical computerized tomography, positron emission tomography and monoclonal antibody scans for evaluation of lymph node metastases in patients with prostate specific antigen relapse after treatment for localized prostate cancer. *J Urol.* 1999;162:1322.
49. Turlakow A, Larson SM, Coakley F, et al. Local detection of prostate cancer by positron emission tomography with 2-fluorodeoxyglucose: comparison of filtered back projection and iterative reconstruction with segmented attenuation correction. *Q J Nucl Med.* 2001;45:235.
50. Nuñez R, Macapinlac HA, Yeung HW, et al. Combined 18F-FDG and 11C-methionine PET scans in patients with newly progressive metastatic prostate cancer. *J Nucl Med.* 2002;43:46.
51. Morris MJ, Akhurst T, Osman I, et al. Fluorinated deoxyglucose positron emission tomography imaging in progressive metastatic prostate cancer. *Urology.* 2002;59:913.
52. Sanz G, Robles JE, Giménez M, et al. Positron emission tomography with 18fluorine-labelled deoxyglucose: utility in localized and advanced prostate cancer. *BJU Int.* 1999;84:1028.
53. Schöder H, Herrmann K, Gönen M, et al. 2-[18F] fluoro-2-deoxyglucose positron emission tomography for the detection of disease in patients with prostate-specific antigen relapse after radical prostatectomy. *Clin Cancer Res.* 2005;11:4761.
54. DeGrado TR, Coleman RE, Wang S, et al. Synthesis and evaluation of 18F-labeled choline as an oncologic tracer for positron emission tomography: initial findings in prostate cancer. *Cancer Res.* 2001;61:110.
55. Cimitan M, Bortolus R, Morassut S, et al. [18F]fluorocholine PET/CT imaging for the detection of recurrent prostate cancer at PSA relapse: experience in 100 consecutive patients. *Eur J Nucl Med Mol Imaging.* 2006;33:1387.
56. Oyama N, Miller TR, Dehdashti F, et al. 11C-acetate PET imaging of prostate cancer: detection of recurrent disease at PSA relapse. *J Nucl Med.* 2003;44:549.
57. Wachter S, Tomek S, Kurtaran A, et al. 11C-acetate positron emission tomography imaging and image fusion with computed tomography and magnetic resonance imaging in patients with recurrent prostate cancer. *J Clin Oncol.* 2006;24:2513.
58. Albrecht S, Buchegger F, Soloviev D, et al. (11)C-acetate PET in the early evaluation of prostate cancer recurrence. *Eur J Nucl Med Mol Imaging.* 2007;34:185.
59. Sandblom G, Sörensen J, Lundin N, et al. Positron emission tomography with C11-acetate for tumor detection and localization in patients with prostate-specific antigen relapse after radical prostatectomy. *Urology.* 2006;67:996.
60. Even-Sapir E, Metser U, Flusser G, et al. Assessment of malignant skeletal disease: initial experience with 18F-fluoride PET/CT and comparison between 18F-fluoride PET and 18F-fluoride PET/CT. *J Nucl Med.* 2004;45:272.
61. Grant FD, Fahey FH, Packard AB, et al. Skeletal PET with 18F-fluoride: applying new technology to an old tracer. *J Nucl Med.* 2008;49:68.
62. *National Comprehensive Cancer Network (NCCN) Guidelines.* Available at: www.nccn.org/prostate.
63. Zagars GK, Pollack A, von Eschenbach AC. Prostate cancer and radiation therapy–the message conveyed by serum prostate-specific antigen. *Int J Radiat Oncol Biol Phys.* 1995;33:23.
64. Cox JD, Gallagher MJ, Hammond EH, et al. Consensus statements on radiation therapy of prostate cancer: guidelines for prostate re-biopsy after radiation and for radiation therapy with rising prostate-specific antigen levels after radical prostatectomy. American Society for Therapeutic Radiology and Oncology Consensus Panel. *J Clin Oncol.* 1999;17:1155.
65. Connolly JA, Shinohara K, Presti JC Jr, Carroll PR. Local recurrence after radical prostatectomy: characteristics in size, location, and relationship to prostate-specific antigen and surgical margins. *Urology.* 1996;47:225.
66. Pazona JF, Han M, Hawkins SA, et al. Salvage radiation therapy for prostate specific antigen progression following radical prostatectomy: 10-year outcome estimates. *J Urol.* 2005;174:1282.
67. Buskirk SJ, Pisansky TM, Schild SE, et al. Salvage radiotherapy for isolated prostate specific antigen increase after radical prostatectomy: evaluation of prognostic factors and creation of a prognostic scoring system. *J Urol.* 2006;176:985.
68. Ward JF, Zincke H, Bergstralh EJ, et al. Prostate specific antigen doubling time subsequent to radical prostatectomy as a prognosticator of outcome following salvage radiotherapy. *J Urol.* 2004;172:2244.
69. Stephenson AJ, Scardino PT, Kattan MW, et al. Predicting the outcome of salvage radiation therapy for recurrent prostate cancer after radical prostatectomy. *J Clin Oncol.* 2007;25:2035.
70. Macdonald OK, D'Amico AV, Sadetsky N, et al. Predicting PSA failure following salvage radiotherapy for a rising PSA post-prostatectomy: from the CaPSURE database. *Urol Oncol.* 2008;26:271.
71. Trock BJ, Han M, Freedland SJ, et al. Prostate cancer-specific survival following salvage radiotherapy vs observation in men with biochemical recurrence after radical prostatectomy. *JAMA.* 2008;299:2760.
72. Boorjian SA, Karnes RJ, Crispen PL, et al. Radiation therapy after radical prostatectomy: impact on metastasis and survival. *J Urol.* 2009;182:2708.
73. Cotter SE, Chen MH, Moul JW, et al. Salvage radiation in men after prostate-specific antigen failure and the risk of death. *Cancer.* 2011;117:3925.
74. *National Institutes of Health Clinical Trials Database.* http://www.clinicaltrials.gov/SHOW/NCT00541047.
75. Cox JD, Gallagher MJ, Hammond EH, et al. Consensus statements on radiation therapy of prostate cancer: guidelines for

prostate re-biopsy after radiation and for radiation therapy with rising prostate-specific antigen levels after radical prostatectomy. American Society for Therapeutic Radiology and Oncology Consensus Panel. *J Clin Oncol.* 1999;17:1155.

76. King CR, Spiotto MT. Improved outcomes with higher doses for salvage radiotherapy after prostatectomy. *Int J Radiat Oncol Biol Phys.* 2008;71:23.
77. Bernard JR Jr, Buskirk SJ, Heckman MG, et al. Salvage radiotherapy for rising prostate-specific antigen levels after radical prostatectomy for prostate cancer: dose-response analysis. *Int J Radiat Oncol Biol Phys.* 2010;76:735.
78. Tomita N, Kodaira T, Furutani K, et al. Early salvage radiotherapy for patients with PSA relapse after radical prostatectomy. *J Cancer Res Clin Oncol.* 2009;135:1561.
79. Bolla M, van Poppel H, Collette L, et al. Postoperative radiotherapy after radical prostatectomy: a randomised controlled trial (EORTC trial 22911). *Lancet.* 2005;366:572.
80. Thompson IM Jr, Tangen CM, Paradelo J, et al. Adjuvant radiotherapy for pathologically advanced prostate cancer: a randomized clinical trial. *JAMA.* 2006;296:2329.
81. Lawton CA, DeSilvio M, Roach M 3rd, et al. An update of the phase III trial comparing whole pelvic to prostate only radiotherapy and neoadjuvant to adjuvant total androgen suppression: updated analysis of RTOG 94-13, with emphasis on unexpected hormone/radiation interactions. *Int J Radiat Oncol Biol Phys.* 2007;69:646.
82. Pommier P, Chabaud S, Lagrange JL, et al. Is there a role for pelvic irradiation in localized prostate adenocarcinomaŒ Preliminary results of GETUG-01. *J Clin Oncol.* 2007;25:5366.
83. Peterson JL, Buskirk SJ, Heckman MG, et al. Late toxicity after postprostatectomy salvage radiation therapy. *Radiother Oncol.* 2009;93:203.
84. Feng M, Hanlon AL, Pisansky TM, et al. Predictive factors for late genitourinary and gastrointestinal toxicity in patients with prostate cancer treated with adjuvant or salvage radiotherapy. *Int J Radiat Oncol Biol Phys.* 2007;68:1417.
85. Vallancien G, Gupta R, Cathelineau X, et al. Initial results of salvage laparoscopic radical prostatectomy after radiation failure. *J Urol.* 2003;170:1838.
86. Stolzenburg JU, Bynens B, Do M, et al. Salvage laparoscopic extraperitoneal radical prostatectomy after failed high-intensity focused ultrasound and radiotherapy for localized prostate cancer. *Urology.* 2007;70:956.
87. Ward JF, Sebo TJ, Blute ML, Zincke H. Salvage surgery for radiorecurrent prostate cancer: contemporary outcomes. *J Urol.* 2005;173:1156.
88. Paparel P, Cronin AM, Savage C, et al. Oncologic outcome and patterns of recurrence after salvage radical prostatectomy. *Eur Urol.* 2009;55:404.
89. Gheiler EL, Tefilli MV, Tiguert R, Grignon D. Predictors for maximal outcome in patients undergoing salvage surgery for radio-recurrent prostate cancer. *Urology.* 1998;51:789.
90. Sanderson KM, Penson DF, Cai J, et al. Salvage radical prostatectomy: quality of life outcomes and long-term oncological control of radiorecurrent prostate cancer. *J Urol.* 2006;176:2025.
91. Garzotto M, Wajsman Z. Androgen deprivation with salvage surgery for radiorecurrent prostate cancer: results at 5-year followup. *J Urol.* 1998;159:950.
92. Bianco FJ Jr, Scardino PT, Stephenson AJ, et al. Long-term oncologic results of salvage radical prostatectomy for locally recurrent prostate cancer after radiotherapy. *Int J Radiat Oncol Biol Phys.* 2005;62:448.
93. Amling CL, Lerner SE, Martin SK, et al. Deoxyribonucleic acid ploidy and serum prostate specific antigen predict outcome following salvage prostatectomy for radiation refractory prostate cancer. *J Urol.* 1999;161:857.
94. Rogers E, Ohori M, Kassabian VS, et al. Salvage radical prostatectomy: outcome measured by serum prostate specific antigen levels. *J Urol.* 1995;153:104.
95. Moul JW, Paulson DF. The role of radical surgery in the management of radiation recurrent and large volume prostate cancer. *Cancer.* 1991;68:1265.
96. Lerner SE, Blute ML, Zincke H. Critical evaluation of salvage surgery for radio-recurrent/resistant prostate cancer. *J Urol.* 1995;154:1103.
97. Stephenson AJ, Scardino PT, Bianco FJ Jr, et al. Morbidity and functional outcomes of salvage radical prostatectomy for locally recurrent prostate cancer after radiation therapy. *J Urol.* 2004;172:2239.
98. Stephenson AJ, Eastham JA. Role of salvage radical prostatectomy for recurrent prostate cancer after radiation therapy. *J Clin Oncol.* 2005;23:8198.
99. Masterson TA, Stephenson AJ, Scardino PT, Eastham JA. Recovery of erectile function after salvage radical prostatectomy for locally recurrent prostate cancer after radiotherapy. *Urology.* 2005;66:623.
100. Tiguert R, Rigaud J, Lacombe L, et al. Neoadjuvant hormone therapy before salvage radiotherapy for an increasing post-radical prostatectomy serum prostate specific antigen level. *J Urol.* 2003;170:447.
101. Pisters LL, Leibovici D, Blute M, et al. Locally recurrent prostate cancer after initial radiation therapy: a comparison of salvage radical prostatectomy versus cryotherapy. *J Urol.* 2009;182:517.
102. Babaian RJ, Donnelly B, Bahn D, et al. Best practice statement on cryosurgery for the treatment of localized prostate cancer. *J Urol.* 2008;180:1993.
103. Allen GW, Howard AR, Jarrard DF, Ritter MA. Management of prostate cancer recurrences after radiation therapy-brachytherapy as a salvage option. *Cancer.* 2007;110:1405.
104. Grado GL, Collins JM, Kriegshauser JS, et al. Salvage brachytherapy for localized prostate cancer after radiotherapy failure. *Urology.* 1999;53:2.
105. Beyer DC. Salvage brachytherapy after external-beam irradiation for prostate cancer. *Oncology (Williston Park).* 2004;18:151.
106. Theodorescu D, Gillenwater JY, Koutrouvelis PG. Prostatourethral-rectal fistula after prostate brachytherapy. *Cancer.* 2000;89:2085.
107. Aaronson DS, Yamasaki I, Gottschalk A, et al. Salvage permanent perineal radioactive-seed implantation for treating recurrence of localized prostate adenocarcinoma after external beam radiotherapy. *BJU Int.* 2009;104:600-604.
108. Lee B, Shinohara K, Weinberg V, et al. Feasibility of high-dose-rate brachytherapy salvage for local prostate cancer recurrence after radiotherapy: the University of California-San Francisco experience. *Int J Radiat Oncol Biol Phys.* 2007;67:1106.
109. Loblaw DA, Virgo KS, Nam R, et al. Initial hormonal management of androgen-sensitive metastatic, recurrent, or progressive prostate cancer: 2006 update of an American Society of Clinical Oncology practice guideline. *J Clin Oncol.* 2007;25:1596.
110. Moul JW, Wu H, Sun L, et al. Early versus delayed hormonal therapy for prostate specific antigen only recurrence of prostate cancer after radical prostatectomy. *J Urol.* 2004;171:1141.
111. Crook JM, O'Callaghan CJ, Duncan G, et al. Intermittent androgen suppression for rising PSA level after radiotherapy. *N Engl J Med.* 2012;367:895.
112. Seidenfeld J, Samson DJ, Hasselblad V, et al. Single-therapy androgen suppression in men with advanced prostate cancer: a systematic review and meta-analysis. *Ann Intern Med.* 2000;132:566.
113. Picus J, Halabi S, Hussain M. Long term efficacy of peripheral androgen blockade on prostate cancer: results of CALGB 9782. *J Clin Oncol.* 2006;24:234s.
114. Barqawi AB, Moul JW, Ziada A, et al. Combination of low-dose flutamide and finasteride for PSA-only recurrent prostate cancer after primary therapy. *Urology.* 2003;62:872.
115. Brufsky A, Fontaine-Rothe P, Berlane K, et al. Finasteride and flutamide as potency-sparing androgen-ablative therapy for advanced adenocarcinoma of the prostate. *Urology.* 1997;49:913.
116. Oh WK, Manola J, Bittmann L, et al. Finasteride and flutamide therapy in patients with advanced prostate cancer: response

to subsequent castration and long-term follow-up. *Urology.* 2003;62:99.
117. Tay MH, Kaufman DS, Regan MM, et al. Finasteride and bicalutamide as primary hormonal therapy in patients with advanced adenocarcinoma of the prostate. *Ann Oncol.* 2004;15:974.
118. Monk JP, Halabi S, Picus J, et al. Efficacy of peripheral androgen blockade in prostate cancer patients with biochemical failure after definitive local therapy: results of Cancer and Leukemia Group B (CALGB) 9782. *Cancer.* 2012;118:4139.
119. Bañez LL, Blake GW, McLeod DG, et al. Combined low-dose flutamide plus finasteride vs low-dose flutamide monotherapy for recurrent prostate cancer: a comparative analysis of two phase II trials with a long-term follow-up. *BJU Int.* 2009;104:310.
120. Smith M, et al. ASCO-2013 – Abstract #5001.
121. Goodin S, Medina P, Capanna T, et al. Effect of docetaxel in patients with hormone-dependent prostate-specific antigen progression after local therapy for prostate cancer. *J Clin Oncol.* 2005;23:3352.
122. Hainsworth JD, Meluch AA, Spigel DR, et al. Weekly docetaxel/estramustine phosphate in patients with increasing serum prostate-specific antigen levels after primary treatment for prostate cancer: a phase II trial of the Minnie Pearl Cancer Research Network. *Clin Genitourin Cancer.* 2006;4:287.
123. Taplin ME, Xie W, Bubley GJ, et al. Docetaxel, estramustine, and 15-month androgen deprivation for men with prostate-specific antigen progression after definitive local therapy for prostate cancer. *J Clin Oncol.* 2006;24:5408.

18 Metastatic Hormone Sensitive Prostate Cancer

JEAN HOFFMAN-CENSITS
WILLIAM KEVIN KELLY

DESCRIPTION AND OVERVIEW OF ANDROGEN SYNTHESIS AND HORMONAL THERAPY IN PROSTATE CANCER

The luteinizing hormone releasing hormone (LHRH) axis, also called gonadotropin-releasing hormone (GnRH) axis, begins in the central nervous system with the secretion of LHRH from the hypothalamus (1). In the anterior pituitary gland, LHRH stimulates the release of the gonadotropins luteinizing hormone (LH) and follicle-stimulating hormone (FSH). LH and FSH then act on the sertoli and Leydig cells of the testes to stimulate production of enzymes that synthesize testosterone from cholesterol, such as 17-α hydroxylase (CYP 17) (2). Testosterone is then converted to active metabolites dihydrotestosterone and estradiol via 5 α reductase and aromatase (3). The equilibrium of this axis is regulated by negative feedback, and manipulation of this pathway at various steps constitutes the mainstay of treatment for prostate cancer.

Hormonal manipulation to suppress testosterone production is first-line therapy for men with newly diagnosed or recurrent prostate cancer with bony, nodal, or visceral metastasis. This suppression can be achieved through medical manipulation of the LHRH pathway, blockade of the androgen binding or production pathway, or surgical castration (bilateral orchiectomy). More complete androgen suppression using a combination of approaches to block androgens such as medical castration with therapies such as nonsteroidal antiandrogens remains controversial regarding the overall clinical benefit, but does increase the overall morbidity of therapy. Constitutional, endocrine, psychiatric, sexual, and cardiac side effects of androgen suppression can cause a significant impact on quality of life and treatment morbidity. The use of intermittent therapy with periods where testosterone level is permitted to rise to the normal range has been studied and may be a safe and effective means of disease control for some men. Future directions in research targeting the androgen axis will continue to focus on optimization of suppression of androgen function while balancing the toxicity of treatment.

MECHANISM FOR LHRH ANALOGS, LHRH ANTAGONISTS, ANTIANDROGENS

The LHRH Axis and LHRH Agonists

Over 70 years ago, Charles Huggins and colleagues were the first to use orchiectomy in the treatment of men with advanced prostate cancer (4).

In 1946, Huggins published the 5-year outcomes of 21 men and demonstrated that orchiectomy could alter the natural history of prostate cancer and lead to prolonged durable remission in some patients. For this and other work on endocrine-regulated malignancies, Huggins was awarded the Nobel Prize in medicine in 1966. Further work understanding of the hypothalamic-pituitary-gonadal pathways led to the first therapeutic use of LHRH agonists in men with prostate cancer in the 1980s (5).

The LHRH axis, also called GnRH axis, begins in the central nervous system with the secretion of LHRH from the hypothalamus (1).

In the anterior pituitary gland, LHRH stimulates the release of the gonadotropins LH and FSH. LH and FSH then act on the testes leading to the production of testosterone. Leuprolide acetate, goserelin acetate, and other synthetic LHRH analogs stimulate the hypothalamus in a constant rather than pulsatile fashion, leading to the desensitization and downregulation of LHRH receptors, LH and FSH production, and subsequent decrease in systemic circulating testosterone. Synthetic agents differ from native peptide by substitution of D-amino acids in position 6 and addition of bulky hydrophobic groups at the sixth amino acid position. These changes lead to increased stability, higher binding affinity, longer half-life, and approximately 100-fold greater potency than endogenous LHRH (6).

A small randomized study of an early LHRH agonist compared with orchiectomy demonstrated similar testosterone suppression and side-effect profile in both groups (7).

In a larger randomized trial, there was no difference in serum testosterone levels, subjective and objective response rates, and 2-year survival outcomes of 358 previously untreated men with metastatic prostatic carcinoma who received goserelin acetate every 28 days compared with orchiectomy (8). Since that time, medical hormonal manipulation has all but replaced surgical castration for men with advanced prostate cancer.

The concern about LHRH agonist is the well-described initial transient increase in both LH that causes a rise in testosterone levels after initiation of LHRH analogs (9).

Reports of bone pain in the days following initiation of LHRH analog therapy range from 7% to 37%, with rare but reported serious sequelae of testosterone surge, including bladder outlet obstruction, spinal cord compression, and even death. Prophylactic antiandrogen therapy with flutamide nilutamide or bicalutamide initiated in the days to weeks before LHRH agonist administration has been shown to block the effect of this testosterone surge in prospective studies. Men pretreated with nilutamide or flutamide prior to LHRH initiation had similar increased levels of testosterone as their untreated counterparts, but experienced fewer treatment related symptoms and lower levels of PSA when measured in the days following LHRH initiation (10, 11).

Thus for men with demonstrable metastasis beginning LHRH agonist therapy, initial pretreatment with an antiandrogen prior to LHRH agonist initiation, followed by 7 to 14 additional days of antiandrogen, is considered standard of care.

LHRH Antagonists

LHRH antagonists are another class of agents that suppress testosterone, but lack the initial stimulation of LH and FSH; and thus there is no testosterone surge seen with these agents. In a phase III study, abarelix was compared with leuprolide in 269 men with prostate cancer who were suitable for medical castration (12).

Abarelix led to a significantly more rapid decline in testosterone to castrate range compared with leuprolide, with 78% of men medically castrate after 7 days compared with 0% of men treated with leuprolide, though there were no differences in achievement of castrate testosterone levels at days 29 and 85 in either group. Furthermore, none of the men in the abarelix group, compared with 82% of men in the leuprolide acetate group, experienced a testosterone surge at therapy initiation. Due to a black box FDA warning of anaphylaxis with injection, the distribution and use of this agent in the United States was tightly regulated, and the agent was discontinued in 2006.

Degarelix is a potent LHRH antagonist that is an analog of the LHRH decapeptide (pGlu-His-Trp-Ser-Tyr-Gly-Leu-Arg-Pro-Gly-NH_2) incorporating p-ureido-phenylalanines at positions 5 and 6 (13).

Several studies have compared degarelix to leuprolide, further demonstrating the early testosterone lowering superiority of LHRH antagonists compared with agonists. In a 610 patient study of untreated men, two different dosing regimens of monthly degarelix (240 mg SQ for 1 month, followed by monthly maintenance 80 or 160 mg) were tested compared with 7.5 mg IM monthly leuprolide (14).

There were no significant differences in testosterone suppression at 28 days or maintenance of castrate levels of testosterone at 1 year, demonstrating that degarelix was noninferior to leuprolide. Patients treated on the degarelix arms had significantly lower levels of testosterone at day 3 of treatment compared with those receiving leuprolide, as well as lower mean PSA levels at days 14 and 28. Degarelix was associated with higher incidence of injection site reactions and chills, but lower incidence of urinary tract infections and arthralgias in comparison to leuprolide acetate.

To address the question of whether a change in LHRH analog from leuprolide to degraelix would have an impact on safety endpoints or clinical outcomes, Crawford and colleagues conducted a crossover continuation of this study (15).

Men on the leuprolide arm who completed 1 year of therapy and agreed to continue on study were re-randomized to one of the two degarelix dosing schemes, while consenting men in the degarelix cohort continued treatment with the prior assigned dose. The primary objective was a safety evaluation, and secondary outcome measures included testosterone and PSA measurements. Three hundred and eighty five of the 504 men who completed the original study enrolled in the extension phase, 135 of whom switched from leuprolide acetate to degarelix. Although a higher incidence of injection site reactions was seen during the first year following switch to degarelix, there were no increases in the rates of adverse events by years 3 and 4 on study when compared with the year on leuprolide. At a median follow up of 27.5 months, testosterone remained suppressed at < 20 ng/dL in both groups, but there was a significant improvement in PSA progression free survival (PFS) in men who had switched from leuprolide acetate to degarelix, compared with no change in PSA PFS in the men continuing degarelix. Lack of a leuprolide acetate only arm makes interpretation of these data somewhat confusing, and there is no current indication for rotating these agents with differing mechanisms for medical castration.

Two studies suggest degarelix may have benefit over LHRH agonists in relief of lower urinary tract symptoms. Compared to goserelin acetate and bicalutamide, degarelix led to a greater degree of improvement in International Prostate Symptom Scores (IPSS) in men with intermediate and high-risk prostate cancer treated for 12 weeks prior to planned radiotherapy (16).

In a similar study in men with locally advanced prostate cancer with significant lower urinary tract symptoms, there were significantly more men with improvement in IPSS scores at 12 weeks treated with degarelix as compared with goserilin and bicalutamide, though this study was closed early due to poor accrual (17).

Though not definitive, these studies suggest that single agent degarelix may have superior clinical benefit compared with combination LHRH agonist with androgen blockade for certain symptoms. Because many men with advanced prostate cancer suffer from lower urinary tract complaints, these data may also translate into improvement in symptom management for men with metastatic disease as well.

Antiandrogens

First generation nonsteroidal antiandrogens have been combined with LHRH agonists and orchiectomy with the goal of maximal androgen blockade (MAB). After studies with conflicting response data were reported, a meta-analysis in 1999 reported on studies conducted in the decade prior. Nine prospective randomized studies enrolled 4,128 patients with advanced prostate cancer, with pooled estimates of 10% improvement in overall survival combining flutamide with LHRH agonist or orchiectomy, over medical or surgical castration alone (18).

Updated meta-analyses, including those where individual patient data were compared, versus reported trial outcomes, suggest no significant differences in combined androgen blockade, and in some cases increased toxicity (19,20). In a multicenter phase III study of LHRH agonist combined with either bicalutamide 80 mg daily or placebo in Japanese men, there was a significant benefit in estimated 5-year overall survival of MAB compared with LHRH agonist alone (75.3% vs. 63.4%, hazard ratio, 0.78; 95% confidence interval, 0.60–0.99; P = .0498) without significant increase in toxicity (21,22).

Patients with measured nadir PSA < 1 ng/mL had a prolonged survival compared with those who did not, and more patients treated with MAB achieved this low nadir PSA, compared with those receiving LHRH agonist monotherapy (81.4 vs. 33.7%). Given all of these data, however, convincing survival data are lacking, and an answer as to whether first line versus sequential use of MAB is better are yet to be determined.

A currently enrolling multicenter cooperative group study may in part answer this question, through evaluation of overall survival in men starting first line therapy with LHRH agonist combined with either bicalutamide, or the CYP 17,20 lyase inhibitor TAK-700, a second generation antiandrogen with increased potency over bicalutamide (NCT01809691). This two arm study is not designed to evaluate the impact of first-line versus sequential use of MAB for either arm and, with no LHRH alone arm, lacks a modern prospective comparator.

Chemohormonal Therapy

Results from the randomized trial (ECOG 3805) of docetaxel chemotherapy with ADT versus ADT alone in men with newly metastatic prostate cancer were recently presented in 2014, with practice changing implications (98). Seven hundred and ninety men accrued between 2006 and 2012 within 4 months of starting ADT for recurrent or metastatic prostate cancer were randomized 1:1 to docetaxel 75 mg/m^2 every 3 weeks for 6 cycles + ADT vs ADT alone. Incidences of neuropathy and neutropenic fever were low, with one patient death on the docetaxel arm. After disease progression, 123 patients on ADT alone received docetaxel. The median overall survival (OS) for patients treated with ADT alone was 42.3 months versus 52.7 months in those on the ADT+ docetaxel arm (P = .0006, HR 0.63). For patients defined as having high volume disease at baseline (visceral metastasis and or 4 or more bone metastasis), the median survival difference was even more pronounced with OS for patients treated with ADT alone 32.2 months versus 49.2 months in those on the ADT+ docetaxel arm (P = .0012, HR 0.62). In the subgroup analysis of patients with low volume disease (not meeting high volume criteria), survival medians have not yet been reached. Thus for men with newly metastatic high volume prostate cancer, the addition of 6 cycles of docetaxel within 4 months of starting ADT should be considered as a standard treatment option in the chemo-fit patient. For others it is reasonable to discuss the upfront addition of docetaxel, however the absolute benefit of early docetaxel versus the addition of docetaxel at castration resistant progression or beyond second line antiandrogen therapy has not been defined.

PSA and Testosterone Values as Predictors of Outcome

The Food and Drug Administration (FDA) defines castration as a serum testosterone level < 50 ng/dL based on radioimmunoassay evaluation, though many men will achieve testosterone levels of < 20 ng/dL on LHRH analogs (23).

Possible better outcomes of LHRH antagonist therapy or MAB over LHRH agonists alone may be explained by differences in achievable testosterone suppression. In a retrospective series of 129 men starting hormone therapy for metastatic prostate cancer, men with higher measured testosterone at 6 months had a risk of cancer-specific death 1.33 times higher than counterparts with lower 6-month testosterone measures (24).

The authors reported that lower testosterone levels also correlated with lower mean PSA levels at 6 months and that these lower PSA values were also predictive of improved survival. Morote and colleagues reported that, in a retrospective series of men with nonmetastatic prostate cancer starting androgen deprivation therapy, that time to androgen-independent disease progression was significantly shorter in those with higher measures of testosterone (25).

During three consecutive measures of testosterone over 6 months of therapy, those with testosterone values rising > 32 ng/dL experienced a mean androgen independent progression free survival of 88 months versus 137 months for those whose testosterone remained < 32 ng/dL. In a subsequent single–center prospective study of 32 men starting hormone therapy, those achieving testosterone level < 32 ng/dL at 9 months experienced a longer time to incidence of castrate resistant disease than those with measured testosterone > 32 ng/dL (33.1 vs. 12.5 months) (26).

In a prospective multicenter study of 153 men starting androgen deprivation therapy for biochemical recurrence only or metastatic disease, a serum testosterone level at 6 months of < 20 ng/dL was associated with a lower risk of death than levels > 30 to 50 (27).

Though accurate measurement of testosterone can be hard to achieve, there appears to be evidence that maintenance of levels in the castrate range, specifically with levels < 32 ng/dL, may translate into clinical benefit and good prognosis of outcomes.

Various studies have also shown that nadir PSA measurement during the first year of androgen deprivation therapy may also be predictive of outcomes. In a single-center retrospective study, nadir PSA < 1.1 was an independent predictor of survival in men with locally advanced and metastatic prostate cancer starting ADT (28).

In a larger multicenter retrospective study of 747 men starting ADT for biochemical recurrence following surgery or radiotherapy, PSA nadir of > 0.2 ng/mL after 8 months of ADT versus < 0.2 was associated with higher prostate cancer–specific mortality, 49% versus 2% estimated at 7 years (29).

The prognostic value of PSA level within the first year of starting ADT was also demonstrated by Hussain et al. in the prospective Southwest Oncology Group 9346 trial, which randomized 1,345 men with newly diagnosed metastatic prostate cancer to continuous versus intermittent ADT if they achieved a PSA nadir of < 4 ng/mL at month 7 of therapy (30).

The authors demonstrated that median survival was significantly longer in men who achieved a PSA < 0.2 ng/mL, compared with those with PSA > 0.2 to 4 ng/mL, versus those with PSA > 4 ng/mL, corresponding to 75, 44, and 13 month survival, respectively. Finally, in another retrospective series, Choueri and colleagues demonstrated that men who achieved their PSA nadir in 6 months or less had shorter overall survival than those whose PSA continued to fall beyond 6 months of therapy initiation, suggesting that PSA kinetics, in addition to absolute nadir value, may also be predictive of outcomes in men starting hormone therapy for advanced prostate cancer (31).

Rationale for Intermittent Therapy

Though guideline recommendations support castration as first-line therapy for metastatic prostate cancer, therapeutic castration is also commonly used in men with biochemical recurrence and local disease. Given the clinical heterogeneity of prostate cancer and medical comorbidities of this older population, the absolute benefit to risk assessment of castration for any individual is not always clear. Furthermore, preclinical models suggest continuous androgen suppression may accelerate change to a castrate resistant phenotype when compared with intermittent androgen deprivation in in vitro and animal studies (32).

Thus, evaluation of intermittent versus continuous androgen deprivation has been the subject of multiple studies.

The Finn Prostate study evaluated iADT versus cADT in a heterogeneous population of men with locally advanced and metastatic prostate cancer, and found no significant differences in time to progression or cancer-specific survival between the arms (33).

Recently, two large well-designed prospective studies with long-term follow-up in distinct disease states have been published, which may better define the patient populations suitable for intermittent androgen deprivation (iADT). Crook and colleagues evaluated castrate naive men without evidence of radiographic metastasis who had undergone primary or salvage radiotherapy for prostate cancer, with rising PSA > 3 ng/mL (34).

All enrolled patients underwent induction with an LHRH agonist and an antiandrogen for 8 months. Those initially randomized to iADT who achieved PSA < 4 ng/mL at 8 months commenced a nontherapy interval, with combined hormone therapy restarted when PSA reached 10 ng/mL or with evidence of clinical progression. At a median follow up of 6.9 years, overall survival of men undergoing iADT was 8.8 years, and 9.1 years in those undergoing continuous ADT (cADT), which met the noninferiority endpoint for iADT compared with cADT. Although there were no differences in quality of life prior to randomization, men on the iADT arm reported significantly better symptom scores while on trial, including significantly better measures of hot flashes, libido, and urinary symptoms, as well as a trend toward better symptom scores pertaining to fatigue.

In an intergroup study by Hussain and colleagues, 3,040 men with hormone sensitive metastatic prostate cancer underwent induction ADT for 7 months, of whom 1,749 achieved PSA decline to < 4 and were randomized to iADT versus cADT (35).

At a median follow up of 9.8 years, the authors could not conclude that iADT was noninferior to cADT with respect to overall survival. Statistically significant improvements in erectile function and mental health were reported in the iADT cohort.

Three recent meta-analyses have been published with focus on various outcomes of prospective iADT versus cADT studies. In a meta-analysis of nine published and unpublished studies comparing continuous to intermittent androgen deprivation, the authors reported no differences in overall survival based on treatment group (36).

Noted trends toward increase in prostate cancer deaths in the iADT groups were balanced by increased nonprostate cancer–related mortality in patients treated continuously, supporting research to better define discrete populations who will benefit from ADT. Similarly, in an analysis of seven trials comprising 4,675 patients, iADT was felt not to be inferior to cADT in regard to overall survival, with notation that on iADT arms, more time was spent castrate than noncastrate. There was a trend for improvement in quality of life scores as related to sexual function on iADT in some of the studies. In an analysis of eight studies comprising 4,664 men, there was again no difference in overall survival between groups, but a small, nonsignificant trend toward worse disease specific survival (37).

Systemic Effects of Castration

For many men with advanced or recurrent prostate cancer, the recommendation for androgen deprivation will be lifelong. Awareness of possible side effects can help patients and physicians work to modify expected toxicities of this chronic therapy.

Weight/Metabolic Changes

Men with nonmetastatic prostate cancer starting androgen deprivation therapy experience a brisk change in body composition that can be measurable as early as 6 months into therapy. A prospective study of men on chronic ADT, those starting ADT, and healthy controls demonstrated that men starting ADT had significant increases in body fat mass and percent body fat (1.16% +/– 0.23%, $P < .0001$) and losses in lean body mass at 6 months (38).

After 24 months, these changes were even more evident, with men initiating ADT experiencing a loss of lean body mass from baseline (–2.27% +/– 0.61%, $P = .001$), with a more profound loss of lean body mass compared with healthy controls followed for 24 months. In a prospective study specifically designed to asses changes in weight following initiation of ADT, 257 men who were starting ADT, men with prostate cancer history not on therapy, and healthy men were age and comorbidity matched and followed for 36 months (39).

Compared with untreated and healthy controls, men on ADT gained significantly more weight, with a maximum increase of 2.57 kg at 24 months, with change most pronounced in men < 65 years of age.

In addition to changes is weight and body mass composition, ADT has also been associated with impaired diabetes control. In an observational cohort study of diabetic men with prostate cancer starting ADT or being followed off hormone therapy, 2,237 pairs were matched by age and comorbid factors and followed through the Veterans Affairs (VA) health system (40).

At 1 year of observation, mean hemoglobin A1c measured in men on ADT had risen, indicative of worse diabetic control, compared with men on no therapy, for whom HgbA1c was stable to lower. These changes in HgbA1c levels from baseline were statistically significant between populations.

Cognitive Changes

In addition to weight and metabolic changes, many men report subjective changes in memory and cognition on ADT. Studies of the effects of testosterone on cognition in animals and in hypogonadal men support these observations in men initiating ADT, and have been expertly reviewed (41).

To better characterize these symptoms, Mohile et al. performed extensive neuropsychological testing in 32 participating men > 50 years old who were initiating ADT for adjuvant, nonmetastatic, or metastatic asymptomatic indications. The authors reported no significant detriment in performance of cognitive testing 6 months following ADT initiation, and in fact, measures of visuospatial planning improved for men with normal cognitive function at baseline. Forty-five percent of enrolled men had impairments in two or more neuropsychiatric tests at baseline, indicative of possibly unrecognized mild cognitive impairment in this typically older population. In a Canadian study, men over 50 years old starting ADT for prostate cancer, compared with those with prostate cancer not starting ADT, and healthy controls were assessed using a neuropsychologic testing at baseline, 6, and 12 months (42).

Subtle declines in memory were noted at 12 months in the ADT group but could not be confirmed, and the authors thus concluded that there was no clear evidence of a detrimental effect of ADT on cognitive function.

In a observational prospective VA medical center study, 15 men with localized prostate cancer or with biochemical recurrence starting ADT and 15 men with localized prostate cancer undergoing expectant observation underwent a battery of baseline and 6 month follow-up neuropsychological and functional MRI testing (fMRI) (43).

There were no differences in neuropsychological testing scores between groups and no significant change from baseline to 6-month measures within the groups. However, there were significant differences at 6 months noted on fMRI testing both at rest and during a cognitive control task, with men receiving ADT having significantly lower rates of activation in brain regions associated with cognitive control, though definitive conclusions cannot be drawn from this small series. Finally, a review of nine mostly prospective controlled studies concluded that there are likely subtle declines in measures of cognition that occur following ADT, and that methods and particular areas of measurement may impact study outcomes and conclusions (41).

Cardiovascular Changes

Cardiovascular disease remains the most common cause of nonprostate cancer–associated death among men with prostate cancer. Given the age and comorbid complexity of this population, many have investigated whether there is a causative association between ADT and cardiovascular morbidity and mortality, and the topic remains controversial. Men with preexisting comorbidities, the elderly, and those with poor functional status undergoing treatment for localized intermediate- and high-risk cancers may not be offered surgery, thus skewing the population of men with reports of cardiovascular morbidity on ADT to a likely sicker population. There is little data on cardiovascular risk and ADT in the noncastrate metastatic population, but many thoughtfully designed and large studies have been done to evaluate this association in various prostate cancer disease states.

To better determine if there is association between ADT and cardiac risk, Medicare analyses using SEER data that capture claims for men 66 and older have been reported. In an analysis of over 73,000 men with locoregional prostate cancer diagnosed between 1992 to 1999, over 18,000 of whom were treated with ADT, rates of diabetes, coronary heart disease, myocardial infarction, and sudden cardiac death were significantly higher (adjusted HRs 1.44, 1.16, 1.11, 1.16, respectively) in those treated with ADT compared with untreated men (44).

Saigal and colleagues identified over 22,000 men with newly diagnosed prostate cancer between 1992 and 1996, with 21% of those starting ADT for various disease states (45).

One multivariable analysis, after accounting for age, prostate cancer grade, stage and treatment, race, comorbidity score, socioeconomic status, and prior cardiac disease, showed that men on ADT had a 1.2 times increased risk of cardiovascular events than men with prostate cancer not on ADT. In men with reported cardiovascular disease preceding prostate cancer diagnosis, the risk of cardiovascular events following ADT was twice that of men with no reported cardiac comorbidity. In an observational study of over 37,000 veterans with locoregional prostate cancer diagnosed between 2001 and 2004, incidences of diabetes, coronary heart disease, myocardial infarction, sudden cardiac death, and stroke were significantly higher (adjusted HRs 1.28, 1.19, 1.28, 1.35, 1.22) in the 39% of men treated with ADT compared with untreated men (44).

The CaPSURE registry (Cancer of the Prostate Strategic Urologic Research Endeavor) is a database of men with prostate cancer of varied disease states and treatments from mostly community urology practices nationwide, with incorporated patient-reported comorbidity data (46).

Over 7,000 men diagnosed with localized prostate cancer between 1995 and 2007 were analyzed based on type of treatment received, including surgery, radiotherapy with or without ADT, ADT alone, or surveillance/watchful waiting (s/ww). Men treated with either ADT alone or s/ww had significantly higher incidences of cardiovascular mortality (HRs 1.94 and 2.46, respectively) than those treated with surgery or radiotherapy. These significant differences in cardiovascular mortality were not sustained when adjusted for cancer-specific factors such as PSA and Gleason score, as well as comorbid diabetes, hypertension, coronary disease, and demographics.

A 2011 meta-analysis of 4,141 patients from eight randomized controlled trials of high-risk localized prostate cancer patients treated with either short-term (3–6 months) or long-term (> 5 years) ADT with surgery or radiotherapy demonstrated no increased risk of cardiovascular death in men treated with ADT compared with untreated men (11.0% vs. 11.2%) (47).

However, it did show an improvement in prostate cancer–specific as well as all-cause mortality in those treated with ADT, better defining the cardiac mortality risk to benefit relationship of ADT in this defined population with localized high-risk cancer. The authors and commentators stress that data from this clinical trial population is not necessarily reflective of all patients, as those with severe preexisting cardiovascular disease would likely have been excluded from prospective trials (48).

Furthermore, without preplanned stratification by risk, this meta-analysis cannot exclude an excess risk of increased cardiovascular mortality in a small percentage of men. This point was reinforced in a retrospective review of over 14,000 men treated with brachytherapy, of which nearly 43% also received ADT, and of whom 9% had previous myocardial infarction or congestive heart failure and were selected for review (49).

In this group of men with preexisting cardiac disease treated in the community, there was an increased risk of all-cause mortality in those who received ADT compared with those not treated with ADT (adjusted HR 1.76). In a Danish population-based observational study of 31,571 men with prostate cancer of all disease states, ADT was again associated with increased risk of MI and stroke (adjusted HRs 1.31 and 1.19), but this risk was not compounded in the 11% of men with preexisting MI or stroke (50).

Finally, a SEER database review of over 185,000 men with locoregional prostate cancer described an association between use of ADT and increased incidence of MI and diabetes (adjusted HRs 1.09 and 1.33) (51).

Regardless of ADT treatment, increased risk of MI was seen in men with comorbid previous MI, CHF, peripheral arterial disease, stroke, hypertension, COPD, and renal disease.

Several of the studies above separately analyzed men who had undergone orchiectomy, with findings both consistent with, and neutral, regarding increased ADT risk (44, 50–52).

However, with only a minority of patients in these series, between 0.8% and 7% of subjects, having had orchiectomy with the remainder medically castrate, these data are likely underpowered to inform a clear relationship to cardiac risk from orchiectomy. Two studies regarding cardiac risk and the LHRH antagonist degarelix have been published. In an analysis of cardiovascular events reported in degarelix studies, the authors reviewed data on 1,704 patients from 9 prospective trials and found no significant increase in cardiovascular event rates in the years before and after degarelix initiation (53).

However, in the subset with prior reported cardiac disease, the cardiovascular event rate was significantly higher following degarelix treatment (HR 1.98). In a prospective study comparing 12 months of degarelix to leuprolide acetate in which incidence of cardiac events was an endpoint, ischemic heart disease was the most commonly reported event, but the incidence did not differ statistically by treatment arm (14, 54).

The underlying pathophysiology for such increase is likely complex. At least two groups have shown that even with short course ADT, measures of arterial stiffness increase (55, 56).

Sexual Function

Most men treated with ADT have had primary therapy with radical prostatectomy and/or radiotherapy. The effects of ADT on sexual function are thus often additive to preexisting surgery or radiation-induced changes. Postprostatectomy, most men have at least transient complaints, but others suffer long-term erectile dysfunction, urinary incontinence, decrease in penile size, Peyronie disease, and altered ejaculatory function (57).

A small prospective study of sexually active men initiating ADT showed statistically significant declines in measures of nocturnal tumescence following ADT initiation that correlated with declines in testosterone and sexual function (58).

ADT leads to a brisk decline in testosterone levels, with resulting decrease in libido and impotence in the majority, but not all patients, underscoring the complexity of sexual function (59–61).

More significant changes in sexual function following ADT initiation were noted in men under 70 and in nondiabetics, suggesting that men without preexisting sexual dysfunction or age-related testosterone decline may have the most pronounced changes in their sexual satisfaction following ADT (62).

More insidious changes, such as weight gain, gynecomastia, fatigue, and loss of body hair can contribute to emotional distress and impact intimacy and sexuality (57).

A small study of education intervention at ADT initiation, consisting of written materials and a counseling session, compared with usual care was suggestive that enhanced education focused on ADT side effects may preserve feelings of intimacy among coupled men who are starting ADT (63).

Bone Health

SEER data reveal that in men over 66 years of age with prostate cancer, ADT is associated with an increased fracture rate compared with untreated men in the same population, leading to significant morbidity and even mortality (64, 65).

In patients without metastatic disease, ADT use was associated with a 34% increased risk of fracture, with increased risk associated with higher cumulative ADT exposure. Despite guideline recommendations, pretreatment DEXA for osteoporotic risk assessment is underutilized, despite high fracture risk in this population (66, 67).

The greatest loss of bone mineral density (BMD) appears to be noted during the first year of ADT, with data to support various pharmacological and nonpharmacological interventions that can lead to improved BMD (66, 68).

In a prospective study of intermittent androgen deprivation therapy in men with biochemical recurrence alone, Yu and colleagues demonstrated that while BMD fell an average of 3.4% during the initial 9-month period of ADT, it also recovered by 1.4 % during the first period off ADT, indicating that iADT may protect bone health in men appropriate for this treatment paradigm. Various studies have demonstrated that pharmacologic intervention with bisphosphonates, selective estrogen receptor modulators, and RANK ligand inhibitors can improve parameters of bone health in men undergoing ADT (69, 70).

In a randomized study of pamidronate 60 mg every 12 weeks compared with placebo in castrate naïve men starting ADT, men treated with pamidronate experienced significantly less bone loss at 48 weeks compared with men in the control group (71).

Studies of 4 mg of zolendronic acid given quarterly to men initiating ADT compared with those on placebo demonstrate consistent improvements in BMD during the first year of ADT, compared with stable BMD or bone loss in control groups (72, 73).

Finally, the effects of denosumab, a monoclonal antibody against the receptor activator of nuclear factor-kB ligand (RANK-ligand), at 60 mg every 6 months in men on ADT were reported. Compared with those receiving placebo, men on ADT treated with denosumab had an increase in BMD in the lumbar spine at a 24-month endpoint, and a decrease in new fractures at 36 months (74).

Hot Flashes

Hot flashes or vasomotor symptoms are reported in up to 80% of men receiving ADT, tend to be persistent during the course of therapy, and are associated with measures of disease-related distress (75, 76).

Although the exact etiology of these flashes is unclear, neurotransmitter dysregulation due to testosterone suppression and interference with hypothalamic control of thermoregulation is thought to be the driving mechanism (77).

Low-dose estrogen therapy and progesterone treatments with agents such as megace have met with success in ameliorating symptoms in small studies, but concern regarding effects on cancer control limit their use (78, 79).

In a prospective blinded French study, men on ADT for 6 months with complaints of hot flashes were randomized to medroxyprogesterone, cyproterone (a steroid with antiandrogenic, antigonadotropic, and progestin-like activity), or the selective serotonin release inhibitor (SSRI) venlafaxine (80).

All men reported a significant decrease in hot flash symptoms compared with baseline, with more pronounced decreases in the medroxyprogesterone and cyproterone treated men. Gabapentin at dosed at 300, 600, or 900 mg daily or placebo was evaluated in a prospective randomized study, with a dose-dependent decrease in symptoms noted compared with baseline after 4 weeks on therapy (81).

In an 8-week extension of this study, men titrated from lower doses or placebo to 900 mg of gabapentin daily experienced symptomatic improvement, but more GI side effects than the placebo treated men (82).

Separate placebo controlled studies of venlafaxine, fluoxetine, paroxetine, and sertraline have all demonstrated improvement in hot flash frequency by at least 50% in 21% to 57% of men within weeks of initiating these SSRIs on trial. In a randomized study, the authors reported a decrease in hot flash incidence of 65% in men treated with pregabalin 75 mg twice daily versus placebo, and felt that this dose optimally controlled symptoms compared with treatment-induced toxicity noted on 150 mg twice daily (83).

Novel Agents to Avoid Hormonal Manipulation

For men with history of prostate cancer treated definitively with surgery, radiotherapy, or both, a rising PSA in the absence of overt radiographic metastasis defines a failure of local therapy, but may predate the onset of clinically significant metastasis by many years. Short PSA doubling time (PSADT), particularly 3 months or less and in some studies up to 15 months or less, predicts for short metastasis free survival and prostate cancer–specific death, and thus initiation of ADT is recommended for these men and for those with high PSA (> 50) (84–87).

However, for those with prolonged PSADT, particularly those with PSADT of 15 months or greater, options other than ADT are reasonable to consider, as time to development of clinically significant metastasis could be years from the onset of biochemical failure. As described, the side effects of ADT can be profound, thus men with biochemical failure following definitive local therapy represent a population for whom there are limited therapeutic options and novel nonhormone agents can be studied. Large studies of peripheral androgen blockade with finasteride and dutasteride have demonstrated improvement in measures of PSA kinetics and are generally well tolerated (88, 89).

Currently, a prospective phase II cooperative group study of bicalutamide in conjunction with the AKT inhibitor MK2206 is ongoing (NCT01251861).

A variety of other agents have been evaluated in men with biochemical recurrence following definitive local therapy, with the majority of studies utilizing PSA kinetics and change in PSADT as endpoints given the lack of measurable disease. A phase II study of the tyrosine kinase inhibitor imatinib was promising but discontinued because of toxicity (90).

The antiangiogenic and immunomodulatory agent lenalidomide has been studied, with evidence of effect on PSA kinetics, with dose-dependent effect on PSA and toxicity measures (91).

The cyclooxygenase-2 inhibitor celecoxib has been evaluated either alone or in combination in multiple studies also with modest impact on PSA measures with modest toxicity profile (92–94).

Lin and colleagues evaluated the cardiac glycoside digoxin with prolongation of PSADT noted in 47% of 15 enrolled patients and favorable toxicity profile (95).

Finally, studies of natural products such as acai juice as well as pomegranate extract have demonstrated slowing of PSADT, encouraging findings for this population for whom there is particular interest in the evaluation nontoxic agents (96, 97).

■ REFERENCES

1. Harrison GS, Wierman ME, Nett TM, Glode LM. Gonadotropin-releasing hormone and its receptor in normal and malignant cells. *Endocr Relat Cancer.* 2004;11(4):725-748. doi: 10.1677/erc.1.00777.
2. Hayes FJ, Seminara SB, Decruz S, Boepple PA, Crowley WF Jr. Aromatase inhibition in the human male reveals a

hypothalamic site of estrogen feedback. *J Clin Endocrinol Metab.* 2000;85(9):3027–3035. doi: 10.1210/jcem.85.9.6795.

3. Miller WL. Molecular biology of steroid hormone synthesis. *Endocr Rev.* 1988;9(3):295–318. doi: 10.1210/edrv-9-3-295.
4. Huggins C. Prostatic cancer treated by orchiectomy; the five year results. *JAMA.* 1946;131:576–581.
5. Moreau J, Delavault P, Blumberg J. Luteinizing hormone-releasing hormone agonists in the treatment of prostate cancer: a review of their discovery, development, and place in therapy. *Clin Ther.* 2006;28(10):1485–1508. doi: http://dx.doi.org/10.1016/j.clinthera.2006.10.018.
6. Conn PM, Crowley WF. Gonadotropin-releasing hormone and its analogues. *N Engl J Med.* 1991;324(2):93-103. doi: 10.1056/NEJM199101103240205.
7. Parmar H, Phillips RH, Lightman SL, Edwards L, Allen L,Schally AV. Randomised controlled study of orchidectomy vs long-acting D-trp-6-LHRH microcapsules in advanced prostatic carcinoma. *Lancet.* 1985;2(8466):1201–1205.
8. Kaisary AV, Tyrrell CJ, Peeling WB,Griffiths K. Comparison of LHRH analogue (zoladex) with orchiectomy in patients with metastatic prostatic carcinoma. *Br J Urol.* 1991;67(5):502–508. doi: 10.1111/j.1464-410X.1991.tb15195.x.
9. Brawer MK. Challenges with luteinizing hormone-releasing hormone agonists: flare and surge. *Rev Urol.* 2004;6(suppl 7):S12-S18.
10. Kuhn J, Billebaud T, Navratil H, et al. Prevention of the transient adverse effects of a gonadotropin-releasing hormone analogue (buserelin) in metastatic prostatic carcinoma by administration of an antiandrogen (nilutamide). *N Engl J Med.* 1989;321(7):413–418. doi: 10.1056/NEJM198908173210701.
11. Noguchi K, Uemura H, Harada M, et al. Inhibition of PSA flare in prostate cancer patients by administration of flutamide for 2 weeks before initiation of treatment with slow-releasing LH-RH agonist. *Int J Clin Oncol.* 2001;6(1):29–33.
12. McLeod D, Zinner N, Tomera K, et al. A phase 3, multicenter, open-label, randomized study of abarelix versus leuprolide acetate in men with prostate cancer. *Urology.* 2001;58(5):756–761. doi: http://dx.doi.org/10.1016/S0090-4295(01)01342–5.
13. Jiang G, Stalewski J, Galyean R, et al. GnRH antagonists: a new generation of long acting analogues incorporating p-ureido-phenylalanines at positions 5 and 6. *J Med Chem.* 2001;44(3):453–467.
14. Klotz L, Boccon-Gibod L, Shore ND, et al. The efficacy and safety of degarelix: a 12-month, comparative, randomized, open-label, parallel-group phase III study in patients with prostate cancer. *BJU Int.* 2008;102(11):1531–1538. doi: 10.1111/j.1464-410X.2008.08183.x.
15. Crawford ED, Tombal B, Miller K, et al. A phase III extension trial with a 1-arm crossover from leuprolide to degarelix: comparison of gonadotropin-releasing hormone agonist and antagonist effect on prostate cancer. *J Urol.* 2011;186(3):889–897. doi: http://dx.doi.org/10.1016/j.juro.2011.04.083.
16. Mason M, Maldonado Pijoan X, Steidle C, et al. Neoadjuvant androgen deprivation therapy for prostate volume reduction, lower urinary tract symptom relief and quality of life improvement in men with intermediate- to high-risk prostate cancer: a randomised non-inferiority trial of degarelix versus goserelin plus bicalutamide. *Clin Oncol.* 2013;25(3):190–196. doi: http://dx.doi.org/10.1016/j.clon.2012.09.010.
17. Axcrona K, Aaltomaa S, da Silva CM, et al. Androgen deprivation therapy for volume reduction, lower urinary tract symptom relief and quality of life improvement in patients with prostate cancer: Degarelix vs goserelin plus bicalutamide. *BJU Int.* 2012;110(11):1721–1728. doi: 10.1111/j.1464-410X.2012.11107.x.
18. Bennett CL, Tosteson TD, Schmitt B, Weinberg PD, Ernstoff MS, Ross SD. Maximum androgen-blockade with medical or surgical castration in advanced prostate cancer: a meta-analysis of nine published randomized controlled trials and 4128 patients using flutamide. *Prostate Cancer Prostatic Dis.* 1999;2(1):4–8. doi: 10.1038/sj.pcan.4500265.
19. Lukka H, Waldron T, Klotz L, et al. Maximal androgen blockade for the treatment of metastatic prostate cancer–a systematic review. *Curr Oncol.* 2006;13(3):81–93.
20. Maximum androgen blockade in advanced prostate cancer: an overview of the randomised trials. prostate cancer trialists collaborative group. *Lancet.* 2000;355(9214):1491–1498.
21. Akaza H, Hinotsu S, Usami M, et al. Combined androgen blockade with bicalutamide for advanced prostate cancer. *Cancer.* 2009;115(15):3437–3445. doi: 10.1002/cncr.24395.
22. Akaza H, Yamaguchi A, Matsuda T, et al. Superior anti-tumor efficacy of bicalutamide 80 mg in combination with a luteinizing hormone-releasing hormone (LHRH) agonist versus LHRH agonist monotherapy as first-line treatment for advanced prostate cancer: interim results of a randomized study in Japanese patients. *Jpn J Clin Oncol.* 2004;34(1):20–28. doi: 10.1093/jjco/hyh001.
23. van der Sluis TM, Bui HN, Meuleman EJH, et al. Lower testosterone levels with luteinizing hormone-releasing hormone agonist therapy than with surgical castration: new insights attained by mass spectrometry. *J Urol.* 2012;187(5):1601–1607. doi: http://dx.doi.org/10.1016/j.juro.2011.12.063.
24. Perachino M, Cavalli V, Bravi F. Testosterone levels in patients with metastatic prostate cancer treated with luteinizing hormone-releasing hormone therapy: prognostic significance? *BJU Int.* 2010;105(5):648–651. doi: 10.1111/j.1464-410X.2009.08814.x.
25. Morote J, Orsola A, Planas J, et al. Redefining clinically significant castration levels in patients with prostate cancer receiving continuous androgen deprivation therapy. *J Urol.* 2007;178(4):1290–1295. doi: http://dx.doi.org/10.1016/j.juro.2007.05.129.
26. Dason S, Allard CB, Tong J,Shayegan B. Defining a new testosterone threshold for medical castration: results from a prospective cohort series. *Can Urol Assoc J.* 2013;7(5-6):E263-E267. doi: 10.5489/cuaj.471; 10.5489/cuaj.471.
27. Bertaglia V, Tucci M, Fiori C, et al. Effects of serum testosterone levels after 6 months of androgen deprivation therapy on the outcome of patients with prostate cancer. *Clin Genitourin Cancer.* 2013;11(3):325.el-330.e1. doi: 10.1016/j.clgc.2013.01.002; 10.1016/j.clgc.2013.01.002.
28. Kwak C, Jeong SJ, Park MS, Lee E, Lee SE. Prognostic significance of the nadir prostate specific antigen level after hormone therapy for prostate cancer. *J Urol.* 2002;168(3):995–1000.
29. Stewart AJ, Scher HI, Chen M, et al. Prostate-specific antigen nadir and cancer-specific mortality following hormonal therapy for prostate-specific antigen failure. *J Clin Oncol.* 2005;23(27):6556–6560.
30. Hussain M, Tangen CM, Higano C, et al. Absolute prostate-specific antigen value after androgen deprivation is a strong independent predictor of survival in new metastatic prostate cancer: data from southwest oncology group trial 9346 (INT-0162). *J Clin Oncol.* 2006;24(24):3984–3990.
31. Choueiri TK, Xie W, D'Amico AV, et al. Time to prostate-specific antigen nadir independently predicts overall survival in patients who have metastatic hormone-sensitive prostate cancer treated with androgen-deprivation therapy. *Cancer.* 2009;115(5):981–987. doi: 10.1002/cncr.24064.
32. Sato N, Gleave ME, Bruchovsky N, et al. Intermittent androgen suppression delays progression to androgen-independent regulation of prostate-specific antigen gene in the LNCaP prostate tumour model. *J Steroid Biochem Mol Biol.* 1996;58(2):139–146. doi: http://dx.doi.org/10.1016/0960-0760(96)00018-0.
33. Salonen AJ, Taari K, Ala-Opas M, Viitanen J, Lundstedt S,Tammela TLJ. The FinnProstate study VII: Intermittent versus continuous androgen deprivation in patients with advanced prostate cancer. *J Urol.* 2012;187(6):2074–2081. doi: http://dx.doi.org/10.1016/j.juro.2012.01.122.
34. Crook JM, O'Callaghan CJ, Duncan G, et al. Intermittent androgen suppression for rising PSA level after radiotherapy. *N Engl J Med.* 2012;367(10):895–903. doi: 10.1056/NEJMoa1201546.
35. Hussain M, Tangen CM, Berry DL, et al. Intermittent versus continuous androgen deprivation in prostate cancer. *N Engl J Med.* 2013;368(14):1314–1325. doi: 10.1056/NEJMoa1212299.

36. Niraula S, Le LW, Tannock IF. Treatment of prostate cancer with intermittent versus continuous androgen deprivation: a systematic review of randomized trials. *J Clin Oncol.* 2013;31(16):2029–2036. doi: 10.1200/JCO.2012.46.5492.
37. Tsai H, Penson DF, Makambi KH, Lynch JH, Van Den Eeden SK, Potosky AL. Efficacy of intermittent androgen deprivation therapy vs conventional continuous androgen deprivation therapy for advanced prostate cancer: a meta-analysis. *Urology.* 2013;82(2):327–334. doi: http://dx.doi.org/10.1016/j.urology.2013.01.078.
38. van Londen GJ, Levy ME, Perera S, Nelson JB,Greenspan SL. Body composition changes during androgen deprivation therapy for prostate cancer: a 2-year prospective study. *Crit Rev Oncol.* 2008;68(2):172–177. doi: http://dx.doi.org/10.1016/j.critrevonc.2008.06.006.
39. Timilshina N, Breunis H,Alibhai SMH. Impact of androgen deprivation therapy on weight gain differs by age in men with nonmetastatic prostate cancer. *J Urol.* 2012;188(6):2183–2189. doi: http://dx.doi.org/10.1016/j.juro.2012.08.018.
40. Keating NL, Liu P, O'Malley AJ, Freedland SJ,Smith MR. Androgen-deprivation therapy and diabetes control among diabetic men with prostate cancer. *Eur Urol.* 2014;65:816–824. doi: http://dx.doi.org/10.1016/j.eururo.2013.02.023.
41. Nelson CJ, Lee JS, Gamboa MC, Roth AJ. Cognitive effects of hormone therapy in men with prostate cancer. *Cancer.* 2008;113(5):1097–1106. doi: 10.1002/cncr.23658.
42. Alibhai SMH, Breunis H, Timilshina N, et al. Impact of androgen-deprivation therapy on cognitive function in men with nonmetastatic prostate cancer. *J Clin Oncol.* 2010;28(34):5030–5037. doi: 10.1200/JCO.2010.30.8742.
43. Chao HH, Uchio E, Zhang S, et al. Effects of androgen deprivation on brain function in prostate cancer patients—a prospective observational cohort analysis. *BMC Cancer.* 2012;12:371. doi: 10.1186/1471-2407-12-371; 10.1186/1471-2407-12-371.
44. Keating NL, O'Malley AJ, Smith MR. Diabetes and cardiovascular disease during androgen deprivation therapy for prostate cancer. *J Clin Oncol.* 2006;24(27):4448–4456. doi: 10.1200/JCO.2006.06.2497.
45. Saigal CS, Gore JL, Krupski TL, et al. Androgen deprivation therapy increases cardiovascular morbidity in men with prostate cancer. *Cancer.* 2007;110(7):1493–1500. doi: 10.1002/cncr.22933.
46. Punnen S, Cooperberg MR, Sadetsky N,Carroll PR. Androgen deprivation therapy and cardiovascular risk. *J Clin Oncol.* 2011;29(26):3510–3516. doi: 10.1200/JCO.2011.35.1494.
47. Nguyen PL, Je Y, Schutz FA, et al. Association of androgen deprivation therapy with cardiovascular death in patients with prostate cancer: a meta-analysis of randomized trials. *JAMA.* 2011;306(21):2359–2366. doi: 10.1001/jama.2011.1745; 10.1001/jama.2011.1745.
48. Kelly WK,Gomella LG. Androgen deprivation therapy and competing risks. *JAMA.* 2011;306(21):2382-2383. doi: 10.1001/jama.2011.1791; 10.1001/jama.2011.1791.
49. Nguyen PL, Chen M, Beckman JA, et al. Influence of androgen deprivation therapy on all-cause mortality in men with high-risk prostate cancer and a history of congestive heart failure or myocardial infarction. *Int J Radiat Oncol Biol Phys.* 2012;82(4):1411–1416. doi: http://dx.doi.org/10.1016/j.ijrobp.2011.04.067.
50. Jespersen CG, Nørgaard M, Borre M. Androgen-deprivation therapy in treatment of prostate cancer and risk of myocardial infarction and stroke: a nationwide Danish population-based cohort study. *Eur Urol.* 2014;65:704–709. doi: http://dx.doi.org/10.1016/j.eururo.2013.02.002.
51. Keating NL, O'Malley AJ, Freedland SJ, Smith MR. Does comorbidity influence the risk of myocardial infarction or diabetes during androgen-deprivation therapy for prostate cancer? *Eur Urol.* 2013;64(1):159–166. doi: http://dx.doi.org/10.1016/j.eururo.2012.04.035.
52. Keating NL, O'Malley AJ, Freedland SJ, Smith MR. Diabetes and cardiovascular disease during androgen deprivation therapy: observational study of veterans with prostate cancer. *J Natl Cancer Inst.* 2010;102(1):39–46. doi: 10.1093/jnci/djp404.
53. Smith MR, Klotz L, van der Meulen E, Colli E, Tankó LB. Gonadotropin-releasing hormone blockers and cardiovascular disease risk: analysis of prospective clinical trials of degarelix. *J Urol.* 2011;186(5):1835–1842. doi: http://dx.doi.org/10.1016/j.juro.2011.07.035.
54. Smith MR, Klotz L, Persson B, Olesen TK, Wilde AAM. Cardiovascular safety of degarelix: Results from a 12-month, comparative, randomized, open label, parallel group phase III trial in patients with prostate cancer. *J Urol.* 2010;184(6):2313–2319. doi: http://dx.doi.org/10.1016/j.juro.2010.08.012.
55. Smith JC, Bennett S, Evans LM, et al. The effects of induced hypogonadism on arterial stiffness, body composition, and metabolic parameters in males with prostate cancer. *J Clin Endocrinol Metab.* 2001;86(9):4261–4267. doi: 10.1210/jc.86.9.4261.
56. Dockery F, Bulpitt CJ, Agarwal S, Donaldson M,Rajkumar C. Testosterone suppression in men with prostate cancer leads to an increase in arterial stiffness and hyperinsulinaemia. *Clin Sci (Lond).* 2003;104(2):195–201. doi: 10.1042/CS20020209.
57. Higano CS. Sexuality and intimacy after definitive treatment and subsequent androgen deprivation therapy for prostate cancer. *J Clin Oncol.* 2012;30(30):3720–3725. doi: 10.1200/JCO.2012.41.8509.
58. Marumo K, Baba S,Murai M. Erectile function and nocturnal penile tumescence in patients with prostate cancer undergoing luteinizing hormone-releasing hormone agonist therapy. *Int J Urol.* 1999;6(1):19–23. doi: 10.1046/j.1442-2042.1999.06128.x.
59. Mazzola CR, Mulhall JP. Impact of androgen deprivation therapy on sexual function. *Asian J Androl.* 2012;14(2):198–203. doi: 10.1038/aja.2011.106; 10.1038/aja.2011.106.
60. Potosky AL, Reeve BB, Clegg LX, et al. Quality of life following localized prostate cancer treated initially with androgen deprivation therapy or no therapy. *J Natl Cancer Inst.* 2002;94(6):430–437. doi: 10.1093/jnci/94.6.430.
61. Wibowo E, Wassersug RJ. The effect of estrogen on the sexual interest of castrated males: Implications to prostate cancer patients on androgen-deprivation therapy. *Crit Rev Oncol.* 2013;87(3):224–238.doi:http://dx.doi.org/10.1016/j.critrevonc.2013.01.006.
62. DiBlasio CJ, Malcolm JB, Derweesh IH, et al. Patterns of sexual and erectile dysfunction and response to treatment in patients receiving androgen deprivation therapy for prostate cancer. *BJU Int.* 2008;102(1):39–43. doi: 10.1111/j.1464-410X.2008.07505.x.
63. Walker LM, Hampton AJ, Wassersug RJ, Thomas BC, Robinson JW. Androgen deprivation therapy and maintenance of intimacy: a randomized controlled pilot study of an educational intervention for patients and their partners. *Contemp Clin Trials.* 2013;34(2):227–231. doi: http://dx.doi.org/10.1016/j.cct.2012.11.007.
64. Beebe-Dimmer JL, Cetin K, Shahinian V, et al. Timing of androgen deprivation therapy use and fracture risk among elderly men with prostate cancer in the united states. *Pharmacoepidemiol Drug Saf.* 2012;21(1):70–78. doi: 10.1002/pds.2258.
65. Shahinian VB, Kuo Y, Freeman JL,Goodwin JS. Risk of fracture after androgen deprivation for prostate cancer. *N Engl J Med.* 2005;352(2):154–164. doi: 10.1056/NEJMoa041943.
66. Alibhai SM, Mohamedali HZ, Gulamhusein H, et al. Changes in bone mineral density in men starting androgen deprivation therapy and the protective role of vitamin D. *Osteoporos Int.* 2013;24:2571–2579. doi: 10.1007/s00198-013-2343-4.
67. Morgans AK, Smith MR, O'Malley AJ,Keating NL. Bone density testing among prostate cancer survivors treated with androgen-deprivation therapy. *Cancer.* 2013;119(4):863–870. doi: 10.1002/cncr.27830.
68. Zhumkhawala A, Gleason JM, Cheetham TC, et al. Osteoporosis management program decreases incidence of hip fracture in patients with prostate cancer receiving androgen deprivation therapy. *Urology.* 2013;81(5):1010–1017. doi: http://dx.doi.org/10.1016/j.urology.2012.11.066.

69. Smith MR, Morton RA, Barnette KG, et al. Toremifene to reduce fracture risk in men receiving androgen deprivation therapy for prostate cancer. *J Urol.* 2013;189(suppl 1):S45–S50. doi: http://dx.doi.org/10.1016/j.juro.2012.11.016.
70. Klotz LH, McNeill IY, Kebabdjian M, Zhang L, Chin JL. A phase 3, double-blind, randomised, parallel-group, placebo-controlled study of oral weekly alendronate for the prevention of androgen deprivation bone loss in nonmetastatic prostate cancer: the cancer and osteoporosis research with alendronate and leuprolide (CORAL) study. *Eur Urol.* 2013;63(5):927–935. doi: http://dx.doi.org/10.1016/j.eururo.2012.09.007.
71. Smith MR, McGovern FJ, Zietman AL, et al. Pamidronate to prevent bone loss during androgen-deprivation therapy for prostate cancer. *N Engl J Med.* 2001;345(13):948–955. doi: 10.1056/NEJMoa010845.
72. Smith MR, Eastham J, Gleason DM, Shasha D, Tchekmedyian S, Zinner N. Randomized controlled trial of zoledronic acid to prevent bone loss in men receiving androgen deprivation therapy for nonmetastatic prostate cancer. *J Urol.* 2003;169(6):2008–2012. doi: http://dx.doi.org/10.1097/01.ju.0000063820.94994.95.
73. Kapoor A, Gupta A, Desai N, Ahn H. Effect of zoledronic acid on bone mineral density in men with prostate cancer receiving gonadotropin-releasing hormone analog. *Prostate Cancer.* 2011;2011:176164. doi: 10.1155/2011/176164; 10.1155/2011/176164.
74. Smith MR, Egerdie B, Toriz NH, et al. Denosumab in men receiving androgen-deprivation therapy for prostate cancer. *N Engl J Med.* 2009;361:745–755. doi: 10.1056/NEJMoa0809003.
75. Thompson CA, Shanafelt TD,Loprinzi CL. Andropause: symptom management for prostate cancer patients treated with hormonal ablation. *Oncologist.* 2003;8(5):474–487. doi: 10.1634/theoncologist.8-5-474.
76. Ulloa EW, Salup R, Patterson SG, Jacobsen PB. Relationship between hot flashes and distress in men receiving androgen deprivation therapy for prostate cancer. *Psychooncology.* 2009; 18(6):598–605. doi: 10.1002/pon.1427.
77. Jones JM, Kohli M, Loprinzi CL. Androgen deprivation therapy-associated vasomotor symptoms. *Asian J Androl.* 2012;14(2): 193–197. doi: 10.1038/aja.2011.101; 10.1038/aja.2011.101.
78. Gerber GS, Zagaja GP, Ray PS, Rukstalis DB. Transdermal estrogen in the treatment of hot flushes in men with prostate cancer. *Urology.* 2000;55(1):97–101. doi: http://dx.doi.org/10.1016/S0090-4295(99)00370-2.
79. Loprinzi CL, Michalak JC, Quella SK, et al. Megestrol acetate for the prevention of hot flashes. *N Engl J Med.* 1994;331(6): 347–352. doi: 10.1056/NEJM199408113310602.
80. Irani J, Salomon L, Oba R, Bouchard P, Mottet N. Efficacy of venlafaxine, medroxyprogesterone acetate, and cyproterone acetate for the treatment of vasomotor hot flushes in men taking gonadotropin-releasing hormone analogues for prostate cancer: a double-blind, randomised trial. *Lancet Oncol.* 2010;11(2): 147–154. doi: http://dx.doi.org/10.1016/S1470-2045(09)70338-9.
81. Loprinzi CL, Dueck AC, Khoyratty BS, et al. A phase III randomized, double-blind, placebo-controlled trial of gabapentin in the management of hot flashes in men (N00CB). *Ann Oncol.* 2009;20(3):542–549. doi: 10.1093/annonc/mdn644.
82. Moraska AR, Atherton PJ, Szydlo DW, et al. Gabapentin for the management of hot flashes in prostate cancer survivors: A longitudinal continuation study-NCCTG trial N00CB. *J Support Oncol.* 2010;8(3):128–132.
83. Loprinzi CL, Qin R, Baclueva EP, et al. Phase III, randomized, double-blind, placebo-controlled evaluation of pregabalin for alleviating hot flashes, N07C1. *J Clin Oncol.* 2010;28(4): 641–647. doi: 10.1200/JCO.2009.24.5647.
84. Antonarakis ES, Feng Z, Trock BJ, et al. The natural history of metastatic progression in men with prostate-specific antigen recurrence after radical prostatectomy: long-term follow-up. *BJU Int.* 2012;109(1):32–39. doi: 10.1111/j.1464-410X.2011.10422.x.
85. Freedland SJ, Humphreys EB, Mangold LA, et al. Risk of prostate cancer-specific mortality following biochemical recurrence after radical prostatectomy. *JAMA.* 2005;294(4):433–439. doi: 10.1001/jama.294.4.433.
86. Antonarakis ES, Chen Y, Elsamanoudi SI, et al. Long-term overall survival and metastasis-free survival for men with prostate-specific antigen-recurrent prostate cancer after prostatectomy: analysis of the center for prostate disease research national database. *BJU Int.* 2011;108(3):378–385. doi: 10.1111/j.1464-410X.2010.09878.x.
87. Freedland SJ, Humphreys EB, Mangold LA, et al. Death in patients with recurrent prostate cancer after radical prostatectomy: Prostate-specific antigen doubling time subgroups and their associated contributions to all-cause mortality. *J Clin Oncol.* 2007;25(13):1765–1771. doi: 10.1200/JCO.2006.08.0572.
88. Monk JP, Halabi S, Picus J, et al. Efficacy of peripheral androgen blockade in prostate cancer patients with biochemical failure after definitive local therapy. *Cancer.* 2012;118(17):4139–4147. doi: 10.1002/cncr.26732.
89. Schröder F, Bangma C, Angulo JC, et al. Dutasteride treatment over 2 years delays prostate-specific antigen progression in patients with biochemical failure after radical therapy for prostate cancer: Results from the randomised, placebo-controlled avodart after radical therapy for prostate cancer study (ARTS). *Eur Urol.* 2013;63(5):779–787. doi: http://dx.doi.org/10.1016/j.eururo.2012.11.006.
90. Lin AM, Rini BI, Weinberg V, et al. A phase II trial of imatinib mesylate in patients with biochemical relapse of prostate cancer after definitive local therapy. *BJU Int.* 2006;98(4):763–769. doi: 10.1111/j.1464-410X.2006.06396.x.
91. Keizman D, Sinibaldi VJ, Carducci MA, et al. Phase I/II double-blinded randomized study to determine the tolerability and efficacy of two different doses of lenalidomide (len) in biochemically relapsed prostate cancer (BRPC) (M0) patients (pts). 2010 ASCO Meeting Abstracts. *J Clin Oncol.* 2010;28:15s (suppl; abstr 4554).
92. Pruthi RS, Derksen JE, Moore D, et al. Phase II trial of celecoxib in prostate-specific antigen recurrent prostate cancer after definitive radiation therapy or radical prostatectomy. *Clin Cancer Res.* 2006;12(7):2172–2177. doi: 10.1158/1078-0432.CCR-05-2067.
93. Srinivas S,Feldman D. A phase II trial of calcitriol and naproxen in recurrent prostate cancer. *Anticancer Res.* 2009;29(9):3605–3610.
94. Goodin S, Stein MN, Shih W, et al. A phase II study of atorvastatin and celecoxib in patients with rising PSA following local therapy for prostate cancer (PC). 2012 ASCO Meeting Abstracts. *J Clin Oncol.* 2012;30 (suppl 5; abstr 89).
95. Lin J, Hoffman-Censits JH, Duffy D, et al. A pilot phase II study of digoxin in patients with recurrent prostate cancer as evident by a rising PSA. 2013 ASCO Meeting Abstracts. *J Clin Oncol.* 2013;31 (suppl; abstr 5061).
96. Paller CJ, Ye X, Wozniak P, et al. A phase II study of pomegranate extract for men with rising prostate-specific antigen following primary therapy. 2011 ASCO Meeting Abstracts. *J Clin Oncol.* 2011;29(suppl; abstr 4522).
97. Kessler E, Su L, Lu X, et al. Apoptotic activity in patient serum while on an acai juice product in the setting of a slowly rising PSA. 2013 ASCO Meeting Abstracts. *J Clin Oncol.* 2013;31(suppl; abstr e16055).
98. Sweeney C, Chen YH, Carducci M, et al. Impact on overall survival (OS) with chemohormonal therapy versus hormonal therapy for hormone-sensitive newly metastatic prostate cancer (mPrCa): An ECOG-led phase III randomized trial. 2014 ASCO Meeting Abstracts. *J Clin Oncol.* 2014;32 (suppl; abstr LBA2)

19.1 Metastatic Castrate-Resistant Prostate Cancer: Mechanisms of Hormone Escape

SUSAN F. SLOVIN

INTRODUCTION

Prostate cancer evolution has been portrayed as a variety of different dynamic models or clinical states (1) that transition into behaviorally distinct diseases with unique sensitivities to different agents. Within the last 2 years, five new treatments have been incorporated into the clinical states with the discerning line of treatment demarcation for starting a specific drug treatment depending on whether or not the patient had received docetaxel to after failing hormonal therapy(ies). Among these treatments is the first cellular product therapy, sipuleucel-T (Provenge®) (2), second-line post-docetaxel chemotherapies with cabazitaxel (Jevtana®) (3), radium-223 (Algeta®) (4), and two androgen receptor (AR)-targeted oral agents, enzalutamide (Xtandi®) (5) and abiraterone (Zytiga®) (6). All of these new drugs conveyed a 3- to 4-month survival benefit much in keeping with the standard chemotherapy docetaxel. Unlike its other treatment counterparts, sipuleucel-T still remains as a treatment for patients with asymptomatic or minimally symptomatic castrate metastatic disease often given in the prechemotherapy window. Although cabazitaxel, radium-223, enzalutamide, and abiraterone have all been approved in the post-docetaxel setting, recent phase III clinical findings have now received approval from regulatory agencies to use the AR-directed therapies earlier in the prechemotherapy setting (7, 8). The flexibility of treatment options in the pre- and post-docetaxel arenas has delighted many oncologists and urologists as the treatment armamentarium has markedly expanded and patients could be delayed from going on to "life-altering" treatment with chemotherapy sometimes delaying referrals from the urologist to the medical oncologist.

Although clinical trials are still addressing how to best strategize the order in which AR-directed therapies are given and whether they are best used as single agents, or given together, or in combination with chemotherapy, biologics, or immune-based therapies, there remains one issue that continues to unite all these therapies, that is, how does the disease become resistant to these drugs and how can resistance be avoided? The assumption has naively been that prostate cancer is a heterogeneous disease with cells that are of a lethal or indolent phenotype but whose proportions change over time through a variety of selection mechanisms. However, as the anatomy of AR has become more unraveled, our understanding how to best target this gene, its cofactors, and splice variants is taking the forefront to assist in how to develop agents that can target one or more sites within AR.

ANATOMY OF THE ANDROGEN RECEPTOR

Understanding how to best develop AR-directed agents and to use them optimally has been gleaned by a comprehensive understanding of AR. AR is a member of the steroid hormone receptor family; other family members consist of the estrogen, progesterone, mineralocorticoid, and glucocorticoid receptors (GRs) (9). AR is a 919-aminoacid protein encoded from approximately 180-kb gene that is located at chromosome Xq11-12. It is composed of three major functional domains and several activation functional units that control its activity (Figure 19.1.1) (10). The *N*-terminal domain (NTD) (11–13) is the largest portion of the receptor that is highly unstructured and contains one of the two activation function (AF1) motifs. The second functional region is the DNA-binding domain (DBD), which contains two zinc fingers. These zinc fingers have different functions, first interacts with the androgen-response element (14–16) and the second facilitates dimerization (14, 16). A flexible hinge region connects the DBD to the ligand-binding domain (LBD), where a second transcriptional activation function (AF2) resides (17–19). AR is localized in the cytoplasm and usually remains inactive but does have some intimacy with heat shock proteins HSP90, HSP70, HSP56, and HSP27 (20, 21), which prevents it from entering the nucleus (22–24). It is well known that AR expression is elevated in castration-resistant prostate cancer (CRPC) (10, 25, 26);

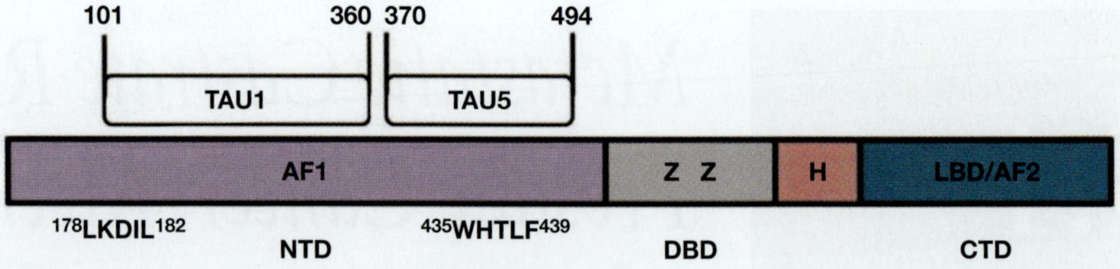

FIGURE 19.1.1 Anatomy of the androgen receptor (AR). Diagram depicting full-length androgen receptor (ARFL) and AR variants. Variants fall into two categories based on structure: truncated variants (e.g., AR-V7) and exon-skipping variants (e.g., AR^{v567es}). DBD, DNA-binding domain; LBD, ligand-binding domain; AF, activation function; TAU, transcriptional activation uni; core motifs LKD1L and WHTLF regulate androgen-independent and androgen-independent AR activity, respectively. The number of amino acids in AR is variable and based on the assumed length of 919 amino acids. Variations in the length of AR are frequent due to a variable number of glutamines.

Source: From Ref. (10). Van der Steen T, Tindall DJ, Huang H. Posttranslational modification of the androgen receptor in prostate cancer. *Int J Mol Sci.* 2013;14:14833–14859. Reproduced with permission of publisher.

this may be reflective of a hypersensitivity to androgens (27–29), or represent constitutive activity (30), or activation by other noncanonical pathways (21). A potential mechanism of resistance to standard hormonal therapy may lie in the fact that there is intratumoral production thereby activating AR in an intracrine manner (31). Constitutively active AR splice variants have been identified (32–37) and may be clinically relevant given their expression not only on prostate cancer cell lines and xenografts but also on human tumors (38, 39). These AR variants (AR-Vs) remain of scientific and clinical interest as they are not dependent on androgens for activation as they do have LBDs (40, 41). These basic observations have laid the groundwork for drug discovery that will be seen below.

Recent data have demonstrated that AR signaling cascades contribute to the development of early and late metastatic disease. Multiple downstream AR targets and important AR cofactors have been identified, which can impact on both the AR pathway and the associated clinical metastatic phenotypes. Androgens work through AR signaling with the antitumor effect of antiandrogens limited to 18 to 24 months before resistance occurs. Current hormone therapy for prostate cancer targets the LBD of the AR using drugs that lower serum testosterone, which are often given with competitive AR antagonists (Figure 19.1.2). Ligand-reducing therapy alone is not curative. Studies at the University of Washington have shown that ligand-reducing therapies, that is, antiandrogens alone or in concert with a gonadotropin-releasing hormone (GnRH) agonist/antagonist, only reduce the intratumoral androgens by 75% at a time when androgen levels in the blood are in the castrate range (42). In this androgen-depleted environment, cells that have survived androgen depletion undergo adaptive changes that inhibit castration-induced cell death, rendering them more resistant. The finding of continued expression of AR target genes such as PSA and TMPRSS2 shows that the levels of androgen that remain are sufficient to signal through the receptor.

Role of AR in Metastatic Disease

AR facilitates the metastatic process and/or maintenance of metastatic disease. There have now been significant changes in the AR cistrome as a function of disease progression, often attributed to altered expression of critical AR cofactors. Multiple investigative studies have revealed major roles for AR in promoting prometastatic events through several different mechanisms. These include (a) differential chemokine receptor/ligand function; (b) altered function of tumor-associated AR cofactors (e.g., FOXA1, cyclin D1b, and SWI/SNF); and (c) formation of prometastatic, AR-dependent gene fusions and downstream effectors (e.g., SOX9) (43). Chemokine receptors have been shown to be regulated by AR (44, 45). The chemokine receptors belong to the G protein-coupled receptor (GPCR) family of proteins with over 20 known members within this family. Each member has a conserved structure consisting of a seven-pass transmembrane monomer and a soluble cytoplasmic tail (43, 46, 47).

Data by Nelson et al. (48, 49) and others (50, 51) have demonstrated that AR, even under the influence of a GnRH agonist and an antiandrogen, can still be active with the tumor despite achieving castrate levels of testosterone in the serum to less than 10 ng/dL (Figure 19.1.3). This confirms that although patients appear to be responding to their hormonal therapy early on, intratumoral resistance slowly develops over time. The recent discovery that AR signaling persists during systemic castration via intratumoral production of androgens has led to the successful development and approval of AR-directed therapies including abiraterone acetate and enzalutamide. The upregulation of enzymes involved in androgen biosynthesis such as AKR1C3 occurred within the tumor microenvironment (31, 42, 52–54); other studies that evaluated androgen levels and mRNA levels of relevant androgen synthesis enzymes have proposed that prostate cancer bone metastases can convert adrenal androgens to

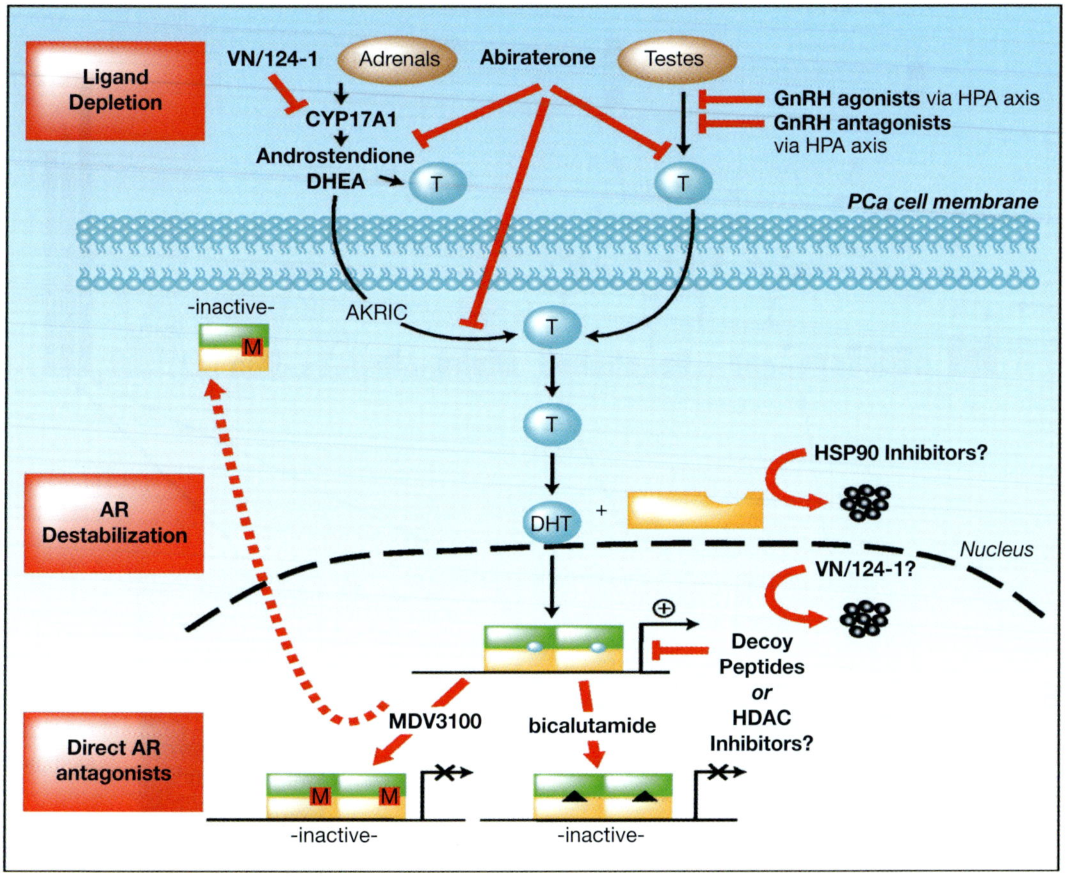

FIGURE 19.1.2 The androgen receptor (AR) pathways. Multiple mechanisms that can destabilize AR may be achieved through HSP90 inhibitors or inhibitors of HSP90–HDAC association. Alternatively, peptides have been used to disrupt the AR N-C-terminal interaction that could reduce AR association with chromatin, in addition to peptides derived from AR corepressors. The AR-directed agent, enzalutamide, precludes both AR–DNA association and AR nuclear accumulation, whereas abiraterone, a selective CYP17 inhibitor, suppresses both testicular and adrenal androgen synthesis via blockade of 17α-hydroxylase and C17,20-lyase enzymes in the adrenal steroid synthetic pathway.

Source: From Ref. (43). Knudsen KE, Scher HI. Starving the addiction: new opportunities for durable suppression of AR signaling in prostate cancer. *Clin Cancer Res* 2009;15:4792–4798. Reproduced with permission of publisher.

testosterone and dihydrotestosterone (DHT) (42, 54). One study has suggested that metastatic castration-resistant prostate cancer (mCRPC) is dependent on the conversion of precursor androstenedione to 5α-androstenedione, which is then converted to the active form of testosterone, DHT, and bypassing the prior conversion to testosterone. Interestingly, according to a recent report by Chang et al. (55), other mechanisms may include amplification of the *HSD17B3* gene by the metastatic prostate cancer with sustained copy number loss of the *HSD17B2* gene, which could in turn lead to diminished conversion of testosterone to the less active androstenedione (56). The heterogeneous expression of various steroidogenic enzymes within the tumor microenvironment has been identified in patients with mCRPC by Mitsiades et al. (57). These observations suggested that a blockade of a combination of enzymes is involved in androgen biosynthesis and hence their blockade by more directed antiandrogens may be a therapeutic pathway. Data by Efstathiou et al. (58) had confirmed this by demonstrating that abiraterone acetate could suppress testosterone concentrations in blood and the tumor microenvironment to less than picograms per milliliter. Although our understanding of the critical pathways involved in AR signaling and amplification has broadened, resistance can occur within 3 to 6 months after starting these agents (de novo resistance) and others may become resistant later (acquired resistance), that is, more than 6 months.

Hofland et al. (59) quantified the steroidogenic mRNA expression in a panel of experimental models of human prostate and in human normal and cancerous tissues (Table 19.1.1). Examining a wide variety of prostate cases, they could not detect the simultaneous expression of all enzymes necessary for de novo synthesis of androgens from cholesterol to testosterone. Intraprostatic production of DHT was found to occur starting from androstenedione due to the presence of AKRIC3 and SRD5A1. Intratumoral ARKIC3 was upregulated in patients receiving hormonal therapy, in addition to the presence of overexpressed AR, thereby suggesting a mechanism whereby castration-resistant disease could evolve. Therefore, it was suggested that the substrate for AKRIC3-encoded enzyme

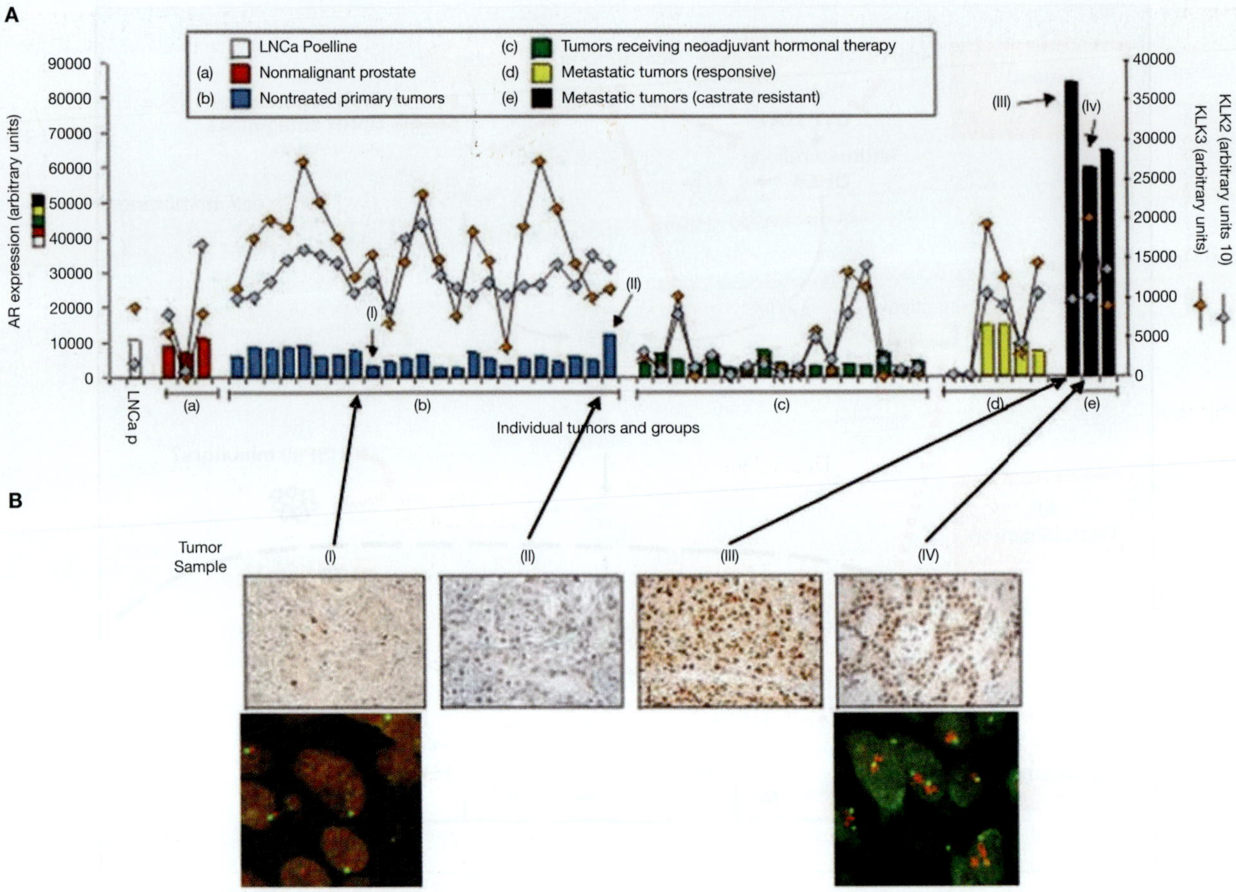

FIGURE 19.1.3 Expression of AR mRNA and protein in castrate-metastatic samples (A), including amplification of the gene by AR FISH (B).

Source: From Ref. (50). Holzbeierlein J, Lal P, La Tulippe E, et al. Gene expression analysis of human prostate carcinoma during hormonal therapy identifies androgen-responsive genes and mechanisms of therapy resistance. *Am J Path.* 2004;164:217–227. Reproduced with permission of publisher.

would be adrenally derived androstenedione given its presence in the serum in nanomolar range. The authors conclude that enzymes for the de novo synthesis of androgens are poorly expressed in normal humans and in prostate cancer samples including lymph nodes as well as in animal models. The increased expression of 5RD5A1 during tumor progression was compared with AKRI3, which increases during hormonal therapy. The implication is that these expression changes can lead the cancer to convert circulating steroids of adrenal origin to testosterone and DHT locally. Recent work by Schoenborn et al. (60) has defined genetic subgroups of prostate cancers with high levels of inter- and intratumoral heterogeneity.

Development of AR Resistance

Terminologies regarding androgen or "hormone" resistance have changed over the years. Historically, if a patient who had been on either a GnRH agonist alone or in combination with an antiandrogen such as flutamide, bicalutamide, or nilutamide failed treatment as indicated by a rise in prostate specific antigen (PSA) after achieving a nadir PSA of less than 0.05 ng/dL, the patient was deemed as "hormone refractory," meaning that the likelihood of responding to additional hormones was minimal or nil. These nonsteroidal antiandrogens are reversible inhibitors that bind to the LBD of AR with low affinity relative to androgens and offer incomplete transcriptional inhibition. All these drugs bind to AR, but the affinity of binding may be variable (61). It was then found by others (61) that a patient could undergo a "withdrawal" response by discontinuing the current antiandrogen and observing whether the cessation of the current antiandrogen could cause a decline in PSA or disease. This "antiandrogen withdrawal" response was further validated to be true in many patients, with the attempt to try another antiandrogen if the achieved response was no longer maintained (62). Patients have often been given two or even three antiandrogens with continued sensitivity to each albeit for shorter periods of time. This led to the understanding that patients were not truly "refractory" to hormonal manipulations but were resistant to the current hormonal treatment without being resistant to future antiandrogens.

To understand the mechanisms contributing to treatment resistance, mRNA expression profiles of prostate cancers representing untreated and posthormone-treated primary tumors and castration-resistant metastatic disease have been performed. This analysis showed persistent expression of AR mRNA and protein

Table 19.1.1 Chart of cell lines used to study AR characteristics of prostate cancer cell lines and xenografts

	Androgen dependence	AR status	Origin
Cell lines			
LNCaP	Responsive	AR+	Lymph node
VCaP	Responsive	AR+	Bone
DuCaP	Responsive	AR+	Dura
PC346C	Responsive	AR+	PC346
Xenografts			
PC82	Dependent	AR+	Prostate
PC295	Dependent	AR+	Lymph node
PC310	Dependent	AR+	Prostate
PC346	Responsive	AR+	TURP
PC346B	Responsive	AR+	TURP
PC374	Responsive	AR+	Skin
PC133	Independent	AR-	Bone
PC135	Independent	AR-	Prostate
PC324	Independent	AR-	TURP
PC339	Independent	AR-	TURP
PC346I	Unresponsive	AR+	PC346
PC346BI	Unresponsive	AR+	PC346B
PC374F	Unresponsive	AR+	PC374

Source: Modified from Ref. (59). Hofland J, van Weerden WM, Dits NFJ, et al. Evidence of limited contribution for intratumoral steroidogenesis in prostate cancer. *Cancer Res.* 2010;70(3):1256–1264. Reproduced with permission of publisher.

in the castrate-metastatic samples (A), including amplification of the gene by AR fluorescence in situ hybridization (FISH) (B) (40). AR expression in the residual tumor following ligand-directed ADT alone showed reduced but persistent AR gene expression. More importantly, the AR and AR gene expression levels were reduced relative to untreated primary tumors, many of the posthormone-treated samples continued to express AR target genes (e.g., PSA, prostatic acid phosphatase, prostate-specific transglutaminase [TGP], kallikrein 1 [KLK1], and TMPRSS2) (40, 51). An association was also shown between the level of PSA mRNA and protein expression and biochemical relapse (51).

The study of targeting the AR and the AR signaling axis has been limited by the lack of pretherapy biopsies, the arrayed samples were provided from whole prostate tissue that was not microdissected, and the absence of quantification of androgen levels in prostate tissue. Nonetheless, recent clinical observations, molecular profiling studies, and laboratory work support the concept of AR signaling as a mechanism of oncogenic growth.

Despite multiple mechanisms by which resistance can develop, studies of cell lines and prostate cancers indicate that several alternative splice forms of the AR (63–65) may explain the complementary resistance of newer AR-directed therapies such as enzalutamide and abiraterone (Figure 19.1.4). These AR-Vs have somewhat different structures. Although each variant lacks portions of the LBD, the AR-Vs have different structure. The lack of a LBD predicts a greater likelihood of a constitutively active receptor. The elevated expression of AR splice variants was also found to be associated with a more rapid disease recurrence following surgery for localized disease, when compared with patients with lower expression of the variant (64, 65). Splice variant forms were not seen in primary prostate cancers. Many investigators have felt that such data may suggest that the presence of constitutively active splice variants of the AR arises following castration may play a major role

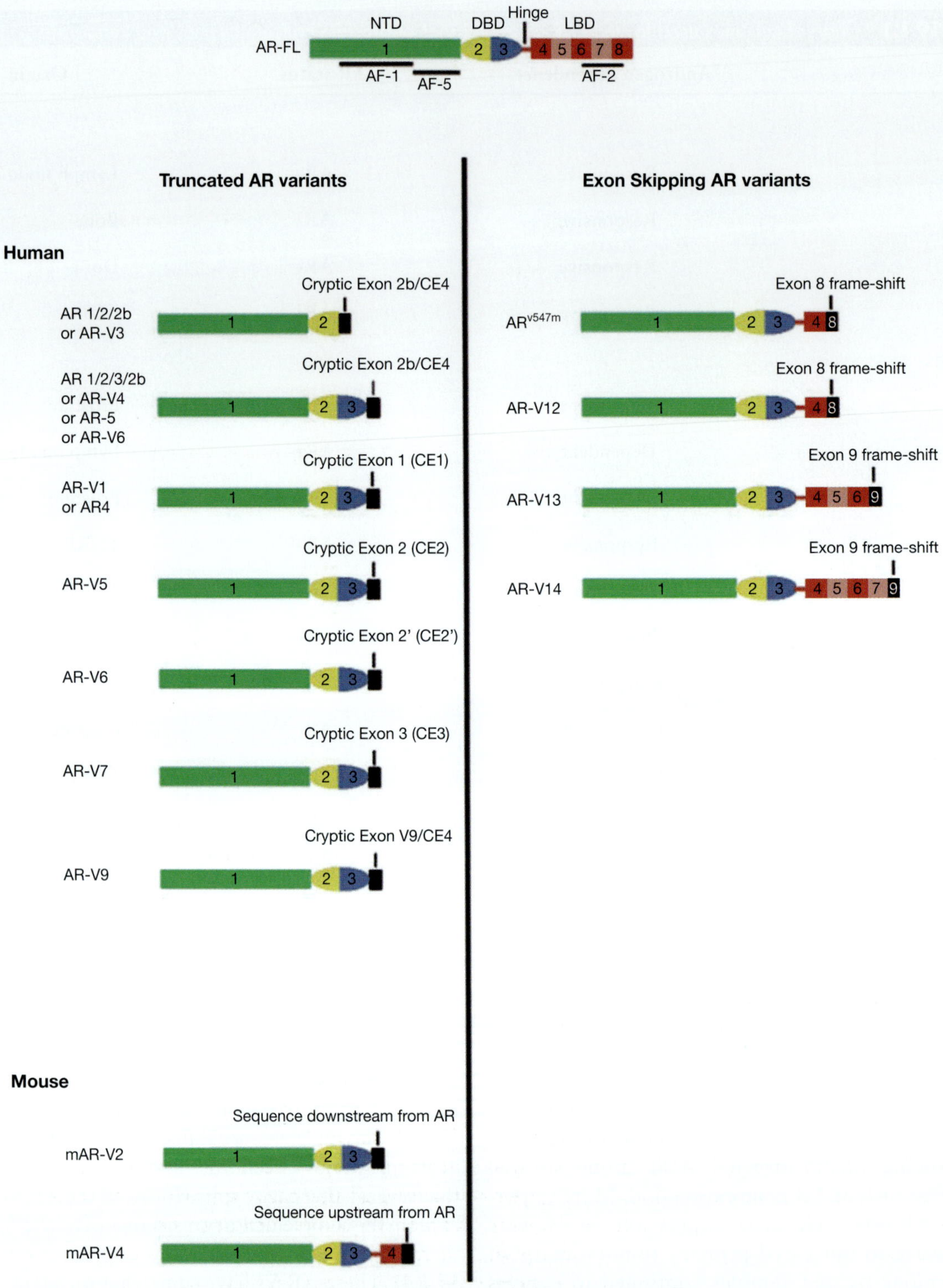

FIGURE 19.1.4 Illustration of splice variants. Depiction of full-length AR with AR variants. The AR variants fall into two categories based on structure: truncated variants, that is, AR-V7, and exon-skipping variants, that is, AR^{v567es}.

Source: From Ref. (76). Li Y, Chan SC, Brand LJ, Hwang TH, Silverstein KA, Dehm SM. Androgen receptor splice variants mediate enzalutamide resistance in castration-resistant prostate cancer cell lines. *Cancer Res.* 2013;73(2):483–489. Reproduced with permission of publisher.

in prostate cancer progression. Recent data by Cai et al. (66) reported the identification and characterization of a previously unrecognized AR splice variant that comprised the full sequences of exons 1 to 4 and the full sequence of exon 8, skipping exons 5, 6, and 7 (denoted as AR^{v567es}). Not only was it constitutively active but also increased the expression of full-length AR in the absence of ligand. This alternative splicing event appeared to have led to a frame shift, so that 10 amino acids that the authors felt to be unique were encoded for and followed by a stop codon that resulted in an AR-V protein that is 180 amino acids shorter than the AR protein. This variant, unlike other reported AR splice variants, retained the hinge region, a feature deemed necessary for complete nuclear translocation of the AR (66) and hence transcription and activation.

The potential clinical ramifications were further evaluated by Cai et al. (66), who interrogated a variety of tissues including lymph node, lung, liver, and bone obtained from men who died of castrate metastatic prostate cancer. Over 50% of the specimens that contained detectable AR transcripts were positive for one or more of the constitutively active variants. The presence of AR^{v567es} was not distributed in a random fashion among the patients but rather the variant clustered within a patient's specimens. As expected, not all specimens within a patient were positive for an AR-V, consistent with a hypothesis of ongoing splicing activity that generates AR-Vs. Additional examination of specimens for the presence of two other AR-Vs recently reported to affect survival in prostate cancer, AR3 and AR-V7 (31, 64). AR^{v567es} was the most common of the three variants examined, and several specimens contained more than one AR-V. Additionally, the authors found that nearly all the specimens that contained one or more of the variants also contained full-length AR, which was not surprising. These observations are in keeping with the multiple mechanisms by which AR remains activated despite castration.

Concepts of Innate (de Novo) and Acquired Resistance

The approval of enzalutamide, an antiandrogen that blocks translocation of AR to the nucleus, and abiraterone, a CYP17,21-lyase inhibitor that targets androgen steroidogenesis have provided an alternative to the current antiandrogens that have been used for over 20 years. Their respective mechanism of action remains unique (5, 6), yet despite the use of these drugs both post-docetaxel and now in the pre-docetaxel space, resistance to one drug does not necessarily preclude resistance to the other, although there are data from de Bono' group to suggest that failure in the prechemotherapy space may portend rapid failure to docetaxel (67, 68).

While the elucidation of the exact mechanism of action by which resistance occurs given the many possible means by which it can occur, data from clinical trials may suggest unique patterns by which one may be able to glean how patients become resistant to these AR-directed agents. In a review by Rathkopf and Scher (69), the authors suggest that they may have an "innate" resistance when a patient is exposed to a drug versus an "acquired" resistance that is seen in patients who have been through hormonal multiple agents over time. This is suggested by those patients who underwent treatment with enzalutamide who demonstrated three consecutive PSA declines following treatment. These patients were shown to have prolonged radiographic progression-free survival (PFS) with a median unreached versus those who had no sequential declines and whose median PFS remains less than 6 months. It is likely that individual patterns to different AR-directed agents will declare themselves over time. Multiple authors have attributed failure on enzalutamide and abiraterone with changes in AR splice forms, which lack the LBD in addition to non-AR mechanisms that may be unknown. Hu et al. (70) looked at a subset of CRPC xenograft models treated with enzalutamide and noted that there appeared to be an "adaptive shift" away from full-length AR to the AR splice variant. This suggested that castration was important in contributing toward drug resistance in prostate cancer progression. Given these concerns, attempts to develop drugs that target these splice variants is of potential interest. One example is EPI-001, which has caused decrease AR gene expression and inhibited tumor growth in LNCaP xenograft models (71). Another approach is derived from the observations that the first- and second-generation antiandrogens bind to the C-terminus of the LBD and that targeting the regulatory NTD may be needed for transcription in the presence or absence of ligand (72).

Splice Variants

Recent data presented by Antonarakis et al. (73) looked at the presence of AR splice variant, AR-V7, on circulating tumor cells (CTCs) and its potential correlation with primary resistance to enzalutamide and to abiraterone (Zytiga), an inhibitor of 17α-hydroxylase/C17,20-lyase (CYP17A1), an enzyme that is expressed in testicular, adrenal, and prostatic tumor tissues. Using quantitative reverse transcriptase polymerase chain reaction on CTCs obtained prospectively from patients with castrate metastatic prostate cancer treated with either enzalutamide or abiraterone, the investigators interrogated the CTCs for the presence or absence of AR-V7. In two well-balanced cohorts of 31 patients treated with either enzalutamide or abiraterone, 39% and 19% had detectable AR-V7 on CTCs, respectively. Correlation of AR-V7 expression with PSA was also examined with the finding that among men who received enzalutamide, those who had AR-V7-positive CTCs, had inferior PSA response rates (0% vs. 52.6%, $P = .004$) as well as inferior outcomes in PFS (median 2.1 vs. 6.1 months, $P < .001$) and PSA-PFS (median 1.4 vs. 5.9 months, $P < .001$) compared with AR-V7-negative patients, respectively. Similar findings were seen for men who had been treated with abiraterone with PFS (median 2.3 vs. not reached) for those with AR-V7 positivity versus those who were AR-V7 negative, respectively. The authors concluded that even with adjusting for full-length AR expression levels, the negative prognostic impact of this splice variant was maintained (73). Although patient number was small, there is significant potential for AR-V7 to be useful as a biomarker that may be predictive of response or conversely predictive of resistance to AR-targeted drugs. The implications of these results remains far-reaching as it may provide further guidance into how to best develop other AR-targeted inhibitors by exploring the AR NTD.

There are several hypotheses as to how splice variants emerge (74). This includes possible genomic rearrangements, the other, through alternative splice events. Several cell lines and xenograft models with AR-Vs have been used to study mechanism of splice variants. This technology has facilitated the observation that intragenic re-arrangement of the AR gene may account for the presence of AR-V7 or AR^{v567es} (75, 76). The authors then used FISH and deep sequencing and discovered that individual prostate cancer cells can express either AR-full length (FL) or AR-Vs but not both. This has implications that suggest that it may be that full-length AR or AR-Vs exist in a unique subset of cancer cells and that during castration and the inhibition of ligand-drive AR-FL, there is the emergence of these AR-V clones that will propel the tumor into rapid growth. Alternative splicing represents a second means for generating splice variants. In malignancies, differential splicing of pre-mRNA is a frequent mechanism used by the cell to generate protein variants that have oncogenic activity (77–79). Plymate and coworkers (80) have demonstrated that transcriptional-associated alternative splicing generates AR-V7 in the human prostate cancer cell line, VCaP, but not in the LNCaP cell line. Interestingly, no intragenic rearrangement or inversion of the AR gene was noted in either of these cell lines (76). However, LNCaP harbors a PTEN mutation and a mutation in the LBD of the AR that increases the promiscuity of ligands that can activate the AR (81, 82), whereas LnCaP cells have a TMPRSS2-ERG fusion with increased copy number of AR-FL marked increase in the copy number of AR-FL (83, 84).

Glucocorticoid Receptor and Acquired Resistance to AR-Directed Therapy

Despite the success of AR-targeted agents, resistance, irrespective of its mechanism remains a persistent program and attempts to find other means by which AR overdrive can be circumvented and resistance prevented are a priority. Reports by Sawyers' group (85, 86) and others (87, 88) have identified an AR point mutation as one resistance mechanism. This was determined by using drug-resistant sublines following prolonged exposure to enzalutamide or a second-generation compound ARN-509. This group has gone on to evaluate a more prevalent mechanism of tumor resistance namely by circumventing AR blockade via upregulation of the GR. Using a variety of tumor models using LNCaP/AR xenograft tumors that have become resistant despite treatment with AR-directed drugs such as enzalutamide and second-generation AR antagonist, ARN-509, the most upregulated gene in the resistance tumors was the *GR* (NR3C1). Interestingly, the *GR* gene shares overlapping target specificity with AR (88). Among other genes that were upregulated was serum glucocorticoid induced kinase (*SGK1*) that is a known AR- and GR-induced target gene. Those that were the most repressed and included androgen-induced genes PMEPA1, SNAI2, KCNN2, LONRF1, and SPOCK1, whereas several known androgen-repressed genes *UGT2b15, PMP22, CAMk2N1, and UGT2B17 were the most upregulated. To determine whether GR expression was associated with clinical antiandrogen resistance, GR expression was evaluated in bone metastases obtained from patients before and then at 8 weeks after starting enzalutamide. GR was quantitated by immunohistochemistry (IHC), and the percentage of GR-positive tumor cells was correlated with clinical response. Those who had benefit from therapy more than 6 months were defined as "good" responders, whereas those treatment was discontinued in less than 6 months were deemed "poor" responders. The "good" responders had greater than 50% PSA declines; however, in the "poor" responders, aside from a single patient who had greater than 50% PSA decline compared with others within that group, GR positivity was noted low. Three of twenty-two tumors had evidence of high GR expression at baseline, and all three had poor clinical response. At 8 weeks, the mean percentage of GR-positive cells was higher than baseline levels in both response groups but was significantly increased in the poor responders (29% vs. 8%, P = .02). The percentage of GR-positive cells at 8 weeks was also higher in poor compared to good responders. GR induction appeared to be associated a more limited PSA decrease. These clinical findings are of interest in that they more than suggest a correlation between GR expression and clinical responsiveness to enzalutamide. This also strongly suggests that AR inhibition may induce GR expression in some but not all patients. Poor PSA declines may also correlate with GR expression. Whether this was due to transcriptional regulation of a particular canonical AR target gene that was under regulation by the GR remains to be determined.

The role of GR has been further interrogated using a unique tumor xenograft derived from enzalutamide-resistant tumors with high GR expression. This LNCaP/AR resistant to enzalutamide xenograft (LREX) cell line (86) is representative of high GR expression and has been used to study the role of GR expression. Intracellular AR staining of these cells were not substantially different from those in control cell lines such as CS1 (derived from a vehicle tumor). In a series of experiments designed to explore AR and GR transcriptomes, expression profiling was performed using LREX cells and treating them with DHT or dexamethasone in the presence of absence of enzalutamide. The expression signatures of AR and GR were then defined as all genes with absolute expression change greater than 1.6-fold after 1 nM DHT or 100 nM Dex treatment. Fifty-two genes were common to both AR and GR signature genes; however, a heatmap analysis of these genes confirmed significant overlap in DHT-versus Dex-induced gene expression. Dex-induced gene expression was not impacted on by enzalutamide. The authors felt that GR activity could bypass the AR inhibition induced by enzalutamide through a distinct and likely significant overlapping transcriptome. The implications for these studies are far reaching as they may provide a mechanism of resistance that is associated with a transition from AR- to GR-driven transcriptional activity and even the possibility that there may be substantial overlap between AR- and GR-binding sites in these resistant cells. The authors caution that these transcriptional differences may not be based solely by DNA binding (85, 86). Therefore, in going forward with future drug development, it will need to be kept in mind that adaptive resistance via what Sawyers' calls "AR-mediated negative feedback of GR expression" can occur in addition to typical clonal selection (85–89). The implications of the GR extend to current treatment strategies as well. Corticosteroids are a mainstay in prostate cancer treatment, used to control pain, nausea, and improve clinical well-being, and can impact on overall survival (90). More recently, it is given with abiraterone at a physiologic dose of 5 mg given twice daily by mouth to prevent side effects of fatigue, hypokalemia, and hypertension. These data showing that GR has a role in drug resistance can be extrapolated to the potential that corticosteroids might promote tumor progression in men whose tumors express GR. The recent phase III trial by Scher et al. (5) demonstrated that while patients in the AFFIRM trial had a survival benefit with enzalutamide, those patients who had been maintained on longstanding prednisone/Decadron seemed to have worse survival.

Role of AR in Metastatic Disease

AR facilitates the metastatic process and/or maintenance of metastatic disease. There have now been significant changes in the AR cistrome as a function of disease progression, often attributed to altered expression of critical AR cofactors. Multiple investigative studies have revealed major roles for AR in promoting prometastatic events through several different mechanisms. These include (a) differential chemokine receptor/ligand function; (b) altered function of tumor-associated AR cofactors (e.g., FOXA1, cyclin D1b, and SWI/SNF); and (c) formation of prometastatic, AR-dependent gene fusions and downstream effectors (e.g., SOX9) (43). Chemokine receptors have been shown to be regulated by AR (44, 45). The chemokine receptors belong to the GPCR family of proteins with over 20 known members within this family. Each member has a conserved structure consisting of a seven-pass transmembrane monomer and a soluble cytoplasmic tail (43, 46, 47).

Clinical Implications: Where Do We Go From Here?

A majority of tumors express both ligand-dependent and constitutively active splice receptors (66). Androgens play a pivotal role in prostate cancer growth and remain the central focus for target drug development. Other agents are under scrutiny and include novel androgen biosynthesis inhibitors such as orteronel (TAK-700) (91) as well as ARN-509 (91), ODM-201 (92), and agents with a dual mechanism of action (galeterone) (93, 94). Although many of these drugs represent second- or third-generation agents from the original compounds, TAK-700 failed to meet its primary endpoint of OS but showed a benefit in radiographic PFS. Recent studies by Lallous et al. (95) tested compounds designed to bind alternative sites on the LBD surface and have shown promising levels of in vitro inhibition of AR transcriptional activity. Targeting the AF2 and BF3 surfaces of the AR to develop a new class of inhibitors can be used alternatively or complementarily to current prostate cancer and CRPC therapies. Using an in silico drug discovery approach integrated with biological validation, we identified several potent small molecule inhibitors selectively targeting the AR AF2 and the BF3 sites (95).

Although no AR-V-specific drugs are available, there are other naturally derived compounds such as EPI-001 or mahanine that can inhibit AR-FL and AR-Vs, which are under evaluation (71, 96, 97). Many investigators feel that drugs that can target AR-Vs should be initiated at the same time as androgen deprivation therapy as this provides a window of time when AR-Vs are likely to emerge as opposed to awaiting a change of therapy due to castration resistance. The latter may confer the presence of mutation changes in the LBD of the AR of the evolution of a completely atypical and aggressive form of prostate cancer, that is, small cell or neuroendocrine, which will be unresponsive to convention AR-targeted agents. Despite various limitations, there is significant progress in our understanding of the mechanisms of resistance in prostate cancer with many future opportunities for successful AR-targeting agents to impact on the disease.

■ REFERENCES

1. Scher HI, Heller G. Clinical states in prostate cancer: towards a dynamic model of disease progression. *Urology*. 2000;55:323-327.
2. Kantoff PW, Higano CS, Shore ND, et al. Sipuleucel-T immunotherapy for castration-resistant prostate cancer. *N Engl J Med*. 2010;363(5):411-422.
3. de Bono JS, Oudard S, Ozguroglu M, et al. Prednisone plus cabazitaxel or mitoxantrone for metastatic castration-resistant prostate cancer progressing after docetaxel treatment: a randomised open-label trial. *Lancet*. 2010;376(9747):1147-1154.
4. Parker C, Nilsson S, Heinrich D, et al. Alpha emitter radium-223 and survival in metastatic prostate cancer. *N Engl J Med*. 2013;369(3):213-223.
5. Scher HI, Fizazi K, Saad F, et al. Increased survival with enzalutamide in prostate cancer after chemotherapy. *N Engl J Med*. 2012;367(13):1187-1197.
6. de Bono JS, Logothetis CJ, Molina A, et al. Abiraterone and increased survival in metastatic prostate cancer. *N Engl J Med*. 2011;364(21):1995-2005.

7. Ryan CJ, Smith MR, de Bono JS, et al. Abiraterone in metastatic prostate cancer without previous chemotherapy. *N Engl J Med.* 2013;368(2):138-148.
8. Beer TM, Armstrong AJ, Rathkopf DE, et al. Enzalutamide in metastatic prostate cancer before chemotherapy. *N Engl J Med.* 2014;371(5):424-433. doi: 10.1056/NEJMoa1405095..
9. Bourguet W, Germain P, Gronemeyer H. Nuclear receptor ligand-binding domains: three-dimensional structures, molecular interactions and pharmacological implications. *Trends Pharmacol Sci.* 2000;21:381-388.
10. Van der Steen T, Tindall DJ, Huang H. Posttranslational modification of the androgen receptor in prostate cancer. *Int J Mol Sci.* 2013;14:14833-14859.
11. Ding D, Xu, L, Menon M, Reddy GP, Barrack ER. Effect of GGC (glycine) repeat length polymorphism in the human androgen receptor on androgen action. *Prostate.* 2005;62:133-139.
12. Ding D, Xu L, Menon M, et al. Effect of a short cag (glutamine) repeat on human androgen receptor function. *Prostate.* 2004;58:23-32.
13. Ferro P, Catalano M.G, Dell'Eva R, Fortunati N, Pfeffer U. The androgen receptor cag repeat: a modifier of carcinogenesis? *Mol Cell Endocrinol.* 2002;193:109-120.
14. Wong CI, Zhou ZX, Sar M, Wilson EM. Steroid requirement for androgen receptor dimerization and DNA binding. Modulation by intramolecular interactions between the nh2-terminal and steroid-binding domains. *J Biol Chem.* 1993;268:19004-19012.
15. Kasper S, Rennie PS, Bruchovsky N, et al. Cooperative binding of androgen receptors to two DNA sequences is required for androgen induction of the probasin gene. *J Biol Chem.* 1994;269:31763-31769.
16. Shaffer PL, Jivan A, Dollins DE, Claessens F, Gewirth DT. Structural basis of androgen receptor binding to selective androgen response elements. *Proc Natl Acad Sci USA.* 2004;101:4758-4763.
17. He B, Gampe RT Jr, Kole AJ, et al. Structural basis for androgen receptor interdomain and coactivator interactions suggests a transition in nuclear receptor activation function dominance. *Mol Cell.* 2004;16:425-438.
18. Hur E, Pfaff SJ, Payne ES, Grøn H, Buehrer BM, Fletterick RJ. Recognition and accommodation at the androgen receptor coactivator binding interface. *PLoS Bio.* 2004;2:E274.
19. Estebanez-Perpina E, Moore JM, Mar E, et al. The molecular mechanisms of coactivator utilization in ligand-dependent transactivation by the androgen receptor. *J Biol Chem.* 2005;280:8060-8068.
20. Veldscholte J, Berrevoets CA, Zegers ND, van der Kwast TH, Grootegoed JA, Mulder E. Hormone-induced dissociation of the androgen receptor-heat-shock protein complex: use of a new monoclonal antibody to distinguish transformed from nontransformed receptors. *Biochemistry.* 1992;31:7422-7430.
21. Zhu ML, Kyprianou N. Androgen receptor and growth factor signaling cross-talk in prostate cancer cells. *Endocr Relat Cancer.* 2008;15:841-849.
22. Pratt WB. Interaction of hsp90 with steroid receptors: organizing some diverse observations and presenting the newest concepts. *Mol Cell Endocrinol.* 1990;74:C69-C76.
23. Smith DF,Sullivan WP, Marion TN, et al. Identification of a 60-kilodalton stress-related protein, p60, which interacts with hsp90 and hsp70. *Mol Cell Biol.* 1993;13:869-876.
24. Smith DF, Toft DO. Steroid receptors and their associated proteins. *Mol Endocrinol.* 1993;7:4-11.
25. Buchanan G, Irvine RA, Coetzee GA, Tilley WD. Contribution of the androgen receptor to prostate cancer predisposition and progression. *Cancer Metastasis Rev.* 2001;20:207-223.
26. Feldman BJ, Feldman D. The development of androgen-independent prostate cancer. *Nat Rev Cancer.* 2001;1:34-45.
27. Heemers HV, Tindall DJ. Androgen receptor (AR) coregulators: a diversity of functions converging on and regulating the AR transcriptional complex. *Endocr Rev.* 2007;28:778-808.
28. Debes JD, Tindall DJ. Mechanisms of androgen-refractory prostate cancer. *N Engl J Med.* 2004;351:1488-1490.
29. Askew EB, Gampe RT Jr, Stanley TB, Faggart JL, Wilson EM. Modulation of androgen receptor activation function 2 by testosterone and dihydrotestosterone. *J Biol Chem.* 2007;282:25801-25816.
30. Bergerat JP, Ceraline J. Pleiotropic functional properties of androgen receptor mutants in prostate cancer. *Hum Mutat.* 2009;30:145-157.
31. Locke JA, Guns ES, Lubik AA, et al. Androgen levels increase by intratumoral *de novo* steroidogenesis during progression of castration-resistant prostate cancer. *Cancer Res.* 2008;68:6407-6415.
32. Haile S, Sadar MD. Androgen receptor and its splice variants in prostate cancer. *Cell Mol Life Sci.* 2011;68:3971-3981.
33. Ceraline J, Cruchant MD, Erdmann E, et al. Constitutive activation of the androgen receptor by a point mutation in the hinge region: a new mechanism for androgen-independent growth in prostate cancer. *Int J Cancer.* 2004;108:152-157.
34. Libertini SJ, Tepper CG, Rodriguez V, Asmuth DM, Kung HJ, Mudryj M. Evidence for calpain-mediated androgen receptor cleavage as a mechanism for androgen independence. *Cancer Res.*2007;67:9001-9005.
35. Hornberg E, Ylitalo EB, Crnalic S, et al. Expression of androgen receptor splice variants in prostate cancer bone metastases is associated with castration-resistance and short survival. *PLoS One.* 2011;6:e19059. doi: 10.1371/journal.pone.0019059.
36. Harada N, Inoue K, Yamaji R, Nakano Y, Inui H. Androgen deprivation causes truncation of the C-terminal region of androgen receptor in human prostate cancer LNCaP cells. *Cancer Sci.* 2012;103:1022-1027.
37. Dehm SM, Schmidt LJ, Heemers HV, Vessella RL, Tindall DJ. Splicing of a novel androgen receptor exon generates a constitutively active androgen receptor that mediates prostate cancer therapy resistance. *Cancer Res.* 2008;68:5469-5477.
38. Sun S, Sprenger CC, Vessella RL, et al. Castration resistance in human prostate cancer is conferred by a frequently occurring androgen receptor splice variant. *J Clin Invest.* 2010;120:2715-2730.
39. Zhang X, Morrissey C, Sun S, et al. Androgen receptor variants occur frequently in castration resistant prostate cancer metastases. *PLoS One.* 2011;6:e27970.
40. Carrión-Salip D, Panosa C, Menendez JA, et al. Androgen-independent prostate cancer cells circumvent EGFR inhibition by overexpression of alternative HER receptors and ligands. *Int J Oncol.* 2012;41(3):1128-1138.
41. Dehm SM, Tindall DJ. Ligand-independent androgen receptor activity is activation function-2-independent and resistant to antiandrogens in androgen refractory prostate cancer cells. *J Biol Chem.* 2006;281:27882-27893.
42. Montgomery RB, Mostaghel EA, Vessella R, et al. Maintenance of intratumoral androgens in metastatic prostate cancer: a mechanism for castration-resistant tumor growth. *Cancer Res.* 2008;68(11):4447-4454. doi: 10.1158/0008-5472.CAN-08-0249.
43. Knudsen KE, Scher HI. Starving the addiction: new opportunities for durable suppression of AR signaling in prostate cancer. *Clin Cancer Res.* 2009;15:4792-4798.
44. Frigo DE, Sherk AB, Wittmann BM, et al. Induction of Kruppel-like factor 5 expression by androgens results in increased CXCR4-dependent migration of prostate cancer cells in vitro. *Mol Endocrinol.* 2009;23:1385-1396.
45. Shulby SA, Dolloff NG, Stearns ME, Meucci O, Fatatis A. CX3CR1-fractalkine expression regulates cellular mechanisms involved in adhesion, migration, and survival of human prostate cancer cells. *Cancer Res.* 2004;64:4693-4698.
46. Furusato B, Mohamed A, Uhlen M, Rhim JS. CXCR4 and cancer. *Pathol Int.* 2010;60:497-505.
47. Sun X, Cheng G, Hao M, et al. CXCL12/CXCR4/CXCR7 chemokine axis and cancer progression. *Cancer Metastasis Rev.* 2010;29:709-722.

48. Nelson PS, Clegg N, Arnold H, et al. The program of androgen-responsive genes in neoplastic prostate epithelium. *Proc Natl Acad Sci USA*. 2002;99:11890-11895.
49. Nelson PS. Molecular states underlying androgen receptor activation: a framework for therapeutics targeting androgen signaling in prostate cancer. *J Clin Oncol*. 2012;30:644-646.
50. Holzbeierlein J, Lal P, La Tulippe E, et al. Gene expression analysis of human prostate carcinoma during hormonal therapy identifies androgen-responsive genes and mechanisms of therapy resistance. *Am J Path*. 2004;164:217-227.
51. Ryan CJ, Smith A, Lal P, et al. Persistent prostate-specific antigen expression after neoadjuvant androgen depletion: an early predictor of relapse or incomplete androgen suppression. *Urology*. 2006;68(4):834-839.
52. Karantanos T, Corn PG, Thompson TC. Prostate cancer progression after androgen deprivation therapy: mechanisms of castrate resistance and novel therapeutic approaches. *Oncogene*. 2013;32(49):5501-5511.
53. Mohler JL, Gregory CW, Ford OH III, et al. The androgen axis in recurrent prostate cancer. *Clin Cancer Res*. 2004;10:440-448.
54. Stanbrough M, Bubley GJ, Ross K, et al. Increased expression of genes converting adrenal androgens to testosterone in androgen-independent prostate cancer. *Cancer Res*. 2006;66:2815-2825.
55. Chang KH, Li R, Papari-Zareei M, et al. Dihydrotestosterone synthesis bypasses testosterone to drive castration-resistant prostate cancer. *Proc Natl Acad Sci USA*. 2011;108(33):13728-13733.
56. Saloniemi T, Jokela H, Strauss L, Pakarinen P, Poutanen M. The diversity of sex steroid action: novel functions of hydroxysteroid (17⊠) dehydrogenases as revealed by genetically modified mouse models. *J Endocrinol*. 2012;212(1):27-40.
57. Mitsiades N, Sung CC, Schultz N, et al. Distinct patterns of dysregulated expression of enzymes involved in androgen synthesis and metabolism in metastatic prostate cancer tumors. *Cancer Res*. 2012;72(23):6142-6152.
58. Efstathiou E, Titus M, Tsavachidou D, et al. Effects of abiraterone acetate on androgen signaling in castrate-resistant prostate cancer in bone. *J Clin Oncol*. 2012;30(6):637-643.
59. Hofland J, van Weerden WM, Dits NFJ, et al. Evidence of limited contribution for intratumoral steroidogenesis in prostate cancer. *Cancer Res*. 2010;70(3):1256-1264.
60. Schoenborn JR, Nelson P, Fang M. Genomic profiling defines subtypes of prostate cancer with the potential for therapeutic stratification. *Clin Cancer Res*. 2013;19(15):4058-4066.
61. Bluemn EG, Nelson PS. The androgen/androgen receptor axis in prostate cancer. *Curr Opin Oncol*. 2012;24:251-257.
62. Scher HI, Kelly WK. Flutamide withdrawal syndrome: its impact on clinical trials in hormone-refractory prostate cancer. *J Clin Oncol*.1993;11(8):1566-1572.
63. Guo Z, Yang X, Sun F, et al. A novel androgen receptor splice variant is up-regulated during prostate cancer progression and promotes androgen depletion-resistant growth. *Cancer Res*. 2009;69(6):2305-2313.
64. Hu R, Dunn TA, Wei S, et al. Ligand-independent androgen receptor variants derived from splicing of cryptic exons signify hormone-refractory prostate cancer. *Cancer Res*. 2009;69(1):16-22.
65. Steinkamp MP, O'Mahony OA, Brogley M, et al. Treatment-dependent androgen receptor mutations in prostate cancer exploit multiple mechanisms to evade therapy. *Cancer Res*. 2009;69(10):4434-4442.
66. Cai C, Chen S, Ng P, et al. Intratumoral de novo steroid synthesis activates androgen receptor in castration-resistant prostate cancer and is upregulated by treatment with CYP17A1 inhibitors. *Cancer Res*. 2011;71(20):6503-6513.
67. Haelens A, Tanner T, Denayer S, Callewaert L, Claessens F. The hinge region regulates DNA binding, nuclear translocation, and transactivation of the androgen receptor. *Cancer Res*. 2007;67(9):4514-4523.
68. Mezynski J, Pezaro C, Bianchini D, et al. Antitumour activity of docetaxel following treatment with the CYP17A1 inhibitor abiraterone: clinical evidence for cross-resistance? *Ann Oncol*. 2012;23(11):2943-2947.
69. Rathkopf D, Scher HI. Androgen receptor antagonists in castration-resistant prostate cancer. *Cancer J*. 2013;19(1):43-49.
70. Hu T, Lu C, Mostaghel EA, et al. Distinct transcriptional programs mediated by the ligand-dependent full-length androgen receptor and it splice variants in castration-resistant prostate cancer. *Cancer Res*. 2012;72(14):3457-3462.
71. Andersen RJ, Mawj NR, Wang J, et al. Regression of castrate-recurrent prostate cancer by a small-molecule inhibitor of the amino-terminus domain of the androgen receptor. *Cancer Cell*. 2010;17(6):535-546.
72. Jenster G, van der Korput HA, van Vroonhoven C, van der Kwast TH, Trapman J, Brinkmann AO. Domains of the human androgen receptor involved in steroid binding, transcriptional activation, and subcellular localization. *Mole Edocrinol*. 1991;5(10):1396-1404.
73. Antonarakis ES, Lu C, Wag H, et al. Androgen receptor splice variant, and resistance to enzalutamide and abiraterone in men with metastatic castration-resistant prostate cancer (mCRPC) [abstract 5001]. *Proc Am Soc Clin Oncol*. 2014;32(5s).
74. Sprenger CCT, Plymate SR. The link between androgen receptor splice variants and castration-resistant prostate cancer. *Horm Canc*. 2014;5(4):207-217. doi:10.1007/s12672-014-0177-y.
75. Nyquist MD, Li Y, Hwang TH, et al. TALEN-engineered AR gene rearrangements reveal endocrine uncoupling of androgen receptor in prostate cancer. *Proc Natl Acad Sci USA*. 2013;110(43):17492-17497.
76. Li Y, Chan SC, Brand LJ, Hwang TH, Silverstein KA, Dehm SM. Androgen receptor splice variants mediate enzalutamide resistance in castration-resistant prostate cancer cell lines. *Cancer Res*. 2013;73(2):483-489.
77. Chen M, Manley JL. Mechanisms of alternative splicing regulation: insights from molecular and genomics approaches. *Nat Rev Mol Cell Biol*. 2009;10(11):741-754.
78. Chen M, Zhang J, Manley JL. Turning on a fuel switch of cancer: hnRNP proteins regulate alternative splicing of pyruvate kinase mRNA. *Cancer Res*. 2010;70(22):8977-8980.
79. Keren H, Lev-Maor G, Ast G. Alternative splicing and evolution: diversification, exon definition and function. *Nat Rev Genet*. 2010;11(5):345-355.
80. Liu LL, Xie N, Sun S, Plymate S, Mostaghel E, Dong X. Mechanisms of the androgen receptor splicing in prostate cancer cells. *Oncogene*. 2014;33(24):3140-3150. doi: 10.1038/onc.2013.284.
81. Veldscholte J, Ris-Stalpers C, Kuiper G, et al. A mutations in the ligand-binding domain of the androgen receptor of the human LNCaP cells affects steroid binding characteristics and response to antiandrogens. *Biochem Biophys Res Commun*. 1990;173(2):534-540.
82. Lin J, Adam R, Santiestevan E, Freeman MR. The phosphatidylimositol 3'-kinase pathway is a dominant growth factor-activated cell survival pathway in LNCaP human prostate carcinoma cells. *Cancer Res*. 1999;59(12):2891-2897.
83. Loberg RD, St John LN, Day LL, Neeley CK, Pienta KJ. Development of the VCaP androgen-independent model of prostate cancer. *Urol Oncol*. 2006;24(2):161-168.
84. Korenchuk S, Lehr JE, Mclean L, et al. VCaP, a cell-based model system of human prostate cancer. *In Vivo*. 2001;15(2):163-168.
85. Arora VK, Schenkein E, Murali R, et al. Glucocorticoid receptor confers resistance to antiandrogens by bypassing androgen receptor blockade. *Cell*. 2013;155(6):1309-1322.
86. Balbas MD, Evans MJ, Hosfield DJ, et al. Overcoming mutation-based resistance to antiandrogens with rational drug design. *Elife*. 2013;2:e00499.
87. Joseph JD, Lu N, Qian J, et al. A clinically relevant androgen receptor mutation confers resistance to 2nd generation anti-androgen enzalutamide and ARN-509. *Cancer Discov*. 2013;3(9):1020-1029.
88. Korpal M, Korn JM, Gao X, et al. An F876L mutation in androgen receptor confers genetic and phenotypic resistance to MDV3100 (enzalutamide). *Cancer Discov*. 2013;3(9):1030-1043.

89. Mangelsdorf DJ, Thummel C, Beato M, et al. The nuclear receptor superfamily: the second decade. *Cell.* 1995;83(6):835-839.
90. Tannock I, Gospodarowicz M, Meakin W, Panzarella T, Stewart L, Rider W. Treatment of metastatic prostate cancer with low-dose prednisone: evaluation of pain and quality of the as pragmatic indices of response. *J Clin Oncol.* 1989; 7:590-597.
91. Results from a phase 3, randomized, double-blind, multicenter, placebo-controlled trial of orteronel (TAK-700) plus prednisone in patients with metastatic castration-resistant prostate cancer (mCRPC) that has progressed during or following docetaxel-based therapy (ELM-PC 5 Trial) [abstract 7]. *Clin Adv Hematol Oncol.* 2014;12(4 suppl 11):6–7.
92. Rathkopf DE, Morris MJ, Fox JJ, et al. Phase I study of ARN-509, a novel antiandrogen, in the treatment of castration-resistant prostate cancer. *J Clin Oncol.* 2013;31(28):3525-3530.
93. Neuzillet Y, Flamand V, Lebdai S, Villers A, Lebret T. Prostate cancer and new hormonal treatments: mechanism of action and main clinical results. *Prog Urol.* 2013;23(suppl 1):S34-S43.
94. Yu Z, Cai C, Gao S, Simon NI, Shen HC, Balk SP. Galeterone prevents androgen receptor binding to chromatin and enhances degradation of mutant androgen receptor. *Clin Cancer Res.* 2014;20(15):4075-4085.
95. Lallous N, Dalal K, Cherkasov A, Rennie PS. Targeting alternative sites on the androgen receptor to treat castration-resistant prostate cancer. *Int J Mol Sci.* 2013;14(6):12496-12519.
96. Sadar MD. Small molecule inhibitors targeting the "achilles' heel" of androgen receptor activity. *Cancer Res.* 2011;71(4):1208-1213.
97. Myung JK, Banuelos CA, Fernandez JG, et al. An androgen receptor N-terminal domain antagonist for treating prostate cancer. *J Clin Invest.* 2013;123(7):2948-2960.19.4.1

19.2 Metastatic Castrate-Resistant Prostate Cancer: Role of Chemotherapy and Multifaceted Treatment Paradigms

ABDEL HAI ALQWASMI
NICHOLAS G. ZAORSKY
ULKA VAISHAMPAYAN

■ INTRODUCTION

Despite all the advances in recent years, metastatic carcinoma of the prostate remains a terminal and morbid disease. About 10% to 20% of men with prostate cancer present with metastatic disease, and in many others, metastases develop despite initial treatment with surgery or radiotherapy (1). Androgen deprivation therapy remains the mainstay of front-line therapy for advanced prostate cancer. Nevertheless, this treatment is not curative and patients invariably develop progressive disease. Castrate-resistant disease implies any disease progression (prostate-specific antigen [PSA] only progression or progression of existing metastases or development of new metastasis) despite being on adequate androgen deprivation therapy. The field of advanced prostate cancer has undergone a rapid overhaul in the last 5 years. A paradigm shift has occurred with multiple novel agents addressing distinct pathways and demonstrating powerful efficacy in a disease state that previously had a large unmet need.

Currently, multiple agents have demonstrated efficacy and tolerability in metastatic castrate-resistant prostate cancer (mCRPC). The judicious use of the multiple available agents with finesse of sequencing and concomitant palliative care has made living with mCRPC a reasonable and tolerable experience. The expertise of multiple specialties can ensure an optimal outcome, not only in terms of improving life expectancy but also in helping to lead a full productive life. To deliver the variety of treatments ranging from immunotherapy to bone-targeted radiation therapy, the involvement of multiple specialties in the care of patient with advanced prostate cancer has become imperative. In addition, the psychological reassurance to patients and families of having continued help and support available from multiple specialties can never be underestimated.

■ MECHANISMS OF CASTRATE RESISTANCE

Several mechanisms of castration resistance have been proposed. These may be dependent or independent of continued activation of the androgen receptor through several pathways.

Adrenal androgen production has long been recognized as a potential source of androgen production despite surgical or chemical castration. Adrenal androgen synthesis inhibitors such as ketoconazole provided a proof of principle about the significance of adrenal androgens in castrate-resistant prostate cancer (CRPC) (2). Several studies showed that despite castrate levels of serum testosterone, testosterone levels remain sufficiently elevated in the prostate cancer microenvironment, suggesting an autocrine pathway of androgen production and receptor activation (3, 4). Androgen receptor hypersensitivity and/or overexpression have been described in prostatic tumor cells (5, 6). All these will lead to a ligand-dependent activation of the androgen receptor independent of the serum testosterone level.

Several other ligand-independent mechanisms were described including mutations in androgen receptor, overexpression of coactivators, activation by growth factors or cytokine signaling, cross-talk with other transcription factors, and epigenetic posttranslational modifications (7, 8).

In addition, activation of the PI3K/Akt/mammalian target of rapamycin pathway has been strongly implicated in prostate cancer progression and is believed to be an independent driver of prostatic cancer cell growth, metastasis, and castrate resistance development (9).

Typically agents affecting the hormone therapy pathway are unlikely to be effective in this setting, and chemotherapy has a higher likelihood of being active. The clinical management of patients with CRPC remains challenging, as several of these mechanisms may be involved simultaneously in any given patient.

■ TREATMENT OPTIONS

Since the Food and Drug Administration (FDA) approval of mitoxantrone for the treatment of CRPC in 1996, many new advances have been made in our understanding of the disease and in therapeutic options. Treatment strategies can be broadly categorized as chemotherapy, hormonal therapy, immunotherapy, and bone-targeted therapy (Figure 19.2.1). Table 19.2.1 summarizes the FDA-approved agents that have demonstrated survival advantage in mCRPC. Figure 19.2.2 illustrates selected agents inhibiting the biosynthesis of androgens.

Chemotherapy

Mitoxantrone was the first chemotherapeutic agent to show significant improvement in pain and quality of life for patients with symptomatic CRPC (10). There was a palliative benefit noted, but no overall survival (OS) advantage with the use of mitoxantrone (10, 11), and for years, cytotoxic chemotherapy was considered to be relatively ineffective in men with CRPC. The appearance of docetaxel-based chemotherapy changed that thinking.

In the landmark, TAX-327 trial, docetaxel plus prednisone was compared to mitoxantrone plus prednisone in men with mCRPC. The median survival was 18.9 months

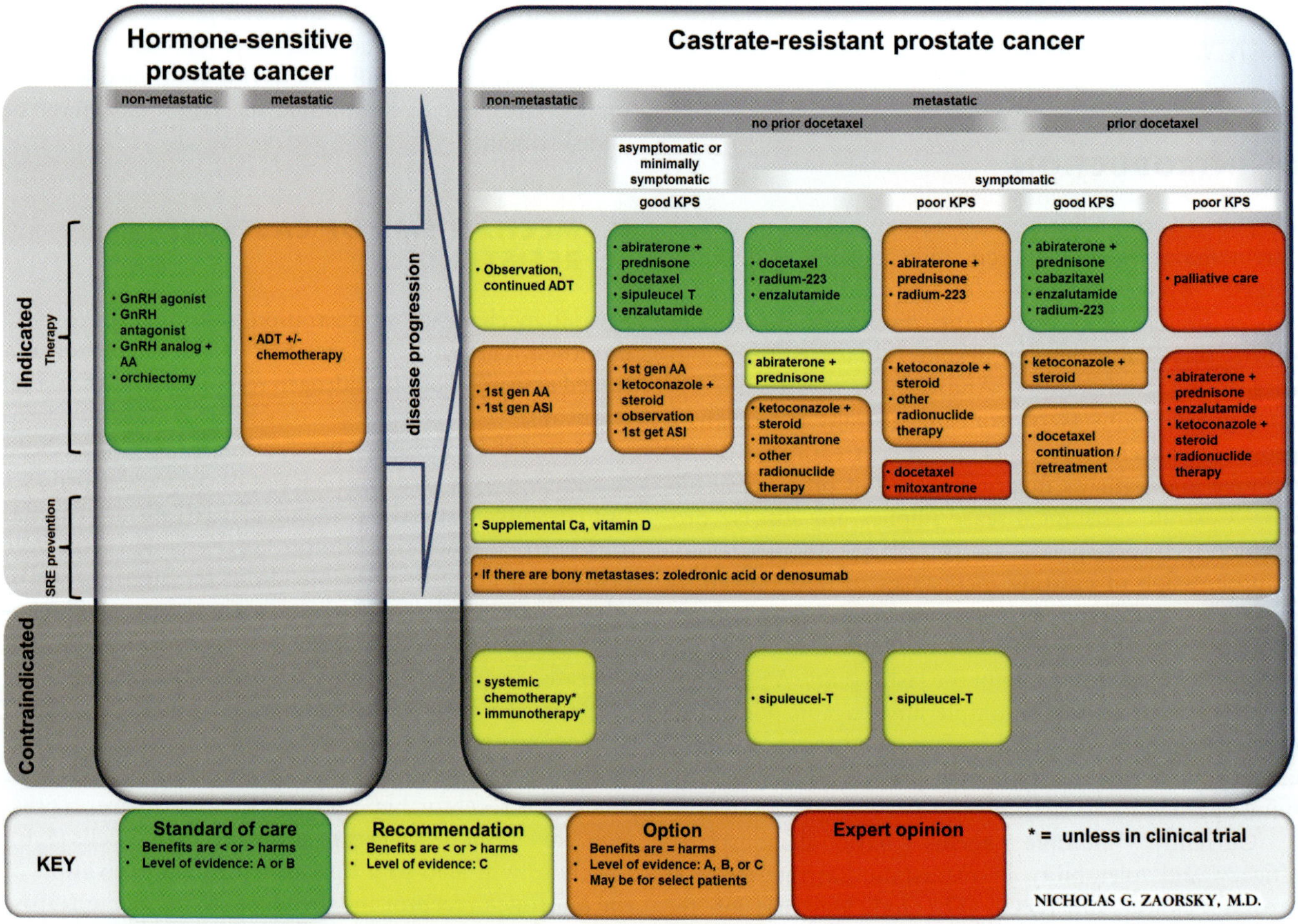

FIGURE 19.2.1 Treatment options for metastatic castrate-resistant prostate cancer (CRPC).

Abbreviations: AA = anti-androgen (e.g. flutamide, bicalutamide, nilutamide); ADT = androgen deprivation therapy (i.e. GnRH analog or orchiectomy); ASI = androgen synthesis inhibitor (1st generation ASIs include ketoconazole, glucocorticoids); GnRH = gonadotropin-releasing hormone; KPS = Karnofsky performance status; SRE = skeletal-related event.

Note: Recommendations adapted from Cookson MS, et al. Castration-Resistant Prostate Cancer: AUA Guideline. Presented at the American Urological Association Annual Meeting; May 4–8, 2013; San Diego, California.

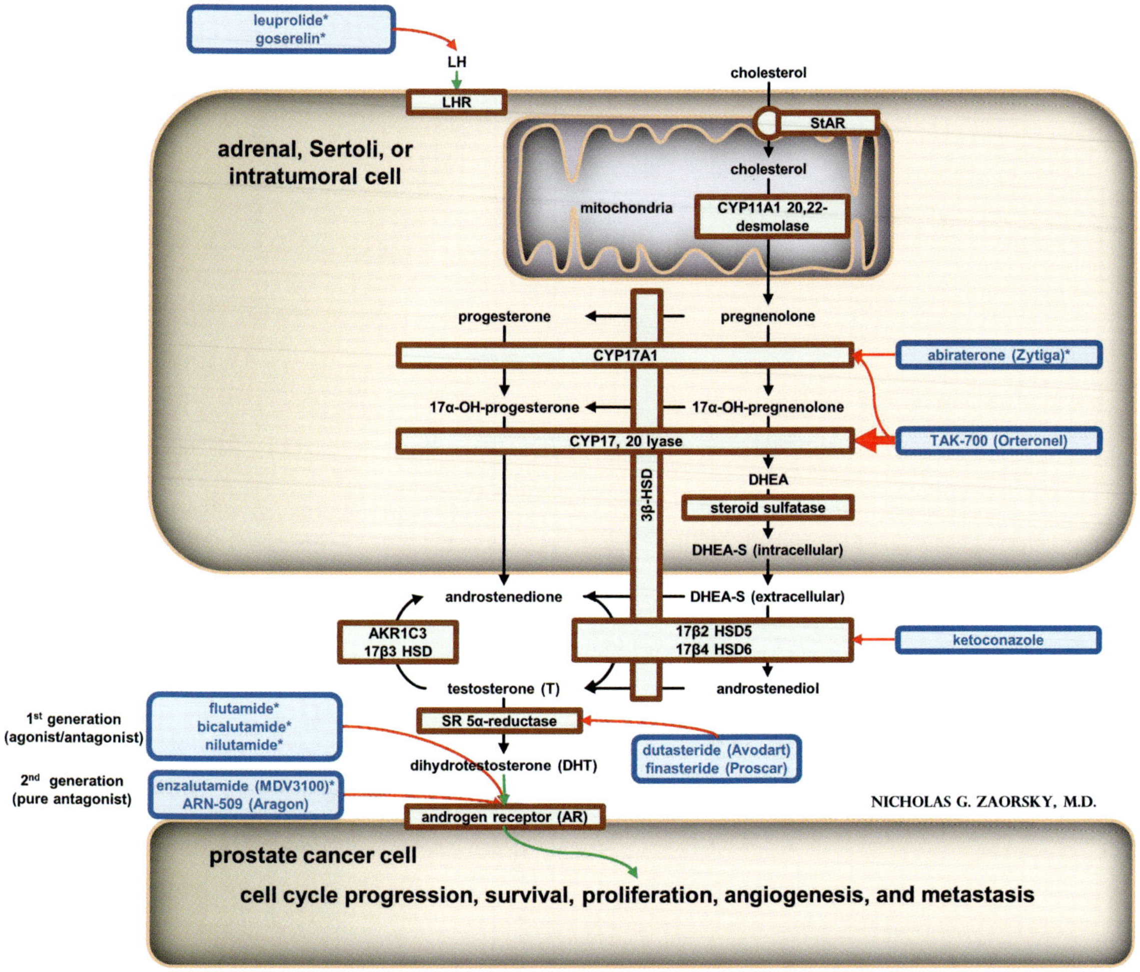

FIGURE 19.2.2 Selected agents inhibiting the biosynthesis of androgens. Enzymes (brown boxes) are key in the synthesis (indicated by black arrows) on androgens, including testosterone (T) and dihydrotestosterone (DHT). Novel agents (rounded blue rectangles) inhibit (red arrows) particular enzymes in the pathways or block the stimulatory effects (green arrows) of hormones. * = FDA approved for the treatment of prostate cancer as of 2013.

Source: Figure adapted from Zaorsky, et al. Multimodality therapy for patients with high-risk prostate cancer: current status and future directions. *Semin Oncol.* 2013;40(3):308–321.

in docetaxel group versus 16.5 months in the mitoxantrone group (hazard ratio [HR] for death 0.76, 95% confidence interval [CI] 0.62–0.94; *P* = .009). There was a significant reduction of PSA levels, improvement in pain, and quality-of-life improvement in the docetaxel group compared to mitoxantrone (12). The survival advantage persisted with extended follow-up (13). In the Tax-327 trial, docetaxel was given either as 75 mg/m^2 every 21 days or 30 mg/m^2 weekly, for 5 of 6 weeks. The OS was significantly improved in the docetaxel regimen administered every 21 days compared to the mitoxantrone and prednisone regimen. However, OS in the weekly docetaxel arm was not superior to the treatment with mitoxantrone. Incidence of severe (grade 3 or 4) neutropenia was substantially higher in the group receiving docetaxel every 3 weeks (9.6%) compared to weekly docetaxel or mitoxantrone (0.6% and 6.6%, respectively). A recently published phase III trial of 361 patients compared the standard every 3 weeks docetaxel to biweekly docetaxel at a dose of 50 mg/m^2. Median time to treatment failure was significantly longer in the 2-weekly group than in the 3-weekly group (5.6 months, 95% CI 5.0–6.2 vs. 4.9 months, 95% CI 4.5–5.4; HR 1.3, 95% CI 1.1–1.6, *P* = .014) (14). OS was a secondary end point and was also statistically increased in the patients receiving 2-weekly docetaxel (median survival 19.5 months vs. 17.0 months; HR 1.4, 95% CI 1.1–1.8; *P* = .021). The incidence of grade 3 or 4 neutropenia and febrile neutropenia was significantly higher in the 3-weekly group (53%) than in the 2-weekly group (36%) (14). About 10% and 5% of the patients on the biweekly and triweekly arms required dose delays, respectively. The results of this trial permit the consideration of a 50 mg/m^2 dose of docetaxel every 2 weeks as an alternative regimen in mCRPC with improved tolerability without compromising outcomes.

The efficacy of docetaxel in mCRPC has led to several trials trying to combine docetaxel with other agents

Table 19.2.1 FDA-approved agents with survival advantage in mCRPC

Trial, References	Study Population	Study Arm	Pred Use	Size (R)	OS	PFS	PSA RR (%)	Adverse Events of Interest (%)		
				Chemotherapy						
Tax 327, Tannock et al. (12)	CRPC with no prior chemotherapy		5 mg bid	1,006 (1:1:1)				Neutropenia[a]	Fatigue	Neuropathy
		Docetaxel 75 mg/m² Q3 wk			18.9	NR	45	9.6	16	9
		Docetaxel 30 mg/m² Q wk			17.4	NR	48	0.6	14.8	7.3
		Mitoxantrone 12 mg/m² Q3 wk			16.5	NR	32	6.6	10.4	2.1
TROPIC, de Bono et al. (24)	CRPC post-docetaxel		10 mg daily	755 (1:1)				Neutropenia[a]	Fatigue	Diarrhea
		Cabazitaxel 25 mg/m² Q3 wk			15.1	2.8	39	82	37	47
		Mitoxantrone 12 mg/m² Q3 wk			12.7	1.4	18	58	27	11
				Hormonal Therapy						
COU-AA-301, de Bono et al. (100)	CRPC post-docetaxel		5 mg bid	1,195 (2:1)				Fluid retention	LFT elevation	Hypokalemia
		Abiraterone 1,000 mg daily			14.8	5.6	29	31	10	17
		Placebo			10.9	3.6	6	22	8	8
COU-AA-302, Ryan et al. (38)	CRPC pre-docetaxel. No or mild symptoms		5 mg bid	1,088 (2:1)				Fluid retention	LFT elevation	Hypokalemia
		Abiraterone 1,000 mg daily			NRea	11.1	62	28	12	17
		Placebo			27.2	5.6	24	24	5	13

(continued)

Table 19.2.1 FDA-approved agents with survival advantage in mCRPC (*continued*)

Trial, References	Study Population	Study Arm	Pred Use	Size (R)	OS	PFS	PSA RR (%)	Adverse Events of Interest (%)		
AFFIRM, Scher et al. (41)	CRPC post-docetaxel		Not a must	1,199 (2:1)				Seizure	Fatigue	Hot Flash
		Enzalutamide 160 mg daily			18.4	8.3	54	<1	34	20
		Placebo			13.6	3	2	0	29	10
				Immunotherapy						
Small et al. (68)	Asymptomatic, no visceral metastasis, most were chemo naïve.		Forbidden	127 (2:1)				Rigors	Pyrexia	Tremor
		Sipuleucel-T 3 infusion Q3 wk			25.9	2.7	NR	60	29	10
		Placebo			21.4	2.3	NR	9	2	0
Kantoff et al. (70)	No or mild symptoms, mostly Gleason ≤ 7, most chemo-naïve		Forbidden	512 (2:1)				Chills	Pyrexia	Headache
		Sipuleucel-T 3 infusion Q3 wk			25.8	3.7	2.6	54	29	16
		Placebo			21.7	3.6	1.3	13	14	5
				Bone-targeted therapy						
ALSYMPCA, Parker et al. (85)	Symptomatic mCRPC with no visceral metastasis, post-decetaxel		NR	921 (2:1)					Neutropenia[a]	Thrombo-cytopenia[a]
		Rad-223 IV Q4 wk for 6 cycles				14	NR	NR	1.8	4
		Placebo				11.2	NR	NR	0.8	2

Abbreviations: NR, not reported; NRea, not reached; OS, median overall survival (mo); PFS, median progression-free survival (mo); Pred, prednisone; PSA RR, prostate-specific antigen response rate; (R), randomization.

[a]Grade 3 or more,

in an attempt to improve on the efficacy profile. These combination therapies failed to enhance the efficacy of the docetaxel and prednisone regimen administered every 21 days at a dose of 75 mg/m^2. Estramustine phosphate is a nitrogen mustard derivative of estradiol-17β-phosphate that showed activity as monotherapy for CRPC (15). The Southwest Oncology Group trial randomized patients to receive either estramustine and docetaxel combination or mitoxantrone and prednisone. The study revealed a benefit in OS favoring the docetaxel-based regimen (16). The OS was comparable to that seen with docetaxel and prednisone, but the toxicity concerns with increased risk of thromboembolic events led to abandonment of estramustine use by clinicians (15). Vascular endothelial growth factor (VEGF)-targeted therapies, such as either bevacizumab (17) or aflibercept (18), when combined with docetaxel, were associated with greater toxicity and no improvement in survival. Multiple other combinations were tested with either no clinical benefit or even an inferior outcome. These include combinations with GVAX (prostate cancer vaccine) (19), DN-101 (high-dose calcitriol) (20), and atrasentan (endothelin receptor antagonist) (21).

The FDA approval of docetaxel and prednisone in mCRPC in 2005, and the widespread use, led to an increasing population of advanced prostate cancer patients who did not have any therapeutic options when their disease progressed after docetaxel therapy. A number of agents were evaluated in this setting and have now demonstrated robust efficacy to gain FDA approval in this setting. The control arm in these studies consisted of either placebo or mitoxantrone and prednisone.

Satraplatin, an oral platinum, was evaluated in the second-line setting with results of improved response rates, progression-free survival, and favorable toxicity profile, but unfortunately lack of a survival benefit in a double-blind, placebo-controlled phase III trial (22).

Cabazitaxel is a novel tubulin-binding taxane that showed preclinical and clinical activity in docetaxel-resistant prostate cancer (23). An open-label phase III trial randomized patients with mCRPC who progressed during or after treatment with a docetaxel-containing regimen, to cabazitaxel (25 mg/m^2 intravenously [IV] every 21 days) plus prednisone (5 mg twice daily orally) or mitoxantrone plus prednisone. HR for death of men treated with cabazitaxel compared to those taking mitoxantrone was 0.70 (95% CI 0.59–0.83, $P < .0001$). The most common clinically significant grade 3 or higher adverse events were neutropenia (cabazitaxel 82% vs. mitoxantrone 58%) and diarrhea (6% vs. < 1%). The median survival was 15.1 months in the cabazitaxel group and 12.7 months in the mitoxantrone group (24). With the high incidence of febrile neutropenia and seven deaths related to sepsis (2%), primary prophylaxis with granulocyte colony-stimulating factor use was introduced and was mandatory on the cabazitaxel arm of the study. Despite the OS benefit noted with cabazitaxel, a careful discussion of toxicities is needed when cabazitaxel is offered as a treatment option for a patient.

Several other chemotherapies have been used in the treatment of CRPC but do not currently have an established role in either the first- or the second-line setting. Other agents with limited activity include paclitaxel, capecitabine, 5-fluorouracil, gemcitabine, topotecan, cyclophosphamide, and ixabepilone (25–30).

Concurrent palliative and supportive therapy is critical in optimizing chemotherapy in patients with metastatic prostate cancer. Antiemetics and premedications to avert hypersensitivity reactions are some key components of care during administration of either docetaxel or cabazitaxel. Close monitoring for cytopenias and dose modifications as necessary for neuropathy related to docetaxel and for diarrhea and cytopenias related to cabazitaxel should be an integral part of the chemotherapy care. Primary growth factor prophylaxis is strongly recommended for cabazitaxel chemotherapy, and secondary prophylaxis should be considered for either chemotherapy agent if febrile neutropenia occurs. Patient and family awareness and education of toxicity of chemotherapy enables prompt attention and better outcomes with chemotherapy.

Hormone Therapy

Hormone refractory prostate cancer is the old terminology used to describe CRPC. The change in terminology reflects our deeper understanding of resistance mechanisms and the emerging data that CRPC cells evolve after traditional androgen deprivation and continue to be responsive to hormonal manipulations. Testicular androgen deprivation (by orchiectomy or gonadotrophin-releasing hormone agonists or antagonists) therapies have shown powerful activity in advanced metastatic prostate cancer, but this sensitivity seemed to maintain for a finite period of time (median 18–24 months) (31). Continuation of androgen deprivation is recommended even beyond development of castrate-resistant disease. A multivariate analysis found observational evidence that continued testicular androgen deprivation was associated with a modest survival benefit of 2 to 6 months (32).

New Hormonal Therapies

Abiraterone acetate is a potent, selective, and irreversible inhibitor of cytochrome P450 (17) alpha (CYP17) (33, 34). CYP17 is a critical enzyme in testosterone synthesis and inhibiting CYP17 will lead to blocking of androgen synthesis by the adrenal glands and testes and within the prostate tumor. In a phase III trial published in 2011, 1,195 patients with CRPC who had received prior docetaxel therapy were randomly assigned in a 2:1 ratio to receive 5 mg of prednisone twice daily with either 1,000 mg of abiraterone acetate or placebo. Study drug was given once daily at least 1 hour before or 2 hours after a meal. Concomitant use of steroids was mandated to ameliorate the symptoms resulting from mineralocorticoid excess. The study was terminated at the interim analysis as OS, and other secondary endpoints exceeded the preplanned criteria for study termination (35). The final analysis of this trial showed that the median OS for the abiraterone acetate group was 15.8 months compared to 11.2 months in the placebo group (HR 0.74, 95% CI 0.64–0.86; $P < .0001$). Median time to PSA progression was 8.5 months in the abiraterone acetate group versus 6.6 months in the placebo group (HR 0.63; $P < .0001$), and median radiologic progression-free survival was 5.6 months versus 3.6 months (HR 0.66; $P < .0001$). A total of 29.5% of patients in the abiraterone acetate group had a PSA response versus 5.5% in the placebo group ($P < .0001$). Abiraterone acetate was well tolerated. Mineralocorticoid excess–related adverse events (hypokalemia, hypertension, and fluid retention) were reported in a higher proportion in the abiraterone acetate group than in the placebo group but were easily managed medically with appropriate patient monitoring. Deaths due to adverse events occurred in similar proportions of patients in the two groups (13% in the abiraterone acetate group vs. 16% in the placebo group), as did deaths due to cardiac adverse events (1% both groups) (36). Subsequent analysis showed that in patients with clinically significant pain at baseline, abiraterone acetate plus prednisone resulted in significantly more palliation (45% of patients vs. 28.8%; $P = .0005$) and faster palliation of pain intensity than did prednisone only. In the overall population, median time to occurrence of first skeletal-related event was significantly longer in the abiraterone acetate arm compared to placebo arm (25.0 months vs. 20.3 months; $P = .0001$) (37).

More recently abiraterone acetate was tested in pre-docetaxel metastatic CRPC. In 1,088 patients with asymptomatic or minimally symptomatic metastatic CRPC, we randomly assigned to receive abiraterone acetate plus prednisone or placebo plus prednisone. The primary endpoints were radiographic progression-free survival and OS. The study was again terminated at the interim analysis. The median radiographic progression-free survival was 16.5 months with abiraterone acetate–prednisone and 8.3 months with prednisone alone (HR 0.53; $P < .001$). There was a trend for increased OS but did not cross efficacy boundaries (median not reached for abiraterone acetate–prednisone, vs. 27.2 months for prednisone alone; HR 0.75; 95% CI 0.61–0.93; $P = .01$). Abiraterone acetate–prednisone was superior to prednisone alone with respect to time to initiation of cytotoxic chemotherapy, opiate use for cancer-related pain, PSA progression, and decline in performance status. Grade 3 or 4 mineralocorticoid-related adverse events and abnormalities on liver function testing were more common with abiraterone acetate plus prednisone but easily manageable (38).

Enzalutamide is an oral androgen receptor signaling inhibitor that binds to androgen receptors and reduces the efficiency of the receptor nuclear translocation, and impairs both DNA binding to androgen response elements and recruitment of coactivators. It was chosen for clinical development on the basis of activity in prostate-cancer models with overexpression of the androgen receptor (39,40).

The AFFIRM trial randomized 1,199 men with CRPC who received prior docetaxel therapy in a 2:1 ratio to receive oral enzalutamide at a dose of 160 mg per day or placebo. The primary end point was OS. The use of prednisone or other glucocorticoids was permitted but not required, and the study drug was given without regard to food intake. The study was stopped after a planned interim analysis. The median OS was 18.4 months in the enzalutamide group versus 13.6 months in the placebo group (HR for death in the enzalutamide group 0.63; 95% CI 0.53–0.75; $P < .001$). Enzalutamide was also significantly superior to placebo in all secondary endpoints including the soft-tissue response rate (29% vs. 4%, $P < .001$), the quality-of-life response rate (43% vs. 18%, $P < .001$), the time to PSA progression (8.3 vs. 3.0 months; HR 0.25; $P < .001$), radiographic progression-free survival (8.3 vs. 2.9 months; HR 0.40; $P < .001$), the proportion of patients with a reduction in PSA by 50% or more (54% vs. 2%, $P < .001$), and the time to the first skeletal-related event (16.7 vs. 13.3 months; HR 0.69; $P < .001$). Treatment was well tolerated. Eight percent of the patients in the enzalutamide arm discontinued treatment due to adverse events compared to 10% in the placebo group. The following frequent adverse events were more common with enzalutamide: fatigue, diarrhea, hot flash, headache, and musculoskeletal pain. Five patients (0.6%) treated with enzalutamide developed a seizure compared to none in the placebo arm. No significant difference was noted in cardiac disorders or abnormalities in liver function test (41). PREVAIL was a phase III study that compared enzalutamide to placebo in men with metastatic CRPC that were chemotherapy naïve. 1,717 patients were randomized. The coprimary endpoints were radiographic progression-free survival and OS. The study was stopped after an interim analysis showed clear benefit of enzalutamide. 29% reduction in the risk of death was associated with enzalutamide use over placebo (HR 0.71; 95% CI, 0.60 to 0.84; $P < .001$). The rate of radiographic progression-free survival at 12 months was 65% among patients treated with enzalutamide, as compared with 14% among patients receiving placebo (HR 0.19; 95% CI, 0.15 to 0.23; $P < .001$). The benefit of enzalutamide was demonstrated with respect to all secondary endpoints, including the time until the initiation of cytotoxic chemotherapy (HR 0.35), the time until the first skeletal-related event (HR 0.72), a complete or partial soft-tissue response (59% vs. 5%), the time until PSA progression (HR 0.17), and a rate of decline of at least 50% in PSA (78% vs. 3%). Fatigue and hypertension were the most common relevant adverse events (42). Enzalutamide was recently FDA approved for chemotherapy naïve metastatic CRPC patients.

Secondary Hormonal Manipulations

Several other hormonal therapies exist to manipulate androgen synthesis and/or binding to androgen receptor. These agents should be primarily considered in the slowly progressing asymptomatic or minimally symptomatic patient population. Nevertheless, they may be useful in postponing other interventions with greater toxicity. Those can induce biochemical or clinical responses, but no OS benefit has been demonstrated.

Antiandrogens (bicalutamide, flutamide, nilutamide) block the binding of dihydrotestosterone to androgen receptor. Those can be used in combination with medical or surgical orchiectomy as part of a combined androgen blockade for the initial treatment of men with advanced prostate cancer but they also showed activity in patients with CRPC. These agents differ by the dosing frequency and the side-effect profile; common side effects include diarrhea, gynecomastia, loss of libido, and hot flashes. Hepatotoxicity is uncommon, but liver enzymes need to be monitored while on treatment. PSA response rate (more than 50% reduction in baseline PSA level) is reported in about 25% of patients (43–47). No study directly compared these agents in the castrate setting, but progression on one antiandrogen does not confer resistance to other antiandrogens and responses were reported in that setting (48–50).

Antiandrogen withdrawal refers to discontinuation of antiandrogen upon disease progression for patients on combined androgen blockade or antiandrogen monotherapy. Clinical and biochemical responses can be seen in patients on combined androgen blockade as initial therapy or as a later line of therapy for castrate disease. Antiandrogen withdrawal can result in a PSA response rate of 10% to 20%. This is often short lived with median response duration of about 3 months (51–53). The mechanism of this phenomenon is not well understood, but androgen receptor mutations or gene amplification might lead in an altered response resulting in the antiandrogen behaving as an activator, not inhibitor (54–57).

Ketoconazole is an azole antifungal agent that inhibits adrenal androgen synthesis; this inhibitory effect was discovered after gynecomastia developed in some patients taking it as an antifungal agent (58). Ketoconazole inhibits many enzymes in the steroid synthesis pathway including CYP17 (34, 59). Ketoconazole has poor bioavailability in high gastric pH and thus should be taken on an empty stomach and the use of antacids should be avoided (60).

PSA response rates in phase II ketoconazole trials ranged from 40% to 62%, with median duration of response lasting between 3.3 and 7 months (61). A large, phase III trial randomized 260 patients with CRPC to either antiandrogen withdrawal only or antiandrogen withdrawal plus ketoconazole at 400 mg TID. PSA response was 11% in the antiandrogen withdrawal arm compared to 27% in the combined modality arm ($P = .0002$). Twenty-one percent of patients receiving ketoconazole had grade 3 and 4 toxicities. [The most common grade 3 or more toxicities were neurologic 4%, malaise or fatigue 3%, and hepatic toxicity 2% (51).] Rates of discontinuing high-dose ketoconazole due to toxicity range from 7% to 20%. Common side effects include nausea and vomiting, skin rash, fatigue, and neurotoxicity. Adrenal insufficiency can also happen. Thus, ketoconazole is usually administered with concurrent corticosteroids (61).

Data about the effectiveness of steroids in CRPC are largely derived from clinical trials at which steroids served as the control arm. Steroids were used in different doses and formulations (prednisone 7.5–20 mg daily, dexamethasone 0.5–2.25 mg daily, hydrocortisone 40–45 mg daily) with notable objective responses and PSA decline (62). Steroids can inhibit adrenocorticotropic hormone (ACTH) production resulting in a decrease in adrenal steroid synthesis including the adrenal androgens. Other possible mechanisms of action include alterations in transcriptional regulation of specific genes responsible for tumor growth and signaling via interaction with the glucocorticoids receptor (63, 64).

Diethylstilbestrol (DES) is a synthetic ethinyl estrogen. It is one of the oldest therapies used to treat advanced prostate cancer but its use was limited by the increased cardiovascular toxicity (65). It suppresses luteinizing hormone secretion by providing a negative feedback on the hypothalamic–pituitary axis. It can also suppress Leydig cells and inhibit the secretion of androgenic steroids. It can also compete with androgens for the androgen receptor (66). DES at 1 mg daily can show a PSA decline in 38% to 79% of patients treated with CRPC with about 7- to 9-month mean time to progression (66).

Immunotherapy

Sipuleucel-T is an immunotherapy product designed to stimulate T-cell immunity to prostatic acid phosphatase (PAP), an antigen expressed in the majority of prostate cancers but not in nonprostate tissue. Specifically, sipuleucel-T is composed of autologous antigen-presenting cells (dendritic cells) cultured with a fusion protein termed PA2024. PA2024 consists of PAP linked to granulocyte-macrophage colony-stimulating factor (67). Peripheral blood mononuclear cells are obtained by leukapheresis and are then exposed ex vivo to PA2024. These activated cells are then infused back into the patient approximately 3 days after the original harvesting. Dendritic cell infusions are repeated for a total of three treatments at 2-week intervals (68).

In a placebo-controlled phase III trial, 127 asymptomatic patients with metastatic CRPC were randomly assigned in a 2:1 ratio to sipuleucel-T or placebo. Median survival was 25.9 months for sipuleucel-T and 21.4 months for placebo ($P = .01$, log-rank; HR 1.70; 95% CI 1.13–2.56). Treatment remained a strong independent predictor of OS after adjusting for prognostic factors. The median for time to disease progression for sipuleucel-T was 11.7 weeks compared with 10.0 weeks for placebo (P = .052). Sipuleucel-T therapy was well tolerated (68). Another phase III trial showed a trend toward increased survival with sipuleucel-T, although it was not statistically significant (69).

A larger phase III trial with OS as the primary end point assigned 512 patients in a 2:1 ratio to receive either sipuleucel-T or placebo (70). Most of the patients (75%) had a Gleason score ≤ 7 and they were either asymptomatic or minimally symptomatic. More than 80% had an Eastern Cooperative Oncology Group (ECOG) performance status of zero. Median survival was 25.8 months in the sipuleucel-T group versus 21.7 months in the placebo group. This 4.1 months difference translates into a relative reduction of 22% in the risk of death in the sipuleucel-T group compared with the placebo group (HR 0.78; 95% CI 0.61–0.98; P = .03). The median time to objective disease progression was 3.7 months in the sipuleucel-T group and 3.6 months in the placebo group (HR 0.95; 95% CI 0.77–1.17; P = .63). One patient in the sipuleucel-T group had a partial objective response. Among patients with PSA assessments after baseline, reductions of at least 50% on two visits at least 4 weeks apart were observed in 2.6% in the sipuleucel-T group, compared with 1.3% in the placebo group. Adverse events that were more frequently reported in the sipuleucel-T group than in the placebo group included chills, fever, and headache (70).

Management of Bone Metastases

Skeletal osteoblastic lesions are the most common site of metastasis in prostate cancer. They can cause pain, pathologic fractures, spinal cord compression, and hypercalcemia and are associated with shorter OS and a decreased quality of life (71, 72). Treatment can include osteoclast inhibition with bisphosphonates or denosumab, or bone-targeted radiopharmaceuticals.

Bisphosphonates

Zoledronic acid is the only bisphosphonate approved by the FDA for treatment of progressive bone metastasis in patients with CRPC. When given at 4 mg IV every 3 weeks versus placebo for 15 months, 11% fewer patients had any skeletal-related events when compared to placebo (CI = −20.3% to −1.8%; P = .021). Skeletal-related events were defined as any of the following: pathologic bone fractures, spinal cord compression, surgery to bone, radiation therapy to bone, or a change of antineoplastic therapy to treat bone pain. Median time to first skeletal-related event was 321 days for patients who received placebo and was not reached for patients who received zoledronic acid (P = .011). Increasing pain was reported more in the placebo group, but there were no differences in disease progression, performance status, or quality-of-life scores among both groups (73). This benefit seems to persist when treatment is continued beyond 15 months and even after the occurrence of a skeletal event (74).

When studied in hormone-sensitive prostate cancer, zoledronic acid prevented bone loss (75) but did not result in any significant difference in the time to first skeletal-related event or OS when compared to placebo (76).

Denosumab

Denosumab is a human monoclonal antibody against RANK ligand. RANK ligand is the main driver of osteoclast formation, function, and survival (77). A phase III study randomized 1,904 patients with CRPC and bone metastasis to receive denosumab at 120 mg subcutaneous or zoledronic acid 4 mg IV both given every 4 weeks. Patients in the denosumab arm had fewer skeletal-related events compared to zoledronic acid arm (HR 0.82, 95% CI 0.71–0.95; P = .0002 for noninferiority; P = .008 for superiority). Median time to first on-study skeletal-related event was 20.7 months with denosumab compared with 17.1 months with zoledronic acid. There was no statistically significant difference in either OS or time to disease progression. Hypocalcemia was significantly more frequent with denosumab compared with zoledronic acid (13% vs. 6%, P < .0001). More patients in the denosumab arm had osteonecrosis of the jaw, but this was not statistically significant (2.3% vs. 1.3%, P = .09) (78).

When given to men with nonmetastatic CRPC, denosumab significantly increased bone metastasis–free survival by a median of 4.2 months compared with placebo (HR 0.85, P = .028). OS did not differ between groups. This modest benefit came at the expense of having more hypocalcemia and osteonecrosis of the jaw in the denosumab arm compared to placebo (2% vs. < 1% and 5% vs. none, respectively). Denosumab is not FDA approved for this indication (79).

Bone-Targeted Radiopharmaceuticals

Bone-seeking radionuclides target the bones adjacent to tumor metastatic lesions due to selective increased metabolic activity and emit high-dose radiation to selectively kill tumor cells (80). Beta-emitting radioisotopes (such as samarium-153 and strontium-89) have been used for decades for palliation of pain associated with bone metastasis but did not show any survival advantage and their use was limited by myelosuppression (81, 82).

Radium-223 is an alpha particle–emitting radiopharmaceutical. Compared to beta particles, alpha particles provide a much more densely ionizing type of radiation and have a shorter range that limits toxicity (83). ALSYMPCA is a phase III trial that compared Radium-223 dichloride given as six doses administered IV every 4 weeks versus placebo in men with CRPC and symptomatic bone metastasis. Men with visceral metastasis were excluded. No intention to use cytotoxic chemotherapy in the 6 months following enrollment was required as well as a positive bone scan showing two or more hot spots. All patients had and received previous docetaxel chemotherapy, refused docetaxel, or were ineligible for docetaxel (84). The trial enrolled 921 patients and was stopped after the interim analysis showed significant improvement in OS and other secondary end point. Updated analysis demonstrated a 3.6-month survival advantage (14.9 vs. 11.3 months, respectively). In addition, the frequency of skeletal-related events was reduced in the Radium-223 group, and the median time to a skeletal-related event increased (15.6 vs. 9.8 months). Radium-223 was well tolerated with low rates of grade 3/4 neutropenia (1.8% vs. 0.8%) and thrombocytopenia (4% vs. 2%) (85). Radium-223 received FDA approval for treatment of men with CRPC and bone metastasis with no visceral metastasis in May 2013.

■ NOVEL AGENTS WITH PROMISING EFFICACY IN CRPC

TAK-700 (Orteronel) is a reversible CYP17 inhibitor with preferential inhibition of 17,20-lyase over 17α-hydroxylase activity. This may reduce the need for corticosteroid supplementation, as secondary mineralocorticoid excess induced by CYP17 inhibition may be more dependent on 17α-hydroxylase (86,87). In a phase I/II trial for men with metastatic CRPC with no prior chemotherapy, four different doses were tested in the phase II part (300 mg BID, 400 mg BID + prednisone 5 mg BID, 600 mg BID + prednisone, or 600 mg QD). PSA response rate (63%, 52%, 41%, and 62%, respectively) and side-effect profile was similar to that seen with abiraterone acetate. Prednisone seems not to have any effect on efficacy (88). Orteronel combination with docetaxel and prednisone appeared tolerable and showed a strong PSA and partial tumor response in another phase II trial (89). A phase III trial in post-docetaxel setting was terminated early for failing to meet its primary endpoint of OS (90). Another phase III trial in chemo-naïve patients showed significant improvement in radiographic progression free survival associated with orteronel use compared to placebo (median 13.8 vs 8.7 months; $P < .00001$). The co-primary endpoint of OS was not met (31.4 vs 29.5 months; $P = .314$) (91).

ARN-509 is a competitive androgen receptor inhibitor that is believed to be more potent than enzalutamide (92). A phase II study showed that ARN-509 has a very high PSA response rate in treatment of naïve mCRPC (88%) and retained some activity in abiraterone acetate–treated mCRPC with a PSA response rate of 29%. No seizures were reported (93).

PROSTVAC-VF is a PSA-targeted vaccine that was evaluated in a randomized blinded phase II study in 125 men with mCRPC. Men with visceral metastasis, cancer-related pain requiring narcotics, prior chemotherapy, or PSA > 7 were excluded. The primary end point was PFS and was similar in PROSTVAC-VF arm and placebo arm. However, PROSTVAC-VF patients had improved OS over placebo (25.1 vs. 16.6 months, HR 0.56, $P = .0061$) (94). A phase III trial is ongoing (95). Some novel agents with promising efficacy agents are summarized in Table 19.2.2.

Antibody drug conjugates are a new type of targeted therapy that links a cancer-specific antibody to a cytotoxic drug hence enabling delivery of high doses of chemotherapy to tumor cells, minimizing systemic toxicity, and maximizing tumor cell death (96). Phase I trials using SLC44A4, prostate-specific membrane antigen, and six-transmembrane epithelial antigen of the prostate-1 (STEAP1) as targets have recently been reported with evidence of antitumor activity (97–99).

Within systemic therapy, chemotherapy has been the mainstay of systemic therapy for the past 2 decades. Mitoxantrone and prednisone regimen initially

■ Table 19.2.2 Novel agents with promising phase II data for the treatment of CRPC

Drug	Mechanism of Action	Dose and Schedule	Size	Results	Side Effects
TAK-700 (Orteronel) (88)	CYP17 inhibitor	300 mg BID, 400 mg BID + prednisone 5 mg BID, 600 mg BID + prednisone, or 600 mg QD	96	PSA response rate: 63%, 52%, 41%, and 62%, respectively Out of 43: 6 PR, 23 SD, 9 PD	Fatigue (72%), nausea (44%), and constipation (31%)
ARN-509 (93)	AR antagonist	240 mg/day oral. Two arms reported. A: treatment naïve, B: abiraterone pretreated.	46 (1:1)	PSA response rate: A: 88%, B: 29%.	Fatigue (30%), abdominal pain (24%), nausea (22%), and diarrhea (17%)

(*continued*)

Table 19.2.2 Novel agents with promising phase II data for the treatment of CRPC (continued)

Drug	Mechanism of Action	Dose and Schedule	Size	Results	Side Effects
PROSTVAC-VF (94)	PSA targeted vaccine	Administered on days 1, 14, 28, 56, 84, 112, and 140. GM-CSF was used. Had a placebo arm.	125 (2:1)	Median PFS: 3.8 mo in the vaccine arm and 3.7 mo in placebo ($P = .6$) Median OS: 25.1 mo in the vaccine and 16.6 mo in placebo ($P = .0061$)	Injection site reactions (12%–58%), fatigue (42%), chills (14.6%), pyrexia (18.3%), nausea (20.7%), and dizziness (12.2%)
Cabozantinib (101)	Tyrosine kinase inhibitor (MET and VEGFR2 inhibitor)	100 mg daily with dose adjustment vs. placebo in CRPC postchemo	31 (1:1)	Median PFS: 23.9 wk in cabozantinib arm and 5.9 wk in placebo (HR 0.12; $P < .001$)	Most common grade 3 adverse events were fatigue (16%), hypertension (12%), and hand-foot syndrome (8%).
Ipilumimab (102)	Anti CTLA-4 monoclonal antibody	10 mg/kg every 3 wk × 4 doses ± radiotherapy	50	PSA response rate 16% CR 2%, SD 12%	Diarrhea (54%), colitis (22%), rash (32%), and pruritus (20%)
Dasatinib (103)	SRC tyrosine kinase inhibitor	100 mg or 70 mg twice daily	47	No progression at week 12 in 43% Reduction in bone alkaline phosphatase in 60%	Grade 3 included: fatigue (10%), pleural effusion (2%), diarrhea (4%), and leukopenia (4%)
OGX-427 (104)	Heat shock protein 27 inhibitor	600 mg IV × 3 loading doses followed by 1,000 mg IV weekly plus prednisone vs. placebo plus prednisone	22 reported so far (1:1)	PSA decline by at least 30%: 55% in OGX arm vs. 20% in placebo	Grade 1–2 infusion reactions in 45% of patients receiving OGX One patient developed hemolytic uremic syndrome

Abbreviations: AR, androgen receptor; CR, complete response; OS, overall survival; PD, progressive disease; PFS, progressive-free survival; PR, partial response; SD, stable disease.

demonstrated palliative benefit, followed by OS benefit shown by docetaxel and prednisone. Finally, cabazitaxel and prednisone regimen also demonstrated OS benefit post-docetaxel in metastatic CRPC. The interspersing and sequencing of chemotherapy within the numerous other agents now approved for metastatic CRPC requires further study. Focus on quality of life and multidisciplinary input into supportive care will enhance chemotherapy outcomes and optimize toxicities.

REFERENCES

1. Vogelzang NJ. One hundred thirteen men with hormone-refractory prostate cancer died today. *J Clin Oncol*. 1996;14:1753–1755.
2. Witjes FJ, Debruyne FM, Fernandez del MP, Geboers AD. Ketoconazole high dose in management of hormonally pretreated patients with progressive metastatic prostate cancer. Dutch South-Eastern Urological Cooperative Group. *Urology*. 1989;33:411–415.
3. Nishiyama T, Hashimoto Y, Takahashi K. The influence of androgen deprivation therapy on dihydrotestosterone levels in the prostatic tissue of patients with prostate cancer. *Clin Cancer Res*. 2004;10:7121–7126.
4. Montgomery RB, Mostaghel EA, Vessella R, et al. Maintenance of intratumoral androgens in metastatic prostate cancer: a mechanism for castration-resistant tumor growth. *Cancer Res*. 2008;68:4447–4454.
5. Bubendorf L, Kononen J, Koivisto P, et al. Survey of gene amplifications during prostate cancer progression by high-throughout fluorescence in situ hybridization on tissue microarrays. *Cancer Res*. 1999;59:803–806.
6. Koivisto P, Kononen J, Palmberg C, et al. Androgen receptor gene amplification: a possible molecular mechanism for androgen deprivation therapy failure in prostate cancer. *Cancer Res*. 1997;57:314–319.
7. Nadiminty N, Gao AC. Mechanisms of persistent activation of the androgen receptor in CRPC: recent advances and future perspectives. *World J Urol*. 2012;30:287–295.

8. Tsao CK, Galsky MD, Small AC, Yee T, Oh WK. Targeting the androgen receptor signalling axis in castration-resistant prostate cancer (CRPC). *BJU Int.* 2012;110:1580–1588.
9. Bitting RL, Armstrong AJ. Targeting the PI3K/Akt/mTOR pathway in castration-resistant prostate cancer. *Endocr Relat Cancer.* 2013;20:R83–R99.
10. Tannock IF, Osoba D, Stockler MR, et al. Chemotherapy with mitoxantrone plus prednisone or prednisone alone for symptomatic hormone-resistant prostate cancer: a Canadian randomized trial with palliative endpoints. *J Clin Oncol.* 1996;14:1756–1764.
11. Kantoff PW, Halabi S, Conaway M, et al. Hydrocortisone with or without mitoxantrone in men with hormone-refractory prostate cancer: results of the cancer and leukemia group B 9182 study. *J Clin Oncol.* 1999;17:2506–2513.
12. Tannock IF, de WR, Berry WR, et al. Docetaxel plus prednisone or mitoxantrone plus prednisone for advanced prostate cancer. *N Engl J Med.* 2004;351:1502–1512.
13. Berthold DR, Pond GR, Soban F, de WR, Eisenberger M, Tannock IF. Docetaxel plus prednisone or mitoxantrone plus prednisone for advanced prostate cancer: updated survival in the TAX 327 study. *J Clin Oncol.* 2008;26:242–245.
14. Kellokumpu-Lehtinen PL, Harmenberg U, Joensuu T, et al. 2-weekly versus 3-weekly docetaxel to treat castration-resistant advanced prostate cancer: a randomised, phase 3 trial. *Lancet Oncol.* 2013;14:117–124.
15. Ravery V, Fizazi K, Oudard S, et al. The use of estramustine phosphate in the modern management of advanced prostate cancer. *BJU Int.* 2011;108:1782–1786.
16. Petrylak DP, Tangen CM, Hussain MH, et al. Docetaxel and estramustine compared with mitoxantrone and prednisone for advanced refractory prostate cancer. *N Engl J Med.* 2004;351:1513–1520.
17. Kelly WK, Halabi S, Carducci M, et al. Randomized, double-blind, placebo-controlled phase III trial comparing docetaxel and prednisone with or without bevacizumab in men with metastatic castration-resistant prostate cancer: CALGB 90401. *J Clin Oncol.* 2012;30:1534–1540.
18. Tannock I, Fizazi K, Ivanov S, et al. Double-blind randomized trial of aflibercept versus placebo with docetaxel and prednisone for treatment of metastatic castration-resistant prostate cancer (mCRPC) [abstract 5002]. *ASCO* Annual Meeting 2013. *J Clin Oncol.* 2013;31 (suppl).
19. Small E, Demkow T, Gerritsen WR, et al. A phase III trial of GVAX immunotherapy for prostate cancer in combination with docetaxel versus docetaxel plus prednisone in symptomatic, castration-resistant prostate cancer (CRPC) [abstract 07]. ASCO—GU Cancers Symposium. 2009.
20. Scher HI, Jia X, Chi K, et al. Randomized, open-label phase III trial of docetaxel plus high-dose calcitriol versus docetaxel plus prednisone for patients with castration-resistant prostate cancer. *J Clin Oncol.* 2011;29:2191–2198.
21. Quinn DI, Tangen CM, Hussain M, et al. SWOG S0421: phase III study of docetaxel (D) and atrasentan (A) versus docetaxel and placebo (P) for men with advanced castrate resistant prostate cancer (CRPC) [abstract 4511]. *J Clin Oncol.* 2012;30(suppl).
22. Sternberg CN, Petrylak DP, Sartor O, et al. Multinational, double-blind, phase III study of prednisone and either satraplatin or placebo in patients with castrate-refractory prostate cancer progressing after prior chemotherapy: the SPARC trial. *J Clin Oncol.* 2009;27:5431–5438.
23. Aller AW, Kraus LA, Bissery M-C. In vitro activity of TXD258 in chemotherapeutic resistant tumor cell lines [abstract]. *Proc Am Assoc Cancer Res.* 2000;41.
24. de Bono JS, Oudard S, Ozguroglu M, et al. Prednisone plus cabazitaxel or mitoxantrone for metastatic castration-resistant prostate cancer progressing after docetaxel treatment: a randomised open-label trial. *Lancet.* 2010;376:1147–1154.
25. Vaughn DJ, Brown AW Jr, Harker WG, et al. Multicenter phase II study of estramustine phosphate plus weekly paclitaxel in patients with androgen-independent prostate carcinoma. *Cancer.* 2004;100:746–750.
26. Berlin JD, Propert KJ, Trump D, et al. 5-Fluorouracil and leucovorin therapy in patients with hormone refractory prostate cancer: an Eastern Cooperative Oncology Group phase II study (E1889). *Am J Clin Oncol.* 1998;21:171–176.
27. Morant R, Bernhard J, Maibach R, et al. Response and palliation in a phase II trial of gemcitabine in hormone-refractory metastatic prostatic carcinoma. Swiss Group for Clinical Cancer Research (SAKK). *Ann Oncol.* 2000;11:183–188.
28. Hudes GR, Kosierowski R, Greenberg R, et al. Phase II study of topotecan in metastatic hormone-refractory prostate cancer. *Invest New Drugs.* 1995;13:235–240.
29. Saxman S, Ansari R, Drasga R, et al. Phase III trial of cyclophosphamide versus cyclophosphamide, doxorubicin, and methotrexate in hormone-refractory prostatic cancer. A Hoosier Oncology Group study. *Cancer.* 1992;70:2488–2492.
30. Hussain M, Tangen CM, Lara PN Jr, et al. Ixabepilone (epothilone B analogue BMS-247550) is active in chemotherapy-naive patients with hormone-refractory prostate cancer: a Southwest Oncology Group trial S0111. *J Clin Oncol.* 2005;23:8724–8729.
31. Hussain M, Tangen CM, Berry DL, et al. Intermittent versus continuous androgen deprivation in prostate cancer. *N Engl J Med.* 2013;368:1314–1325.
32. Taylor CD, Elson P, Trump DL. Importance of continued testicular suppression in hormone-refractory prostate cancer. *J Clin Oncol.* 1993;11:2167–2172.
33. Barrie SE, Potter GA, Goddard PM, Haynes BP, Dowsett M, Jarman M. Pharmacology of novel steroidal inhibitors of cytochrome P450(17) alpha (17 alpha-hydroxylase/C17–20 lyase). *J Steroid Biochem Mol Biol.* 1994;50:267–273.
34. Potter GA, Barrie SE, Jarman M, Rowlands MG. Novel steroidal inhibitors of human cytochrome P45017 alpha (17 alpha-hydroxylase-C17,20-lyase): potential agents for the treatment of prostatic cancer. *J Med Chem.* 1995;38:2463–2471.
35. de Bono JS, Logothetis CJ, Molina A, et al. Abiraterone and increased survival in metastatic prostate cancer. *N Engl J Med.* 2011;364:1995–2005.
36. Fizazi K, Scher HI, Molina A, et al. Abiraterone acetate for treatment of metastatic castration-resistant prostate cancer: final overall survival analysis of the COU-AA-301 randomised, double-blind, placebo-controlled phase 3 study. *Lancet Oncol.* 2012;13:983–992.
37. Logothetis CJ, Basch E, Molina A, et al. Effect of abiraterone acetate and prednisone compared with placebo and prednisone on pain control and skeletal-related events in patients with metastatic castration-resistant prostate cancer: exploratory analysis of data from the COU-AA-301 randomised trial. *Lancet Oncol.* 2012;13:1210–1217.
38. Ryan CJ, Smith MR, de Bono JS, et al. Abiraterone in metastatic prostate cancer without previous chemotherapy. *N Engl J Med.* 2013;368:138–148.
39. Tran C, Ouk S, Clegg NJ, et al. Development of a second-generation antiandrogen for treatment of advanced prostate cancer. *Science.* 2009;324:787–790.
40. Jung ME, Ouk S, Yoo D, et al. Structure-activity relationship for thiohydantoin androgen receptor antagonists for castration-resistant prostate cancer (CRPC). *J Med Chem.* 2010;53:2779–2796.
41. Scher HI, Fizazi K, Saad F, et al. Increased survival with enzalutamide in prostate cancer after chemotherapy. *N Engl J Med.* 2012;367:1187–1197.
42. Beer TM, Armstrong AJ, Rathkopf DE et al. Enzalutamide in metastatic prostate cancer before chemotherapy. *N Engl J Med* 2014;371:424-433.
43. Labrie F, Dupont A, Giguere M, et al. Benefits of combination therapy with flutamide in patients relapsing after castration. *Br J Urol.* 1988;61:341–346.

44. Miyake H, Hara I, Eto H. Clinical outcome of maximum androgen blockade using flutamide as second-line hormonal therapy for hormone-refractory prostate cancer. *BJU Int.* 2005;96:791–795.
45. Manikandan R, Srirangam SJ, Pearson E, Brown SC, O'Reilly P, Collins GN. Diethylstilboestrol versus bicalutamide in hormone refractory prostate carcinoma: a prospective randomized trial. *Urol Int.* 2005;75:217–221.
46. Fossa SD, Slee PH, Brausi M, et al. Flutamide versus prednisone in patients with prostate cancer symptomatically progressing after androgen-ablative therapy: a phase III study of the European organization for research and treatment of cancer genitourinary group. *J Clin Oncol.* 2001;19:62–71.
47. Kassouf W, Tanguay S, Aprikian AG. Nilutamide as second line hormone therapy for prostate cancer after androgen ablation fails. *J Urol.* 2003;169:1742–1744.
48. Suzuki H, Okihara K, Miyake H, et al. Alternative nonsteroidal antiandrogen therapy for advanced prostate cancer that relapsed after initial maximum androgen blockade. *J Urol.* 2008;180:921–927.
49. Scher HI, Liebertz C, Kelly WK, et al. Bicalutamide for advanced prostate cancer: the natural versus treated history of disease. *J Clin Oncol.* 1997;15:2928–2938.
50. Davis NB, Ryan CW, Stadler WM, Vogelzang NJ. A phase II study of nilutamide in men with prostate cancer after the failure of flutamide or bicalutamide therapy. *BJU Int.* 2005;96:787–790.
51. Small EJ, Halabi S, Dawson NA, et al. Antiandrogen withdrawal alone or in combination with ketoconazole in androgen-independent prostate cancer patients: a phase III trial (CALGB 9583). *J Clin Oncol.* 2004;22:1025–1033.
52. Small EJ, Srinivas S. The antiandrogen withdrawal syndrome. Experience in a large cohort of unselected patients with advanced prostate cancer. *Cancer.* 1995;76:1428–1434.
53. Sartor AO, Tangen CM, Hussain MH, et al. Antiandrogen withdrawal in castrate-refractory prostate cancer: a Southwest Oncology Group trial (SWOG 9426). *Cancer.* 2008;112:2393–2400.
54. Taplin ME, Rajeshkumar B, Halabi S, et al. Androgen receptor mutations in androgen-independent prostate cancer: Cancer and Leukemia Group B Study 9663. *J Clin Oncol.* 2003;21:2673–2678.
55. Taplin ME, Bubley GJ, Ko YJ, et al. Selection for androgen receptor mutations in prostate cancers treated with androgen antagonist. *Cancer Res.* 1999;59:2511–2515.
56. Suzuki H, Ueda T, Ichikawa T, Ito H. Androgen receptor involvement in the progression of prostate cancer. *Endocr Relat Cancer.* 2003;10:209–216.
57. Palmberg C, Koivisto P, Kakkola L, Tammela TL, Kallioniemi OP, Visakorpi T. Androgen receptor gene amplification at primary progression predicts response to combined androgen blockade as second line therapy for advanced prostate cancer. *J Urol.* 2000;164:1992–1995.
58. Pont A, Williams PL, Loose DS, et al. Ketoconazole blocks adrenal steroid synthesis. *Ann Intern Med.* 1982;97:370–372.
59. Loose DS, Kan PB, Hirst MA, Marcus RA, Feldman D. Ketoconazole blocks adrenal steroidogenesis by inhibiting cytochrome P450-dependent enzymes. *J Clin Invest.* 1983;71:1495–1499.
60. Blum RA, D'Andrea DT, Florentino BM, et al. Increased gastric pH and the bioavailability of fluconazole and ketoconazole. *Ann Intern Med.* 1991;114:755–757.
61. Yap TA, Carden CP, Attard G, de Bono JS. Targeting CYP17: established and novel approaches in prostate cancer. *Curr Opin Pharmacol.* 2008;8:449–457.
62. Fakih M, Johnson CS, Trump DL. Glucocorticoids and treatment of prostate cancer: a preclinical and clinical review. *Urology.* 2002;60:553–561.
63. Kassi E, Moutsatsou P. Glucocorticoid receptor signaling and prostate cancer. *Cancer Lett.* 2011;302:1–10.
64. Nishimura K, Nonomura N, Satoh E, et al. Potential mechanism for the effects of dexamethasone on growth of androgen-independent prostate cancer. *J Natl Cancer Inst.* 2001;93:1739–1746.
65. Malkowicz SB. The role of diethylstilbestrol in the treatment of prostate cancer. *Urology.* 2001;58:108–113.
66. Bosset PO, Albiges L, Seisen T, et al. Current role of diethylstilbestrol in the management of advanced prostate cancer. *BJU Int.* 2012;110:E826–E829.
67. Small EJ, Fratesi P, Reese DM, et al. Immunotherapy of hormone-refractory prostate cancer with antigen-loaded dendritic cells. *J Clin Oncol.* 2000;18:3894–3903.
68. Small EJ, Schellhammer PF, Higano CS, et al. Placebo-controlled phase III trial of immunologic therapy with sipuleucel-T (APC8015) in patients with metastatic, asymptomatic hormone refractory prostate cancer. *J Clin Oncol.* 2006;24:3089–3094.
69. Higano CS, Schellhammer PF, Small EJ, et al. Integrated data from 2 randomized, double-blind, placebo-controlled, phase 3 trials of active cellular immunotherapy with sipuleucel-T in advanced prostate cancer. *Cancer.* 2009;115:3670–3679.
70. Kantoff PW, Higano CS, Shore ND, et al. Sipuleucel-T immunotherapy for castration-resistant prostate cancer. *N Engl J Med.* 2010;363:411–422.
71. Oefelein MG, Ricchiuti V, Conrad W, Resnick MI. Skeletal fractures negatively correlate with overall survival in men with prostate cancer. *J Urol.* 2002;168:1005–1007.
72. Scher HI, Chung LW. Bone metastases: improving the therapeutic index. *Semin Oncol.* 1994;21:630–656.
73. Saad F, Gleason DM, Murray R, et al. A randomized, placebo-controlled trial of zoledronic acid in patients with hormone-refractory metastatic prostate carcinoma. *J Natl Cancer Inst.* 2002;94:1458–1468.
74. Saad F, Chen YM, Gleason DM, Chin J. Continuing benefit of zoledronic acid in preventing skeletal complications in patients with bone metastases. *Clin Genitourin Cancer.* 2007;5:390–396.
75. Polascik TJ, Given RW, Metzger C, et al. Open-label trial evaluating the safety and efficacy of zoledronic acid in preventing bone loss in patients with hormone-sensitive prostate cancer and bone metastases. *Urology.* 2005;66:1054–1059.
76. Smith MR, Halabi S, Ryan CJ et al. Randomized controlled trial of early zoledronic acid in men with castration-sensitive prostate cancer and bone metastases: results of CALGB 90202 (alliance). *J Clin Oncol* 2014;32:1143–1150.
77 Lacey DL, Boyle WJ, Simonet WS, et al. Bench to bedside: elucidation of the OPG-RANK-RANKL pathway and the development of denosumab. *Nat Rev Drug Discov.* 2012;11:401–419.
78. Fizazi K, Carducci M, Smith M, et al. Denosumab versus zoledronic acid for treatment of bone metastases in men with castration-resistant prostate cancer: a randomised, double-blind study. *Lancet.* 2011;377:813–822.
79. Smith MR, Saad F, Coleman R, et al. Denosumab and bone-metastasis-free survival in men with castration-resistant prostate cancer: results of a phase 3, randomised, placebo-controlled trial. *Lancet.* 2012;379:39–46.
80. Brady D, Parker CC, O'Sullivan JM. Bone-targeting radiopharmaceuticals including radium-223. *Cancer J.* 2013;19:71–78.
81. Sartor O, Reid RH, Hoskin PJ, et al. Samarium-153-Lexidronam complex for treatment of painful bone metastases in hormone-refractory prostate cancer. *Urology.* 2004;63:940–945.
82. Quilty PM, Kirk D, Bolger JJ, et al. A comparison of the palliative effects of strontium-89 and external beam radiotherapy in metastatic prostate cancer. *Radiother Oncol.* 1994;31:33–40.
83. Nilsson S, Larsen RH, Fossa SD, et al. First clinical experience with alpha-emitting radium-223 in the treatment of skeletal metastases. *Clin Cancer Res.* 2005;11:4451–4459.
84. Parker C, Nilsson S, Heinrich D, et al: Alpha emitter radium-223 and survival in metastatic prostate cancer. *N Engl J Med.* 2013; 369:213–223.
85. Parker C, Nilsson S, Heinrich D, et al. Updated analysis of the phase III, double-blind, randomized, multinational study of radium-223

chloride in castration-resistant prostate cancer (CRPC) patients with bone metastases (ALSYMPCA) [abstract LBA4512]. ASCO Meeting Abstracts. *J Clin Oncol.* 2012;30(suppl).
86. Kaku T, Hitaka T, Ojida A, et al. Discovery of orteronel (TAK-700), a naphthylmethylimidazole derivative, as a highly selective 17,20-lyase inhibitor with potential utility in the treatment of prostate cancer. *Bioorg Med Chem.* 2011;19:6383–6399.
87. Yamaoka M, Hara T, Kusaka M. Overcoming persistent dependency on androgen signaling after progression to castration-resistant prostate cancer. *Clin Cancer Res.* 2010; 16:4319–4324.
88. Agus DB, Stadler WM, Shevrin DH, et al. Safety, efficacy, and pharmacodynamics of the investigational agent TAK-700 in metastatic castration-resistant prostate cancer (mCRPC): updated data from a phase I/II study [abstract 98]. ASCO Meeting Abstracts 2011;4531. *J Clin Oncol.* 2012;30(suppl 5).
89. Petrylak D, Gandhi JG, Clark WR, et al. A phase I/II study of safety and efficacy of orteronel (TAK-700), an oral, investigational, nonsteroidal 17,20-lyase inhibitor, with docetaxel and prednisone (DP) in metastatic castration-resistant prostate cancer (mCRPC): updated phase II results [abstract 59]. ASCO Meeting Abstracts 2013. *J Clin Oncol.* 2013;31(suppl 6).
90. Results from a phase 3, randomized, double-blind, multicenter, placebo-controlled trial of orteronel (TAK-700) plus prednisone in patients with metastatic castration-resistant prostate cancer (mCRPC) that has progressed during or following docetaxel-based therapy (ELM-PC 5 Trial). *Clin Adv Hematol Oncol* 2014;12:6–7.
91. De Wit R, Fizazi K, Jinga V et al. Phase 3, randomized, placebo-controlled trial of orteronel (TAK-700) plus prednisone in patients (pts) with chemotherapy-naïve metastatic castration-resistant prostate cancer (mCRPC) (ELM-PC 4 trial). *J Clin Oncol.* 2014; 32:5s, (suppl; abstr 5008).
92. Clegg NJ, Wongvipat J, Joseph JD, et al. ARN-509: a novel antiandrogen for prostate cancer treatment. *Cancer Res.* 2012;72:1494–1503.
93. Rathkopf DE, Antonarakis ES, Shore ND, et al. ARN-509 in men with metastatic castration-resistant prostate cancer (mCRPC) [abstract 48]. ASCO Meeting Abstracts 2013. *J Clin Oncol.* 2013;31(suppl 6).
94. Kantoff PW, Schuetz TJ, Blumenstein BA, et al. Overall survival analysis of a phase II randomized controlled trial of a poxviral-based PSA-targeted immunotherapy in metastatic castration-resistant prostate cancer. *J Clin Oncol.* 2010;28:1099–1105.
95. *A Randomized, Double-Blind, Phase 3 Efficacy Trial of PROSTVAC-V/F +(GM-CSF in Men With Asymptomatic or Minimally Symptomatic Metastatic Castrate-Resistant Prostate Cancer (Prospect).* http://clinicaltrials.gov/ct2/show/NCT01322490. 2013.
96. Bander NH, Czuczman MS, Younes A. Antibody-drug conjugate technology development for hematologic disorders. *Clin Adv Hematol Oncol.* 2012;10:1–16.
97. Petrylak DP, Kantoff PW, Mega AE, et al. Prostate-specific membrane antigen antibody drug conjugate (PSMA ADC): a phase I trial in metastatic castration-resistant prostate cancer (mCRPC) previously treated with a taxane [abstract 119]. ASCO 2013 Annual Meeting 2013; Abstract No: 5017. *J Clin Oncol.* 2013;31(suppl 6).
98. Danila DC, Szmulewitz RZ, Higano CS, et al. A phase I study of the safety and pharmacokinetics of DSTP3086S, an anti-STEAP1 antibody-drug conjugate (ADC), in patients (pts) with metastatic castration-resistant prostate cancer (CRPC) [abstract 5020]. ASCO Annual Meeting 2013. *J Clin Oncol.* 2013;31(suppl).
99. Morris MJ, Bruce JY, Reyno LM, et al. Phase I trial of ASG-5ME in metastatic castration-resistant prostate cancer (CRPC) [abstract 4568]. *J Clin Oncol.* 2012;30(suppl).
100. de Bono JS, Logothetis CJ, Molina A, et al. Abiraterone and increased survival in metastatic prostate cancer. *N Engl J Med.* 2011;364:1995–2005.
101. Smith DC, Smith MR, Sweeney C, et al. Cabozantinib in patients with advanced prostate cancer: results of a phase II randomized discontinuation trial. *J Clin Oncol.* 2013;31:412–419.
102. Slovin SF, Higano CS, Hamid O, et al. Ipilimumab alone or in combination with radiotherapy in metastatic castration-resistant prostate cancer: results from an open-label, multicenter phase I/II study. *Ann Oncol.* 2013;24:1813–1821.
103. Yu EY, Wilding G, Posadas E, et al. Phase II study of dasatinib in patients with metastatic castration-resistant prostate cancer. *Clin Cancer Res.* 2009;15:7421–7428.
104. Chi KN, Hotte SJ, Ellard S, et al. A randomized phase II study of OGX-427 plus prednisone versus prednisone alone in patients with chemotherapy-naive metastatic castration-resistant prostate cancer [abstract 121]. *J Clin Oncol.* 2012;30(suppl 5).

19.3 Metastatic Castrate-Resistant Prostate Cancer: Role of Androgen Signaling Inhibitors

AUSTIN POOLE
AJJAI ALVA
JULIA BATTEN
NEERAJ AGARWAL

INTRODUCTION

Medical castration with androgen deprivation therapy (ADT) with either a gonadotropin-releasing hormone (GnRH) antagonist or, less commonly, surgical castration with orchiectomy remains the cornerstone of treatment for metastatic prostate cancer. Responses, however, are not durable with a median duration of response of approximately 18 months (1). Almost all men eventually develop castrate-resistant prostate cancer (CRPC) and die of their disease (2). Over the last decade, it has been recognized that, despite the failure of ADT, most prostate tumors maintain some dependence on androgen and/or androgen receptor (AR) signaling for proliferation (3). Indeed, a significant fraction of patients with metastatic prostate cancer respond to the sequential administration of secondary hormone manipulation, following disease progression on ADT (4). Additionally, molecular pathways independent of androgen signaling may be invoked by prostate cancer to facilitate tumor progression. Subsequently, drugs have been developed targeting these pathways, many of which have received recent regulatory approval. Herein, we will focus on the drugs targeting androgen-dependent and -independent AR signaling pathways, which have recently been approved or have reached advanced stages of development in clinical trials.

MOLECULAR MECHANISM UNDERLYING PROGRESSION OF METASTATIC PROSTATE CANCER

Many mechanisms have been hypothesized to underlie the progression of metastatic prostate cancer and can be best addressed by understanding the role of endocrine and intracrine, androgens, and the AR in the different states of metastatic prostate cancer.

Prostate cancer is fueled by the androgen-axis, even after progression on ADT (Figure 19.3.1). Accordingly, the progression of metastatic prostate cancer may evolve through various molecular states of AR activity (5, 6). The first state in most patients is the endocrine androgen and AR-dependent state. The hallmark of this state is that the AR is stimulated by testicular testosterone, and disease is typically controlled by medical or surgical castration. Other states include (a) intracrine androgen-dependent and AR-dependent state, whereby the AR is activated by intratumoral androgens, (b) the androgen/ligand-independent and AR-dependent state, where AR activation appears to be independent of ligand binding and is due to either AR splice variants (AR-Vs) or to cross-talk with other pathways (e.g., Src kinase, c-Met, epidermal growth factor, Ras-Raf kinase pathway, PI3K-Akt pathway, fibroblast growth factor, insulin-like growth factors), and (c) the androgen/ligand-independent and AR-independent state, where AR signalling is no longer primarily responsible for tumor progression.

Intratumoral Androgen Synthesis

With castrate levels of serum testosterone, the adrenal glands are the predominant source of androgens. Prostate cancer cells adapt to castration by the intratumoral synthesis of androgens or by the conversion of adrenal

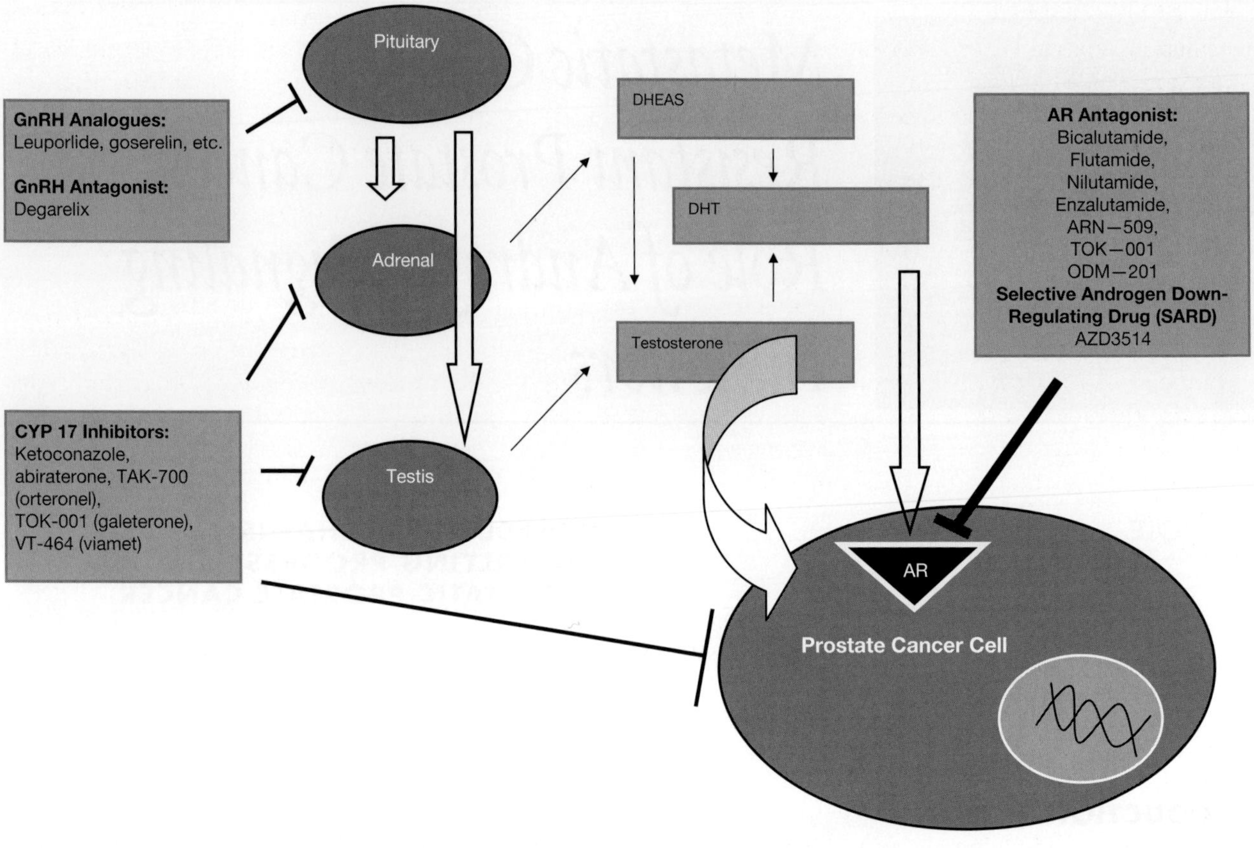

FIGURE 19.3.1 Drugs targeting androgen synthesis and androgen receptor, currently approved and those in clinical stages of development. Thick arrows denote stimulation, flat lines denote inhibition, and thin arrows denote synthesis.

androgens to testosterone and dihydrotestosterone (DHT) and, subsequently, derive a growth advantage (7). This may explain why the concentration of intratumoral testosterone in metastatic prostate tumors in men with CRPC are two to three times higher than in men who have never received ADT, despite the fact that men naïve to ADT have much higher serum testosterone levels (4, 8). Additionally, castrate-resistant cell lines have been shown to synthesize much higher levels of androgens than androgen-dependent cell lines and are capable of directly converting radioactive cholesterol into testosterone in vitro (9). Furthermore, many enzymes involved in androgen synthesis are highly up-regulated in CRPC compared to androgen-sensitive prostate cancer (8). In particular, the CYP17 enzymes, CYP17 hydroxylase, and CYP17,20 lyase are the pivotal enzymes in androgen synthesis and catalyze the conversion of pregnenolone and progesterone to the weak androgen steroids, dehydroepiandrosterone (DHEA) and androstenedione, respectively. Both DHEA and androstenedione are eventually converted to testosterone and, subsequently, to the most potent androgen, DHT. In addition, it was recently demonstrated that the upregulation of 3β-hydroxysteroid dehydrogenase type 1 (3βHSD1), which mediates the conversion of DHEA to DHT, has been implicated in the progression of CRPC (10). A gain-of-stability mutation was shown to render 3βHSD1 resistant to ubiquitination and degradation, resulting in its profound accumulation in the cytoplasm and subsequent accelerated conversion of DHEA to DHT with persistent activation of the AR.

Aberrant AR Signaling

Multiple mechanisms facilitate the aberrant AR signaling underlying disease progression in CRPC including (a) somatic mutations of the *AR* gene, (b) increased *AR* gene expression, and (c) *AR* gene rearrangement, among others (11).

Somatic AR mutations occur under the selection pressure of ADT and/or antiandrogens and lead to promiscuous ARs. These mutations have been shown to be activated by antiandrogens, such as bicalutamide, as well as other endogenous steroids, including progesterone or deoxycorticosterone (3, 12, 13). These have been implicated in the withdrawal syndrome associated with antiandrogen therapy, where tumor regression and prostate-specific antigen (PSA) decline have been correlated with the cessation of treatment with AR antagonists (14). This mechanism may also explain why prostate cancer that progresses on one AR antagonist may respond favorably to another AR antagonist (15).

Explaining this phenomenon, sequencing studies have also shown a prevalence of mutations in both the ligand binding domain and the N-terminal domain of the AR coding region (12). Using a reporter-based mutagenesis screen, a novel AR mutant (AR F876L) was recently identified in enzalutamide-sensitive cell lines and in xenograft models after prolonged exposure to enzalutamide (16). Acquisition of the AR F876L mutation converts enzalutamide and ARN-509 into AR agonists and induces treatment resistance in vitro, as well as in vivo (16–18). Using structural modeling, AR F876L has been shown to allow AR helix (helix 12) repositioning to an agonist-like conformation that permits coactivation recruitment in enzalutamide-treated tumor cells. Interestingly, bicalutamide remained an antagonist in these AR-mutant cells. Notably, DR103, a recently developed molecule, has been shown to restore the position of helix 12 into the antagonist form, which subsequently inhibited the growth of prostate cancer cell lines that expressed both wild-type and F876L-mutant AR (16).

An increased *AR* gene expression occurs, due to *AR* gene amplification, an increased rate of transcription of the *AR* gene, or increased stability of the AR transcript (9, 19). *AR* gene rearrangement is a relatively recently reported mechanism underlying aberrant AR signaling and results in constitutively active truncated AR-Vs (20). AR-Vs lead to AR protein variants which are capable of mediating ligand-independent AR signaling, leading to prostate cancer progression.

Novel mechanisms underlying aberrant AR signaling continue to be unraveled. Recently, long noncoding RNAs (lncRNAs) have been implicated in aberrant AR signaling. Two lncRNAs (PRNCR1 and PCGEM1) were shown to be highly overexpressed in CRPC. These lncRNAs bind successively to both truncated and full-length ARs and strongly enhance both ligand-dependent and -independent AR activation. Furthermore, targeting of lncRNAs by antisense RNA in CRPC cell lines strongly suppressed tumor xenograft growth in vivo (21).

■ AGENTS TARGETING ANDROGEN SYNTHESIS

Ketoconazole

Ketoconazole, a cytochrome P-450 inhibitor, is an imidazole antifungal agent that has a weak and nonspecific inhibitory affect on several enzymes involved in androgen synthesis, including CYP17. Although ketoconazole has never been shown to improve survival, it was been frequently used in the past as a part of secondary hormonal manipulation, following the onset of CRPC (22). The use of ketoconazole, however, is associated with multiple drug interactions, as well as significant toxicities, due to nonspecific inhibition of cytochrome P-450. This, coupled with the advent of effective novel CYP17 inhibitors, has made ketoconazole a suboptimal treatment option (23).

Abiraterone Acetate

Abiraterone acetate (AA), a pregnenolone analogue, and its metabolite, abiraterone, are selective irreversible inhibitors of CYP17 α hydroxylase and CYP17,20 lyase: both required for androgen biosynthesis (Figures 19.3.1 and 19.3.2). Remarkably, within just a few years after the discovery that the intratumoral expression of CYP17A1 (17α-hydroxylase/17,20-lyase) was an alternative means of increasing androgen levels within the tumor microenvironment, AA received regulatory approval for the treatment of metastatic castration-resistant prostate cancer (mCRPC) in April 2011.

In vitro studies have demonstrated that abiraterone is a more potent inhibitor of the CYP17 enzyme when compared to ketoconazole (24). In a phase II study, the efficacy and safety of AA in combination with prednisone was studied in 58 men with progressive CRPC who experienced a prior treatment failure with docetaxel-based chemotherapy (25). Patients received AA at a dose of 1,000 mg daily, along with prednisone, 5 mg twice a day, to reduce abiraterone-induced hyperaldosteronism. The primary outcome was a ≥ 50% decline in PSA, which was achieved in 36% of patients. The addition of prednisone reduced the incidence of mineralocorticoid-related toxicity. This was followed by phase III studies in patients with CRPC in the post- and predocetaxel settings (Table 19.3.1).

In the first phase III trial, COU AA-301, 1,195 patients with metastatic CRPC, who received prior docetaxel or two lines of chemotherapy, were randomized in a 2:1 fashion to receive 5 mg of prednisone twice daily with either 1,000 mg of AA (797 patients) or placebo (398 patients) (26). A prespecified interim analysis demonstrated a survival benefit of AA over placebo (14.8 months vs. 10.9 months; hazard ratio [HR] 0.65; 95% confidence interval [CI] 0.54–0.77; $P < .001$), resulting in subsequent crossover of all eligible patients in the placebo group to receive abiraterone. Adverse effects were associated with secondary mineralocorticoid excess, including hypertension, hypokalemia, and edema, which were manageable with the addition of a mineralocorticoid antagonist or a corticosteroid. The final analysis prior to the crossover demonstrated that at a median follow up of 20.2 months, the median overall survival (OS) with AA was significantly better than placebo (15.8 months vs. 11.2 months; HR 0.74; 95% CI 0.64–0.86; $P < .0001$) (Table 19.3.1) (27).

The favorable results seen with AA do not appear to be limited to post docetaxel mCRPC. Another phase III study, COU AA-302, evaluated 1,088 men with mCRPC who had never received chemotherapy. Patients were randomized (1:1) to receive either AA with prednisone or placebo with prednisone (28). The co-primary endpoints were radiographic progression-free survival (rPFS) and OS. At the planned interim analysis, the study was unblinded after 43% of the expected deaths had occurred. The median rPFS was significantly improved in the abiraterone–prednisone group compared to the placebo–prednisone group (16.5 months vs. 8.3 months; HR 0.53; 95% CI 0.45–0.62; $P < .001$). OS was also improved with abiraterone–prednisone (median not reached vs. 27.2 months for placebo–prednisone; HR 0.75; 95% CI 0.61–0.93; *P* = .01) but did not cross the efficacy boundary. Notably, all secondary endpoints, including the time to initiation of cytotoxic chemotherapy, opiate use for cancer-related pain, PSA progression, and decline in performance status, were improved with abiraterone–prednisone compared to placebo–prednisone. Based on these results, AA was also approved for the treatment of mCRPC in the prechemotherapy setting in December 2012. While the COU AA-302 trial allowed only asymptomatic or minimally symptomatic men and excluded those with visceral metastasis, the data from COU AA-301 suggests that patients with visceral disease may also benefit from AA in the chemo-naive setting (29).

Orteronel (TAK 700)

Orteronel, a novel naphthylmethylimidazole derivative, is a next-generation CYP17 inhibitor with higher selectivity for CYP17,20 lyase than CYP17 hydroxylase (i.e., for androgen as opposed to corticosteroid synthesis) and does not appear to cause secondary mineralcorticoid excess (Figures 19.3.1 and 19.3.2) (30).

Orteronel was investigated in a phase I/II study in men with progressive, chemotherapy-naive mCRPC (31). In the phase I portion, 26 men received orteronel at doses of 100 to 600 mg twice daily or at 400 mg twice daily, along with prednisone 5 mg twice daily. No dose-limiting toxicities were observed. In the phase II portion, 97 men were treated with orteronel in four different dose cohorts: 300 mg twice daily (n = 23), 400 mg twice daily + prednisone 5 mg twice daily (n = 24), 600 mg twice daily + prednisone (n = 26), or 600 mg daily without prednisone (n = 24). Forty-five of 84 evaluable patients (54%) achieved a ≥ 50% decline in PSA. At a 12-week follow-up analysis, the median levels of testosterone, DHEA-S, and the level of mean circulating tumor cells were decreased in all groups. Unconfirmed partial responses were reported in 10 of 51 evaluable phase II patients (20%). The most common grade ≥ 3 adverse effects were fatigue, hypokalemia, hyperglycemia, and diarrhea.

In an another phase II trial in men with nonmetastatic CRPC with biochemical recurrence, treatment with orteronel 300 mg twice daily without prednisone resulted in PSA response rates of ≥ 50% in 76% of men after 12 weeks of treatment with minimal toxicities (32).

The promising data from these early clinical trials led to two phase III, randomized, placebo controlled trials comparing the efficacy of orteronel 400 mg orally BID with placebo in chemotherapy-naïve patients and in patients who previously progressed on docetaxel (Table 19.3.1). Despite earlier promising results, the data from the phase III trial of men with mCRPC (n = 1099) who had received prior docetaxel therapy showed that treatment with orteronel with prednisone did not

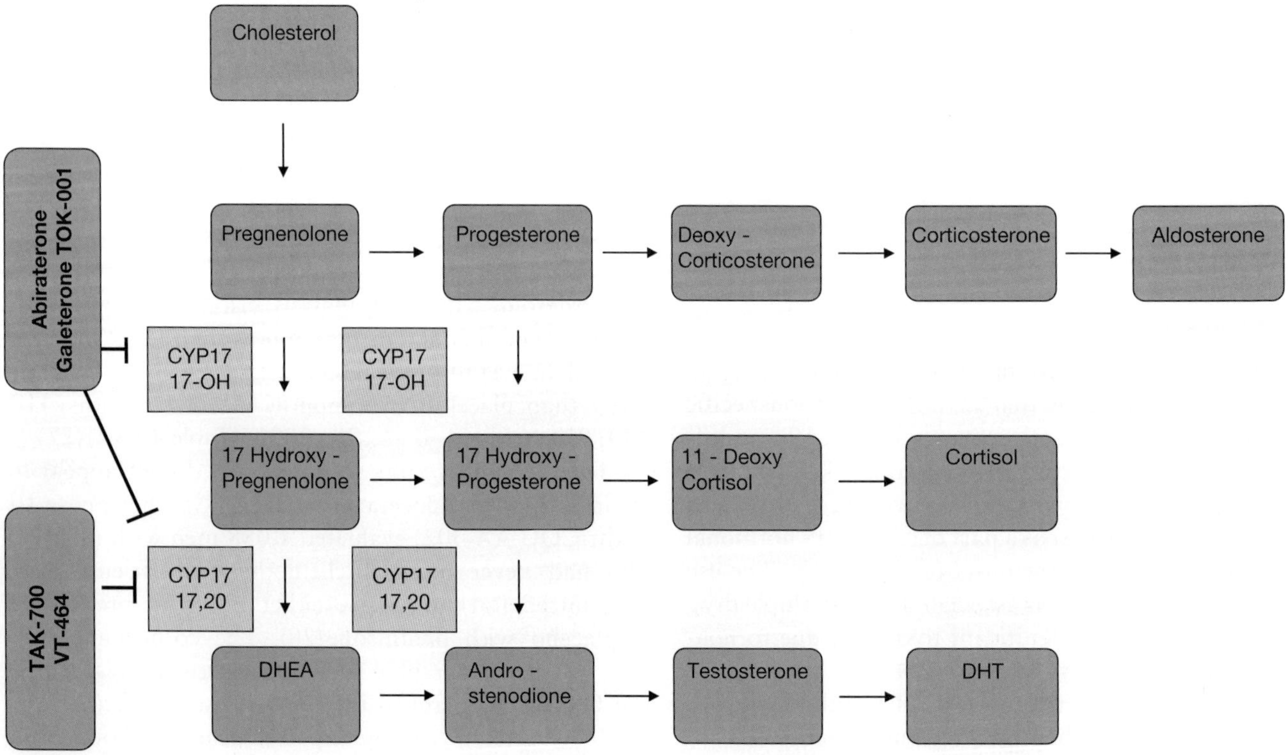

FIGURE 19.3.2 Steroid synthesis pathway and the sites of action of novel agents, recently approved and those in clinical development. *Abbreviations*: CYP17, cytochrome P450 17 α-hydroxylase-C17,20-lyase; ACTH, adrenocorticotrophic hormone; DHEA, dihydroepiandrostenedione; DHT, dihydrotestosterone.

Table 19.3.1 Recently reported and ongoing phase III clinical trials investigating agents targeting androgen signaling in CRPC

Molecular Target	Arms	Population	Primary End Point	Comments	Clinical Trial ID (clinicaltrials.gov)
CYP17: 17 hydroxylase; 17,20 lyase activity	AA + P Placebo + P	Docetaxel pretreated	OS	Median OS with AA was significantly better than placebo (15.8 mo vs. 11.2 mo) (COU-AA-301)	NCT00638690
CYP17: 17 hydroxylase; 17,20 lyase activity	AA + P Placebo + P	Chemo-naïve	OS, rPFS	Median rPFS was significantly improved with AA + P (16.5 mo vs. 8.3 mo). OS improved but did not cross efficacy boundary (COU AA-302)	NCT00887198
CYP17: 17,20 lyase; 17 hydroxylase activity	TAK-700 (orteronel) + P Placebo + P	Docetaxel pretreated	OS	No improvement demonstrated in OS, but with significant improvement in rPFS (a secondary end point). Posttrial treatment with abiraterone may have confounded OS data.	NCT01193257
CYP17: 17,20 lyase; 17 hydroxylase activity	TAK-700 (orteronel) + P Placebo + P	Chemo-naïve	OS, rPFS	Accrual: completed; results: pending	NCT01193244
AR	Enzalutamide Placebo	Chemo-naïve	OS, rPFS	Significant improvement in rPFS with enzalutamide over placebo. Median OS was 32.4 mo in the enzalutamide arm vs. 30.2 mo in the placebo arm constituting a 29% reduction in risk of death (PREVAIL)	NCT01212991
AR	Enzalutamide Placebo	Prior chemotherapy	OS	Increased median OS compared to the placebo group (18.4 mo vs. 13.6 mo) (AFFIRM)	NCT00974311
AR	ARN-509 Placebo	Nonmetastatic chemo-naive	Metastasis-free survival	Accrual: ongoing (SPARTAN)	NCT01946204
AR and CYP17	Enzalutamide ± abiraterone acetate and prednisone	Chemo-naïve	OS	Accrual: ongoing	NCT01949337

Abbreviations: AA, abiraterone acetate; AR, androgen receptor; CRPC, castrate-resistant prostate cancer; mCRPC, metastatic castration-resistant prostate cancer; OS, overall survival; P, prednisone; PFS, progression-free survival; rPFS, radiographic progression-free survival.

demonstrate an improvement in OS when compared to the control arm of prednisone alone (17 months vs. 15.2 months, HR 0.886, *P* = .1898)(33). There was, however, an advantage with orteronel plus prednisone for the secondary end point of rPFS (8.3 months vs. 5.7 months, HR 0.76, *P* = .00038). In addition, no safety concerns were reported. It is possible that the impact of orteronel on OS may have been confounded by posttrial treatment with AA, which received Food and Drug Administration approval at the time the trial was accruing patients. Indeed, substantial regional differences were seen in the OS benefit according to the availability of AA: median OS (orteronel vs. placebo) was 20.9 versus 16.9 months (HR 0.889) in North America (*n* = 112), 18.3 versus 17.8 months (HR 1.048) in Europe (*n* = 590), and 15.3 versus 10.1 months (HR 0.709) in the rest of the world (*n* = 397). Another phase III trial in the pre-docetaxel setting has recently completed accrual (Table 19.3.1).

VT-464 (Viamet)

Viamet is a novel oral CYP17 inhibitor with a higher selectivity for 17,20-lyase over 17-hydroxylase (Figures 19.3.1 and 19.3.2). This selectivity was demonstrated in comparison of the activity of VT-464 to that of AA both in vitro and in the adult male castrate rhesus monkeys. VT-464 was 10-fold more selective for human CYP17 lyase over hydroxylase inhibition, resulting in androgen suppression, but, importantly, no increases of up-stream steroids or evidence of cortisol suppression. In contrast, abiraterone was sixfold more selective for hydroxylase over lyase inhibition resulting in increased up-stream steroid and cortisol suppression. Thus, VT-464 provides an opportunity to be potentially used without concomitant steroids(34). Currently, VT 464 is undergoing phase I development.

■ AGENTS TARGETING THE ANDROGEN RECEPTOR

Conventional Antiandrogens

Antiandrogens work by competitively inhibiting the binding of testosterone and DHT with the AR. Currently approved antiandrogens in the United States include bicalutamide, flutamide, and nilutamide, all of which are nonsteroidal antiandrogens. In the setting of mCRPC, antiandrogens are used for secondary hormonal manipulation. Monotherapy with antiandrogens (without GnRH agonist) is not recommended because of concerns for inferior survival when compared to GnRH agonist therapy alone(23).

Enzalutamide

Enzalutamide, formerly referred to as MDV3100, is a novel a thiohydantoin AR antagonist that binds to the androgen binding site of the AR with a greater relative affinity than bicalutamide (Figure 19.3.1). Enzalutamide reduces the efficiency of nuclear translocation of the AR, DNA binding to androgen response elements, and the recruitment of coactivators by the AR(35).

In a phase I/II study of 140 men with mCRPC, antitumor effects were seen at all doses (30 mg to 600 mg daily), including decreases in serum PSA of ≥ 50% in 56% patients, soft tissue responses in 22% of patients, stabilization of bone disease in 56% of patients, and conversion from unfavorable to favorable circulating tumor cell counts in 49% of patients(36). The maximum tolerated dose for sustained treatment (> 28 days) was 240 mg. Enzalutamide was generally well tolerated, with fatigue as the most common dose-dependent grade 3 to 4 side effect. These data led to placebo-controlled phase III trials, the AFFIRM and PREVAIL trials, in the post-docetaxel setting and in chemo-naive patients with metastatic CRPC, respectively (Table 19.3.1).

In the AFFIRM phase III trial, 1,199 men with mCRPC who had received prior chemotherapy were randomized (2:1) to receive oral enzalutamide at 160 mg daily versus placebo, with OS being the primary end point(37). The study was stopped after the planned interim analysis, when 520 deaths occurred. In patients randomized to enzalutamide, there was a significant increase in the median OS when compared to the placebo group (18.4 months vs. 13.6 months; HR 0.63; 95% CI 0.53–0.75; *P* < .001). This led to the regulatory approval of enzalutamide in August 2012. Enzalutamide was also superior over placebo with respect to all secondary endpoints, including PSA progression, rPFS, quality-of-life response rate, time to PSA progression, and soft-tissue response rate. Overall, enzalutamide was well tolerated with fatigue, diarrhea, and hot flashes more common in the enzalutamide group. Seizures were also reported in five (0.6%) patients, with the majority of these cases associated with underlying predisposing factors. Of note, enzalutamide does cross the blood–brain barrier and decreases the seizure threshold in a small number of predisposed patients. It has been hypothesized that this may be due to inhibition of the gamma-aminobutyric acid–gated chloride channel(38).

In the PREVAIL trial, 1,717 chemo-naïve patients with mCRPC were randomized (1:1) to enzalutamide 160 mg daily or placebo. OS and rPFS were the co-primary endpoints(39). The rate of rPFS at 12 months was 65% among patients treated with enzalutamide, as compared with 14% among patients receiving placebo (81% risk reduction; HR in the enzalutamide group, 0.19; 95% CI 0.15 to 0.23; *P* < .001). The median OS was also improved, with a 29% reduction in risk of death (HR 0.71; 95% CI 0.60 to 0.84; *P* < .001). The estimated median OS was 32.4 months (mo) (95% CI, 31.5–upper limit not yet reached in the enzalutamide arm) versus 30.2 mo (95% CI, 28–upper limit not yet reached) in the placebo arm.

The superiority of enzaluamide over placebo was shown with respect to all secondary end points: the time until the initiation of cytotoxic chemotherapy (HR 0.35), the time until the first skeletal-related event (HR 0.72), a complete or partial soft-tissue response (59% vs. 5%), the time until PSA progression (HR 0.17), and a rate of decline of at least 50% in PSA (78% vs. 3%) ($P < .001$ for all comparisons). The most common clinically relevant adverse events associated with enzalutamide were fatigue and hypertension. Seizure events were reported in two patients, one in each arm. Currently, there are two ongoing studies evaluating the role of enzalutamide prior to cytotoxic chemotherapy in men with CRPC after failure with primary ADT, in the metastatic and nonmetastatic settings (Table 19.3.1).

ARN-509

ARN-509 is a novel small molecule AR antagonist that is structurally and mechanistically similar to enzalutamide. In a murine xenograft model of mCRPC, ARN-509 showed greater antitumor activity than enzalutamide, for any given dose and plasma concentration. Furthermore, ARN-509 achieved significantly lower steady-state brain levels than those observed with enzalutamide, suggesting a potential lower risk for seizures (40). In a phase I/II study of 24 men with metastatic CRPC, ARN-509 was found to be safe and well tolerated with promising PSA responses. (55% patients had ≥ 50% PSA declines.) There was also pharmacodynamic evidence of AR antagonism, with fluoro-dihydro-testosterone (FDHT)–positron emission tomography imaging demonstrating AR blockade at 4 weeks across multiple doses. Of the seven dose levels investigated, a dose of 240 mg daily was selected for the phase II portion (41). The most common treatment-related grade 1 to 2 side effects were fatigue (38%), nausea (29%), and pain (24%). A phase II evaluation showed that, at 12 weeks, the PSA response was 91% in therapy-naïve, 60% in post-AA mCRPC patients, and 89.5% in nonmetastatic CRPC patients (42, 43). Currently, a phase III trial of ARN-509 is accruing men with nonmetastatic CRPC (Table 19.3.1).

ODM-201

This is a novel and a potent oral AR antagonist that does not penetrate the blood–brain barrier in preclinical models (Figure 19.3.1). In a phase I/II study, treatment with ODM-201 was well tolerated and was associated with a high level of activity in mCRPC, including those with prior treatment with docetaxel and a CYP17 inhibitor (44). Overall, 136 patients were recruited (phase I: 24; phase II: 112) and treated at three twice daily dose levels: 100, 200, and 700 mg. No dose-limiting toxicity was found. Seventy-eight of 108 (70%) evaluable patients experienced a PSA decline during the first 12 weeks, including a > 50% PSA drop in 44 of the 108 (41%). No seizures were observed (44). An updated analysis of clinical efficacy of ODM-201 in this trial was recently reported. Of 136 patients, 124 were eligible for the evaluation of imaging responses. Objective responses in soft tissue (complete response + partial response + stable disease) and bone lesions (improved + stable), respectively, were observed in (a) patients without prior exposure to chemotherapy or a CYP17 inhibitor (n = 37, 85% and 82%); (b) patients with prior exposure to chemotherapy but not to a CYP inhibitor (n = 32, 60% and 62%); and (c) patients with prior treatment with a CYP17 inhibitor only (n = 55, 59% and 54%). Remarkably, imaging responses were seen in a majority of patients with prior treatment with a CYP17 inhibitor (45).

AZD3514

This is a first in class, selective androgen receptor down regulator (SARD), which inhibits both androgen-dependent and -independent AR signaling (Figure 19.3.1). This is an oral agent that modulates AR signaling through two distinct mechanisms: first, through inhibition of ligand-driven nuclear translocation of the AR and second through down regulation of AR levels, likely by reducing the rate of synthesis. Preclinically, AZD3514 has been shown to have antitumor activity in both androgen-sensitive and castration-resistant prostate tumors (46). In a first-in-man phase I trial, 49 men with CRPC were treated with escalating dose levels of AZD3514 (47). Encouraging responses were observed, even in those with prior disease progression on AA. These included PSA decline of ≥ 30% in 11 of 49 men (23%), PSA decline of ≥ 50% in 7 of 49 men (14%), and objective soft tissue responses in 2 of 26 men (8%) with measurable disease. No dose-limiting toxicities were seen, and the most common toxicities were nausea and vomiting, managed with oral antiemetics.

■ AGENTS TARGETING ANDROGEN SYNTHESIS AND AR

TOK-001 (Galeterone)

TOK-001 is a rationally designed inhibitor of androgen biosynthesis that is structurally similar to abiraterone. Like abiraterone, TOK-001 directly inhibits CYP17, as well as the AR, but TOK-001 has the additional unique ability to down regulate AR expression by binding with the AR and reducing AR protein levels (Figures 19.3.1 and 19.3.2) (48). In mouse xenograft models, TOK-001 reduced tumor growth more effectively than castration and bicalutamide (48). In a phase I study (ARMOR1) of chemo-naïve men with CRPC, TOK-001 was well tolerated and demonstrated clinical activity, with 22% of 49 patients demonstrating a > 50% PSA decline and an additional 26% with PSA declines of 30% to 50% (49).

Based on these encouraging preliminary results, a two-part phase II study (ARMOR2) designed to confirm the dose of reformulated oral galeterone (part 1) and to demonstrate safety and efficacy in four distinct CRPC patient cohorts (part 2) has been initiated and is expected to enroll 136 patients. Preliminary results of part 1 of the study were recently reported (50). Metastatic and nonmetastatic treatment naïve CRPC patients were enrolled to three dose cohorts of 1,700, 2,550, or 2,400 mg daily. Additionally, an AA refractory group of patients were treated with a starting dose of 2,550 mg daily. A once-daily galeterone dose of 2,550 mg was selected for part 2 based on safety, efficacy, and pharmacokinetic data. Of 39 patients followed up for at least 12 weeks across all doses, 79% experienced a PSA response of ≥ 30% and 67% achieved a PSA response of ≥ 50%. Notably, galeterone showed activity in three patients with prior disease progression on AA, with one achieving a PSA response of 30% and two experiencing stabilization of PSA. Galeterone was well tolerated with majority (94%) of adverse effects being grade 1 and 2. There were no reports of mineralocorticoid excess and no patient required prednisone.

■ CONCLUSIONS

Improved understanding of the molecular biology underlying progression of CRPC over the last two decades has led to the discovery of novel molecular pathways and targets. This has led to a proliferation of therapeutic agents for treatment of metastatic CRPC. In a short span of 3 years, many novel drugs have been approved for use, revolutionizing the treatment paradigm in mCRPC. Amidst this changing landscape of treatment options in metastatic CRPC, more changes are on the horizon as many ongoing trials are likely to result in regulatory approval of newer agents. Unfortunately, despite all these therapeutic advances, current therapy has only conferred modest gains in survival outcomes and the disease remains, ultimately, incurable. Working against improved outcomes are heterogenous mechanisms of drug resistance. Advances, therefore, are required in the identification of predictive biomarkers and the need for personalized treatments of patients with CRPC both initially and at the time of disease progression. This will ultimately improve outcomes by employing a model with drug regimens targeting molecular pathways specific to a given patient's tumor rather than a model consisting of nonspecific treatment for all. An example of this is demonstrated with the onset of resistance to AA, which can occur as a result of upregulation of CYP17A1 expression and/or the induction of ligand-independent AR variants, among other mechanisms (51). This upregulation alone provides the rationale for using a more potent CYP17A1 inhibitor. In addition, the induction of a ligand-independent AR variant alone provides the rationale for using enzalutamide. From the perspective of personalized medicine, the identification of both of these drug resistance pathways in an individual provides the rationale for combining both strategies. Indeed, clinical trials are evaluating rational combinations of biologic agents based on a better understanding of tumor biology, which may, subsequently, lead to approval of these combinatorial regimens, for example, AA combined with PI3K/Akt inhibitors or combined with enzalutamide (Table 19.3.1).

The first step toward personalizing mCRPC treatment is the development of innovative clinical trials consisting of pretreatment genomic characterization of the tumor, followed by adaptive randomization of each patient to a particular treatment arm based on the underlying genomic signatures of their individual tumors. Until predictive biomarkers are identified and validated, the sequencing of all approved agents demonstrated to extend survival should be attempted based on patient-specific clinical factors. No effort should be spared in providing access to clinical trials evaluating promising new agents or the use of previously approved agents in tumors with known susceptibility.

■ REFERENCES

1. Crawford ED, Eisenberger MA, McLeod DG, et al. A controlled trial of leuprolide with and without flutamide in prostatic carcinoma. *N Engl J Med*. 1989;321:419–424.
2. Agarwal N, Hussain M. Management of hormone-sensitive metastatic prostate cancer. *Hematol Oncol Clin North Am*. 2013;27:1221–1241, viii.
3. Taplin ME, Rajeshkumar B, Halabi S, et al. Androgen receptor mutations in androgen-independent prostate cancer: Cancer and Leukemia Group B Study 9663. *J Clin Oncol*. 2003;21:2673–2678.
4. Chen Y, Clegg NJ, Scher HI. Anti-androgens and androgen-depleting therapies in prostate cancer: new agents for an established target. *Lancet Oncol*. 2009;10:981–991.
5. Nelson PS. Molecular states underlying androgen receptor activation: a framework for therapeutics targeting androgen signaling in prostate cancer. *J Clin Oncol*. 2012;30:644–646.
6. Zhang TY, Agarwal N, Sonpavde G, et al. Management of castrate resistant prostate cancer-recent advances and optimal sequence of treatments. *Curr Urol Rep*. 2013;14:174–183.
7. Titus MA, Schell MJ, Lih FB, et al. Testosterone and dihydrotestosterone tissue levels in recurrent prostate cancer. *Clin Cancer Res*. 2005;11:4653–4657.
8. Montgomery RB. Maintenance of intratumoral androgens in metastatic prostate cancer: a mechanism for castration-resistant tumor growth. *Cancer Res*. 2008;68:4447–4454.
9. Dillard PR, Lin MF, Khan SA. Androgen-independent prostate cancer cells acquire the complete steroidogenic potential of synthesizing testosterone from cholesterol. *Mol Cell Endocrinol*. 2008;295:115–120.
10. Chang KH, Li R, Kuri B, et al. A gain-of-function mutation in DHT synthesis in castration-resistant prostate cancer. *Cell*. 2013;154:1074–1084.
11. Agarwal N, Di Lorenzo G, Sonpavde G, Bellmunt J. New agents for prostate cancer. *Ann Oncol*. 2014 [Epub ahead of print].
12. Steinkamp MP, O'Mahony OA, Brogley M, et al. Treatment-dependent androgen receptor mutations in prostate cancer exploit multiple mechanisms to evade therapy. *Cancer Res*. 2009;69:4434–4442.
13. Feldman BJ, Feldman D. The development of androgen-independent prostate cancer. *Nat Rev Cancer*. 2001;1:34–45.
14. Hara T, Miyazaki J, Araki H, et al. Novel mutations of androgen receptor: a possible mechanism of bicalutamide withdrawal syndrome. *Cancer Res*. 2003;63:149–153.
15. Suzuki H, Okihara K, Miyake H, et al. Alternative nonsteroidal antiandrogen therapy for advanced prostate cancer that

relapsed after initial maximum androgen blockade. *J Urol.* 2008;180:921–927.

16. Balbas MD, Evans MJ, Hosfield DJ, et al. Overcoming mutation-based resistance to antiandrogens with rational drug design. *Elife.* 2013;2:e00499.
17. Joseph JD, Lu N, Qian J, et al. A clinically relevant androgen receptor mutation confers resistance to second-generation antiandrogens enzalutamide and ARN-509. *Cancer Discov.* 2013;3:1020–1029.
18. Korpal M, Korn JM, Gao X, et al. An F876L mutation in androgen receptor confers genetic and phenotypic resistance to MDV3100 (enzalutamide). *Cancer Discov.* 2013;3:1030–1043.
19. Edwards J, Krishna NS, Grigor KM, Bartlett JM. Androgen receptor gene amplification and protein expression in hormone refractory prostate cancer. *Br J Cancer.* 2003;89:552–556.
20. Li Y, Chan SC, Brand LJ, Hwang TH, Silverstein KA, Dehm SM. Androgen receptor splice variants mediate enzalutamide resistance in castration-resistant prostate cancer cell lines. *Cancer Res.* 2013;73:483–489.
21. Yang L, Lin C, Jin C, et al. lncRNA-dependent mechanisms of androgen-receptor-regulated gene activation programs. *Nature.* 2013;500:598–602.
22. Small EJ, Halabi S, Dawson NA, et al. Antiandrogen withdrawal alone or in combination with ketoconazole in androgen-independent prostate cancer patients: a phase III trial (CALGB 9583). *J Clin Oncol.* 2004;22:1025–1033.
23. Small EJ, Vogelzang NJ. Second-line hormonal therapy for advanced prostate cancer: a shifting paradigm. *J Clin Oncol.* 1997;15:382–388.
24. Haidar S, Ehmer PB, Barassin S, et al. Effects of novel 17alpha-hydroxylase/C17, 20-lyase (P450 17, CYP 17) inhibitors on androgen biosynthesis in vitro and in vivo. *J Steroid Biochem Mol Biol.* 2003;84:555–562.
25. Danila DC, Morris MJ, de Bono JS, et al. Phase II multicenter study of abiraterone acetate plus prednisone therapy in patients with docetaxel-treated castration-resistant prostate cancer. *J Clin Oncol.* 2010;28:1496–1501.
26. de Bono JS, Logothetis CJ, Molina A, et al. Abiraterone and increased survival in metastatic prostate cancer. *N Engl J Med.* 2011;364:1995–2005.
27. Fizazi K, Scher HI, Molina A, et al. Abiraterone acetate for treatment of metastatic castration-resistant prostate cancer: final overall survival analysis of the COU-AA-301 randomised, double-blind, placebo-controlled phase 3 study. *Lancet Oncol.* 2012;13:983–992.
28. Ryan CJ, Smith MR, de Bono JS, et al. Abiraterone in metastatic prostate cancer without previous chemotherapy. *N Engl J Med.* 2013;368:138–148.
29. Goodman OB, Flaig TW, Molina A, et al. Exploratory analysis of the visceral disease (VD) patient subset in COU-AA-301, a phase III study of abiraterone acetate (AA) in metastatic castration-resistant prostate cancer (mCRPC) [abstract 14]. *J Clin Oncol.* 2013;31 (suppl 6).
30. Kaku T, Hitaka T, Ojida A, et al. Discovery of orteronel (TAK-700), a naphthylmethylimidazole derivative, as a highly selective 17,20-lyase inhibitor with potential utility in the treatment of prostate cancer. *Bioorg Med Chem.* 2011;19:6383–6399.
31. Dreicer R, Maclean D, Suri A, et al. Phase I/II trial of orteronel (TAK-700)–an investigational 17,20-lyase inhibitor—in patients with metastatic castration-resistant prostate cancer. *Clin Cancer Res.* 2014;20:1335–1344.
32. Hussain M, Corn P, Michaelson D, et al. Activity and safety of the investigational agent orteronel in men with nonmetastatic castration-resistant prostate cancer and rising prostate-specific antigen: results of a phase 2 study. 27th Annual European Association of Urology; February 24–28, 2012: Poster 124; Paris, France.
33. Dreicer R, Jones R, OudardS, et al. Results from a phase 3, randomized, double-blind, multicenter, placebo-controlled trial of orteronel (TAK-700) plus prednisone in patients with metastatic castration-resistant prostate cancer (mCRPC) that has progressed during or following docetaxel-based therapy (ELM-PC 5 trial) [abstract 7]. *J Clin Oncol.* 2014;32(suppl 4).
34. Eisner JR, Abbott DH, Bird IM, et al. VT-464: a novel, selective inhibitor of P450c17(CYP17)-17,20 lyase for castration-refractory prostate cancer (CRPC) [abstract 7]. *J Clin Oncol.* 2012;30.
35. Tran C, Ouk S, Clegg NJ, et al. Development of a second-generation antiandrogen for treatment of advanced prostate cancer. *Science.* 2009;324:787–790.
36. Scher HI, Beer TM, Higano CS, et al. Antitumour activity of MDV3100 in castration-resistant prostate cancer: a phase 1-2 study. *Lancet.* 2010;375:1437–1446.
37. Scher HI, Fizazi K, Saad F, et al. Increased survival with enzalutamide in prostate cancer after chemotherapy. *N Engl J Med.* 2012;367:1187–1197.
38. Scher HI, Fizazi K, Saad F, et al. Increased survival with enzalutamide in prostate cancer after chemotherapy. *N Engl J Med.* 2012;367:1187–1197.
39. Beer TM, Armstrong AJ, Rathkopf DE, et al. Enzalutamide in metastatic prostate cancer before chemotherapy. *N Engl J Med.* 2014;371:424–33.
40. Clegg NJ, Wongvipat J, Joseph JD, et al. ARN-509: a novel antiandrogen for prostate cancer treatment. *Cancer Res.* 2012;72:1494–1503.
41. Rathkopf DE, DanilaDC, MorrisMJ, et al. Phase I/II safety and pharmacokinetic (PK) study of ARN-509 in patients with metastatic castration-resistant prostate cancer (mCRPC): phase I results of a Prostate Cancer Clinical Trials Consortium study [abstract 43]. *J Clin Oncol.* 2012;30(suppl 5).
42. Rathkopf DE, Antonarakis ES, Shore ND, et al. ARN-509 in men with metastatic castration-resistant prostate cancer. ESMO Congress; September 2012; Vienna, Austria. Abstract 964 TIP.
43. Smith MR, Antonarakis ES, Ryan CJ, et al. ARN-509 in men with high-risk non-metastatic castration reistant prostate cancer. ESMO Congress; September 2012; Vienna, Austria. Abstract 920P.
44. Fizazi K, Bono P, Jones RH, et al. An open-label, phase I/II safety, pharmacokinetic, and proof-of concept study of ODM-201 in patients with progressive metastatic castration-resistant prostate cancer (CRPC). European Cancer Congress 2013; September 27–October 1, 2013; Amsterdam, the Netherlands. Abstract2853.
45. Garcia JA, Kataja VV, James ND, et al. Bone and soft tissue response from a phase I/II study with ODM 201 in metastatic castration-resistant prostate cancer (mCRPC) [abstract 102]. *J Clin Oncol.* 2014;32(suppl 4).
46. Loddick SA, Ross SJ, Thomason AG, et al. AZD3514: a small molecule that modulates androgen receptor signaling and function in vitro and in vivo. *Mol Cancer Ther.* 2013;12:1715–1727.
47. Omlin A, Jones RJ, van der Noll R, et al. A first-in-human study of the oral selective androgen receptor down-regulating drug (SARD) AZD3514 in patients with castration-resistant prostate cancer (CRPC) [abstract 4511]. *J Clin Oncol.* 2013;31(suppl).
48. Vasaitis T, Belosay A, Schayowitz A, et al. Androgen receptor inactivation contributes to antitumor efficacy of 17{alpha}-hydroxylase/17,20-lyase inhibitor 3beta-hydroxy-17-(1H-benzimidazole-1-yl)androsta-5,16-diene in prostate cancer. *Mol Cancer Ther.* 2008;7:2348–2357.
49. Montgomery RB, Eisenberger MA, Rettig M, et al. Phase I clinical trial of galeterone (TOK-001), a multifunctional antiandrogen and CYP17 inhibitor in castration resistant prostate cancer (CRPC) [abstract 4665]. *J Clin Oncol.* 2012;30(suppl).
50. Taplin ME, Montgomery RB; ARMOR2 Group. ARMOR2: galeterone in progressive CRPC patients who have failed oral therapy [abstract 71]. *J Clin Oncol.* 2014;32(suppl 4).
51. Mostaghel EA, Marck BT, Plymate SR, et al. Resistance to CYP17A1 inhibition with abiraterone in castration-resistant prostate cancer: induction of steroidogenesis and androgen receptor splice variants. *Clin Cancer Res.* 2011;17:5913–5925.

19.4.1 *Radiation and the Immune System*

ANDREW SHARABI
CHARLES DRAKE

■ INTRODUCTION

Classically, the effects of radiotherapy are believed to induce killing of tumor cells through direct and indirect DNA damage leading to cell cycle arrest and mitotic catastrophe (1). Effective tumor control is obtained by reaching a dose high enough to induce sufficient lethal DNA damage in every tumor cell clone within the radiation field. For prostate cancer, radiotherapy dose escalation has been shown in multiple randomized trials to improve biochemical progression-free survival (2–4), likely as a result of eradicating residual prostate cancer clones. However, there is now a growing body of literature suggesting that in addition to DNA damage, radiation may modulate the immune system and induce antitumor immune responses (5–16). Recent data have shown that radiotherapy can activate antigen-presenting cells and induce T cell–mediated antitumor immune responses (8,10–14). Furthermore, multiple groups have shown that when radiotherapy is combined with immunotherapy, there can be enhanced systemic responses outside of the radiation field, termed abscopal effects (6,16–20). Here, we review the literature related to the general effects of radiotherapy on the immune system as well as the role of combining radiotherapy with immunotherapy. We divide the actions of radiotherapy into direct effects acting on cells of the immune system versus indirect effects acting on the tumor cells.

■ RADIATION AND THE IMMUNE SYSTEM

Traditionally, radiotherapy has been believed to have a negative effect on the immune system, potentially by directly killing or inactivating leukocytes within the radiation field (21). Evidence of this immunosuppressive effect comes from studies of whole body irradiation or large radiotherapy fields encompassing substantial proportions of bone marrow or lymphoid organs (22,23). However, recent studies have countered these findings and instead suggest that high-dose focused radiotherapy has the potential to enhance and boost immune responses. The mechanism behind this enhancement is not fully understood but believed to involve the release of tumor antigens during inflammatory cell death, activation of dendritic cells, and/or recruitment of effector T-cell populations. The effects of radiotherapy on the immune system and antitumor immune responses can be divided into direct effects versus indirect effects. Here, we refer to direct effects as the impact of radiotherapy directly on cells of the immune system (i.e., antigen-presenting cell [APC], T cells, B cells). We categorize indirect effects as immunomodulation brought about by radiation on tumor cells.

Professional APC includes dendritic cells, macrophages, and B cells. Among APCs, dendritic cells are the most potent due to their extensive dendrite morphology and high concentration of major histocompatibility complex (MHC)–antigen complexes and co-stimulatory molecules including CD80, CD86, and CD70. This is important because MHC–antigen complexes are the signal 1 required for T-cell activation. Signal 2 represents the co-stimulatory cell surface molecules (e.g., CD80, CD86), which are also required for initial T-cell licensing and activation. Thus, many groups have used dendritic cell vaccines as an approach to boost antitumor immune responses. However, aggressive prostate cancers develop multiple mechanisms of overcoming and suppressing the immune system, including decreased antigen expression, expression and secretion of inhibitory surface molecules or cytokines, and recruitment of suppressor populations (24–27). Furthermore, in the setting of central and peripheral self-tolerance, the repertoire of antigen-specific cytotoxic T cells may already be deleted, anergic, or converted and tolerized (28). Thus, major hurdles must be overcome to induce a robust and efficacious immune response in the face of considerable inhibitory regulation.

One of the first studies to investigate the role of the immune system in the effects of radiotherapy was published in 1979 by Stone et al. (29). This study used fibrosarcoma tumors induced in over 500 mice to address the question whether the status of the host immune system impacts the dose of radiotherapy required to control fibrosarcoma tumors. Four groups of mice were studied. Two groups of mice had their immune systems suppressed by either whole body radiation (WBI) or thymectomy at 8 weeks of age followed by WBI and reconstitution with whole bone marrow cells. A third group of mice had their immune systems stimulated with attenuated *Corynebacterium parvum*. The authors reported significant differences in the dose of radiotherapy required to control 50% of the tumors between the groups. Control mice required a dose of 3,040 rads (confidence interval [CI] 2,850–3,240, $n = 296$), where immunosuppressed mice required higher doses of 5,080 rads (CI 4,760–5,430, $n = 55$) or 6,450 rads (CI 6,200–6,710, $n = 80$). Furthermore, mice with activated immune systems required a significantly lower dose of 1,530 rads (CI 1,160–2,020, $n = 142$) to control the tumors. They then performed rechallenge experiments using mice that were cured from the initial treatment and observed multiple spontaneous rejections in all groups except the mice immunosuppressed with WBI. This early work provides substantial evidence that the status of the host immune system plays an important role in the therapeutic effects of radiotherapy.

More recent studies have elaborated on these findings, isolating the cell populations required for this effect and identifying mechanistic effects of radiation on tumor cells and cells of the immune system. For example, Lugade et al. used a mouse model of B16 melanoma expressing the model antigen ovalbumin and reported that mice irradiated with 15 Gy ×1 or 5 Gy ×3 had increased tumor-associated antigen presentation and T-cell activation in the draining lymph node (15). Additionally, radiotherapy resulted in an increase in tumor infiltrating lymphocytes, which they showed was most likely due to increased trafficking of T cells to the tumor (15). Interestingly, the single dose of 15 Gy was superior in inducing these immune responses when compared to the fractionated schedule, although it is known from radiobiology principles and biologically equivalent dose calculations that 15 Gy ×1 is not equivalent to 5 Gy ×3. Nevertheless, this study was one of the first to demonstrate that radiotherapy alone is capable of inducing antigen-specific antitumor immune responses.

Mechanistically, Reits et al. from the National Cancer Institute (NCI) studied the effects of radiotherapy on MHC class I antigen presentation (14). They showed that radiotherapy alone increased the cell surface expression of MHC class I on melanoma cells in a dose-dependent manner. This is a critical finding because MHC class I is the molecule directly recognized by classical cytotoxic CD8 T cells. Molecularly, they reported that radiotherapy resulted in increased degradation of existing cellular proteins that increased the intracellular peptide pool (14). Subsequent activation of mammalian target of rapamycin (MTOR) then resulted in enhanced protein translation and antigen presentation. Intriguingly, they also demonstrated that radiotherapy can result in the production of novel proteins with distinct epitopes loaded into MHC class I, which are recognizable by CD8 T cells (14). This study provides important mechanistic rationale for the ability of radiotherapy to enhance tumor-associated antigen presentation.

If radiotherapy increases the expression of MHC on the surface of tumor cells, this raises the following question: Are irradiated human tumor cells more susceptible to cytotoxic T cells and immune-mediated cell death? This question was addressed in a study published in *Cancer Research* by Garnett et al. (30). The authors analyzed the effects of radiotherapy on 23 human cell lines, including 12 colon, 7 lung, and 4 prostate lines. They found that at 72 hours after irradiation, 91% of the cell lines (21 of 23) increased expression of cell surface molecules involved in immune-mediated cytotoxicity, including Fas, major histocompatibility complex (MHC), and intercellular adhesion molecule 1 (ICAM-1). They then showed that radiotherapy significantly increased the susceptibility of tumor cells to immune-mediated cell death from antigen-specific CD8 T cells using cytotoxicity assays. These findings provide powerful evidence for the ability of radiotherapy to increase the susceptibility of tumor cells to immune-mediated recognition and cell death.

The importance of CD8 T cells was also addressed by the groups of Ralph Weichselbaum and Yang-Xin Fu from University of Chicago in a study entitled: "Therapeutic Effects of Ablative Radiation on Local Tumor Require CD8^{+} T Cells: Changing Strategies for Cancer Treatment" (13). In this study, the authors used a B16 melanoma model to study the ability of radiotherapy to induce antigen-specific antitumor immune responses. Wild-type C57B/6 mice were injected SQ with 10^5 B16 melanoma cells and treated 14 days later with 15 Gy with or without CD8 T-cell depletion using 200 µg of anti-CD8 antibody 0, 4, and 8 days after radiation therapy (RT). They reported that the mice receiving RT plus CD8 depletion had significantly increased tumor size and decreased survival compared to RT alone group ($P < .007$ at day 14 and $P < .001$, respectively) (13). They subsequently went on to show that radiotherapy enhanced the proliferation of antigen-specific T cells in the tumor draining lymph node. This effect was not seen using chemotherapy alone and was diminished in the chemotherapy combined with radiotherapy group compared to radiotherapy alone. These findings run counter to the classical teaching that the effects of radiotherapy are mediated via DNA damage alone in either tumor cells or tumor stroma. Instead, they suggest a new paradigm where CD8 T cells may be induced by radiotherapy and contribute to tumor control.

Studies have also been undertaken looking at the direct effects of radiotherapy on APCs of the immune system. Gupta et al. analyzed the effects of a single dose of 10 Gy on dendritic cell function and how that correlated with the efficacy of radiotherapy (8). By using a MC38 colorectal cancer model and a B16 melanoma model, they reported that the ability of radiotherapy to control tumor growth was actually dependent on both CD8 T cells and CD11c+ dendritic cells, but not on CD4 T cells or macrophages. In other words, depletion of CD8 cells or CD11c cells blocked the ability of radiation to slow tumor growth. They subsequently showed that a single dose of 10 Gy increased activation and expression of co-stimulatory molecules CD86 and CD70 on the cell surface of dendritic cells. Given that dendritic cells play a critical upstream role in cross-presentation of tumor antigens and induction of adaptive immune responses, it is logical that they too would play a key role in the immune-modulating effects of radiotherapy.

Taken together these corroborating studies from multiple different groups provide solid evidence for the ability of radiotherapy to induce antitumor immune responses and that these immune responses may contribute to tumor control. Furthermore, these findings open up exciting new avenues for research and provide mechanistic rational for combining radiotherapy with immunotherapy.

■ CELL-BASED IMMUNOTHERAPY AND RADIATION

Recently, the field of immunotherapy has gained significant interest as basic science discoveries have been translated to Food and Drug Administration (FDA)–approved clinical therapies. It is now widely accepted that the immune system plays a critical role in tumor biology, as described by the three Es of cancer immunoediting: elimination, equilibrium, and escape (31). The term elimination represents the classical paradigm of immunosurveillance, where the immune system is seeking and eradicating cells that have undergone malignant transformation. Equilibrium represents a dynamic state potentially lasting years where malignant cells under internal and external stress adapt and respond to survive while interacting and modulating the immune system. Tumor escape denotes a phase where select cancer cells have overcome barriers to continued growth and can proliferate and spread in an immunocompetent host. As these interactions between the immune system and cancer cells become better understood, additional targets and strategies for immunomodulation have been discovered and translated for clinical benefit.

After many years of basic science and clinical research, Sipuleucel-T (Provenge, Dendreon Corp.) was approved by FDA in 2010 for prostate cancer and was the first therapeutic dendritic cell–based vaccine approved for any cancer type. Sipuleucel-T is a dendritic cell vaccine generated from the patient's autologous peripheral blood mononuclear cells (PBMCs). It is FDA approved for minimally symptomatic metastatic castrate-resistant prostate cancer (mCRPC). PBMC are cultured ex vivo with a prostatic acid phosphatase (PAP)–granulocyte-macrophage colony-stimulating factor (GM-CSF) fusion and are then re-infused back into the patient. PAP is an enzyme that functions to dephosphorylate macromolecules in human prostate tissues and is an antigenic biomarker of prostate cancer (32). GM-CSF is a powerful hematopoietic growth factor with pleotropic ability to enhance dendritic cell maturation and function by activating key signaling pathways including canonical nuclear factor-κB, JAK/STAT, and mitogen-activated protein kinases (MAPK) (33). Thus, the aim of this fusion protein is to induce an antigen-specific antitumor immune response against PAP with GM-CSF providing cytokine co-stimulation.

Along these lines, GM-CSF has also been used in studies combined with radiotherapy to evaluate for any potential synergy. In a study by Wada et al., transgenic adenocarcinoma of the mouse prostate (TRAMP) mice were used to study the effects of radiotherapy combined with a GM-CSF cell–based vaccine on development of antitumor immune responses (34). TRAMP mice spontaneously develop prostate adenocarcinoma and serve as an excellent autochthonous mouse model for prostate cancer. In this study, the TRAMP mice were engineered to express the model antigen hemaglutinin (HA) under a prostate-specific probasin promoter for the purposes of tracking antigen-specific immune responses (ProHA/TRAMP mice). Interestingly, ProHA/TRAMP mice treated with stereotactic radiotherapy in combination with the GM-CSF–secreting cell-based vaccine showed decreased tumor bulk and pathologic grade compared to radiotherapy or immunotherapy alone (34). Additionally, the combined treatment improved survival of the mice in a metastatic model and also increased the ratio of CD8 and CD4 T-effector to T-regulatory cells within the prostate tumors. Note that in this study, the radiotherapy was delivered precisely using computed tomography–based image guidance present on the small animal radiation research platform (SARRP). By using the SARRP, the authors also investigated the effect of radiation dose on the presence of HA-specific T cells within the prostate tumors and found that 12 Gy ×1 appeared to be the optimal for this mouse model. This study supports the use of radiotherapy combined with immunotherapy for potentiating immune responses and improving local control. These data also highlight the importance of timing and radiotherapy dose effects, which deserve further investigation.

■ CHECKPOINT BLOCKADE COMBINED WITH RADIOTHERAPY—THE ABSCOPAL EFFECT

Much of the recent attention that immunotherapy has received has centered on clinical results from studies incorporating checkpoint blockade. The immune system is very powerful and when dysregulated can cause severe damage to the host as evidenced by autoimmune disease or cytokine storm. Thus, to maintain homeostasis, powerful mechanisms and checkpoints must exist to control and negatively regulate the immune system. Checkpoint blockade mainly refers to the use of monoclonal antibodies that target these negative regulators and block their function. In other words, blocking or removing the brakes on the immune system leads to increased activation. One of the most powerful regulatory mechanisms that dampens or shuts down T-cell responses are immune checkpoint receptor molecules expressed on the T-cell surface, including cytotoxic T-lymphocyte antigen 4 (CTLA-4) and programmed cell death 1 (PD-1) (35,36) (Figure 19.4.1.1). Monoclonal antibodies against CTLA-4 and PD-1 now have demonstrated clinical efficacy in multiple different tumor types and are currently in phase III development in non–small-cell lung carcinoma (NSCLC), renal cell carcinoma, and melanoma (37,38).

When radiotherapy is combined with checkpoint blockade, there is growing preclinical data in animal models as well as clinical case reports of robust immune responses and durable systemic tumor control (17–20). Interestingly, this provocative evidence suggests that antitumor immune responses induced by radiotherapy can act at distant sites outside of the radiation field, termed the abscopal effect (Figure 19.4.1.2). Originally coined by Dr. R. H. Mole in 1953, the abscopal effect refers to an effect of radiation outside the radiation field ("Ab" means "away," while "scopal" refers to the "target," thus away from target)(39). Silvia Formenti and Sandra Demaria from New York University have pioneered combining radiotherapy with checkpoint blockade and have investigated the abscopal effect in animal models and clinical

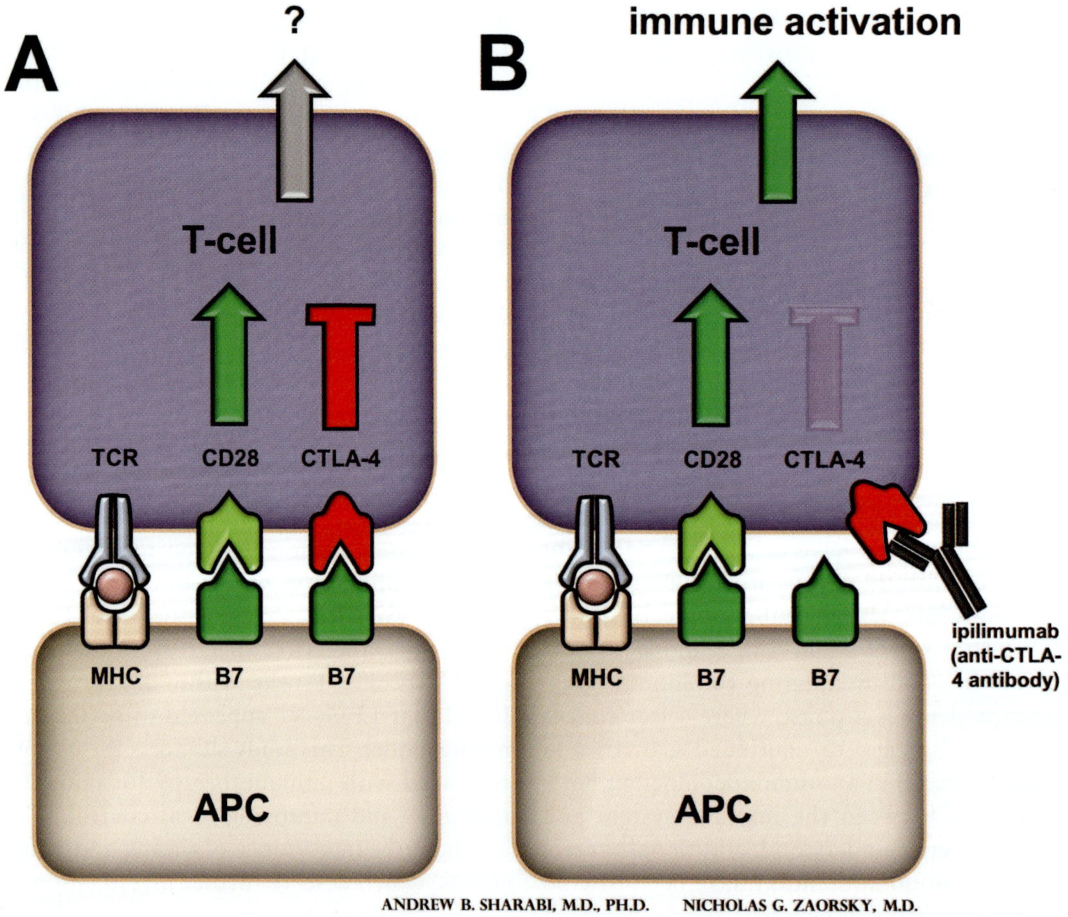

FIGURE 19.4.1.1 One of the most powerful regulatory mechanisms which dampens or shuts down T-cell responses are immune checkpoint receptor molecules expressed on the T-cell surface (e.g., cytotoxic T-lymphocyte antigen 4 [CTLA-4]). (A) Binding of B7 (on an antigen-presenting cell [APC]) to CTLA-4 (on a T cell) abrogates immune activation (inhibitory [red] signal and stimulatory [green arrow] signal result in neutral response [grey arrow]). (B) An anti-CTLA-4 antibody (e.g., ipilimumab) prevents binding of B7 to CTLA-4, thereby decreasing the abrogation (faded red signal).

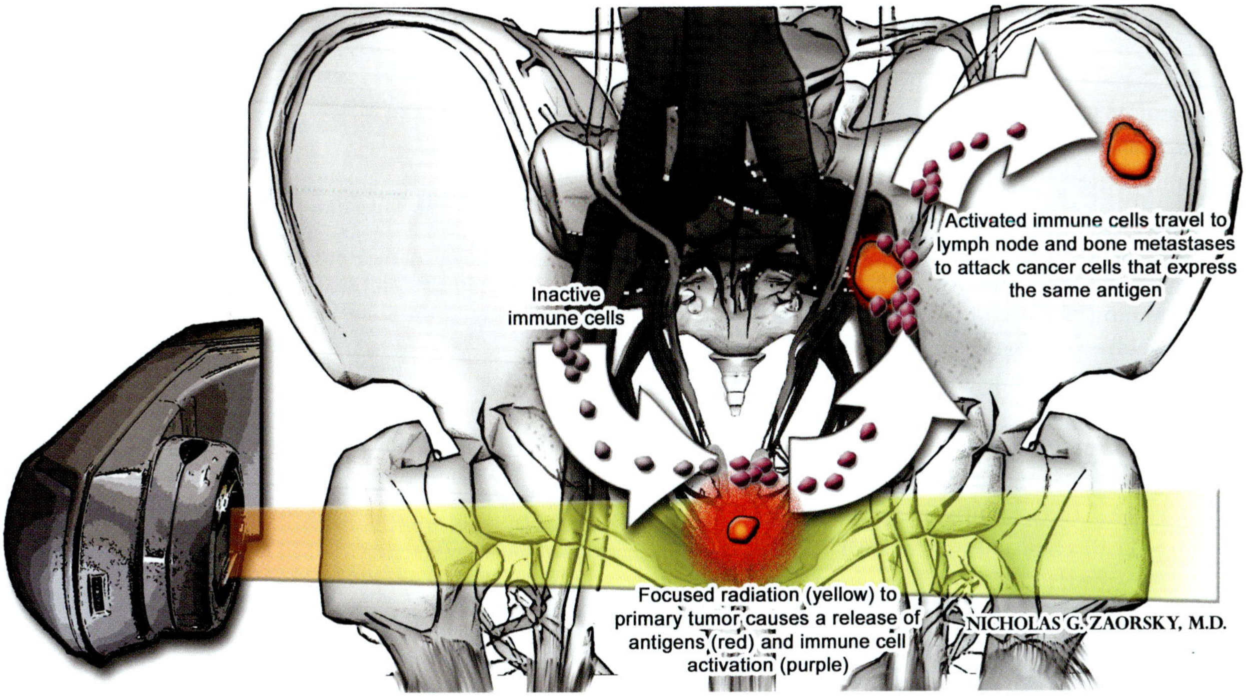

FIGURE 19.4.1.2 Antitumor immune responses induced by radiotherapy can act at distant sites outside the radiation field, termed the abscopal effect.

trials. In a study published in 2009, Dewan et al. analyzed the effects of CTLA-4 blockade combined with various radiation dose and fractionation schemes on TSA breast carcinoma and MC38 colorectal carcinoma models (20). By using a model developed to test for the abscopal effect, they established tumors in the bilateral flanks of mice and treated the primary tumor with radiotherapy while shielding the secondary opposite tumor. Thus, in this model, any distant or abscopal effects of radiotherapy on the secondary shielded tumor could be evaluated and compared to control or systemic treatment alone. The authors reported that using the 9H10 monoclonal antibody against CTLA-4 alone or radiotherapy alone had no effect on the secondary shielded tumors. However, radiotherapy combined with anti-CTLA-4 Ab resulted in an abscopal effect with significant growth inhibition of the contralateral shielded tumor ($P < .01$) (20). Furthermore, they reported that the inhibition of the secondary contralateral tumors was proportional to the frequency of tumor-specific interferon-gamma-positive CD8 T cells. Interestingly, they evaluated the effect of varying the radiation dose and fractionation used and reported that fractionated radiotherapy of 8 Gy ×3 was significantly more effective in inducing the abscopal effect compared to single dose of 20 Gy ×1. This study serves as a key reference and provides critical preclinical evidence of improved local and distant tumor control when radiotherapy is combined with checkpoint blockade immunotherapy.

A study published by an independent group in Chicago evaluated the effects of radiotherapy combined with blockade of programmed cell death ligand 1 (PD-L1) in TUBO breast carcinoma and MC38 colorectal carcinoma (17). They reported that PD-L1 was upregulated in the tumor microenvironment after irradiation and that anti-PD-L1 antibody (clone 10F.9G2; Bio-X Cell) enhanced the efficacy of radiotherapy (12 Gy ×1), also resulting in an abscopal effect (17). Note that they showed that depleting CD8 T cells abrogated this synergy, demonstrating again the dependence of the immune system for the abscopal effect. Other groups have described similar abscopal effects in different cell types including hepatocellular carcinoma and pancreatic adenocarcinoma (40,41). Thus, further investigation and clinical trials are needed to determine whether these preclinical findings can be reproduced and observed in patients.

In this regard, clinical trials have been performed incorporating anti-CTLA-4 antibody (ipilimumab) with radiotherapy for mCRPC (42,43), based on preclinical evidence of synergistic activity. A phase I/II study evaluated ipilimumab alone or in combination with radiotherapy (8 Gy ×1) for mCRPC (43). Thirty-three patients received ipilimumab at 3, 5, or 10 mg/kg every 3 weeks for four doses or 3 or 10 mg/kg combined with radiotherapy. The high-dose ipilimumab cohort of 10 mg/kg was expanded to 50 patients. Ipilimumab is known to have immune-related adverse events, which were observed, including diarrhea, colitis, rash, and pruritus. There was 16% grade 3/4 colitis and 10% grade 3/4 hepatitis, as well as one treatment-related death. In the group of patients receiving 10 mg/kg ± radiotherapy, they reported that eight patients had a prostate-specific antigen decline of ≥ 50%, one with complete response and six with stable disease. A larger multicenter, randomized, double-blind phase III study randomly assigned patients with mCRPC to receive bone-directed radiotherapy (8 Gy ×1) followed by ipilimumab at 10 mg/kg or placebo every 3 weeks for up to four doses (42). Seven hundred and ninety-nine patients were randomized with 399 in the ipilimumab group and 400 in the placebo group. The authors reported a median overall survival of 11.2 months in the patients receiving ipilimumab (95% CI 9.5–12.7) versus 10.0 months in patients receiving placebo (CI 8.3–11.0) resulting in a hazard ratio of 0.85 (0.72–1.00; P = .053) (42). Common immune-related adverse events include diarrhea, fatigue, anemia, and colitis. These results did not show a significant improvement in overall survival, although there were signs of clinical activity that may warrant further investigation. Note that preclinical data suggest that the ability of radiotherapy to synergize with immunotherapy depends on dose, fractionation, and potentially timing of treatments. Regarding radiotherapy dose, it is possible that doses higher than 8 Gy are needed to induce significant immune responses or possibly combining immunotherapy with anti-CTLA-4 and anti-PD-1/PD-L1 antibodies. Furthermore, the sequencing and fractionation scheme used could also potentially influence immunologic responses, and this area is a focus of active investigation.

■ CONCLUSION

It is becoming clear that the immune system plays a critical role in managing and controlling multiple different tumor types. Harnessing the power of the immune system using immunotherapy is now recognized as a viable cancer treatment that can improve clinical outcomes and lead to durable responses. Although radiotherapy has traditionally been believed to be immunosuppressive, there is now a substantial body of preclinical evidence demonstrating that radiotherapy can induce antigen-specific antitumor immune responses and synergize with immunotherapy. Furthermore, these antitumor immune responses can act at distant sites outside the radiation field and help to improve distant tumor control, termed the abscopal effect. As immunotherapy is developed as a potential fourth pillar of cancer therapy along with surgery, chemotherapy, and radiation, further studies are required to understand how to best incorporate immunotherapy into current treatment paradigms especially with regard to radiation dose, fractionation, and timing.

■ REFERENCES

1. Ward JF. DNA damage produced by ionizing radiation in mammalian cells: identities, mechanisms of formation, and reparability. *Prog Nucleic Acid Res Mol Biol*. 1988;35:95–125.
2. Kuban DA, Tucker SL, Dong L, et al. Long-term results of the M. D. Anderson randomized dose-escalation trial for prostate cancer. *Int J Radiat Oncol Biol Phys*. 2008;70(1):67–74.
3. Zietman AL, DeSilvio ML, Slater JD, et al. Comparison of conventional-dose vs high-dose conformal radiation therapy in clinically localized adenocarcinoma of the prostate: a randomized controlled trial. *JAMA*. 2005;294(10):1233–1239.
4. Pollack A, Zagars GK, Smith LG, et al. Preliminary results of a randomized radiotherapy dose-escalation study comparing 70 Gy with 78 Gy for prostate cancer. *J Clin Oncol*. 2000;18(23):3904–3911.
5. Liang H, Deng L, Chmura S, et al. Radiation-induced equilibrium is a balance between tumor cell proliferation and T cell-mediated killing. *J Immunol*. 2013;190(11):5874–5881.
6. Schaue D, Ratikan JA, Iwamoto KS, McBride WH. Maximizing tumor immunity with fractionated radiation. *Int J Radiat Oncol Biol Phys*. 2012;83(4):1306–1310.
7. Rubner Y, Wunderlich R, Rühle PF, et al. How does ionizing irradiation contribute to the induction of anti-tumor immunity? *Front Oncol*. 2012;2:75.
8. Gupta A, Probst HC, Vuong V, et al. Radiotherapy promotes tumor-specific effector CD8+ T cells via dendritic cell activation. *J Immunol*. 2012;189(2):558–566.
9. Demaria S, Formenti SC. Radiation as an immunological adjuvant: current evidence on dose and fractionation. *Front Oncol*. 2012;2:153.
10. Burnette BC, Liang H, Lee Y, et al. The efficacy of radiotherapy relies upon induction of type i interferon-dependent innate and adaptive immunity. *Cancer Res*. 2011;71(7):2488–2496.
11. Takeshima T, Chamoto K, Wakita D, et al. Local radiation therapy inhibits tumor growth through the generation of tumor-specific CTL: its potentiation by combination with Th1 cell therapy. *Cancer Res*. 2010;70(7):2697–2706.
12. Perez CA, Fu A, Onishko H, Hallahan DE, Geng L. Radiation induces an antitumour immune response to mouse melanoma. *Int J Radiat Biol*. 2009;85(12):1126–1136.
13. Lee Y, Auh SL, Wang Y, et al. Therapeutic effects of ablative radiation on local tumor require CD8+ T cells: changing strategies for cancer treatment. *Blood*. 2009;114(3):589–595.
14. Reits EA, Hodge JW, Herberts CA, et al. Radiation modulates the peptide repertoire, enhances MHC class I expression, and induces successful antitumor immunotherapy. *J Exp Med*. 2006;203(5):1259–1271.
15. Lugade AA, Moran JP, Gerber SA, Rose RC, Frelinger JG, Lord EM. Local radiation therapy of B16 melanoma tumors increases the generation of tumor antigen-specific effector cells that traffic to the tumor. *J Immunol*. 2005;174(12):7516–7523.
16. Demaria S, Ng B, Devitt ML, et al. Ionizing radiation inhibition of distant untreated tumors (abscopal effect) is immune mediated. *Int J Radiat Oncol Biol Phys*. 2004;58(3):862–870.
17. Deng L, Liang H, Burnette B, et al. Irradiation and anti-PD-L1 treatment synergistically promote antitumor immunity in mice. *J Clin Invest*. 2014;124(2):687–695.
18. Formenti SC, Demaria S. Combining radiotherapy and cancer immunotherapy: a paradigm shift. *J Natl Cancer Inst*. 2013;105(4):256–265.
19. Postow MA, Callahan MK, Barker CA, et al. Immunologic correlates of the abscopal effect in a patient with melanoma.pdf. *N Engl J Med*. 2012;366:925–931.
20. Dewan MZ, Galloway AE, Kawashima N, et al. Fractionated but not single-dose radiotherapy induces an immune-mediated abscopal effect when combined with anti-CTLA-4 antibody. *Clin Cancer Res*. 2009;15(17):5379–5388.

21. Merrick A, Errington F, Milward K, et al. Immunosuppressive effects of radiation on human dendritic cells: reduced IL-12 production on activation and impairment of naive T-cell priming. *Br J Cancer.* 2005;92(8):1450–1458.
22. Blomgren H, Edsmyr F, Näslund I, Petrini B, Wasserman J. Distribution of lymphocyte subsets following radiation therapy directed to different body regions. *Clin Oncol.* 1983;9(4):289–298.
23. Raben M, Walach N, Galili U, Schlesinger M. The effect of radiation therapy on lymphocyte subpopulations in cancer patients. *Cancer.* 1976;37(3):1417–1421.
24. Ebelt K, Babaryka G, Figel AM, et al. Dominance of CD4+ lymphocytic infiltrates with disturbed effector cell characteristics in the tumor microenvironment of prostate carcinoma. *Prostate.* 2008;68(1):1–10.
25. Degl'Innocenti E, Grioni M, Capuano G, et al. Peripheral T-cell tolerance associated with prostate cancer is independent from CD4+CD25+ regulatory T cells. *Cancer Res.* 2008;68(1):292–300.
26. Anderson MJ, Shafer-Weaver K, Greenberg NM, Hurwitz AA. Tolerization of tumor-specific T cells despite efficient initial priming in a primary murine model of prostate cancer. *J Immunol.* 2007;178(3):1268–1276.
27. Drake CG, Doody AD, Mihalyo MA, et al. Androgen ablation mitigates tolerance to a prostate/prostate cancer-restricted antigen. *Cancer Cell.* 2005;7(3):239–249.
28. Shafer-Weaver KA, Anderson MJ, Stagliano K, Malyguine A, Greenberg NM, Hurwitz AA. Cutting edge: tumor-specific CD8+ T cells infiltrating prostatic tumors are induced to become suppressor cells. *J Immunol.* 2009;183(8):4848–4852.
29. Stone HB, Peters LJ, Milas L. Effect of host immune capability on radiocurability and subsequent transplantability of a murine fibrosarcoma. *J Natl Cancer Inst.* 1979;63(5):1229–1235.
30. Garnett CT, Palena C, Chakraborty M, Tsang KY, Schlom J, Hodge JW. Sublethal irradiation of human tumor cells modulates phenotype resulting in enhanced killing by cytotoxic T lymphocytes. *Cancer Res.* 2004;64(21):7985–7994.
31. Dunn GP, Old LJ, Schreiber RD. The three Es of cancer immunoediting. *Annu Rev Immunol.* 2004;22:329–360.
32. Hassan MI, Aijaz A, Ahmad F. Structural and functional analysis of human prostatic acid phosphatase. *Expert Rev Anticancer Ther.* 2010;10(7):1055–1068.
33. van de Laar L, Coffer PJ, Woltman AM. Regulation of dendritic cell development by GM-CSF: molecular control and implications for immune homeostasis and therapy. *Blood.* 2012;119(15):3383–3393.
34. Wada S, Harris TJ, Tryggestad E, et al. Combined treatment effects of radiation and immunotherapy: studies in an autochthonous prostate cancer model. *Int J Radiat Oncol Biol Phys.* 2013;87(4):769–776.
35. Scalapino KJ, Daikh DI. CTLA-4: a key regulatory point in the control of autoimmune disease. *Immunol Rev.* 2008;223:143–155.
36. Zha Y, Blank C, Gajewski TF. Negative regulation of T-cell function by PD-1. *Crit Rev Immunol.* 2004;24(4):229–237.
37. Brahmer JR, Tykodi SS, Chow LQ, et al. Safety and activity of anti-PD-L1 antibody in patients with advanced cancer. *N Engl J Med.* 2012;366(26):2455–2465.
38. Hodi FS, O'Day SJ, McDermott DF, et al. Improved survival with ipilimumab in patients with metastatic melanoma. *N Engl J Med.* 2010;363(8):711–723.
39. Mole RH. Whole body irradiation; radiobiology or medicine? *Br J Radiol.* 1953;26(305):234–241.
40. Blanquicett C, Saif MW, Buchsbaum DJ, et al. Antitumor efficacy of capecitabine and celecoxib in irradiated and lead-shielded, contralateral human BxPC-3 pancreatic cancer xenografts: clinical implications of abscopal effects. *Clin Cancer Res.* 2005;11 (24 pt 1):8773–8781.
41. Cao ZA, Daniel D, Hanahan D. Sub-lethal radiation enhances anti-tumor immunotherapy in a transgenic mouse model of pancreatic cancer. *BMC Cancer.* 2002;2:11.
42. Kwon ED, Drake CG, Scher HI, et al. Ipilimumab versus placebo after radiotherapy in patients with metastatic castration-resistant prostate cancer that had progressed after docetaxel chemotherapy (CA184-043): a multicentre, randomised, double-blind, phase 3 trial. *Lancet Oncol.* 2014;15(7):700–712.
43. Slovin SF, Higano CS, Hamid O, et al. Ipilimumab alone or in combination with radiotherapy in metastatic castration-resistant prostate cancer: results from an open-label, multicenter phase I/II study. *Ann Oncol.* 2013;24(7):1813–1821.

Immunotherapy: Agents Targeting Prostate Cancer

19.4.2

GURVEEN KAUR
NAVEED H. AKHTAR
BEERINDER K. SINGH
SCOTT T. TAGAWA

■ INTRODUCTION

It is now recognized that evasion of an effective immune response is a hallmark of cancer (1). During the last decade, insights into the regulation of immune responses in malignancies have facilitated the emergence of novel immunotherapeutic treatment approaches, ranging from activation of innate and adaptive immune responses to neutralizing inhibitory responses (2). Immunotherapy may induce tumor cell death with a relatively high degree of specificity unlike chemotherapy, which has a nonspecific action. Prostate cancer (PC) is an ideal target for immunotherapy because of its indolent nature, which allows adequate time to activate the immune system (3). Identification of PC tumor-associated antigens (TAA) such as prostate-specific antigen (PSA), prostatic acid phosphatase (PAP), prostate stem cell antigen (PSCA), and prostate-specific membrane antigen (PSMA) has provided ideal targets for immunotherapy as they are largely prostate specific and their expression is strongly upregulated in PC, both locally and at metastatic sites (4–6). Targeting these TAAs is usually not associated with significant morbidity and adverse events as the prostate is not an essential organ (7, 8). In addition, early detection of recurrent disease with the help of PSA allows use of immunotherapy in patients with minimal tumor burden (9). This chapter will review various approaches to immunotherapy in the setting of PC (overview in Table 19.4.2.1).

■ THERAPEUTIC CANCER VACCINES

Dendritic Cell Vaccines

Sipuleucel-T (APC8015; Provenge, Dendreon Inc.) was the first therapeutic cancer vaccine approved by the FDA (10). Sipuleucel-T is an active autologous cellular immunotherapy, manufactured specifically for individual patients by isolating the patient's peripheral blood mononuclear cells (PBMCs), including antigen presenting cells (APCs) and T cells by leukapheresis and culturing the freshly isolated PBMCs with a fusion protein PA2024 composed of PAP linked to granulocyte-macrophage-colony stimulating factor (GM-CSF), an APC activator. PAP was selected as a target antigen because it is overexpressed in more than 95% of PCs (11) and epitopes of PAP are recognized by CD8+ T cells (12, 13). Upregulation of CD54 molecule occurs on the surface of APCs after the culture and it can be used as a marker to assess the maturation of APCs and hence theoretically the efficacy of sipuleucel-T (14), with clinical supporting evidence (10, 15). Once infused, the activated APCs tend to activate PAP-specific CD4+ and CD8+T cells, which migrate to the tumor lesions and initiate an antitumor immune response (16). Based on the encouraging results of sipuleucel-T in phase I/II clinical trials, a phase III study randomized 127 patients with minimally symptomatic castration-resistant prostate cancer (CRPC) 2:1 to receive sipuleucel-T or placebo. Although the study did not meet its primary endpoint of time to progression, a secondary endpoint of 4.5 month improvement in overall survival was reported on long-term follow-up (25.9 months vs. 21.4 months; $P = .01$) (17). To confirm these findings, a pivotal-randomized, placebo-controlled, multicenter phase III trial (IMPACT) randomized 512 patients with metastatic CRPC to sipuleucel-T or placebo with a primary end point of overall survival (10). Upon progression, subjects on the placebo arm could receive frozen product. A relative reduction of 22% in the risk of death (hazard ratio 0.78 [0.61–0.98 CI]; $P = .03$) and a 4.1 month improvement in the median survival (25.8 months vs. 21.7 months) was demonstrated, without improvement in PRS was reported (10). Sipuleucel-T is generally well tolerated with low-grade infusion related toxicities (consistent with release of cytokines) such as fevers, rigors, chills, headache, and nausea. Based on a combination of demonstrated effective therapeutic results plus the theory of targeting lower volume disease and increasing efficacy in metastatic disease, a number of additional clinical trials are ongoing (Table 19.4.2.3).

Table 19.4.2.1 Different immunotherapeutic approaches for prostate cancer

Immunologic Approach	Brief Description of Mechanism of Action	Agent
	Therapeutic cancer vaccines	
Dendritic cell vaccine	Autologous PBMCs (dendritic cells) cultured ex vivo against PAP designed to activate T-cells to initiate antitumor response	Sipuleucel-T
Viral vector vaccine	Semi-heterologous prime-boost approach poxviral vaccine result in PSA-specific T-cell activation and tumor cell killing	ProstVac-VF
DNA-based vaccine	PAP-specific CD4+ and CD8+ T-cell proliferation leads to antitumor response	pTVG-HP
Whole tumor cell vaccine	Irradiated replication defective prostate cancer cell lines genetically modified to secrete GM-CSF which activate APCs and hence T-cells to produce antitumor response	GVAX
Peptide-based vaccine	MUC-1 specific T-cell proliferation produces antitumor response	L-BLP25
	Checkpoint inhibitors	
Anti-CTLA-4 monoclonal antibody	Potentiation of T-cell-mediated antitumor response with the blockade of CTLA-4 immune checkpoint	Ipilimumab
Anti-PD-1 monoclonal antibody	Potentiation of antitumor immune response with blockade of PD-1 immune checkpoint	MDX-1106
	Monoclonal antibody–based immunotherapy	
Human monoclonal antibody as single agent	mAb blockade of RANK ligand	Denosumab
Radioimmunotherapy	mAb-directed targeting of beta-emitting radionuclides to PSMA-expressing cells	^{177}Lu-J591
Antibody-drug conjugate (ADC)	mAb directed targeting of toxin to PSMA-expressing cells	PSMA ADC

Viral Vector Vaccines

PSA-Tricom (ProstVac-VF™, developed by National Cancer Institute [NCI] and licensed to Bavarian Nordic, Washington, DC) is a PSA-directed viral vector vaccine. Viruses are selected as vectors because of several reasons: easy to engineer, can carry large amounts of genetic material, and there is good clinical experience with poxvirus vectors in worldwide eradication of small-pox, hence viral vectors can be safely administered without any risk of disruption of host DNA(18). The current vaccination regimen with ProstVac-VF consists of primary vaccination with recombinant poxvirus (vaccinia) vector, which is then followed by multiple booster vaccination with fowlpox vector, a semi-heterologous prime-boost approach(19).

Once injected subcutaneously, the poxvirus vectors should infect epithelial cells, some of which undergo lysis, releasing the encoded antigens and other cellular debris, which are taken up by the nearby immature APCs. The APCs become activated and express the PSA peptide within the MHC and result in PSA-specific T-cell activation(19,20). The newer generation of poxviral vaccines incorporated transgenes for a triad of costimulatory molecules called TRICOM including B7.1, leukocyte function associated antigen-3 (LFA-3), and intercellular adhesion molecule-1 (ICAM-1). Two randomized phase II trials have been carried out using the current version of vaccine in patients with metastatic CRPC (mCRPC) with monthly dosing of the vaccine until disease progression. The first study was a 125 patient placebo-controlled multicenter trial. As seen with sipuleucel-T, with longer-term follow up, the trial reported an overall survival benefit with 25 (30%) of 82 patients alive versus 7 (17%) of 40 controls alive at 3 years. An improvement in the median survival of 8.5 months (25.1 months with PSA-TRICOM vs. 16.6 months with placebo; $P = .0061$) was also observed (21). This was supported by a second study carried out by the NCI in 32 patients reporting a median survival of 26.6 months (22). Based on the promising results from these trials, a phase III study is underway (Table 19.4.2.3).

Encouraging evidence of enhanced antitumor response in various clinical models led to various clinical trials with DNA vaccines, including early phase clinical trials with pVAX/PSA DNA vaccine with GM-CSF and IL-2 adjuvants (23) and pTVG-HP plasmid DNA with GM-CSF (24). Based on the latter, a randomized phase II study has complete recruitment with final results pending (Table 19.4.2.3).

Whole Tumor Cell Vaccines

Initially, whole tumor cell vaccines were produced using the patient's own autologous tumor cells as they contained the patient-specific TAAs, so it precluded the need for antigen preselection. But this method presented with a number of difficulties—labor intensive, required a significant amount of patient tumor tissue, dilution of TAAs by other normal cellular components of tumor cells, and lack of standardization making measurement of vaccine-specific immune responses difficult (25–27). Therefore, because of the above reasons allogeneic tumor cell lines from various tumors, which are faster and easier to prepare, were used to produce whole tumor cell vaccines. GVAX (Cell Genesys, Inc) is a whole tumor cell vaccine consisting of two allogeneic PC cell lines (LNCaP and PC-3), which are irradiated to make them replication defective and genetically modified to produce GM-CSF (26,28,29). Initial studies demonstrated safety with interesting potential immunotherapeutic benefit (26,30), leading to two multicenter, randomized, controlled phase III trials, VITAL-1 and VITAL-2. VITAL-1 compared GVAX with docetaxel and prednisone in asymptomatic metastatic CRPC and VITAL-2 compared GVAX combined with docetaxel versus docetaxel and prednisone in symptomatic mCRPC. Unfortunately, both studies were essentially negative, but the approach of whole tumor vaccine remains of interest.

Peptide-Based Vaccines

Peptide vaccines consist of peptide antigens with appropriate HLA-restricted amino acid sequence. They are often combined with various adjuvants and cytokines to increase their immunogenicity, and substitution of amino acids may be performed to enhance the binding of tumor antigen epitopes with the MHC molecules (31). E75, an immunogenic HLA-A2-restricted peptide derived from the HER-2/neu protein demonstrated safety in high-risk PC patients in a phase I study (32) and is currently being used in a phase II study. L-BLP25, another peptide vaccine targeting exposed core peptides of MUC1 TAA has been used in 16 patients with PSA recurrence following radical prostatectomy and demonstrated MUC1-specific proliferative T-cell responses with a favorable alteration of PSA kinetics in six patients (33). MKC1106-PP is a vaccine composed of plasmid and peptide fragments of preferentially expressed antigen in melanoma (PRAME) and PSMA that demonstrated immune response in 15 of 24 evaluable subjects and stable disease with PSA decline in some of the subjects with PC (34).

■ IMMUNE CHECKPOINT BLOCKADE

Activation of T-cells require two simultaneous but independent signals: interaction between antigen and MHC on the APC plus a costimulatory molecule from the interaction of B7.1 (CD80) and B7.2 (CD86) present on the surface of APCs with the receptor CD28 present on T-cells (35–39). CTLA-4 is a protein homologue of CD28 that binds with B7 ligands with 50- to 200-fold higher affinity and negatively regulates T-cell responses, inhibiting recognition of self-antigens by T-cells and truncating the antitumor immune response (36,39–41). In addition, there are various accessory positive—OX-40 (CD134) (42,43), 4-1BB (CD137) (44), and inducible costimulator (37)–and negative—PD-1, B7-H3, or B7X (39) coregulators—that ultimately govern the fate of activated T-cells. Ipilimumab (MDX-010, Bristol Myers Squibb), a fully human anti-CTLA-4 monoclonal antibody, was approved by the FDA for advanced melanoma in early 2011 (45). Early studies of ipilimumab in PC yielded PSA declines as well as objective clinical responses (46,47). Based on these findings, two randomized phase III trials of ipilimumab have completed accrual in mCRPC (Table 19.4.2.2). The initially reported study included men with progressive mCRPC following docetaxel. Subjects received a single fraction (8 Gy) of radiation to a site of bone metastasis followed by induction, then maintenance ipilimumab or placebo with the primary endpoint of overall survival. Ipilimumab demonstrated a strong trend for survival benefit, but the study was negative overall with a hazard ratio for death of .85 [95% confidence interval .72 – 1.00, $P = .053$] (96). An interesting subset analysis revealed that men without visceral metastases had a survival benefit, leading to the hypothesis that men in the chemo-naïve phase III study may have a benefit from ipilimumab. In addition, several trials are focused on combining this agent with other therapies or using this agent in patients with an earlier

Table 19.4.2.2 Selected completed clinical trials with immunotherapy in prostate cancer patients

Agent	Clinical Trial Phase	Design of Trial (Ref.)	Number of Subjects	Results
Sipuleucel-T	III	Randomized, placebo-controlled trial of sipuleucel-T vs. placebo in asymptomatic mCRPC (D9901) (17)	127	Primary end point (TTP) not met, but secondary endpoint of improvement in overall survival demonstrated
Sipuleucel-T	III	Randomized, placebo-controlled trial of sipuleucel-T vs. placebo in asymptomatic mCRPC (IMPACT) (10)	512	Primary end point of OS met with 4.1 mon improvement in median survival and 22% reduction in the risk of death
Denosumab	III	Randomized, double-blind trial of denosumab vs. placebo in men receiving androgen deprivation therapy (62)	1468	Increased bone mineral density at all sites and a reduction in the incidence of new vertebral fractures
Denosumab	III	Randomized, double-blind study of denosumab vs. zoledronic acid for treatment of bone metastasis in men with mCRPC (63)	1904	Denosumab superior to zoledronic acid for prevention of skeletal-related events
Denosumab	III	Randomized, double-blind, placebo-controlled study of denosumab in men with nonmetastatic CRPC (64)	1432	Targeting of the bone microenvironment can delay bone metastasis in men with CRPC.
ProstVac-VF	II	Randomized, controlled trial of ProstVac-VF in mCRPC (21)	125	Primary endpoint of PFS not met, but 8.5 mon improvement in median OS demonstrated
pTVG-HP	I/IIa	Dose-escalation trial with PAP encoding DNA vaccine in D0 prostate cancer (24)	22	Increased PSA doubling time from a median 6.5 mon pretreatment to 8.5 mon on-treatment
GVAX	III	Randomized, open label trial of GVAX vs. docetaxel in asymptomatic mCRPC (VITAL-1) (93)	621	Unplanned interim analysis showed trial futility
GVAX	III	Randomized, open label trial of GVAX combined with docetaxel vs. docetaxel in symptomatic mCRPC (VITAL-2) (94)	114 (600 planned)	Planned interim analysis showed higher mortality in combined treatment group
Ipilimumab	I/II	Open-label, multicenter trial of ipilimumab alone or in combination with radiotherapy in mCRPC (95)	50	> 50% PSA declines and objective tumor responses reported in eight subjects with manageable adverse events

(continued)

Table 19.4.2.2 Selected completed clinical trials with immunotherapy in prostate cancer patients *(continued)*

Agent	Clinical Trial Phase	Design of Trial (Ref.)	Number of Subjects	Results
Ipilimumab	III	Randomized, placebo-controlled trial comparing low-dose radiation ipilimumab or placebo in mCRPC previously treated with docetaxel chemotherapy (96)	800	Negative for OS, but with strong trend: HR .85 [95% CI .72 – 1.00, $P = .053$]. Hypothesis generating subset analysis demonstrated OS benefit for men without visceral metastases.
^{177}Lu-J591	II	Single dose trial of ^{177}Lu-J591 in mCRPC (85)	47	PSA declines, CTC count declines, and dose response seen with excellent tumor targeting and reversible hematologic toxicity
PSMA ADC	I	Dose escalation study of PSMA ADC in taxane-refractory mCRPC (92)	52	Reductions in PSA or CTCs, particularly at higher doses

stage of disease (48–50). It is noteworthy that blockade of this critical immune checkpoint also resulted in a significant incidence (25%–35%) of clinically important immune-related toxicities, including colitis, neutropenia, dermatitis, pneumonitis, and a variety of endocrine disorders such as hypothyroidism and hypophysitis that may be severe, but are usually controllable when recognized early (51, 52).

Programmed cell death-1 (PD-1) is another immunological checkpoint that has recently been evaluated clinically in various clinical trials. PD-1 interacts with its ligand B7-H1 (PD-L1) and leads to inhibition of T-cell function (53–55). PD-1 blockade has been shown to potentiate antitumor immune response in various animal studies (56–58), which led to human clinical trials. To study the safety, clinical activity, pharmacodynamics, and immunologic correlates, two clinical trials have been completed with anti-PD-1 monoclonal antibodies in patients with different cancers including PC (59, 60). Anti-PD-1 seems to be well tolerated with rare but potentially fatal pneumonitis.

■ MONOCLONAL ANTIBODY–BASED IMMUNOTHERAPY

In 1975, Milstein and Kohler developed a method for isolating monoclonal antibodies (mAb) from hybridoma cells, leading to an intense interest. Through developments in de-immunization of mouse mAb to fully human mAb, many mAb have been approved in oncology. mAb bind to specific antigens and produce therapeutic response in one or more of the following ways: (a) antibody-dependent cellular cytotoxicity (ADCC) and complement dependent cytotoxicity (CDC), (b) blocking the activation signal (targeted therapy), (c) enhancing the development of active antitumor immune response or altering cytokine milieu (immunotherapy), and (d) signaling mediated by cross-linking tumor antigen that leads to cell death (61). The mAb may also be conjugated to act as vehicles to deliver the substances to specific cells based on antigen specificity.

Denosumab is a fully human monoclonal antibody against RANK-ligand and is the first mAb approved for PC indications. In an initial phase III study of low-dose denosumab (60 mg every six months), denosumab was superior to placebo in increasing bone density in men with nonmetastatic PC on androgen deprivation therapy (ADT) and also decreased fracture rate (62). In a phase III trial of patients with metastatic CRPC to bone, high-dose denosumab (120 mg every four weeks) was superior to zoledronic acid in delaying time to skeletal-related events (63). Interestingly, denosumab also significantly increased bone-metastasis-free survival in men with nonmetastatic CRPC, but based upon risk:benefit ratio and lack of overall survival difference, it was not approved by the FDA for this indication (64).

In addition to the mAbs discussed in sections above, additional mAbs have been investigated in human clinical trials. Bevacizumab, a mAb against vascular endothelial growth factor (VEGF), is built upon interesting correlative data and has been tested in combination with docetaxel chemotherapy in men with metastatic CRPC by CALGB investigators. Though an improvement in PFS and response rate was demonstrated, the primary endpoint of OS was negative (65). Several studies have demonstrated the association of IL-6 and PC outcome. Siltuximab is an anti-IL-6 mAb, which has been tested in three trials in PC. A phase I study of siltuximab in combination with docetaxel was tolerated with preliminary evidence of efficacy (66) but a phase II trial of single-agent siltuximab and a randomized trial of mitoxantrone with or without siltuximab did not meet their primary endpoints (67). Additional mAb have also been studied in PC (68–72). One mAb (J591), which has been in human clinical trials the longest, is discussed below.

■ PROSTATE-SPECIFIC MEMBRANE ANTIGEN (PSMA) TARGETED-MONOCLONAL ANTIBODIES

As an example of mAbs with a PC-specific target that have been studied in several different modalities, we will discuss the clinical development of anti-PSMA mAbs, including the J591 mAb. PSMA is a highly specific prostate epithelial cell membrane antigen that is present on most PC cells, with increased expression with higher grade and hormonal therapy (4, 73–79). PSMA represents an ideal target for mAb therapy as it is an integral cell-surface membrane protein and not a secretory protein like other prostate TAAs, such as PSA and PAP, and rapid internalization of the PSMA-antibody complex occurs. J591 is the first IgG anti-PSMA mAb developed for use in PC and it has been deimmunized (humanized) to allow for repeated dosing in patients; targeting (with trace-labeled ^{111}In-J591), safety, and induction of ADCC have been demonstrated (80, 81). In addition to initial single-agent use, J591 has been combined with low-dose IL-2. In a limited study, 17 men with recurrent PC received weekly infusions with J591 plus IL-2 subcutaneously (82). The regimen was generally well tolerated with a trend for those with NK cell expansion and in those with stable disease on treatment.

Because of the specificity of mAbs, they may be utilized as targeting agents for therapy or imaging. Radioimmunotherapy, the labeling of mAbs with radionuclides, has successfully been employed in lymphoma, and has been tested in PC using J591 and other mAbs. Phase I studies of radiolabeled J591 using ^{177}Lu and ^{90}Y provided safety and dosing data, with reversible myelosuppression as the dose-limiting toxicity (as expected with radioimmunotherapy) (83, 84). A phase II trial with a single dose infusion of ^{177}Lu in 47 men with metastatic CRPC confirmed efficacy, with PSA declines, circulating tumor cell count declines, and a dose-response relationship demonstrated (85). Myelosuppression was reported to a significant degree, but grade 4 thrombocytopenia and neutropenia was predictable and reversible. Additional studies of radiolabelled J591 are ongoing, including studies of dose fractionation and combination with docetaxel chemotherapy (86–88). An interesting Department of Defense–sponsored randomized phase II study is investigating the concept of salvage radioimmunotherapy in men with nonmetastatic CRPC with a rising PSA, utilizing the targeting ability of J591 with the physical properties of ^{177}Lu suited for micrometastatic disease (Table 19.4.2.3) (86, 89).

■ **Table 19.4.2.3** Selected ongoing clinical trials with immunotherapy in prostate cancer patients

Agent	Clinical Trial Phase	Design of Trial	Planned Enrollment	Purpose
Sipuleucel-T	II	Randomized, open label trial of sipuleucel-T with concurrent vs. sequential administration of abiraterone acetate in mCRPC (NCT01487863)	60	Plans to assess safety and cumulative sipuleucel-T CD54 upregulation
ProstVac-VF	II	Randomized trial of docetaxel with or without PSA-TRICOM vaccine in mCRPC (NCT01145508)	144	Primary endpoint is to compare the median overall survival
ProstVac-VF	II	Randomized trial combining ProstVac-VF and Flutamide vs. Flutamide alone in nonmetastatic CRPC (NCT00450463)	65	To compare time to treatment failure in the two groups
ProstVac-VF	III	Randomized, double-blind, efficacy trial of ProstVac-VF +/- GM-CSF in mCRPC (NCT01322490)	1200	To determine whether ProstVac alone or in combination with GM-CSF is effective in prolonging overall survival

(*continued*)

Table 19.4.2.3 Selected ongoing clinical trials with immunotherapy in prostate cancer patients *(continued)*

Agent	Clinical Trial Phase	Design of Trial	Planned Enrollment	Purpose
pTVG-HP	II	Pilot randomized two-arm study of a DNA vaccine encoding PAP in nonmetastatic CRPC (NCT00849121)	34	Intends to find out the safety and dosing schedule of vaccine, generation of long-lived immune responses, and prolongation of PSA doubling time
Ipilimumab	III	Randomized, double-blind trial of ipilimumab vs. placebo in asymptomatic or minimally symptomatic chemotherapy-naive mCRPC (NCT01057810)	600	Aims to compare the overall survival
^{177}Lu-J591	II	Randomized trial of ^{177}Lu-J591 and ketoconazole in patients with high-risk castrate biochemically relapsed prostate cancer after local therapy (NCT00859781)	140	To assess PSA response rate and proportion free of radiographically evident metastasis at the end of 18 mon

Targeted therapy to PC cells can also be delivered using antibody-drug conjugates (ADC). MLN2704 and PSMA ADC are examples of ADCs that have been evaluated clinically in PC patients. The initial generation of PSMA-directed ADCs (MLN2704) consisted of maytansinoid 1 (DM1), potent microtubule-depolymerizing compound, conjugated to J591 (90). Demonstration of activity in preclinical study led to phase I dose escalation (n = 23) and a subsequent multicenter phase I/II study (n = 62) with MLN2704 (90, 91). However, treatment was limited by toxicity due to disassociation of DM1 from the mAb, stressing the need for new and improvised linkers to J591 with enhanced tumor targeting. More recently, with an improvement in linker technology, safety and preliminary activity has been demonstrated with PSMA ADC, fully human antibody to PSMA linked to microtubule disrupting agent monomethyl auristatin E (MMAE). Preclinical success led to a phase I dose escalation study of PSMA ADC in taxane-refractory mCRPC, in which 52 patients received escalating doses demonstrating general safety and some PSA declines, leading to a large multicenter phase II study (Table 19.4.2.3) (92).

CONCLUSION

In summary, it is now recognized that the immune system plays an important part in the development and control of cancer. The specificity and potential durability of response makes immunotherapy in oncology quite promising. PC is associated with many favorable properties for immunotherapy and the first therapeutic cancer vaccine to be approved by the FDA was for men with metastatic castration-resistant PC. In addition to vaccines (dendritic cell, viral vectors, tumor cell vaccines, DNA, and peptide-based), blockade of checkpoint inhibitors and monoclonal antibody-based therapy are attractive in PC, and several late-stage clinical trials are completed or underway.

REFERENCES

1. Hanahan D, Weinberg RA. Hallmarks of cancer: the next generation. *Cell.* 2011;144(5):646–674.
2. Drake CG, Jaffee E, Pardoll DM. Mechanisms of immune evasion by tumors. *Adv Immunol.* 2006;90:51–81.
3. Coffey DS, Isaacs JT. Prostate tumor biology and cell kinetics–theory. *Urology.* 1981;17(suppl 3):40–53.
4. Wright GL Jr, Grob BM, Haley C, et al. Upregulation of prostate-specific membrane antigen after androgen-deprivation therapy. *Urology.* 1996;48(2):326–334.
5. Kawakami M, Nakayama J. Enhanced expression of prostate-specific membrane antigen gene in prostate cancer as revealed by in situ hybridization. *Cancer Res.* 1997;57(12):2321–2324.
6. Harada M, Noguchi M, Itoh K. Target molecules in specific immunotherapy against prostate cancer. *Int J Clin Oncol.* 2003;8(4):193–199.
7. Rhodes DR, Barrette TR, Rubin MA, et al. Meta-analysis of microarrays: interstudy validation of gene expression profiles reveals pathway dysregulation in prostate cancer. *Cancer Res.* 2002;62(15):4427–4433.
8. Fong L, Small EJ. Immunotherapy for prostate cancer. *Semin Oncol.* 2003;30(5):649–658.

9. Sharifi N, Gulley JL, Dahut WL. Androgen deprivation therapy for prostate cancer. *JAMA*. 2005;294(2):238–244.
10. Kantoff PW, Higano CS, Shore ND, et al. Sipuleucel-T immunotherapy for castration-resistant prostate cancer. *N Engl J Med*. 2010;363(5):411–422.
11. Jacobs EL, Haskell CM. Clinical use of tumor markers in oncology. *Curr Probl Cancer*. 1991;15(6):299–360.
12. Fong L, Ruegg CL, Brockstedt D, et al. Induction of tissue-specific autoimmune prostatitis with prostatic acid phosphatase immunization: implications for immunotherapy of prostate cancer. *J Immunol*. 1997;159(7):3113–3117.
13. Peshwa MV, Shi JD, Ruegg C, et al. Induction of prostate tumor-specific CD8+ cytotoxic T-lymphocytes in vitro using antigen-presenting cells pulsed with prostatic acid phosphatase peptide. *Prostate*. 1998;36(2):129–138.
14. Sheikh NA, Jones LA. CD54 is a surrogate marker of antigen presenting cell activation. *Cancer Immunol Immunother*. 2008;57(9):1381–1390.
15. Higano CS, Schellhammer PF, Small EJ, et al. Integrated data from 2 randomized, double-blind, placebo-controlled, phase 3 trials of active cellular immunotherapy with sipuleucel-T in advanced prostate cancer. *Cancer*. 2009;115(16):3670–3679.
16. Drake CG. Prostate cancer as a model for tumour immunotherapy. *Nat Rev Immunol*. 2010;10(8):580–593.
17. Small EJ, Schellhammer PF, Higano CS, et al. Placebo-controlled phase III trial of immunologic therapy with sipuleucel-T (APC8015) in patients with metastatic, asymptomatic hormone refractory prostate cancer. *J Clin Oncol*. 2006;24(19):3089–3094.
18. Arlen PM, Kaufman HL, DiPaola RS. Pox viral vaccine approaches. *Semin Oncol*. 2005;32(6):549–555.
19. Madan RA, Arlen PM, Mohebtash M, et al. Prostvac-VF: a vector-based vaccine targeting PSA in prostate cancer. *Expert Opin Invest Drugs*. 2009;18(7):1001–1011.
20. Essajee S, Kaufman HL. Poxvirus vaccines for cancer and HIV therapy. *Expert Opin Biol Ther*. 2004;4(4):575–588.
21. Kantoff PW, Schuetz TJ, Blumenstein BA, et al. Overall survival analysis of a phase II randomized controlled trial of a Poxviral-based PSA-targeted immunotherapy in metastatic castration-resistant prostate cancer. *J Clin Oncol*. 2010;28(7):1099–1105.
22. Gulley JL, Arlen PM, Madan RA, et al. Immunologic and prognostic factors associated with overall survival employing a poxviral-based PSA vaccine in metastatic castrate-resistant prostate cancer. *Cancer Immunol Immunother*. 2010;59(5):663–674.
23. Pavlenko M, Roos AK, Lundqvist A, et al. A phase I trial of DNA vaccination with a plasmid expressing prostate-specific antigen in patients with hormone-refractory prostate cancer. *Br J Cancer*. 2004;91(4):688–694.
24. McNeel DG, Dunphy EJ, Davies JG, et al. Safety and immunological efficacy of a DNA vaccine encoding prostatic acid phosphatase in patients with stage D0 prostate cancer. *J Clin Oncol*. 2009;27(25):4047–4054.
25. Tani K, Azuma M, Nakazaki Y, et al. Phase I study of autologous tumor vaccines transduced with the GM-CSF gene in four patients with stage IV renal cell cancer in Japan: clinical and immunological findings. *Mol Ther*. 2004;10(4):799–816.
26. Small EJ, Sacks N, Nemunaitis J, et al. Granulocyte macrophage colony-stimulating factor–secreting allogeneic cellular immunotherapy for hormone-refractory prostate cancer. *Clin Cancer Res*. 2007;13(13):3883–3891.
27. Schlom J, Arlen PM, Gulley JL. Cancer vaccines: moving beyond current paradigms. *Clin Cancer Res*. 2007;13(13):3776–3782.
28. Dranoff G, Jaffee E, Lazenby A, et al. Vaccination with irradiated tumor cells engineered to secrete murine granulocyte-macrophage colony-stimulating factor stimulates potent, specific, and long-lasting anti-tumor immunity. *Proc Natl Acad Sci U S A*. 1993;90(8):3539–3543.
29. Nguyen MC, Tu GH, Koprivnikar KE, et al. Antibody responses to galectin-8, TARP and TRAP1 in prostate cancer patients treated with a GM-CSF-secreting cellular immunotherapy. *Cancer Immunol Immunother*. 2010;59(9):1313–1323.
30. Higano CS, Corman JM, Smith DC, et al. Phase 1/2 dose-escalation study of a GM-CSF-secreting, allogeneic, cellular immunotherapy for metastatic hormone-refractory prostate cancer. *Cancer*. 2008;113(5):975–984.
31. Slingluff CL Jr, Petroni GR, Chianese-Bullock KA, et al. Immunologic and clinical outcomes of a randomized phase II trial of two multipeptide vaccines for melanoma in the adjuvant setting. *Clin Cancer Res*. 2007;13(21):6386–6395.
32. Hueman MT, Dehqanzada ZA, Novak TE, et al. Phase I clinical trial of a HER-2/neu peptide (E75) vaccine for the prevention of prostate-specific antigen recurrence in high-risk prostate cancer patients. *Clin Cancer Res*. 2005;11(20):7470–7479.
33. North SA, Graham K, Bodnar D, et al. A pilot study of the liposomal MUC1 vaccine BLP25 in prostate specific antigen failures after radical prostatectomy. *J Urol*. 2006;176(1):91–95.
34. Weber JS, Vogelzang NJ, Ernstoff MS, et al. A phase 1 study of a vaccine targeting preferentially expressed antigen in melanoma and prostate-specific membrane antigen in patients with advanced solid tumors. *J Immunother*. 2011;34(7):556–567.
35. Mueller DL, Jenkins MK, Schwartz RH. Clonal expansion versus functional clonal inactivation: a costimulatory signalling pathway determines the outcome of T cell antigen receptor occupancy. *Annu Rev Immunol*. 1989;7:445–480.
36. Chambers CA, Kuhns MS, Egen JG, et al. CTLA-4-mediated inhibition in regulation of T cell responses: mechanisms and manipulation in tumor immunotherapy. *Annu Rev Immunol*. 2001;19:565–594.
37. Frauwirth KA, Thompson CB. Activation and inhibition of lymphocytes by costimulation. *J Clin Invest*. 2002;109(3):295–299.
38. Schwartz RH. T cell anergy. *Annu Rev Immunol*. 2003;21:305–334.
39. Chen L. Co-inhibitory molecules of the B7-CD28 family in the control of T-cell immunity. *Nat Rev Immunol*. 2004;4(5):336–347.
40. Thompson CB, Allison JP. The emerging role of CTLA-4 as an immune attenuator. *Immunity*. 1997;7(4):445–450.
41. Pardoll D, Drake C. Immunotherapy earns its spot in the ranks of cancer therapy. *J Exp Med*. 2012;209(2):201–209.
42. Gramaglia I, Weinberg AD, Lemon M, et al. Ox-40 ligand: a potent costimulatory molecule for sustaining primary CD4 T cell responses. *J Immunol*. 1998;161(12):6510–6517.
43. Weinberg AD, Rivera MM, Prell R, et al. Engagement of the OX-40 receptor in vivo enhances antitumor immunity. *J Immunol*. 2000;164(4):2160–2169.
44. Cheuk AT, Mufti GJ, Guinn BA. Role of 4-1BB:4-1BB ligand in cancer immunotherapy. *Cancer Gene Ther*. 2004;11(3):215–226.
45. Hodi FS, O'Day SJ, McDermott DF, et al. Improved survival with ipilimumab in patients with metastatic melanoma. *N Engl J Med*. 2010;363(8):711–723.
46. O'Mahony D, Morris JC, Quinn C, et al. A pilot study of CTLA-4 blockade after cancer vaccine failure in patients with advanced malignancy. *Clin Cancer Res*. 2007;13(3):958–964.
47. Small EJ, Tchekmedyian NS, Rini BI, et al. A pilot trial of CTLA-4 blockade with human anti-CTLA-4 in patients with hormone-refractory prostate cancer. *Clin Cancer Res*. 2007;13(6):1810–1815.
48. Madan RA, Mohebtash M, Arlen PM, et al. Ipilimumab and a poxviral vaccine targeting prostate-specific antigen in metastatic castration-resistant prostate cancer: a phase 1 dose-escalation trial. *Lancet Oncol*. 2012;13(5):501–508.
49. Antonarakis ES. Combining active immunotherapy with immune checkpoint blockade for the treatment of advanced prostate cancer. *Asian J Androl*. 2012;14(4):520–521.
50. van den Eertwegh AJ, Versluis J, van den Berg HP, et al. Combined immunotherapy with granulocyte-macrophage colony-stimulating factor-transduced allogeneic prostate cancer cells and ipilimumab in patients with metastatic castration-resistant prostate cancer: a phase 1 dose-escalation trial. *Lancet Oncol*. 2012;13(5):509–517.

51. Rosenberg SA, Yang JC, Restifo NP. Cancer immunotherapy: moving beyond current vaccines. *Nat Med*. 2004;10(9):909–915.
52. Weber J. Ipilimumab: controversies in its development, utility and autoimmune adverse events. *Cancer Immunol Immunother*. 2009;58(5):823–830.
53. Dong H, Zhu G, Tamada K, et al. B7-H1, a third member of the B7 family, co-stimulates T-cell proliferation and interleukin-10 secretion. *Nat Med*. 1999;5(12):1365–1369.
54. Freeman GJ, Long AJ, Iwai Y, et al. Engagement of the PD-1 immunoinhibitory receptor by a novel B7 family member leads to negative regulation of lymphocyte activation. *J Exp Med*. 2000;192(7):1027–1034.
55. Hirano F, Kaneko K, Tamura H, et al. Blockade of B7-H1 and PD-1 by monoclonal antibodies potentiates cancer therapeutic immunity. *Cancer Res*. 2005;65(3):1089–1096.
56. Dong H, Strome SE, Salomao DR, et al. Tumor-associated B7-H1 promotes T-cell apoptosis: a potential mechanism of immune evasion. *Nat Med*. 2002;8(8):793–800.
57. Iwai Y, Ishida M, Tanaka Y, et al. Involvement of PD-L1 on tumor cells in the escape from host immune system and tumor immunotherapy by PD-L1 blockade. *Proc Natl Acad Sci U S A*. 2002;99(19):12293–12297.
58. Iwai Y, Terawaki S, Honjo T. PD-1 blockade inhibits hematogenous spread of poorly immunogenic tumor cells by enhanced recruitment of effector T cells. *Int Immunol*. 2005;17(2):133–144.
59. Brahmer JR, Tykodi SS, Chow LQ, et al. Safety and activity of anti-PD-L1 antibody in patients with advanced cancer. *N Engl J Med*. 2012;366(26):2455–2465.
60. Topalian SL, Hodi FS, Brahmer JR, et al. Safety, activity, and immune correlates of anti-PD-1 antibody in cancer. *N Engl J Med*. 2012;366(26):2443–2454.
61. Weiner GJ. Monoclonal antibody mechanisms of action in cancer. *Immunol Res*. 2007;39(1-3):271–278.
62. Smith MR, Egerdie B, Hernandez Toriz N, et al. Denosumab in men receiving androgen-deprivation therapy for prostate cancer. *N Engl J Med*. 2009;361(8):745–755.
63. Fizazi K, Carducci M, Smith M, et al. Denosumab versus zoledronic acid for treatment of bone metastases in men with castration-resistant prostate cancer: a randomised, double-blind study. *Lancet*. 2011;377(9768):813–822.
64. Smith MR, Saad F, Coleman R, et al. Denosumab and bone-metastasis-free survival in men with castration-resistant prostate cancer: results of a phase 3, randomised, placebo-controlled trial. *Lancet*. 2012;379(9810):39–46.
65. Kelly WK, Halabi S, Carducci M, et al. Randomized, double-blind, placebo-controlled phase III trial comparing docetaxel and prednisone with or without bevacizumab in men with metastatic castration-resistant prostate cancer: CALGB 90401. *J Clin Oncol*. 2012;30(13):1534–1540.
66. Hudes G, Tagawa ST, Whang YE, et al. A phase 1 study of a chimeric monoclonal antibody against interleukin-6, siltuximab, combined with docetaxel in patients with metastatic castration-resistant prostate cancer. *Invest New Drugs*. 2013;31(3):669–676.
67. Fizazi K, De Bono JS, Flechon A, et al. Randomised phase II study of siltuximab (CNTO 328), an anti-IL-6 monoclonal antibody, in combination with mitoxantrone/prednisone versus mitoxantrone/prednisone alone in metastatic castration-resistant prostate cancer. *Eur J Cancer*. 2012;48(1):85–93.
68. Marschner N, Ruttinger D, Zugmaier G, et al. Phase II study of the human anti-epithelial cell adhesion molecule antibody adecatumumab in prostate cancer patients with increasing serum levels of prostate-specific antigen after radical prostatectomy. *Urol Int*. 2010;85(4):386–395.
69. Rabbani SA, Ateeq B, Arakelian A, et al. An anti-urokinase plasminogen activator receptor antibody (ATN-658) blocks prostate cancer invasion, migration, growth, and experimental skeletal metastasis in vitro and in vivo. *Neoplasia*. 2010;12(10):778–788.
70. Rosen LS, Hurwitz HI, Wong MK, et al. A phase I first-in-human study of TRC105 (Anti-Endoglin Antibody) in patients with advanced cancer. *Clin Cancer Res*. 2012;18(17):4820–4829.
71. Antonarakis ES, Carducci MA, Eisenberger MA, et al. Phase I rapid dose-escalation study of AGS-1C4D4, a human anti-PSCA (prostate stem cell antigen) monoclonal antibody, in patients with castration-resistant prostate cancer: a PCCTC trial. *Cancer Chemother Pharmacol*. 2012;69(3):763–771.
72. Cathomas R, Rothermundt C, Klingbiel D, et al. Efficacy of cetuximab in metastatic castration-resistant prostate cancer might depend on EGFR and PTEN expression: results from a phase II trial (SAKK 08/07). *Clin Cancer Res*. 2012;18(21):6049–6057.
73. Horoszewicz JS, Kawinski E, Murphy GP. Monoclonal antibodies to a new antigenic marker in epithelial prostatic cells and serum of prostatic cancer patients. *Anticancer Res*. 1987;7(5B):927–935.
74. Israeli RS, Powell CT, Fair WR, et al. Molecular cloning of a complementary DNA encoding a prostate-specific membrane antigen. *Cancer Res*. 1993;53(2):227–230.
75. Israeli RS, Powell CT, Corr JG, et al. Expression of the prostate-specific membrane antigen. *Cancer Res*. 1994;54(7):1807–1811.
76. Wright GL Jr, Haley C, Beckett ML, et al. Expression of prostate-specific membrane antigen in normal, benign, and malignant prostate tissues. *Urol Oncol*. 1995;1(1):18–28.
77. Sweat SD, Pacelli A, Murphy GP, et al. Prostate-specific membrane antigen expression is greatest in prostate adenocarcinoma and lymph node metastases. *Urology*. 1998;52(4):637–640.
78. Mannweiler S, Amersdorfer P, Trajanoski S, et al. Heterogeneity of prostate-specific membrane antigen (PSMA) expression in prostate carcinoma with distant metastasis. *Pathol Oncol Res*. 2009;15(2):167–172.
79. Ananias HJ, van den Heuvel MC, Helfrich W, et al. Expression of the gastrin-releasing peptide receptor, the prostate stem cell antigen and the prostate-specific membrane antigen in lymph node and bone metastases of prostate cancer. *Prostate*. 2009;69(10):1101–1108.
80. Bander NH, Nanus DM, Milowsky MI, et al. Targeted systemic therapy of prostate cancer with a monoclonal antibody to prostate-specific membrane antigen. *Semin Oncol*. 2003;30(5):667–676.
81. Morris MJ, Divgi CR, Pandit-Taskar N, et al. Pilot trial of unlabeled and indium-111-labeled anti-prostate-specific membrane antigen antibody J591 for castrate metastatic prostate cancer. *Clin Cancer Res*. 2005;11(20):7454–7461.
82. Khagi Y, Kaur G, Christos P, et al. Anti-prostate-specific membrane antigen (PSMA) monoclonal antibody J591 plus low dose interleukin-2 (IL-2) in patients with recurrent prostate cancer (PC). *Proceedings of the Annual Meeting of the American Association for Cancer Research, San Diego, CA. 2014; Abst CT304.*
83. Milowsky MI, Nanus DM, Kostakoglu L, et al. Phase I trial of yttrium-90-labeled anti-prostate-specific membrane antigen monoclonal antibody J591 for androgen-independent prostate cancer. *J Clin Oncol*. 2004;22(13):2522–2531.
84. Bander NH, Milowsky MI, Nanus DM, et al. Phase I trial of 177 lutetium-labeled J591, a monoclonal antibody to prostate-specific membrane antigen, in patients with androgen-independent prostate cancer. *J Clin Oncol*. 2005;23(21):4591–4601.
85. Tagawa ST, Milowsky MI, Morris MJ, et al. Phase II study of lutetium-177 labeled anti-prostate-specific membrane antigen (PSMA) monoclonal antibody J591 for metastatic castration-resistant prostate cancer. *Clin Cancer Res*. 2013;19(18):5182–5191.
86. Tagawa ST, Beltran H, Vallabhajosula S, et al. Anti-prostate-specific membrane antigen-based radioimmunotherapy for prostate cancer. *Cancer*. 2010;116(4 suppl):1075–1083.
87. Tagawa ST, Vallabahajosula S, Osborne J, et al. Phase I trial of fractionated-dose ^{177}lutetium radiolabelled anti-prostate-specific membrane antigen (PSMA) monoclonal antibody J591 (^{177}Lu-J591) in patients (pts) with metastatic castration-resistant prostate cancer (metCRPC). *J Clin Oncol*. 2010;28(15s):4667.

88. Beltran H, Vallabhajosula S, Kelly WK. Phase Idose escalation study of Docetaxel/Predisone and fractionated 177Lu-J591for metastatic castrate resistant prostate cancer (metCRPC) [abstract TPS247]. *J Clin Oncol.* 2010;28(15s).
89. Kosuri S, Akhtar NH, Smith M, et al. Review of salvage therapy for biochemically recurrent prostate cancer: the role of imaging and rationale for systemic salvage targeted anti-prostate-specific membrane antigen radioimmunotherapy. *Adv Urol.* 2012;2012:921674.
90. Henry MD, Wen S, Silva MD, et al. A prostate-specific membrane antigen-targeted monoclonal antibody-chemotherapeutic conjugate designed for the treatment of prostate cancer. *Cancer Res.* 2004;64(21):7995–8001.
91. Alley SC, Okeley NM, Senter PD. Antibody-drug conjugates: targeted drug delivery for cancer. *Curr Opin Chem Biol.* 2010;14(4):529–537.
92. Petrylak DP, Kantoff PW, Mega AE, et al. Prostate-specific membrane antigen antibody drug conjugate (PSMA ADC): a phase I trial in metastatic castration-resistant prostate cancer (mCRPC) previously treated with a taxane [abstract 5018]. *J Clin Oncol.* 2013;(suppl).
93. Higano C, Saad F, Somer B, et al. A phase 3 trial of GVAX immunotherapy for prostate cancer vs. docetaxel plus prednisone in asymptomatic, castration-resistant prostate cancer. In: 2009 Genitourinary Cancers Symposium: A multidisciplinary approach; February 26–28, 2009; Orlando, FL.
94. Small EJ, Demkow T, Gerritsen WR. A phase 3 trial of GVAX immunotherapy for prostate cancer in combination with docetaxel vs. docetaxel plus prednisone in asymptomatic, castration-resistant prostate cancer. In: ASCO Genitourinary Cancer Symposium; 2009; Orlando, FL.
95. Slovin SF, Higano CS, Hamid O, et al. Ipilimumab alone or in combination with radiotherapy in metastatic castration-resistant prostate cancer: results from an open-label, multicenter phase I/II study. *Ann Oncol.* 2013;24(7):1813–1821.
96. Kwon ED, Drake CG, Scher HI, et al. Ipilimumab versus placebo after radiotherapy in patients with metastatic castration-resistant prostate cancer that had progressed after docetaxel chemotherapy (CA184-043): a multicentre, randomised, double-blind, phase 3 trial. *Lancet Oncol.* 2014;15(7):700–712.

19.5 Treatment of Bony Metastases: Inhibitors of Bone Resorption

CLARA HWANG
ELISABETH I. HEATH

■ INTRODUCTION

An astute clinician cannot neglect the impact of osseous complications on the morbidity of patients with metastatic prostate cancer. Bone is the predominant metastatic site for most patients, and nearly all patients develop osseous metastases during the course of the disease (1, 2). Furthermore, bone metastases have significant clinical consequences such as severe and intractable bone pain. Spinal metastases with cord compression may result in paralysis and/or incontinence. The poor quality of bone associated with osteoblastic prostate cancer metastases is at risk for pathologic fracture. These skeletal-related events are estimated to affect half of patients with bone metastases and are associated with poorer survival (2, 3). Bone metastases can negatively affect hematopoiesis and calcium balance. Clearly, complications from bone metastases (especially pain, spinal cord compression, and pathologic fracture) have the potential to dramatically affect functional ability and quality of life.

The management of complications from bone metastases can include analgesic management, radiation, and, occasionally, surgery (4). Analgesia (systemic and regional) and radiation can be effective in treating cancer-related pain. Spinal cord compression and pathologic fractures may be managed with surgery and/or radiation therapy. This care can be financially costly. The estimated cost to treat a skeletal-related event is between US$5,000 and US$10,000 (5, 6), while the total financial burden of caring for prostate cancer patients with metastatic bone disease has been estimated at US$1.9 billion (7). Furthermore, treatment of skeletal-related events with surgery, radiation, or analgesic management may not completely reverse pain and debility that has already occurred. The primary role of bone resorption inhibitors is to prevent skeletal-related events and their associated morbidity. This chapter focuses on the use of bone resorption inhibitors in the management of prostatic osseous metastases.

■ UNDERSTANDING THE PATHOPHYSIOLOGY OF SKELETAL-RELATED EVENTS IN PROSTATE CANCER

Bone resorption and formation continuously remodel normal bone throughout life (8). Bone remodeling allows bone to adjust to mechanical stress, repair damage to bone, and regulate calcium homeostasis. Bone formation and bone resorption are carried out by osteoblasts and osteoclasts, respectively (Figure 19.5.1). Osteoblasts are mononucleate cells with typically basophilic cytoplasm. These cells, essentially specialized fibroblasts, differentiate from multipotent stromal progenitor cells. When activated, mature osteoblasts initiate bone formation by producing an extracellular protein matrix called osteoid. Osteoid is composed primarily of cross-linked type I collagen. Formation of this collagen matrix requires cleavage of amino- and carboxy-terminal propeptides from procollagen. Finally, osteoblasts mineralize osteoid by the deposition of hydroxyapatite, a calcium phosphate mineral [$Ca_{10}(PO_4)_6(OH)_2$]. Bone mineralization is dependent on osteoblast alkaline phosphatase (9), as well as on sufficient quantities of calcium and phosphate.

In contrast to bone-forming osteoblasts, osteoclasts are the cells responsible for bone lysis and resorption. Osteoclasts are multinucleated giant cells derived from precursor cells in the monocyte-macrophage lineage. Upon activation, osteoclasts resorb bone through the digestion of calcified bone matrix, ultimately releasing calcium and other matrix degradation products to the bloodstream. Many of these degradation products are collagen derivatives. For example, cross-linked type I collagen degradation products such as NTX (N-terminal telopeptide) and CTX (C-terminal telopeptide) are two commonly measured markers of bone resorption (Figure 19.5.2). Osteoclasts are located within resorption pits in the bone surface, which contact the ruffled membrane of the activated osteoclast. Multiple cytoplasmic vacuoles and vesicles are present within the osteoclast, responsible for delivery of matrix degradation enzymes and transport of bone degradation products. These vesicles and vacuoles lend a foamy appearance to the characteristically eosinophilic cytoplasm.

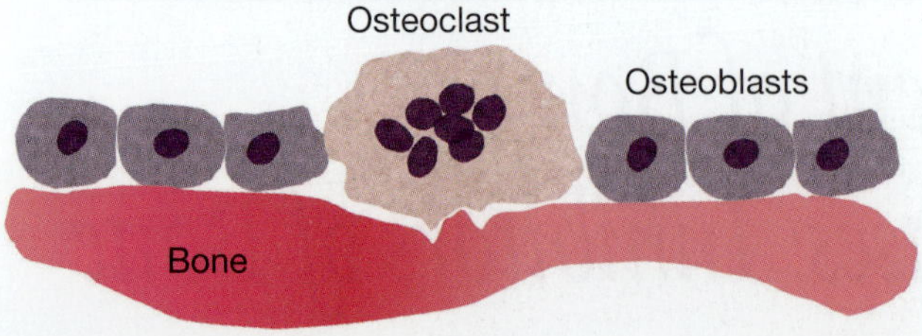

FIGURE 19.5.1 Bone remodeling by osteoclasts and osteoblasts. Osteoclasts are multinucleated giant cells derived from precursor cells in the monocyte-macrophage lineage. Osteoclasts are located within resorption pits in the bone surface, which contact the ruffled membrane of the activated osteoclast. Upon activation, osteoclasts are responsible for bone resorption through the digestion of calcified bone matrix, releasing calcium to the bloodstream. Osteoblasts differentiate from multipotent stromal cells and are responsible for bone formation. Activated osteoblasts synthesize a fibrous matrix that is primarily type I collagen. Osteoblasts also control the mineralization of this matrix by the deposition of hydroxyapatite ($Ca_{10}(PO_4)_6(OH)_2$), depending on the availability of sufficient calcium and phosphate.

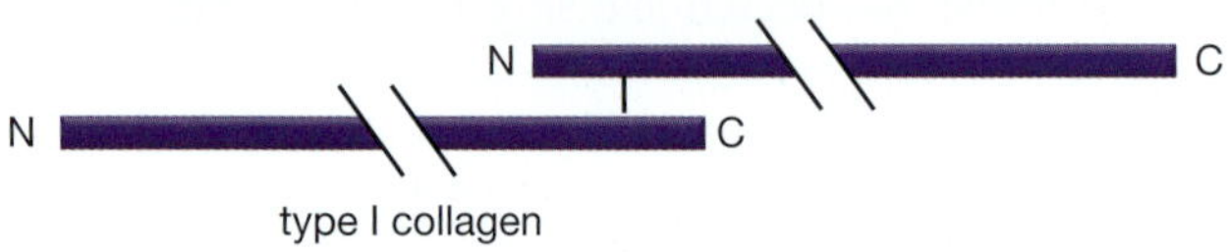

FIGURE 19.5.2 Cross-linked collagen degradation products are markers of bone resorption. Strands of collagen are cross-linked during bone formation. During resorption of mature bone, proteolytic cleavage releases peptide degradation products, which can be measured in the blood and urine. Cross-linked amino-terminal (NTX) and carboxy-terminal telopeptides (CTX) are commonly used markers of bone resorption in clinical trials.

Prostate cancer is classically associated with osteoblastic metastases, which appear sclerotic on bone radiographs (Figure 19.5.3). Molecular interactions between prostate cancer cells and the bone microenvironment preferentially promote migration, attachment, and proliferation in the bone metastatic niche (10). Bone immediately adjacent to prostate cancer metastases is associated with increased osteoid formation and mineralization (11, 12), leading to the sclerotic appearance on radiographs. The mechanisms underlying osteoblastic metastases are presumed to be related to the secretion of osteogenic factors such as endothelin-1 (13). Despite increased mineralization, osteoblastic metastases remain at risk for pathologic fracture because of the inferior quality of bone associated with metastatic lesions. Mature lamellar bone is produced slowly and is characterized by tightly packed linear collagen strands. In contrast, the osteoid produced by osteoblasts in prostate cancer metastases is characterized by randomly oriented collagen fibrils (11), or so-called woven bone (Figure 19.5.4). Woven bone has lower collagen density and poor structural integrity in comparison to lamellar bone. The weakness of woven bone, in combination with the resorption of mature lamellar bone described below, explains the propensity for even osteoblastic metastases to fracture. Overall, fractures account for up to half of skeletal-related events in patients with prostate cancer and the majority of these are nonvertebral fractures (14, 15).

The role of bone resorption inhibitors may initially seem to be unclear in the context of the osteoblastic

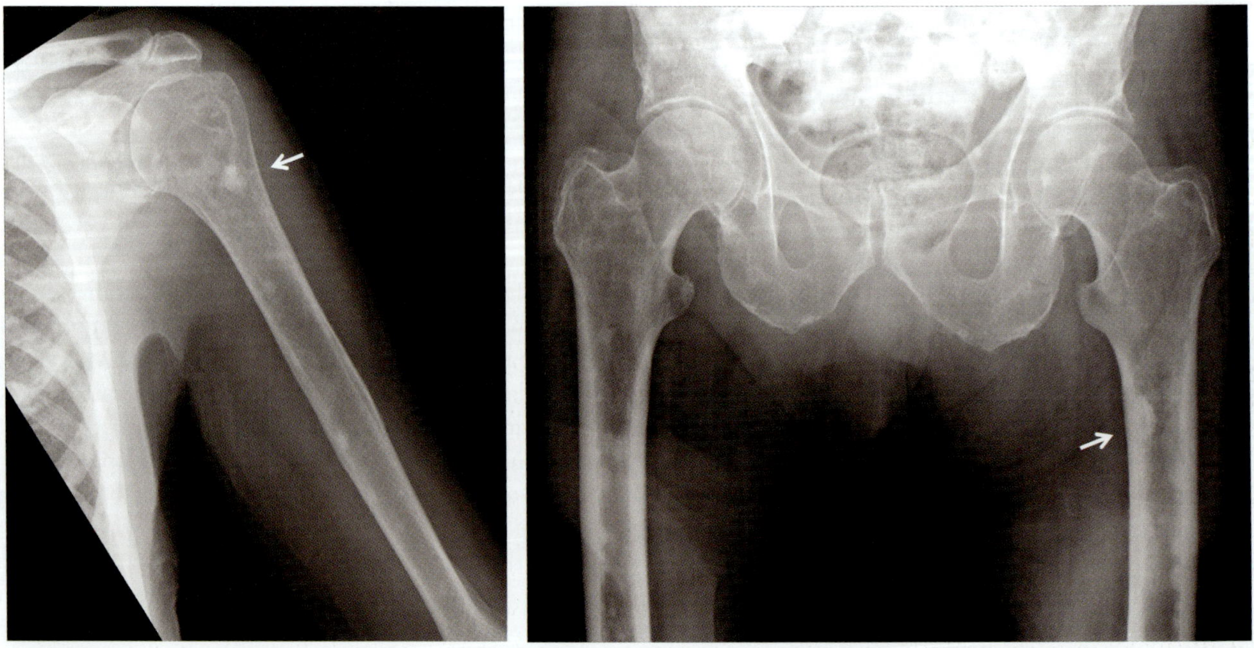

FIGURE 19.5.3 Osteoblastic metastases from prostate cancer. Plain radiographs of the humerus and femur demonstrate diffuse and patchy osseous blastic metastases involving the proximal to mid-humerus and femurs. Additional lesions can be seen in the ribs and pelvis. Unlike lytic bone lesions, which are radiolucent, osteoblastic metastases have a dense sclerotic appearance that is radiopaque.

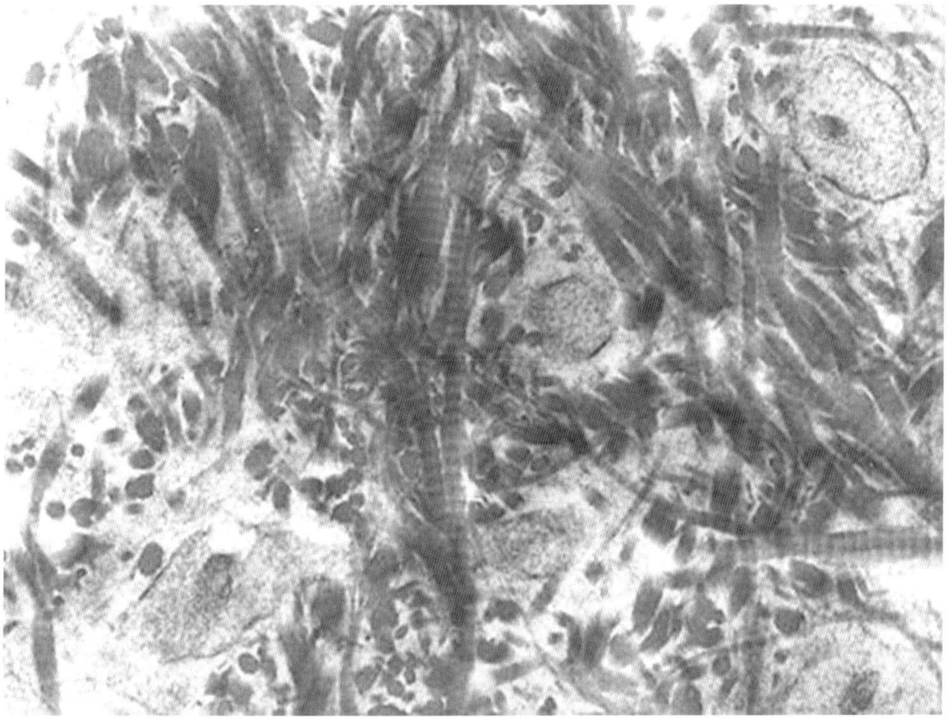

FIGURE 19.5.4 Collagen fibrils of woven bone. Unlike the linearly organized collagen fibrils of lamellar bone, the woven bone associated with osteoblastic metastases have randomly oriented collagen fibrils, which lack structural integrity. *Source:* From Robert M. Hunt, public domain.

appearance of prostate cancer bone lesions. However, several lines of evidence have established that prostate cancer perturbs the process of bone resorption and bone formation (reviewed in 16). Markers of bone resorption, such as cross-linked type I collagen degradation products, are increased in prostate cancer (17–20). Furthermore, biochemical measures of bone resorption correlate with clinically relevant prostate cancer outcomes such as extent of skeletal metastases, risk of skeletal-related events, and survival (reviewed in 21, 22). Careful histologic examination also reveals evidence of bone resorption in the bone in prostate cancer patients (11, 17, 23). In fact, inhibition of bone resorption can in some circumstances prevent the establishment of bone metastases in preclinical prostate cancer models (24). The importance of bone resorption in the pathophysiology of osteoblastic prostatic metastases underlies the clinical relevance of bone resorption inhibitors in the management of prostate cancer patients.

The processes of bone formation and bone resorption are associated with specific biochemical molecules that can be used as surrogate measures of bone turnover (reviewed in 25, 26). Markers of bone turnover are primarily related to the synthesis and degradation of bone mineral and collagen. As described above, bone synthesis by osteoblasts involves bone-specific alkaline phosphatase and processing of procollagen. As such, bone-specific alkaline phosphatase, the amino-terminal (PINP), and the carboxy-terminal propeptides of type I collagen (PICP) are typical markers of bone formation. Similarly, osteoclast enzymes such as tartrate-resistant acid phosphatase and cross-linked collagen degradation products are used as markers of bone resorption.

Markers of both bone resorption and bone formation correlate with clinical endpoints in prostate cancer patients. Total alkaline phosphatase levels, the most widely used clinical marker, predict survival in patients with metastatic prostate cancer (27, 28). Elevated levels of bone-specific alkaline phosphatase and urinary cross-linked type I collagen N-telopeptide correlate with the risk of developing a skeletal-related event, time to first skeletal-related event, progression in bone, and death (15, 29–32). Markers of bone turnover also respond to the initiation of bone resorption inhibitors (33) and may distinguish bone from other sites of metastatic disease. To date, the measurement of most bone turnover markers has not entered general clinical practice but shows promise for predicting and monitoring the treatment of skeletal-related events in prostate cancer.

Clinical attributes also correlate with an increased risk of developing a skeletal-related event in patients with prostate cancer. Skeletal-related events are much more likely to occur after the development of castrate-resistant disease (19, 34). For patients with metastatic prostate cancer, the presence of bone pain and a greater extent of disease in bone predict the occurrence of skeletal-related events (34). Prostate-specific antigen (PSA) and Gleason score did not correlate with the circumstance of skeletal-related events in these studies. Among men without evidence of bone metastases, a study of 331 patients with castrate-resistant nonmetastatic prostate cancer demonstrated that baseline PSA levels and PSA kinetics are associated with time to first bone metastasis (29), confirming results of a previous study (35). The median time to first bone metastasis for patients with nonmetastatic castrate-resistant prostate cancer was reported to be 25 months and 30 months in these studies (29, 35), respectively.

Several other features of the prostate cancer population increase the risk of skeletal complications, primarily by decreasing bone mineralization. Prostate cancer is typically a disease of older men, with a peak incidence in the sixth and seventh decades of life and mortality rates that continue to rise with advancing age (36). Androgen deprivation, although a highly effective first-line therapy for prostate cancer, has a negative impact on bone integrity (37, 38). Androgen deprivation therapy may continue for years, particularly when started early in patients with high-risk localized disease or in the setting of biochemical recurrence (39). Fracture rates increase with a longer duration of androgen deprivation (40). Once patients develop metastatic disease, treatment regimens often include glucocorticoids, either for therapeutic intent or to counteract the glucocorticoid deficiency associated with certain androgen synthesis inhibitors (41–44). Advanced age, the use of hormonal therapy, and the use of glucocorticoids all decrease bone mineralization and increase the fracture risk in men with prostate cancer (45).

The molecular elements that regulate osteoclast and osteoblast function have provided important targets for the treatment of patients with bone metastases (reviewed in 10, 46). The central element that balances the processes of bone formation and resorption is the receptor activator of nuclear factor kappa-B ligand (RANKL) signaling pathway (Figure 19.5.5). RANKL, the key mediator of osteoclastogenesis, is expressed by osteoblast precursors and stromal cells. Soluble and membrane-bound forms of RANKL bind to the receptor activator of nuclear-factor kappa-B (RANK) on osteoclasts and osteoclast precursors to promote osteoclast differentiation, activation, and survival. RANKL can also interact with osteoprotegerin, a soluble decoy receptor that inhibits RANK signaling. Osteoprotegerin thus protects the bone from excess resorption (24, 47). The balance between bone resorption and formation is determined primarily by the ratio of osteoprotegerin to RANKL. Systemic factors that impact this balance include parathyroid hormone, vitamin D, glucocorticoids, and sex steroids; additional local growth factors secreted by tumor and stromal cells such as platelet-derived growth factor, fibroblast growth factor, bone morphogenetic proteins, insulin-like growth factor, and transforming growth factor-beta also influence osteoblast/osteoblast maturation and function.

Clinically, the most important bone-targeting therapies are osteoclast inhibitors, namely bisphosphonates and denosumab. Although osteoblasts seem to play a large role in the pathogenesis of bone metastases from prostate cancer, data from randomized controlled trials with osteoblast inhibitors have been negative to date (48–50). Bisphosphonates derive their clinical activity from their chemical similarity to pyrophosphate (reviewed in 51). As pyrophosphate analogues, bisphosphonates bind hydroxyapatite and accumulate in bone where they inhibit osteoclast activity. When bisphosphonates are incorporated into bone matrix, they are not released until the bone is resorbed, resulting in an extremely long half-life. Zoledronic acid is the most potent inhibitor of bone resorption among the bisphosphonates (by one to four orders of magnitude). In contrast, denosumab, a monoclonal antibody against RANKL, is a bone resorption inhibitor that acts in a similar fashion to osteoprotegerin. Binding and neutralization of RANKL by denosumab inhibits RANKL-mediated osteoclast formation, function, and survival. Both zoledronic acid and denosumab have been shown to have clinical benefits for patients with prostate cancer and will be further discussed.

■ CLINICAL BENEFITS OF BONE RESORPTION INHIBITORS

Antiresorption Agents to Treat Osseous Metastatic Disease

Studies of zoledronic acid were the first to show that inhibition of bone resorption improved outcomes in patients with bone metastases from prostate cancer. As a result, zoledronic acid was the first bone resorption inhibitor approved by the Food and Drug Administration (FDA) for the prevention of skeletal-related events in prostate cancer. This approval was based on the results of a randomized controlled trial of 643 patients comparing zoledronic acid with placebo (14, 52). Initially, two doses of zoledronic acid (4 mg and 8 mg intravenously over 5 minutes every 21 days) were studied. However, concerns regarding nephrotoxicity led to a lengthening of the infusion time from 5 minutes to 15 minutes and a reduction of the 8 mg dose to 4 mg. Patients were treated for 15 months with an optional 9-month extension. Conclusions regarding efficacy were drawn from comparing the 4 mg zoledronic acid with the placebo group. The primary outcome was the proportion of patients with at least one skeletal-related event.

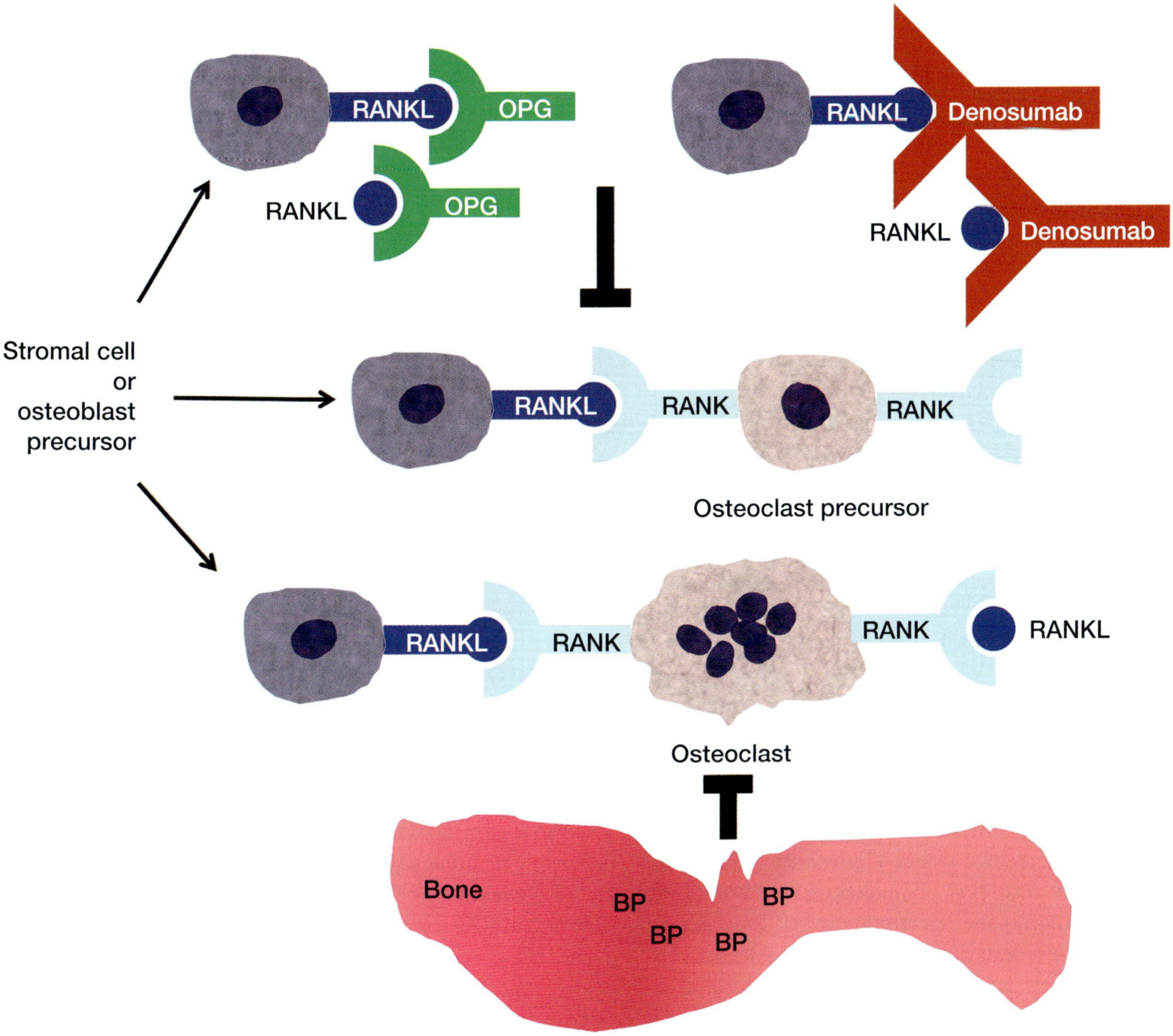

FIGURE 19.5.5 Receptor activator of nuclear factor kappa-B (RANK) and receptor activator of nuclear factor kappa-B ligand (RANKL) signaling. RANKL is expressed by osteoblasts and stromal cells. RANKL binds RANK on osteoclasts and osteoclast procursors, promoting osteoclast differentiation, activation, and survival. Osteoprotegerin (OPG), a soluble decoy receptor, inhibits the interaction between RANK and RANKL, thus protecting the bone from excess resorption. Denosumab, a monoclonal antibody against RANKL, is a bone resorption inhibitor that acts in a similar fashion to OPG. In contrast, bisphosphonates (BP) bind hydroxyapatite, accumulate in bone, and inhibit osteoclast activity there.

The group receiving zoledronic acid had a lower incidence of skeletal-related events compared with placebo (33.2% vs. 44.2%; $P = .021$) in the initial analysis (14), with the benefit persisting in the extended follow-up (38% vs. 49%, $P = .028$) (52). In addition, the administration of zoledronic acid delayed the onset of the first skeletal-related event (488 days vs. 321 days, $P = .009$) and the proportion of patients with symptomatic skeletal-related events (30% vs. 41%, $P = .019$). Zoledronic acid improved outcomes in patients both with and without prior skeletal-related events. The benefit continued during the extension period, with 19% in the zoledronic acid group versus 38% of patients in the placebo group experiencing at least one skeletal-related event during 15 months through 24 months ($P = .017$). Zoledronic acid did not impact time to progression or overall survival.

Zoledronic acid also exerted positive effects on pain and markers of bone turnover. Compared to placebo, treatment of patients with castrate-resistant prostate cancer with zoledronic acid reduces pain from bone metastatic disease as measured by the Brief Pain Inventory pain score (52, 53). Measures of bone resorption and bone formation were evaluated, including N-telopeptide, bone-specific type I collagen cross-links, and alkaline phosphatase. At 15 months, markers of bone turnover were lower in patients treated with zoledronic acid compared to placebo. The urinary N-telopeptide to creatinine ratio (a bone resorption marker) declined 70% after 1 month and remained suppressed.

Similarly, serum bone alkaline phosphatase, an osteoblast marker, remained significantly lower in patients receiving zoledronic acid compared to placebo.

Other than nephrotoxicity observed in the 8-mg zoledronic acid group, side effects reported in this study were generally mild and not significantly different between the zoledronic and placebo groups. Grade 3 nephrotoxicity was observed at a rate of 2% to 3% in the zoledronic acid group compared to 1% in the placebo group. Compared to placebo, the relative risk of renal function deterioration was 1.07 in the 4-mg group and 1.76 in the 8-mg group. The 8-mg zoledronic acid dose is not recommended for this reason. Bone pain was less common in the 4-mg zoledronic acid group (50.5% vs. 61.1%) compared to placebo, consistent with the ability of zoledronic acid to reduce pain from bone metastases (53). Fatigue, anemia, myalgia, fever, edema, and dizziness were slightly higher in the zoledronic acid group; however, there were no differences in the discontinuation rate in the two groups due to adverse events. Osteonecrosis of the jaw was not reported in this study but is a known toxicity of bisphosphonate therapy (54).

Two negative bisphosphonate studies for patients with metastatic castrate-resistant prostate cancer and symptomatic bone metastases have also been reported. The National Cancer Institute of Canada randomized 209 men with castrate-resistant prostate cancer and symptomatic bone metastases to receive either clodronate (1,500 mg intravenously every 3 weeks) or placebo (55). All patients also received mitoxantrone 12 mg/m^2 every 3 weeks in combination with prednisone. Compared to placebo, clodronate did not have significant effects on pain, analgesic use, duration of response, progression-free survival, overall survival, or quality of life. Similarly, treatment with pamidronate did not meet the primary endpoint of pain reduction in prostate cancer patients with symptomatic bone metastases (56). In a combined analysis of two studies, outcomes from 350 men with castrate-resistant metastatic prostate cancer and symptomatic bone lesions who were randomized to receive either pamidronate (90 mg intravenously every 3 weeks) or placebo for 27 weeks were analyzed. The analysis reported no difference in pain scores, analgesic use, or rates of skeletal-related events compared to placebo. Consequently, zoledronic acid is the only bisphosphonate with an indication for treatment of patients with bone metastases and castrate-resistant prostate cancer.

A randomized phase II evaluation of denosumab demonstrated that denosumab is effective at inhibiting bone resorption in patients with a suboptimal response to bisphosphonate therapy (57). Eligible patients had at least one bone metastasis from prostate cancer, other solid tumor, or multiple myeloma and evidence of increased levels of bone resorption despite at least 8 weeks of treatment on intravenous bisphosphonate. For the purpose of eligibility, elevated bone resorption was defined as a urinary N-telopeptide to creatinine ratio of greater than 50 nM bone collagen equivalents/mM creatinine. The study randomized 111 patients to either continue intravenous bisphosphonate or receive one of two schedules of subcutaneous denosumab for 25 weeks. Denosumab was more effective at normalizing multiple markers of bone resorption (58) and also appeared to reduce rates of skeletal-related events. These conclusions also extended to a subset of 50 patients with prostate cancer (59).

The encouraging results of phase II studies led to a trial comparing the administration of denosumab and zoledronic acid in patients with bone metastases from castrate-resistant prostate cancer (60). The study enrolled 1,904 bisphosphonate-naive patients with castrate-resistant prostate cancer and at least one bone metastasis. Patients were randomized to receive either denosumab (120 mg subcutaneously every 28 days) or zoledronic acid (4 mg intravenously every 28 days). Skeletal-related events were defined as the need for radiation or surgery to bone, cord compression, or pathologic fracture. The median time on study was 1 year at the time of first analysis. Compared to zoledronic acid, denosumab delayed the onset of the first skeletal-related event (20.7 months vs. 17.1 months; $P = .008$). The cumulative mean rate of skeletal-related events per patient was also less in the denosumab arm (rate ratio = 0.82; $P = .004$). The most common skeletal-related event was the need for radiation to bone (203 events in the zoledronic acid arm vs. 177 events in the denosumab arm). Pathologic fracture accounted for approximately 40% of skeletal-related events observed on the trial. The rate of vertebral versus nonvertebral fracture was not reported, nor was the proportion of fractures identified solely on the basis of routine radiographic assessment. There were no significant differences in overall survival or time to progression. The results of this trial led to the approval of denosumab by the FDA in 2010 for patients with bone metastases and castrate-resistant prostate cancer.

Patients treated with denosumab had significantly lower levels of bone resorption (urinary N-telopeptide to creatinine ratio) and bone formation (serum bone-specific alkaline phosphatase) than patients treated with zoledronic at 13 weeks. The median absolute decline in urinary N-telopeptide to creatinine ratio was 28.4 nmol/mmol in the zoledronic acid group and 40.3 nmol/mmol in the denosumab group ($P < .0001$). The median absolute decline in bone-specific alkaline phosphatase was 4.8 mcg/L in the zoledronic acid group and 7.9 mcg/L in the denosumab group ($P < .0001$).

Adverse events were similar between the two treatment arms, with only hypocalcemia meeting criteria for statistical significance. Hypocalcemia occurred more commonly with denosumab treatment, and most events were asymptomatic. Grade 3 hypocalcemia occurred in 5% of patients treated with denosumab compared to 1% of patients treated with zoledronic acid ($P < .0001$).

The most common side effects reported were anemia, back pain, anorexia, nausea, fatigue, constipation, and bone pain and were similar between the two treatment arms. Contributing factors to these adverse events (such as tumor progression or toxicity from other therapy) were not discussed. Rates of osteonecrosis of the jaw were reported for both denosumab (2%) and zoledronic acid (1%) groups and were not statistically different ($P = .09$).

In contrast to patients with castrate-resistant prostate cancer, antiresorptive therapy has not been shown to benefit patients with metastatic castration-sensitive disease. Zoledronic acid was evaluated in castrate-sensitive patients in a double-blind placebo-controlled phase III trial (61). Between June 2004 and April 2012, the study randomized 645 men with castrate-sensitive prostate cancer and bone metastases to receive either zoledronic acid (4 mg intravenously every 4 weeks) or placebo. Patients who developed castrate resistance went on to receive open-label zoledronic acid. The target sample size was 680 patients and 470 skeletal-related events; however, the study was terminated early for lack of drug supply. Results were presented in abstract form in 2013. After 284 skeletal-related events, there was no significant difference in time to first skeletal-related event between the two groups (hazard ratio = 0.89; $P = .34$) and no difference in overall survival. A similar study performed with clodronate previously reported no significant difference in bone progression-free survival or overall survival (62). Patients treated with clodronate had more gastrointestinal toxicity compared with patients on placebo. Thus, current evidence does not support the use of bisphosphonate therapy to prevent skeletal-related events in the setting of castrate-sensitive prostate cancer. Denosumab has not been studied for the prevention of skeletal-related events in this population.

Antiresorption Agents in the Absence of Osseous Metastatic Disease: Effects on Bone Mineral Density

There is interest in using antiresorption agents for patients who do not have clinically apparent bone metastases because (a) androgen deprivation therapy places patients at risk for osteoporosis and (b) antiresorption agents have the potential of preventing bone metastases based on preclinical data.

Multiple placebo-controlled studies have demonstrated that bisphosphonate therapy prevents bone mineral density loss and suppresses bone turnover markers in patients receiving androgen deprivation therapy (63–67). Although bisphosphonate therapy has beneficial effects on bone mineral density, the clinical significance of this finding for patients starting androgen deprivation therapy is unclear due to the absence of data supporting a reduction in fracture risk. However, these studies evaluating the role of bisphosphonate therapy were not powered to detect differences in fracture risk.

The effect of denosumab on fracture risk was studied in a phase III double-blind, placebo-controlled trial performed in patients with nonmetastatic, castrate-sensitive prostate cancer on androgen deprivation (68). Eligible patients were at an increased risk of osteoporotic fracture on the basis of age older than or equal to 70 years, low bone mineral density (T score at the lumbar spine, hip, or femoral neck < -1.0), or previous osteoporotic fracture. A total of 1,468 patients were randomized to receive either denosumab (60 mg subcutaneous) or a placebo injection every 6 months for a total of six doses. Calcium and vitamin D supplementation was standard therapy in both treatment arms. Compared to placebo, denosumab increased bone mineral density at the hip, femoral neck, distal third of the radius, and whole body at all time points. Furthermore, denosumab was associated with a reduced risk of vertebral fractures in men receiving androgen deprivation therapy for nonmetastatic prostate cancer compared to placebo (1.5% vs. 3.9% at 36 months, respectively; $P = .006$). The rate of fracture at any site was 5.2% in the denosumab arm compared with 7.2% in the placebo arm, which did not meet criteria for statistical significance ($P = .10$). The rate of multiple fracture at any site was 0.7% in the denosumab arm versus 2.5% in the placebo arm ($P = .006$). Improvement in bone mineral density and fracture risk corresponded to suppression of bone turnover markers (69). Improvement in bone density with denosumab was observed regardless of age, fracture history, bone mineral density, and baseline markers of bone turnover (70). On the basis of these results, denosumab was granted an indication by the FDA in 2011 for improving bone mass in prostate cancer patients on androgen deprivation at high risk for fracture.

Antiresorption Agents in the Absence of Osseous Metastatic Disease: Prevention of Bone Metastases

Data from three randomized phase III studies have led to the conclusion that bisphosphonates are not effective in preventing the development of bone metastases in patients with nonmetastatic prostate cancer. An early trial of zoledronic acid versus placebo in men with castration-resistant nonmetastatic prostate cancer was stopped early because the event rate was lower than expected (35). The low event rate observed in these patients points to an indolent course for many patients with nonmetastatic prostate cancer. The median time to skeletal-related events in the placebo arm was 30 months. The early termination of the study precluded efficacy analyses; however, analyses of the placebo arm identified both high baseline PSA concentration and short PSA doubling time as independently associated with bone-metastasis-free survival. Subsequent trials have used these criteria to identify a high-risk subset of patients more likely to benefit from bone-metastases prevention.

In a later study of 508 men with high-risk hormone-naive or hormone-sensitive nonmetastatic prostate cancer, oral clodronate did not improve symptomatic bone-metastasis-free survival compared with placebo (71). Eligibility criteria included men with T2–T4 prostate cancer within 3 years of diagnosis and without current evidence of metastatic disease. Patients were assigned to receive either clodronate 2,080 mg orally daily versus placebo for 5 years. At a median follow-up of 10 years, 148 events were observed. There were no significant differences between the two groups in the development of metastatic disease, prostate cancer mortality, and overall mortality.

Finally, results of a large randomized trial of zoledronic acid for prevention of bone metastases in men with prostate cancer were presented in March 2013 at the European Association of Urology 28th Annual Congress (72). The study randomized 1,433 men with high-risk nonmetastatic prostate cancer to receive either zoledronic acid (4 mg intravenously every 3 months for 4 years) or standard of care only. High-risk disease was defined as a PSA of at least 20 ng/mL at diagnosis, Gleason sum of 8 to 10, or node-positive disease. Median follow-up was 50 months. There was no difference in the rate of bone metastases between the two groups (13.7% for zoledronic acid vs. 13.0% for the control arm; $P = .721$) and no difference in overall survival.

In contrast to bisphosphonates, more potent osteoclast inhibition with denosumab can prevent the development of bone metastases (73). Denosumab was studied in a large double-blind placebo-controlled randomized phase III study in men with nonmetastatic castrate-resistant prostate cancer. Patients selected for the study had a high risk of developing metastatic disease on the basis of PSA greater than 8 ng/mL and/or a PSA doubling time of less than or equal to 10 months. A total of 1,432 patients were randomized on a 1:1 basis to denosumab (120 mg subcutaneously every 4 weeks) or placebo. Denosumab prolonged bone-metastases-free survival (median 29.5 vs. 25.2 months; hazard ratio = 0.85; $P = .028$), as defined by either time to first bone metastases or death from any cause. Denosumab also delayed the onset of first bone metastasis (median 33.2 vs. 29.5 months; hazard ratio = 0.84; $P = .032$). Most of the bone metastases were asymptomatic at the time of detection (440 of 605 events); however, denosumab administration also decreased the likelihood of developing symptomatic bone metastasis (hazard ratio = 0.67; $P = .01$, median time to symptomatic metastasis not reached). There was no difference in overall survival between the two arms. The two toxicities that differed between the two treatment arms were osteonecrosis of the jaw (5% of patients in the denosumab arm vs. none) and hypocalcemia (2% vs. < 1%). After review of this data, the FDA did not approve denosumab for bone-metastases prevention, citing an insufficient benefit in bone-metastases-free survival to outweigh the risks of treatment (including osteonecrosis of the jaw). Although the results of this trial have yet to be fully implemented in clinical practice, the finding provides proof of principle that potent osteoclast inhibition can prevent the establishment of prostate cancer metastases in bone. It remains to be seen whether further studies on prevention of bone metastases yield a more favorable risk/benefit ratio for antiresorptive therapy.

■ CLINICAL CONSIDERATIONS

As has been discussed, the major on-target toxicities of both zoledronic acid and denosumab are hypocalcemia and osteonecrosis of the jaw. Calcium and vitamin D supplementation is standard in all prostate cancer patients receiving bone resorption inhibitors, and calcium levels should be monitored. Concomitant vitamin D deficiency may be present and potentially exacerbate hypocalcemia. Evaluation of vitamin D levels with additional supplementation as necessary is suggested, especially at northern latitudes. The risk of hypocalcemia is higher with denosumab, particularly in patients with renal dysfunction (creatinine clearance < 30 mL/min or dialysis). Osteonecrosis of the jaw is more common in patients with poor dental health and can be precipitated by dental extractions. Duration and frequency of osteoclast inhibitor therapy are additional risk factors for osteonecrosis of the jaw. Baseline dental evaluation is recommended with preventative dentistry performed prior to therapy. Invasive dental procedures should be avoided while on osteoclast inhibitor therapy if possible, with an individual risk/benefit assessment performed by the dentist and treating oncologist. Patients should be encouraged to maintain optimal dental health and referred to a dentist or an oral surgeon if they develop jaw or tooth complaints. Both denosumab and zoledronic acid are associated with atypical fractures of the femur, including subtrochanteric and diaphyseal femur fractures without significant preceding trauma. Patients reporting pain in the hip, thigh, or groin areas should be assessed for the possibility of femoral fracture with contralateral assessment also recommended.

Nephrotoxicity of these agents appears to be specific to bisphosphonates. Dose reduction of zoledronic acid is recommended for patients with a creatinine clearance less than 60 mL/min. Patients with a creatinine clearance of less than 30 mL/min should not receive zoledronic acid. To avoid nephrotoxicity, the recommended infusion rate is no faster than 4 mg of zoledronic acid over 15 minutes. As previously mentioned, patients with a creatinine clearance of less than 30 mL/min are at risk for hypocalcemia with denosumab administration. However, the dose and frequency of denosumab do not need to be adjusted with renal dysfunction.

Although data suggest that denosumab is a more potent osteoclast inhibitor than zoledronic acid, not all patients with bone metastases experience a skeletal-related event, and not all protocol-defined skeletal events are clinically significant (e.g., a radiographically detected vertebral fracture). It is unknown whether there are lower risk patients in whom osteoclast inhibitor treatment could be delayed, given at reduced dose intensity, or in whom a trial of zoledronic acid would be warranted. Clinical questions also remain regarding the optimal duration of therapy for both zoledronic acid and denosumab. Benefit has been demonstrated in clinical trials with up to 2 years of osteoclast inhibitor therapy for patients with metastatic castrate-resistant prostate cancer; however, the benefit beyond that time frame is uncertain, especially because the risk of osteonecrosis of the jaw also increases with cumulative doses.

COMPARISON BETWEEN ZOLEDRONIC ACID AND DENONSUMAB

There are several salient differences between denosumab and zoledronic, which may influence treatment choices in the setting of osseous metastatic disease. In comparison to zoledronic acid, which is given intravenously over 15 minutes, denosumab is administered as a subcutaneous injection. Denosumab does not accumulate in bone, unlike zoledronic acid. As reported by Fizazi et al. (60), grade 3 and 4 adverse events are more common with denosumab than with zoledronic acid, although there was no significant difference in rates of adverse events that led to discontinuation. The primary driver of this difference was likely the higher rate of grade 3 or higher hypocalcemia seen in denosumab-treated patients (5% vs. 1%). Overall rates of hypocalcemia, an expected on-target toxicity of both denosumab and zoledronic acid, were 13% and 6%, respectively ($P < .0001$). Osteonecrosis of the jaw occurs at similar rates in patients treated with denosumab and zoledronic acid (2% vs. 1%, respectively). In contrast, although adverse events overall were more common with denosumab, denosumab is less likely to precipitate an acute phase reaction compared with zoledronic acid (18% vs. 8%).

Nephrotoxicity is a significant dose-dependent concern with zoledronic acid treatment (74) but has not been reported with denosumab treatment (57). The risk of nephrotoxicity from zoledronic acid increases in the setting of preexisting renal dysfunction and thus was a basis for exclusion from the phase III trial comparing denosumab with zoledronic acid in patients with prostate cancer. No significant difference in nephrotoxicity between the two agents was reported in patients with prostate cancer (60); however, other studies have reported a significantly reduced rate of nephrotoxicity for denosumab compared to zoledronic acid (75). In summary, denosumab is associated with higher rates of hypocalcemia, similar rates of osteonecrosis of the jaw, and lower rates of acute phase reactions and renal dysfunction compared to zoledronic acid.

At the moment, denosumab is costlier than zoledronic acid. Several studies have attempted to assess the relative cost-effectiveness of these two treatments. Over 1 year of treatment, the incremental cost of denosumab treatment compared to zoledronic acid in the United States is approximately $7,000 (76,77). Given the lower skeletal-related event rate on denosumab versus zoledronic acid (60), the incremental cost of preventing one skeletal-related event with denosumab over zoledronic acid was estimated to be $71,027 in the first year and $51,319 over 3 years (77). An independent analysis using a lifetime horizon concluded that the cost to prevent one skeletal-related event with denosumab was $8,567 (78). The time horizon of analysis may have similarly affected estimates of cost per quality-adjusted life-year gained with denosumab treatment which ranged from $49,405 (78) to $1M (76). In comparison, zoledronic acid is associated with an incremental cost of $12,300 per skeletal-related event avoided and $159,200 per quality-adjusted life year compared to placebo (79).

Cost-effectiveness analyses are sensitive to drug costs, which in turn are affected by the new availability of generic competition for zoledronic acid as well as industry-supported patient access schemes. For example, a study in the United Kingdom concluded that denosumab was cost-effective compared to zoledronic acid only with the availability of discounted drug through a patient access scheme (80). The source of research funding may influence research methodology and ultimately, the conclusions of cost-effectiveness studies (81). Regardless of the controversy and uncertainties regarding cost-effectiveness, one thing that is not disputed is the superiority of denosumab compared to zoledronic acid in prevention of skeletal-related events.

CONCLUSION

In summary, cancer-, host-, and treatment-dependent factors place patients with prostate cancer at high risk of skeletal morbidity. Prostate cancer bone metastases typically appear osteoblastic on imaging studies but are characterized by both abnormal bone formation and resorption. This state of increased bone turnover can be measured biochemically in clinical samples such as blood and urine. An understanding of the molecular signaling driving osteoblast and osteoclast function has led to the development of clinically useful treatments to minimize the skeletal-related morbidity. Two inhibitors of bone resorption, namely zoledronic acid and denosumab, are effective at reducing skeletal-related events in patients with metastatic castrate-resistant prostate cancer.

■ REFERENCES

1. Bubendorf L, Schopfer A, Wagner U, et al. Metastatic patterns of prostate cancer: an autopsy study of 1,589 patients. *Hum Pathol.* 2000;31(5):578–583.
2. Sathiakumar N, Delzell E, Morrisey MA, et al. Mortality following bone metastasis and skeletal-related events among men with prostate cancer: a population-based analysis of US Medicare beneficiaries, 1999-2006. *Prostate Cancer Prostatic Dis.* 2011;14(2):177–183.
3. Norgaard M, Jensen AO, Jacobsen JB, et al. Skeletal related events, bone metastasis and survival of prostate cancer: a population based cohort study in Denmark (1999 to 2007). *J Urol.* 2010;184(1):162–167.
4. Lee RJ, Saylor PJ, Smith MR. Treatment and prevention of bone complications from prostate cancer. *Bone.* 2011;48(1):88–95.
5. Groot MT, Boeken Kruger CG, Pelger RC, et al. Costs of prostate cancer, metastatic to the bone, in the Netherlands. *Eur Urol.* 2003;43(3):226–232.
6. Lage MJ, Barber BL, Harrison DJ, et al. The cost of treating skeletal-related events in patients with prostate cancer. *Am J Manag Care.* 2008;14(5):317–322.
7. Schulman KL, Kohles J. Economic burden of metastatic bone disease in the U.S. *Cancer.* 2007;109(11):2334–2342.
8. Hadjidakis DJ, Androulakis, II. Bone remodeling. *Ann N Y Acad Sci.* 2006;1092:385–396.
9. Golub EE, Boesze-Battaglia K. The role of alkaline phosphatase in mineralization. *Curr Opin Orthop.* 2007;18(5):444–448.
10. Roodman GD. Mechanisms of bone metastasis. *N Engl J Med.* 2004;350(16):1655–1664.
11. Clarke NW, McClure J, George NJ. Morphometric evidence for bone resorption and replacement in prostate cancer. *Br J Urol.* 1991;68(1):74–80.
12. Charhon SA, Chapuy MC, Delvin EE, et al. Histomorphometric analysis of sclerotic bone metastases from prostatic carcinoma special reference to osteomalacia. *Cancer.* 1983;51(5):918–924.
13. Nelson JB, Hedican SP, George DJ, et al. Identification of endothelin-1 in the pathophysiology of metastatic adenocarcinoma of the prostate. *Nat Med.* 1995;1(9):944–949.
14. Saad F, Gleason DM, Murray R, et al. A randomized, placebo-controlled trial of zoledronic acid in patients with hormone-refractory metastatic prostate carcinoma. *J Natl Cancer Inst.* 2002;94(19):1458–1468.
15. Brown JE, Cook RJ, Major P, et al. Bone turnover markers as predictors of skeletal complications in prostate cancer, lung cancer, and other solid tumors. *J Natl Cancer Inst.* 2005;97(1):59–69.
16. Keller ET, Brown J. Prostate cancer bone metastases promote both osteolytic and osteoblastic activity. *J Cell Biochem.* 2004;91(4):718–729.
17. Percival RC, Urwin GH, Harris S, et al. Biochemical and histological evidence that carcinoma of the prostate is associated with increased bone resorption. *Eur J Surg Oncol.* 1987;13(1):41–49.
18. Garnero P, Buchs N, Zekri J, et al. Markers of bone turnover for the management of patients with bone metastases from prostate cancer. *Br J Cancer.* 2000;82(4):858–864.
19. Berruti A, Dogliotti L, Bitossi R, et al. Incidence of skeletal complications in patients with bone metastatic prostate cancer and hormone refractory disease: predictive role of bone resorption and formation markers evaluated at baseline. *J Urol.* 2000;164(4):1248–1253.
20. Jung K, Lein M, Stephan C, et al. Comparison of 10 serum bone turnover markers in prostate carcinoma patients with bone metastatic spread: diagnostic and prognostic implications. *Int J Cancer.* 2004;111(5):783–791.
21. Brown JE, Sim S. Evolving role of bone biomarkers in castration-resistant prostate cancer. *Neoplasia.* 2010;12(9):685–696.
22. Saad F, Eastham JA, Smith MR. Biochemical markers of bone turnover and clinical outcomes in men with prostate cancer. *Urol Oncol.* 2012;30(4):369–378.
23. Urwin GH, Percival RC, Harris S, et al. Generalised increase in bone resorption in carcinoma of the prostate. *Br J Urol.* 1985;57(6):721–723.
24. Zhang J, Dai J, Qi Y, et al. Osteoprotegerin inhibits prostate cancer-induced osteoclastogenesis and prevents prostate tumor growth in the bone. *J Clin Invest.* 2001;107(10):1235–1244.
25. Seibel MJ. The use of molecular markers of bone turnover in the management of patients with metastatic bone disease. *Clin Endocrinol (Oxf).* 2008;68(6):839–849.
26. Seibel MJ. Biochemical markers of bone turnover: part I: biochemistry and variability. *Clin Biochem Rev.* 2005;26(4):97–122.
27. Halabi S, Small EJ, Kantoff PW, et al. Prognostic model for predicting survival in men with hormone-refractory metastatic prostate cancer. *J Clin Oncol.* 2003;21(7):1232–1237.
28. Smaletz O, Scher HI, Small EJ, et al. Nomogram for overall survival of patients with progressive metastatic prostate cancer after castration. *J Clin Oncol.* 2002;20(19):3972–3982.
29. Smith MR, Cook R, Lee KA, et al. Disease and host characteristics as predictors of time to first bone metastasis and death in men with progressive castration-resistant nonmetastatic prostate cancer. *Cancer.* 2011;117(10):2077–2085.
30. Smith MR, Cook RJ, Coleman R, et al. Predictors of skeletal complications in men with hormone-refractory metastatic prostate cancer. *Urology.* 2007;70(2):315–319.
31. Cook RJ, Coleman R, Brown J, et al. Markers of bone metabolism and survival in men with hormone-refractory metastatic prostate cancer. *Clin Cancer Res.* 2006;12(11 pt 1):3361–3367.
32. Lein M, Miller K, Wirth M, et al. Bone turnover markers as predictive tools for skeletal complications in men with metastatic prostate cancer treated with zoledronic acid. *Prostate.* 2009;69(6):624–632.
33. Lipton A, Cook R, Saad F, et al. Normalization of bone markers is associated with improved survival in patients with bone metastases from solid tumors and elevated bone resorption receiving zoledronic acid. *Cancer.* 2008;113(1):193–201.
34. Berruti A, Tucci M, Mosca A, et al. Predictive factors for skeletal complications in hormone-refractory prostate cancer patients with metastatic bone disease. *Br J Cancer.* 2005;93(6):633–638.
35. Smith MR, Kabbinavar F, Saad F, et al. Natural history of rising serum prostate-specific antigen in men with castrate nonmetastatic prostate cancer. *J Clin Oncol.* 2005;23(13):2918–2925.
36. Brawley OW. Prostate cancer epidemiology in the United States. *World J Urol.* 2012;30(2):195–200.
37. Shahinian VB, Kuo YF, Freeman JL, et al. Risk of fracture after androgen deprivation for prostate cancer. *N Engl J Med.* 2005;352(2):154–164.
38. Smith MR. Treatment-related osteoporosis in men with prostate cancer. *Clin Cancer Res.* 2006;12(20 pt 2):6315s–6319s.
39. Sharifi N, Gulley JL, Dahut WL. Androgen deprivation therapy for prostate cancer. *JAMA.* 2005;294(2):238–244.
40. Oefelein MG, Ricchuiti V, Conrad W, et al. Skeletal fracture associated with androgen suppression induced osteoporosis: the clinical incidence and risk factors for patients with prostate cancer. *J Urol.* 2001;166(5):1724–1728.

41. Tannock IF, Osoba D, Stockler MR, et al. Chemotherapy with mitoxantrone plus prednisone or prednisone alone for symptomatic hormone-resistant prostate cancer: a Canadian randomized trial with palliative endpoints. *J Clin Oncol.* 1996;14(6):1756–1764.
42. Tannock IF, de Wit R, Berry WR, et al. Docetaxel plus prednisone or mitoxantrone plus prednisone for advanced prostate cancer. *N Engl J Med.* 2004;351(15):1502–1512.
43. de Bono JS, Oudard S, Ozguroglu M, et al. Prednisone plus cabazitaxel or mitoxantrone for metastatic castration-resistant prostate cancer progressing after docetaxel treatment: a randomised open-label trial. *Lancet.* 2010;376(9747):1147–1154.
44. de Bono JS, Logothetis CJ, Molina A, et al. Abiraterone and increased survival in metastatic prostate cancer. *N Engl J Med.* 2011;364(21):1995–2005.
45. Drake MT, Murad MH, Mauck KF, et al. Clinical review. Risk factors for low bone mass-related fractures in men: a systematic review and meta-analysis. *J Clin Endocrinol Metab.* 2012;97(6):1861–1870.
46. Khosla S. Minireview: the OPG/RANKL/RANK system. *Endocrinology.* 2001;142(12):5050–5055.
47. Lacey DL, Timms E, Tan HL, et al. Osteoprotegerin ligand is a cytokine that regulates osteoclast differentiation and activation. *Cell.* 1998;93(2):165–176.
48. Quinn DI, Tangen CM, Hussain M, et al. Docetaxel and atrasentan versus docetaxel and placebo for men with advanced castration-resistant prostate cancer (SWOG S0421): a randomised phase 3 trial. *Lancet Oncol.* 2013;14(9):893-900.
49. Fizazi KS, Higano CS, Nelson JB, et al. Phase III, randomized, placebo-controlled study of docetaxel in combination with zibotentan in patients with metastatic castration-resistant prostate cancer. *J Clin Oncol.* 2013;31(14):1740–1747.
50. Nelson JB, Love W, Chin JL, et al. Phase 3, randomized, controlled trial of atrasentan in patients with nonmetastatic, hormone-refractory prostate cancer. *Cancer.* 2008;113(9):2478-2487.
51. Michaelson MD, Smith MR. Bisphosphonates for treatment and prevention of bone metastases. *J Clin Oncol.* 2005;23(32):8219–8224.
52. Saad F, Gleason DM, Murray R, et al. Long-term efficacy of zoledronic acid for the prevention of skeletal complications in patients with metastatic hormone-refractory prostate cancer. *J Natl Cancer Inst.* 2004;96(11):879–882.
53. Weinfurt KP, Anstrom KJ, Castel LD, et al. Effect of zoledronic acid on pain associated with bone metastasis in patients with prostate cancer. *Ann Oncol.* 2006;17(6):986–989.
54. Woo S-B, Hellstein JW, Kalmar JR. Systematic review: bisphosphonates and osteonecrosis of the jaws. *Ann Intern Med.* 2006;144(10):753–761.
55. Ernst DS, Tannock IF, Winquist EW, et al. Randomized, double-blind, controlled trial of mitoxantrone/prednisone and clodronate versus mitoxantrone/prednisone and placebo in patients with hormone-refractory prostate cancer and pain. *J Clin Oncol.* 2003;21(17):3335–3342.
56. Small EJ, Smith MR, Seaman JJ, et al. Combined analysis of two multicenter, randomized, placebo-controlled studies of pamidronate disodium for the palliation of bone pain in men with metastatic prostate cancer. *J Clin Oncol.* 2003;21(23):4277–4284.
57. Fizazi K, Lipton A, Mariette X, et al. Randomized phase II trial of denosumab in patients with bone metastases from prostate cancer, breast cancer, or other neoplasms after intravenous bisphosphonates. *J Clin Oncol.* 2009;27(10):1564–1571.
58. Body JJ, Lipton A, Gralow J, et al. Effects of denosumab in patients with bone metastases with and without previous bisphosphonate exposure. *J Bone Miner Res.* 2010;25(3):440–446.
59. Fizazi K, Bosserman L, Gao G, et al. Denosumab treatment of prostate cancer with bone metastases and increased urine N-telopeptide levels after therapy with intravenous bisphosphonates: results of a randomized phase II trial. *J Urol.* 2009;182(2):509–515; discussion 515–516.
60. Fizazi K, Carducci M, Smith M, et al. Denosumab versus zoledronic acid for treatment of bone metastases in men with castration-resistant prostate cancer: a randomised, double-blind study. *Lancet.* 2011;377(9768):813–822.
61. Smith MR, Halabi S, Ryan CJ, et al. Efficacy and safety of zoledronic acid in men with castration-sensitive prostate cancer and bone metastases: results of CALGB 90202 (Alliance) [abstract 27]. *J Clin Oncol.* 2013;31(S6).
62. Dearnaley DP, Sydes MR, Mason MD, et al. A double-blind, placebo-controlled, randomized trial of oral sodium clodronate for metastatic prostate cancer (MRC PR05 Trial). *J Natl Cancer Inst.* 2003;95(17):1300–1311.
63. Smith MR, McGovern FJ, Zietman AL, et al. Pamidronate to prevent bone loss during androgen-deprivation therapy for prostate cancer. *N Engl J Med.* 2001;345(13):948–955.
64. Smith MR, Eastham J, Gleason DM, et al. Randomized controlled trial of zoledronic acid to prevent bone loss in men receiving androgen deprivation therapy for nonmetastatic prostate cancer. *J Urol.* 2003;169(6):2008–2012.
65. Klotz LH, McNeill IY, Kebabdjian M, et al. A phase 3, double-blind, randomised, parallel-group, placebo-controlled study of oral weekly alendronate for the prevention of androgen deprivation bone loss in nonmetastatic prostate cancer: the cancer and osteoporosis research with alendronate and leuprolide (CORAL) study. *Eur Urol.* 2013;63(5):927–935.
66. Greenspan SL, Nelson JB, Trump DL, et al. Effect of once-weekly oral alendronate on bone loss in men receiving androgen deprivation therapy for prostate cancer: a randomized trial. *Ann Intern Med.* 2007;146(6):416–424.
67. Choo R, Lukka H, Cheung P, et al. Randomized, double-blinded, placebo-controlled, trial of risedronate for the prevention of bone mineral density loss in nonmetastatic prostate cancer patients receiving radiation therapy plus androgen deprivation therapy. *Int J Radiat Oncol Biol Phys.* 2013;85(5):1239–1245.
68. Smith MR, Egerdie B, Hernandez Toriz N, et al. Denosumab in men receiving androgen-deprivation therapy for prostate cancer. *N Engl J Med.* 2009;361(8):745–755.
69. Smith MR, Saad F, Egerdie B, et al. Denosumab and changes in bone turnover markers during androgen deprivation therapy for prostate cancer. *J Bone Miner Res.* 2011;26(12):2827–2833.
70. Smith MR, Saad F, Egerdie B, et al. Effects of denosumab on bone mineral density in men receiving androgen deprivation therapy for prostate cancer. *J Urol.* 2009;182(6):2670–2675.
71. Mason MD, Sydes MR, Glaholm J, et al. Oral sodium clodronate for nonmetastatic prostate cancer—results of a randomized double-blind placebo-controlled trial: Medical Research Council PR04 (ISRCTN61384873). *J Natl Cancer Inst.* 2007;99(10):765–776.
72. Wirth M, Tammela T, Cicalese V, et al. Prevention of Bone Metastases in Patients with High-risk Nonmetastatic Prostate Cancer Treated with Zoledronic Acid: Efficacy and Safety Results of the Zometa European Study (ZEUS). *Eur Urol*, 2014. http://dx.doi.org/10.1016/j.eururo.2014.02.014.
73. Smith MR, Saad F, Coleman R, et al. Denosumab and bone-metastasis-free survival in men with castration-resistant prostate cancer: results of a phase 3, randomised, placebo-controlled trial. *Lancet.* 2012;379(9810):39–46.
74. Chang JT, Green L, Beitz J. Renal failure with the use of zoledronic acid. *N Engl J Med.* 2003;349(17):1676–1679; discussion 1676–1679.
75. Stopeck AT, Lipton A, Body JJ, et al. Denosumab compared with zoledronic acid for the treatment of bone metastases in patients with advanced breast cancer: a randomized, double-blind study. *J Clin Oncol.* 2010;28(35):5132–5139.
76. Snedecor SJ, Carter JA, Kaura S, et al. Denosumab versus zoledronic acid for treatment of bone metastases in men with castration-resistant prostate cancer: a cost-effectiveness analysis. *J Med Econ.* 2013;16(1):19–29.
77. Xie J, Namjoshi M, Wu EQ, et al. Economic evaluation of denosumab compared with zoledronic acid in hormone-refractory

prostate cancer patients with bone metastases. *J Manag Care Pharm*. 2011;17(8):621–643.

78. Stopeck A, Rader M, Henry D, et al. Cost-effectiveness of denosumab vs zoledronic acid for prevention of skeletal-related events in patients with solid tumors and bone metastases in the United States. *J Med Econ*. 2012;15(4):712–723.
79. Reed SD, Radeva JI, Glendenning GA, et al. Cost-effectiveness of zoledronic acid for the prevention of skeletal complications in patients with prostate cancer. *J Urol*. 2004;171(4):1537–1542.
80. Ford J, Cummins E, Sharma P, et al. Systematic review of the clinical effectiveness and cost-effectiveness, and economic evaluation, of denosumab for the treatment of bone metastases from solid tumours. *Health Technol Assess*. 2013;17(29):1–386.
81. Koo K, Lam K, Mittmann N, et al. Comparing cost-effectiveness analyses of denosumab versus zoledronic acid for the treatment of bone metastases. *Support Care Cancer*. 2013;21(6):1785–1791.

19.6 Treatment of Bone Metastases: Radiopharmaceuticals

HOSSEIN JADVAR

LESLIE BALLAS

DAVID I. QUINN

■ INTRODUCTION

Castration-resistant prostate cancer is universally fatal. More than 90% of patients have bone metastases, which are predominantly osteoblastic (1). There has been a myriad of progress in the therapy of advanced prostate cancer in recent years with novel chemotherapy, immunotherapy, and androgen receptor pathway targeted therapy all demonstrating improvements in survival (2–7). Concurrently, attempts have been made at targeting the bone milieu where most patients manifest their disease. Targeted therapy of the bone with osteoblast-directed endothelin pathway inhibitors such as atrasentan and zibotentan have not proven successful (8, 9). Osteoclast inhibitors in the form of bisphosphonates and rank-ligand inhibition have demonstrated success in delaying skeletal-related events and pain but did not improve survival (10, 11). Radiopharmaceutical agents such as strontium-89 (Sr-89) and samarium-153 (Sm-153) have major palliative impact and delay disease progression but have not improved prostate cancer survival (12–15).

On that basis, a major opportunity existed for a bone-targeted agent that palliates and improves survival. Although molecular agents targeting vascular endothelial growth factor and C-MET pathways have shown promise, the calcium mimetic targeted alpha particle as a radiopharmaceutical, radium-223 (Ra-223), is the first to achieve this goal (16, 17). Radium-223 has unique properties related to delivery to the site of calcium deposition at the interface between prostate cancer and bone and the narrow band and exponential cancer killing ability of alpha particles. Such a therapy is beneficial in both treating and delaying cancer-associated pain and extending survival in castration-resistant prostate cancer patients with symptomatic bone metastases. This chapter discusses the use of radiopharmaceutical agents in the treatment of bone metastases in men with prostate cancer, focusing on Sm-153, Sr-89, and Ra-223, and reviews the use of imaging to assess response to these agents.

■ OLDER BONE-DIRECTED RADIONUCLIDES: Sr-89 AND Sm-153

Bone pain is a common symptom in metastatic cancer and is often not controlled with opioids alone. Radiation, in the form of radiopharmaceuticals, is one treatment modality that has been used to palliate bone pain. Radiopharmaceuticals offer ease in administration, the ability to treat multiple sites of disease at once, and the benefit in therapeutic ratio that comes with a highly specific and localized treatment modality; they localize to areas of high bone turnover and deliver high focal doses of radiation with limited distribution to normal tissues using beta particles.

Candidates for radionuclide therapy have multiple metastases that demonstrate radiotracer uptake on bone scintigraphy and who have competent bone marrow. Practice guidelines by the ACR-ASTRO (18) state that patients should have a complete blood count with platelets within 7 days prior to therapy to determine a competent bone marrow. Platelet count should be greater than 60,000/mL, leukocyte count greater than 2,400/mL, and absolute granulocyte count greater than 2,000/mL. In addition, the patient should have a life span of greater than 3 months, and if the patient has urinary incontinence, the patient should have bladder catheterization to minimize the risk of radiation contamination. Other recommendations include the restriction that the patient should not have received myelosuppressive chemotherapy for 6 to 8 weeks prior to infusion (18). Relative contraindications to the use of bone-targeted radionuclides include soft-tissue pain, unifocal bone lesions, and osteolytic lesions (those that show poor uptake on a bone scan). Absolute contraindications include severe marrow suppression and severe renal dysfunction (19, 20).

Table 19.6.1 Physical characteristics of radiopharmaceuticals in common use in patients with bone metastases from prostate cancer

Radionuclide	Half-Life (days)	Maximum Energy (MeV)	Mean Energy (MeV)	Maximum Range	γ-Emission (keV)
Sm-153	1.9	0.81 (β)	0.229 (β)	4 mm	None
Sr-89	50.5	1.4 (β)	0.583 (β)	7 mm	103
Ra-223	11.4	NA	5.78 (α)	< 10 μm	154

Source: Refs. (58), (108), (109).

Table 19.6.2 Comparative clinical properties of Sm-153, Sr-89, and Ra-223 in patients with advanced prostate cancer

Radionuclide	Delayed Skeletal-Related Events	Palliation	Overall Survival Benefit	Delayed PSA Progression	Surrogate Marker	Marrow Suppression
Sm-153	Not assessed	Yes (37)	No (37)	Yes (14)	Nil	Mild to moderate (37)
Sr-89	Trend (15)	Yes (15)	No (15)	Yes (25)	Nil	Moderate to severe (110)
Ra-223	Yes (17)	Yes (17)	Yes (17)	Yes (62)	Serum alkaline phosphatase (17, 62)	Minimal to mild (17, 62)

Although multiple radionuclides have been studied for use in bone metastases, the most commonly used are Sr-89 and Sm-153 (Tables 19.6.1 and 19.6.2). Each radionuclide targets bone through a different mechanism. Sr-89 is taken up as a calcium analogue, and Sm-153 is chelated to ethylenediamine tetra(methylene phosphonic) acid (EDTMP) and localizes to bone in association with hydroxyapatite. Once chelated, Sm-153 emits beta particles with a maximum energy of 0.81 MeV, an average soft-tissue range of 0.6 mm, and a half-life of 1.9 days. Sr-89 has a maximum energy of 1.47 MeV, an average soft-tissue range of 2.4 mm, and a half-life of 50.5 days (21). The shorter half-life of Sm-153 allows for a faster radiation delivery and rapid clearance from the body after intravenous injection. Delivery of approximately 90% of the total dose of radiation requires approximately 3.5 half-lives or 1 week for Sm-153 and 25 weeks for Sr-89 (19,20).

RANDOMIZED DATA FOR THE CLINICAL USE OF STRONTIUM

Sr-89 has a 10-fold increased localization for metastatic tumor over normal bone (21). Despite nonuniformity in studies regarding the dose-response relationship, a retrospective review found a dose-response relationship with increasing doses of Sr-89 (22). The recommended dose for Sr-89 is 40 to 60 mCi/kg or about 4 mCi for standard weight patients.

Multiple phase III studies have been performed testing the efficacy of Sr-89. Complete pain relief has been reported in between 17.6% and 65.1% of patients at 3 months (23–25) with some pain response in 91% (26). In a systematic review published by Finlay et al., the complete pain response varied between 8% and 77% with a mean value of 32%. The time delay until the onset of treatment effect varied from 4 to 28 days with a mean duration of response lasting 15 months. Decreased analgesic use has been reported in 71% to 81% of patients (27). Compared with placebo in a phase III crossover double-blind trial, Lewington found a complete pain response in the Sr-89 arm and a better clinical response with Sr-89 than with placebo at first assessment ($P < .01$) (28).

Using a pain score, performance status, and analgesic use, Oosterhof et al. compared Sr-89 with local radiation therapy (XRT) and found no difference in the subjective response of patients (13). Porter et al. followed involved-field XRT with Sr-89 and found that at 3 months, a higher proportion of patients who received Sr-89 were pain free (no statistical significance reported). In addition, the patients who received Sr-89 had fewer new sites of pain than those who did not receive Sr-89 (23).

Although the majority of studies showed no overall survival benefit to the addition of Sr-89 to either cisplatin or radiation, Buchali compared Sr-89 with placebo and found a median overall survival to be 46% at 2 years in the Sr-89 group compared with 4% at 2 years in the placebo group (the authors did not report on 10 patients who died of disease in the first 3 months and the study had a small sample size) (29). Pain relief was not different in the two groups.

Toxicity in all of these studies included leukopenia and thrombocytopenia. Just as pain response varied, so too did toxicity. Reports of thrombocytopenia ranged from 30% to 80% with a mean nadir of counts 4 to 8 weeks following injection; grade 3 to 4 leukopenia was reported in < 10% of patients (21).

Based on these randomized control studies, practice guidelines were developed by the Practice Guidelines Initiative Genitourinary Cancer Disease Site Group. They recommended the use of Sr-89 in the setting of castrate-resistant metastatic prostate cancer in which multiple single-XRT fields are not possible. Moreover, they did not recommend Sr-89 as an adjunct to XRT (30).

The addition of Sr-89 to chemotherapy or the reverse has been evaluated in several early phase clinical studies (31–34). The tolerability of different combinations has varied but is acceptable in selected patients. A randomized phase II trial evaluated treatment with ketoconazole, doxorubicin, estramustine, and vinblastine with or without Sr-89 consolidation in men with castration-resistant prostate cancer (35, 36). In this trial of 103 men, 72 of whom were randomized to strontium, the median survival favored the strontium group with a median of 27.7 months compared with 16.8 months in the control group (P = .0014). A follow-up phase III study examining chemotherapy with or without Sr-89 completed accrual in 2012 with results awaited. A phase III TRAPEZE study examined the addition of Sr-89 or zoledronic acid to docetaxel in men with castration-resistant prostate cancer and bone metastases (15). The use of Sr-89 delayed progression-free survival in the context of a prespecified multivariate analysis (hazard ratio = 0.85; P = .036) but did not delay skeletal-related events or improve survival compared to arms containing docetaxel and docetaxel with zoledronic acid (15).

Sr-89 is a useful palliative agent in patients with advanced prostate cancer and bone metastases; however, its use in combination with chemotherapy is not standard care.

■ RANDOMIZED DATA FOR THE CLINICAL USE OF SAMARIUM

Samarium, when complexed with EDTMP, has preferential affinity for metastatic lesions over normal bone (21). Multiple phase I/II studies have examined the dose-response relationship of samarium. Although doses from 0.2 mCi/kg to 2.5 mCi/kg have been evaluated, the recommended dose of Sm-153 is 1.0 mCi/kg. The adverse effects that limited dose escalation were myelosuppression and thrombocytopenia. This was reported in 20% to 42% of patients (27). Pain response in this same population ranged from 72% to 88% (21).

Three phase III studies and one abstract looked at Sm-153 either compared to placebo or compared to smaller doses of samarium. The endpoint for all three studies was pain relief. Olea et al. found overall pain relief of 73%, which was independent of dose (30). Serafini et al. compared 0.5 mCi/kg to 1.0 mCi/kg and placebo in 118 patients with symptomatic bone metastases from a variety of primary tumor sites. In this study, 62% to 72% of patients had pain relief with 1.0 mCi/kg during the first 4 weeks and 31% had complete/marked relief by week 4 while 0.5 mCi/kg was less effective and did not produce sustained pain responses. With 1.0 mCi/kg of samarium, the grade 3 to 4 anemia was 6%, thrombocytopenia was 3%, and leukopenia was 14%. The placebo group reported 35%, 0%, and 0%, respectively. In addition, they examined analgesic use during the same period and found significant correlation between reductions of analgesia and pain scores in the 1.0 mCi/kg cohort (37).

Another phase III study led by Sartor et al. compared 1.0 mCi/kg Sm-153 to nonradioactive lexidronam complexes in a 2:1 ratio in 152 men with advanced castration-resistant prostate cancer. These patients received significant improvement in bone pain and decrease in analgesic use with Sm-153 (P < .05). The patients reported differences favoring Sm-153 in areas of pain descriptor scales, visual analogue scales, and opiate use (20, 30).

The third phase III study by Resche et al. compared Sm-153 at 0.5 mCi/kg with 1.0 mCi/kg for differences in pain relief. There was a significant difference in pain scores between the doses at week 4 (P = .0476). Although the leukocyte nadir and platelets were lower with the 1.0 mCi/kg group, there was no overall survival difference between the two groups. At week 4, pain relief was 70% in the 1.0 mCi/kg group compared with 55% in the 0.5mCi/kg group. All three studies prove that 1.0 mCi/kg of Sm-153 is safe and effective in pain control and should be considered in patients who meet the criteria for radionuclide usage (38).

Sm-153 can be combined with docetaxel in patients with mCRPC with symptomatic improvement and a reasonable duration of cancer control, but thrombocytopenia is dose limiting for Sm-153 retreatment in at least 30% of patients (39). In addition, a French study used Sm-153 in combination to consolidate in patients responding to four cycles of docetaxel-based therapy (14). They observed long-term pain and serum prostate-specific antigen (PSA) control in these patients with minimal toxicity. These findings should ideally be tested in a phase III setting, but this is unlikely given the advent of Ra-223. Sm-153 has clinical efficacy in improving pain and has a reasonable safety profile in patients with advanced prostate cancer; however, it has not shown improved survival (Table 19.6.2).

■ COMPARATIVE EFFICACY OF SR-89 AND SM-153

Liepe et al. compared Re-186, Sm-153, and Sr-89 in terms of impact on pain symptoms, quality of life as assessed with Karnofsky performance status, and bone marrow function. There was no difference reported for toxicity between the different radiopharmaceuticals; 73% of patients had some relief of their pain and there was a trend toward improved performance status at 12 weeks (P = .15) (40). In another study involving the comparison of Sr-89 and Sm-153 in 100 patients with prostate and breast cancer bone metastases, no difference was seen between the two agents regarding analgesic effects (21).

■ ALPHA PARTICLE THERAPY AND RA-223

There are more than 100 alpha-emitting radioisotopes, but most decay too quickly to be useful for targeted radionuclide therapy. Alpha particles are positively charged helium nuclei with a short range of about 50 to 80 μm (vs. several millimeters for beta particles) and high linear transfer energy of about 100 to 200 keV/μm (vs. beta particles 0.2 keV/μm) (Table 19.6.1). The relative biological effect (RBE) of alpha particles is about three- to sevenfold of that for x-ray reference radiation for cell sterilization (41–46). The very high-energy deposition of alpha particles at a very small distance can cause irreversible double-strand DNA breaks. This is in contrast to beta particles, which are often associated with single-strand DNA breaks. Cells are much better equipped to repair single-strand DNA breaks than double-strand DNA breaks (47). Other than DNA breaks, the high localized irradiated energy leads to radiolysis of intracellular water, which results in highly toxic radicals and chemicals that destroy the cell. Since the high energy of alpha particles is given off over a very short range, the targeted cells receive high absorbed radiation doses while adjacent cells (tumor or healthy cells) may receive little or no radiation at all. The conventional MIRD (medical internal radiation dose) dosimetric method may therefore not be appropriate in this setting, and microdosimetric methods have been devised (48). Of further importance in prostate cancer, and also potentially breast cancer, is that the mechanisms of action of 223Ra through ds-DNA breaks and radiolysis are independent of the sex steroid receptor signaling mechanisms leveraged by most hormonal agents. This is potentially important as more exposure to androgen receptor pathway blockade pushes the cells toward an anaplastic state that may have growth kinetics independent of hormone signal and response (49). In this context of therapies such as 223Ra, which act independent of these agents, benefit may increase as the cancer progresses through these treatments.

Although there has been much interest in the use of alpha particles for targeted therapy, only lately this topic has been brought into spotlight by the U.S. Food and Drug Administration (FDA) approval (in May 2013) of 223Ra dichloride for targeted therapy of bone metastases in men with castration-resistant prostate cancer (50).

■ 223RA

Radium is a calcium mimetic and, along with barium and strontium, belongs to the alkali earth metals in the periodic table. On December 26, 1898, the Curies (Marie Curie and her husband Pierre Curie) informed the *l'Académie des Sciences* that they had come upon a very active substance that behaved chemically almost like pure barium and they suggested the name of *radium* (226Ra with a half-life of 1,601 years) for the new element. The Curies and Henri Becquerel shared the Nobel Prize in Physics in 1903 in recognition of the discovery and research on the radioactivity phenomenon (51). One of the radium isotopes, 223Ra, is the first alpha emitter that has undergone formal testing for clinical use. It can be obtained from uranium mill tailings or in generator form from 227Ac ($t_{1/2}$ = 21.8 years) parent through the reaction 227Ac⇒ 227Th ⇒ 223Ra. The half-life of 223Ra is 11.43 days. The emitted energy distribution is 93.5% as alpha particles, 5.78 MeV (average), < 3.6% as beta particles, < 1.1% as γ radiation with 28 MeV combined energy for complete decay including 0.9 MeV as γ radiation (Table 19.6.1).

223Ra targets the hydroxyapatite $[Ca_{10}(P0_4)_6(OH)_2]$ matrix in the bone naturally because it simulates the stoichiometry of calcium. It is interesting that the potential use of 223Ra in therapy was recognized more than a century ago by Dr. Louis Wickham, Director of the Radium Institute in 1909, when he observed that the "radium-therapy . . . has won its place in the therapeutic armamentarium, [as evidence that] that the French discovery of Curie and Madame Curie has borne definite and certain fruit in the medical field" (51,52). It should be noted that radium was used as a source for external beam radiation therapy until the 1960s when cobalt-60 and other more modern techniques prevailed (53,54). Ra-223 was first given intravenously to humans in the 1960s (55,56). Most recently in 2013, Vapiwala and Glatstein observed that "alpha particles in medicine may be newly explored 115 years after their discovery" (57).

Given the self-targeting of 223Ra to areas of active bone remodeling and formation, 223Ra was systematically evaluated for highly localized treatment of osteoblastic bone metastases (58–61). Early phase and dose finding trials with 223Ra led to a randomized phase II trial of the agent given every 4 weeks for four doses or placebo in 64 men with symptomatic bone metastases from prostate cancer who had just completed palliative external beam radiation to bone (62). In this study, primary endpoints were change in bone–alkaline phosphatase concentration and time to skeletal-related events, whereas secondary endpoints included toxic effects, time to PSA progression, and overall survival. Treatment with 223Ra produced a significant reduction in bone alkaline phosphates in serum and a trend toward delay in skeletal-related events with no significant differences in toxicity between the arms. Overall survival favored the 223Ra arm with a hazard ratio of 2.12 ($P = .02$, in a Cox regression model) (62).

In designing the phase III ALSYMPCA trial, investigators selected men with symptomatic, metastatic castration-resistant prostate cancer and gave six treatments of Ra-223 at a dose of 50 Kbq per kilogram of body weight every 4 weeks for six treatments in a ratio of two patients given Ra-223 for each patient who got placebo (17). Patients were required to have declined docetaxel or to have progressed on it or after it and were given best supportive care including secondary hormonal manipulation, analgesia, and osteoclast inhibitor agents during the trial. The primary endpoint was overall survival and the major secondary endpoint was delay in skeletal-related events. At the first interim analysis, 809 patients were evaluated, and there was a significant benefit in favor of Ra-223 for overall survival. An updated analysis involving 921 patients confirmed the survival benefit of Ra-223 (median 14.9 months vs. 11.3 months; hazard ratio = 0.70; 95% CI, 0.58–0.83; $P < .001$). Ra-223 also delayed time to skeletal-related events and was associated with fewer adverse effects and was notably associated with very low rates of myelosuppression (Table 19.6.2). The therapeutic benefit of Ra-223 was seen independent of concurrent bisphosphonate use or prior docetaxel use. Patients with elevated serum alkaline phosphates appeared to benefit more from Ra-223 than those with normal values at baseline. Subsequently, the U.S. FDA approved Ra-223 in May 2013 as treatment for patients with bone metastases from castration-resistant prostate cancer who do not have visceral metastases.

In practice, Ra-223 is now presented as an alternative to docetaxel chemotherapy when prostate cancer becomes castration resistant and progresses on subsequent hormonal therapy, including abiraterone acetate or enzalutamide or both and perhaps also immunotherapy with sipuleucel-T. Ra-223 is also used in patients who have progressed on docetaxel. The ideal timing of Ra-223 in the treatment sequence is the subject of debate. Clinicians currently struggle with the desire to use Ra-223 as an active agent in symptomatic bone metastases but in a window before visceral disease develops. The issue of combination with systemic agents that might control subclinical or treat clinical visceral metastases while Ra-223 acts on bone metastases is of considerable interest. Subsequent trials of Ra-223 will focus on combinations with abiraterone, enzalutamide, and docetaxel. In addition, the question of whether patients can be retreated with Ra-223 again with disease progression subsequent to a first course of treatment will be evaluated in a trial.

■ IMAGING IN THE ASSESSMENT OF BONE METASTASES

Imaging plays an important role in diagnosis and objective assessment of treatment response in metastatic prostate cancer (63–65). Imaging of prostate cancer response in bone is especially challenging given the lack of a single optimal imaging test and the need to interpret changes in the light of clinical and other data. There are several response criteria that have been devised incorporating image-based data in conjunction with other relevant information to guide treatment decisions. Imaging data may be based on anatomic information or may rely on physiologic information. It is well recognized that anatomic-based imaging may be deficient for accurate treatment response evaluation in view of the increasing use of novel cytostatic (rather than cytotoxic) drug regimen and the evidence that has been generated from the use of anatomic–physiologic hybrid imaging systems, often demonstrating that the anatomic response to treatment is discordant to or lags behind the metabolic changes (66,67). While bone scintigraphy and computed tomography remain the mainstay imaging for therapy assessment in metastatic prostate cancer, they are not readily quantifiable and have limited specificity (68). Other imaging methods such as magnetic resonance imaging (MRI) and positron emission tomography (PET) with various radiotracers allow for lesion quantification, which can then be monitored for changes induced by treatment and linked as imaging-based biomarkers to other independent clinical assessment criteria and to outcome parameters.

Computed Tomography

Computed tomography (CT) provides cross-sectional imaging information that can be reformatted to other planes for comprehensive assessment of cortical bony changes. However, CT is insensitive to bone marrow infiltration of disease in which there may be little or no visible structural abnormality of the bone cortex, and there is considerable interobserver variation in the assessment of bone lesions (69). The combination of PET and CT provides a comprehensive evaluation of both structural and metabolic abnormalities such that marrow lesions can be detected through PET when there may be no abnormal CT correlates (70). Osseous metastases from prostate cancer are commonly sclerotic on CT demonstrating high CT density. By examining the change in number of and density of bony lesions, CT can provide general information on the disease process. However, increasing density of osseous lesions may not necessarily indicate worsening of the metastatic disease. Messiou et al. showed that increase in bone sclerosis in the absence of fading bone metastases can be interpreted as "flare" response to treatment that in their study occurred 3 months after treatment in 8% of the patients with castrate-resistant metastatic prostate cancer (71).

Magnetic Resonance Imaging

MRI offers excellent soft-tissue contrast, high spatial resolution, multiplanar imaging, flexible imaging protocols including dynamic contrast enhanced and diffusion-weighted imaging sequences, and no patient exposure to ionizing radiation. Whole-body MRI with 1.5 T or 3.0 T scanners has been proposed as a one-stop shop imaging evaluation of patients with a variety of cancers (72–75).

In the context of bone metastases from prostate cancer, Reischauer et al. evaluated prospectively the utility of diffusion-weighted MRI and functional diffusion maps in monitoring antiandrogen treatment response (13, 76). The mean apparent diffusion coefficients (ADC, a marker of Brownian motion of water molecules in tissue with indirect information on tissue organization at a microscopic level and with tumor displaying restricted free water molecule diffusion or low ADC) for each metastasis were measured prior to and 3 months after therapy and were compared with serum PSA levels. The investigators found that mean ADCs of metastases increased significantly after therapy in comparison to pretreatment values, in concordance with significant decline in serum PSA levels, although marked heterogeneity of response was also noted, reflecting the complex chronologic and spatial evolution of bone metastases undergoing therapy. Similar results have been reported by others (77–79). Despite these early encouraging results, further studies will be needed to delineate the role of whole-body MRI with various sequence protocols in the quantitative assessment of treatment response in patients with metastatic prostate cancer.

Tc99m-Based Bone Scintigraphy

Bone scintigraphy with Tc99m-based radiotracers (e.g., Tc99m-methylene diphosphonate [MDP]) is the most common procedure in the imaging evaluation of patients with prostate cancer, is low cost, and is broadly available. High tracer uptake is typically associated with osteoblastic activity that is commonly associated with prostate cancer. Bone scintigraphy portrays the osteoblastic reaction of bone to the prostate tumor and does not image the tumor itself. It is important to recognize the relative nonspecificity of bone scintigraphy in cancer since radiotracer accumulation may also be seen with benign conditions such as inflammation (e.g., enthesopathy, arthropathy, spondylosis), infection, and fractures (80, 81).

Bone scintigraphy has long been used for evaluation of response to treatment. Successful treatment leads to tumor cell apoptosis, which can induce reactive bony changes (e.g., healing) and hence result in increased radiotracer accumulation or appearance of new lesions despite effective therapy (82). This treatment-related "flare" phenomenon is recognized and can be differentiated from true progression by serial imaging and correlation with pertinent clinical and laboratory information (83). A variety of response criteria such as the Response Evaluation Criteria in Solid Tumors (RECIST 1.0 and 1.1) guidelines are used to evaluate bone metastases in prostate cancer (84–87). Bone metastases are nonmeasurable lesions, and unequivocal resolution or the development of new lesions is considered as evidence of response or progression, respectively. Several institutions have attempted to improve on the standard imaging criteria, but these are not in widespread use (88–91).

Positron Emission Tomography

18F-Sodium Fluoride

18F-sodium fluoride (NaF) PET/CT offers significantly higher sensitivity and specificity for identifying bone metastases in comparison to 99mTc-based bone scintigraphy (92, 93). NaF was introduced in 1962 and approved by the FDA in 1972 (46, 94). There was, however, limited early use due to high-energy imaging technical limitations and widespread availability of Tc-99m-labeled agents. Czernin et al. summarizes the mechanism of 18F-NaF uptake in the bone (47, 95). Almost all the tracer is retained by bone after a single pass of blood with rapid clearance from plasma and urine excretion by the kidneys. The bone uptake is related to chemisorption onto hydroxyapatite matrix surface through 18F exchange for OH to form fluorapatite. Practice guidelines for the use of NaF PET/CT have been published (48, 96).

For evaluation of treatment response, NaF PET/CT is typically analyzed qualitatively, similar to 99mTc-MDP bone scan, based on comparative visual assessment of number, intensity, and extent of lesions before and after therapy. It must be noted that similar to 99mTc-MDP, a treatment-related "flare" phenomenon may also be seen with NaF PET(49,97). With respect to metastatic prostate cancer, only one case series from Britain showed that NaF PET/CT may be useful for semiquantitative assessment of response to alpha particle treatment with 223Ra-dichloride(50,98). Additional studies will be needed to define the role of NaF PET/CT in assessment of therapy response in patients with metastatic prostate cancer. Other PET tracer–based scans including fluoro deoxyglucose, choline, fluorocholine, and fluorodihydrotestosterone may have utility in prostate cancer but require further validation(99–106).

■ USE OF IMAGING TO ASSESS DISEASE CONTROL AND RESPONSE TO RADIOPHARMACEUTICALS

Objective assessment of therapy response in patients with bone metastases from prostate cancer is of prime importance to tailor treatment appropriately to individual patients and to achieve optimal outcome. Radiopharmaceuticals represent a particular challenge for clinicians because they are not associated with responses in traditional markers such as serum PSA. Experience with Sm-153 and Sr-89 suggests that disappearance of lesions on Tc99m-based bone scanning correlates with pain relief and duration of disease control, but prospective data are lacking. In assessing response to Ra-223, early experience suggests that the serum alkaline phosphatase is a more consistent marker of cancer control in bone than PSA(107), and decrease in serum alkaline phosphatase was associated with better survival in the ALSYMPCA trial(17). Experience outside the trial setting with Tc99m-based and NaF PET scan techniques suggests the correlation between symptom control and nonprogression on these scans, but further prospective experience is needed and will be forthcoming from several trials. Importantly, it has become clear that a proportion of patients on Ra-223 will develop progression outside the skeleton as signaled by symptoms and/or rapid rise in serum PSA or circulating tumor cell counts. On that basis, we routinely include imaging with CT or MRI and Tc99m or NaF scanning after three cycles of a six-cycle course of Ra-223 to assess for progression at that time point. Visceral or lymph node progression may mandate the addition of other systemic agents to keep the patient's cancer controlled.

■ CONCLUSION

Bone-directed radiopharmaceuticals have been available to treat prostate cancer with bone metastases for many years. Sm-153 and Sr-89 are useful palliative agents, which may delay time to progression in bone as measured by the time to the next skeletal-related event. The advent of Ra-223 has provided us with an agent that is more specifically targeted to the bone milieu and results in extension of survival as well as palliation and delay in skeletal-related events. Radiological assessment of bone metastases is challenging, and its role in assessing response to radiopharmaceuticals in concert with clinical and other biomarker data is being actively assessed. The approval of Ra-223 comes at a time when a series of other systemic agents has been developed and approved for advanced prostate cancer. The optimal sequencing and combining of these agents is currently unclear and the subject of clinical trials and evolving real-world use.

■ REFERENCES

1. Bubendorf L, Schopfer A, Wagner U, et al. Metastatic patterns of prostate cancer: an autopsy study of 1,589 patients. *Hum Pathol.* 2000;31(5):578–583.
2. Kantoff PW, Higano CS, Shore ND, et al. Sipuleucel-T immunotherapy for castration-resistant prostate cancer. *N Engl J Med.* 2010;363(5):411–422.
3. de Bono JS, Oudard S, Ozguroglu M, et al. Prednisone plus cabazitaxel or mitoxantrone for metastatic castration-resistant prostate cancer progressing after docetaxel treatment: a randomised open-label trial. *Lancet.* 2010;376(9747):1147–1154.
4. de Bono JS, Logothetis CJ, Molina A, et al. Abiraterone and increased survival in metastatic prostate cancer. *N Engl J Med.* 2011;364(21):1995–2005.
5. Ryan CJ, Smith MR, de Bono JS, et al. Abiraterone in metastatic prostate cancer without previous chemotherapy. *N Engl J Med.* 2013;368(2):138–148.
6. Scher HI, Beer TM, Higano CS, et al. Antitumour activity of MDV3100 in castration-resistant prostate cancer: a phase 1-2 study. *Lancet.* 2010;375(9724):1437–1446.
7. Scher HI, Fizazi K, Saad F, et al. Increased survival with enzalutamide in prostate cancer after chemotherapy. *N Engl J Med.* 2012;367:1187–1197.
8. Nelson JB, Fizazi K, Miller K, et al. Phase 3, randomized, placebo-controlled study of zibotentan (ZD4054) in patients with castration-resistant prostate cancer metastatic to bone. *Cancer.* 2012;118:5709–5718.
9. Quinn DI, Tangen CM, Hussain M, et al. Docetaxel and atrasentan versus docetaxel and placebo for men with advanced castration-resistant prostate cancer (SWOG S0421): a randomised phase 3 trial. *Lancet Oncol.* 2013;14(9):893–900.
10. Saad F, Gleason DM, Murray R, et al. A randomized, placebo-controlled trial of zoledronic acid in patients with hormone-refractory metastatic prostate carcinoma. *J Natl Cancer Inst.* 2002;94(19):1458–1468.
11. Fizazi K, Carducci M, Smith M, et al. Denosumab versus zoledronic acid for treatment of bone metastases in men with castration-resistant prostate cancer: a randomised, double-blind study. *Lancet.* 2011;377(9768):813–822.
12. Serafini AN. Samarium Sm-153 lexidronam for the palliation of bone pain associated with metastases. *Cancer.* 2000;88(12 suppl):2934–2939.
13. Oosterhof GO, Roberts JT, de Reijke TM, et al. Strontium(89) chloride versus palliative local field radiotherapy in patients with hormonal escaped prostate cancer: a phase III study of the European Organisation for Research and Treatment of Cancer, Genitourinary Group. *Eur Urol.* 2003;44(5):519–526.

14. Fizazi K, Beuzeboc P, Lumbroso J, et al. Phase II trial of consolidation docetaxel and samarium-153 in patients with bone metastases from castration-resistant prostate cancer. *J Clin Oncol*. 2009;27(15):2429–2435.
15. James ND, Pirrie S, Barton D, et al. *Clinical outcomes in patients with castrate-refractory prostate cancer (CRPC) metastatic to bone randomized in the factorial TRAPEZE trial to docetaxel (D) with strontium-89 (Sr89), zoledronic acid (ZA), neither, or both (ISRCTN 12808747)* [abstract LBA5000]. ASCO Meeting Abstracts. J Clin Oncol. 2013;31(suppl).
16. Smith DC, Smith MR, Sweeney C, et al. Cabozantinib in patients with advanced prostate cancer: results of a phase II randomized discontinuation trial. *J Clin Oncol*. 2013;31(4):412–419.
17. Parker C, Nilsson S, Heinrich D, et al. Alpha emitter radium-223 and survival in metastatic prostate cancer. *N Engl J Med*. 2013;369(3):213–223.
18. Henkin RE, Del Rowe JD, Grigsby PW, et al. ACR-ASTRO practice guideline for the performance of therapy with unsealed radiopharmaceutical sources. *Clin Nucl Med*. 2011;36(8):e72–e80.
19. Sartor O. Overview of samarium sm 153 lexidronam in the treatment of painful metastatic bone disease. *Rev Urol*. 2004;6 suppl 10:S3–S12.
20. Sartor O, Reid RH, Hoskin PJ, et al. Samarium-153-Lexidronam complex for treatment of painful bone metastases in hormone-refractory prostate cancer. *Urology*. 2004;63(5):940–945.
21. Goyal J, Antonarakis ES. Bone-targeting radiopharmaceuticals for the treatment of prostate cancer with bone metastases. *Cancer Lett*. 2012;323(2):135–146.
22. Mertens WC, Stitt L, Porter AT. Strontium 89 therapy and relief of pain in patients with prostatic carcinoma metastatic to bone: a dose response relationship? *Am J Clin Oncol*. 1993;16(3):238–242.
23. Porter AT, McEwan AJ, Powe JE, et al. Results of a randomized phase-III trial to evaluate the efficacy of strontium-89 adjuvant to local field external beam irradiation in the management of endocrine resistant metastatic prostate cancer. *Int J Radiat Oncol Biol Phys*. 1993;25(5):805–813.
24. Quilty PM, Kirk D, Bolger JJ, et al. A comparison of the palliative effects of strontium-89 and external beam radiotherapy in metastatic prostate cancer. *Radiother Oncol*. 1994;31(1):33–40.
25. Turner SL, Gruenewald S, Spry N, Gebski V. Less pain does equal better quality of life following strontium-89 therapy for metastatic prostate cancer. *Br J Cancer*. 2001;84(3):297–302.
26. Sciuto R, Festa A, Rea S, et al. Effects of low-dose cisplatin on 89Sr therapy for painful bone metastases from prostate cancer: a randomized clinical trial. *J Nucl Med*. 2002;43(1):79–86.
27. Finlay IG, Mason MD, Shelley M. Radioisotopes for the palliation of metastatic bone cancer: a systematic review. *Lancet Oncol*. 2005;6(6):392–400.
28. Lewington VJ, McEwan AJ, Ackery DM, et al. A prospective, randomised double-blind crossover study to examine the efficacy of strontium-89 in pain palliation in patients with advanced prostate cancer metastatic to bone. *Eur J Cancer*. 1991;27(8):954–958.
29. Buchali K, Correns HJ, Schuerer M, Schnorr D, Lips H, Sydow K. Results of a double blind study of 89-strontium therapy of skeletal metastases of prostatic carcinoma. *Eur J Nucl Med*. 1988;14(7-8):349–351.
30. Bauman G, Charette M, Reid R, Sathya J. Radiopharmaceuticals for the palliation of painful bone metastasis-a systemic review. *Radiother Oncol*. 2005;75(3):258–270.
31. Akerley W, Butera J, Wehbe T, et al. A multiinstitutional, concurrent chemoradiation trial of strontium-89, estramustine, and vinblastine for hormone refractory prostate carcinoma involving bone. *Cancer*. 2002;94(6):1654–1660.
32. Pagliaro LC, Delpassand ES, Williams D, Millikan RE, Tu SM, Logothetis CJ. A Phase I/II study of strontium-89 combined with gemcitabine in the treatment of patients with androgen independent prostate carcinoma and bone metastases. *Cancer*. 2003;97(12):2988–2994.
33. Ben-Yosef R, Pelled O, Marko R, et al. Establishing schedules for repeated doses of strontium and for concurrent chemotherapy in hormone-resistant patients with prostate cancer: measurement of blood and urine strontium levels. *Am J Clin Oncol*. 2005;28(2):138–142.
34. Nilsson S, Strang P, Ginman C, et al. Palliation of bone pain in prostate cancer using chemotherapy and strontium-89. A randomized phase II study. *J Pain Symptom Manage*. 2005;29(4):352–357.
35. Tu SM, Delpassand ES, Jones D, Amato RJ, Ellerhorst J, Logothetis CJ. Strontium-89 combined with doxorubicin in the treatment of patients with androgen-independent prostate cancer. *Urol Oncol*. 1996;2(6):191–197.
36. Tu SM, Millikan RE, Mengistu B, et al. Bone-targeted therapy for advanced androgen-independent carcinoma of the prostate: a randomised phase II trial. *Lancet*. 2001;357(9253):336–341.
37. Serafini AN, Houston SJ, Resche I, et al. Palliation of pain associated with metastatic bone cancer using samarium-153 lexidronam: a double-blind placebo-controlled clinical trial. *J Clin Oncol*. 1998;16(4):1574–1581.
38. Resche I, Chatal JF, Pecking A, et al. A dose-controlled study of 153Sm-ethylenediaminetetramethylenephosphonate (EDTMP) in the treatment of patients with painful bone metastases. *Eur J Cancer*. 1997;33(10):1583–1591.
39. Autio KA, Pandit-Taskar N, Carrasquillo JA, et al. Repetitively dosed docetaxel and (1)(5)(3)samarium-EDTMP as an antitumor strategy for metastatic castration-resistant prostate cancer. *Cancer*. 2013;119(17):3186–3194.
40. Liepe K, Kotzerke J. A comparative study of 188Re-HEDP, 186Re-HEDP, 153Sm-EDTMP and 89Sr in the treatment of painful skeletal metastases. *Nucl Med Commun*. 2007;28(8):623–630.
41. Mulford DA, Scheinberg DA, Jurcic JG. The promise of targeted {alpha}-particle therapy. *J Nucl Med*. 2005;46(suppl 1):199S–204S.
42. Baidoo KE, Yong K, Brechbiel MW. Molecular pathways: targeted alpha-particle radiation therapy. *Clin Cancer Res*. 2013;19(3):530–537.
43. Vaidyanathan G, Zalutsky MR. Applications of 211At and 223Ra in targeted alpha-particle radiotherapy. *Curr Radiopharm*. 2011;4(4):283–294.
44. Kim YS, Brechbiel MW. An overview of targeted alpha therapy. *Tumour Biol*. 2012;33(3):573–590.
45. Sgouros G. Alpha-particles for targeted therapy. *Adv Drug Deliv Rev*. 2008;60(12):1402–1406.
46. Vaidyanathan G, Zalutsky MR. Targeted therapy using alpha emitters. *Phys Med Biol*. 1996;41(10):1915–1931.
47. Kassis AI. Therapeutic radionuclides: biophysical and radiobiologic principles. *Semin Nucl Med*. 2008;38(5):358–366.
48. Humm JL, Roeske JC, Fisher DR, Chen GT. Microdosimetric concepts in radioimmunotherapy. *Med Phys*. 1993;20 (2 pt 2):535–541.
49. Logothetis CJ, Gallick GE, Maity SN, et al. Molecular classification of prostate cancer progression: foundation for marker-driven treatment of prostate cancer. *Cancer Discov*. 2013;3(8): 849–861.
50. Kluetz PG, Pierce W, Maher VE, et al. Radium Ra 223 dichloride injection: U.S. Food and Drug Administration drug approval summary. *Clin Cancer Res*. 2014;20(1):9–14.
51. Mould RF. The discovery of radium in 1898 by Maria Sklodowska-Curie (1867–1934) and Pierre Curie (1859–1906) with commentary on their life and times. *Br J Radiol*. 1998;71(852):1229–1254.
52. Mould RF, Robison RF, Van Tiggelen R. Louis-Frédéric Wickham (1861-1913): father of radium therapy. *Nowotwory J Oncol*. 2010;60(4):79e–103e.
53. Quick D. Radium in cancer therapy. *Br Med J*. 1930;2(3644): 765–769.
54. Quick D. The influence of radium on cancer therapy. *Can Med Assoc J*. 1954;71(2):103–109.
55. Bishop M, Harrison GE, Raymond WHA, Sutton A, Rundo J. Excretion and retention of radioactive strontium in normal men following a single intravenous injection. *International Journal of*

Radiation Biology and Related Studies in Physics Chemistry and Medicine. 1960;2(2):125–142.

56. Harrison GE, Carr TE, Sutton A, Rundo J. Plasma concentration and excretion of calcium-47, strontium-85, barium-133 and radium-223 following successive intravenous doses to a healthy man. *Nature*. 1966;209(5022):526–527.
57. Vapiwala N, Glatstein E. Fighting prostate cancer with radium-223–not your Madame's isotope. *N Engl J Med*. 2013; 369(3):276–278.
58. Bruland OS, Nilsson S, Fisher DR, Larsen RH. High-linear energy transfer irradiation targeted to skeletal metastases by the alpha-emitter 223Ra: adjuvant or alternative to conventional modalities? *Clin Cancer Res*. 2006;12(20 pt 2):6250s–6257s.
59. Nilsson S, Larsen RH, Fossa SD, et al. First clinical experience with alpha-emitting radium-223 in the treatment of skeletal metastases. *Clin Cancer Res*. 2005;11(12):4451–4459.
60. Henriksen G, Fisher DR, Roeske JC, Bruland OS, Larsen RH. Targeting of osseous sites with alpha-emitting 223Ra: comparison with the beta-emitter 89Sr in mice. *J Nucl Med*. 2003;44(2):252–259.
61. Henriksen G, Breistol K, Bruland OS, Fodstad O, Larsen RH. Significant antitumor effect from bone-seeking, alpha-particle-emitting (223)Ra demonstrated in an experimental skeletal metastases model. *Cancer Res*. 2002;62(11):3120–3125.
62. Nilsson S, Franzen L, Parker C, et al. Bone-targeted radium-223 in symptomatic, hormone-refractory prostate cancer: a randomised, multicentre, placebo-controlled phase II study. *Lancet Oncol*. 2007;8(7):587–594.
63. Roberts CC, Daffner RH, Weissman BN, et al. ACR appropriateness criteria on metastatic bone disease. *J Am Coll Radiol*. 2010;7(6):400–409.
64. Soderlund V. Radiological diagnosis of skeletal metastases. *Eur Radiol*. 1996;6(5):587–595.
65. Bauerle T, Semmler W. Imaging response to systemic therapy for bone metastases. *Eur Radiol*. 2009;19(10):2495–507.
66. Vassiliou V, Andreopoulos D, Frangos S, Tselis N, Giannopoulou E, Lutz S. Bone metastases: assessment of therapeutic response through radiological and nuclear medicine imaging modalities. *Clin Oncol (R Coll Radiol)*. 2011;23(9):632–645.
67. Saylor PJ, Mahmood U, Kunawudhi A, Smith MR, Palmer EL, Michaelson MD. Multitargeted tyrosine kinase inhibition produces discordant changes between 99mTc-MDP bone scans and other disease biomarkers: analysis of a phase II study of sunitinib for metastatic castration-resistant prostate cancer. *J Nucl Med*. 2012;53(11):1670–1675.
68. Morisson C, Jeraj R, Liu G. Imaging of castration-resistant prostate cancer: development of imaging response biomarkers. *Curr Opin Urol*. 2013;23(3):230–236.
69. Gourtsoyianni S, Hwang S, Panicek DM, et al. Reproducibility and clinical correlations of post-treatment changes on CT of prostate cancer bone metastases treated with chemotherapy. *Br J Radiol*. 2012;85(1017):1243–1249.
70. Hicks RJ, Ware RE, Lau EW. PET/CT: will it change the way that we use CT in cancer imaging? *Cancer Imaging*. 2006;6:S52–S62.
71. Messiou C, Cook G, Reid AH, et al. The CT flare response of metastatic bone disease in prostate cancer. *Acta Radiol*. 2011;52(5):557–561.
72. Schmidt GP, Reiser MF, Baur-Melnyk A. Whole-body imaging of the musculoskeletal system: the value of MR imaging. *Skeletal Radiol*. 2007;36(12):1109–1119.
73. Schmidt GP, Reiser MF, Baur-Melnyk A. Whole-body MRI for the staging and follow-up of patients with metastasis. *Eur J Radiol*. 2009;70(3):393–400.
74. Schlemmer HP, Schafer J, Pfannenberg C, et al. Fast whole-body assessment of metastatic disease using a novel magnetic resonance imaging system: initial experiences. *Invest Radiol*. 2005;40(2):64–71.
75. Li C, Liu ZS, Du XM, et al. Clinical value of whole-body magnetic resonance diffusion weighted imaging on detection of malignant metastases. *Chin Med Sci J*. 2009;24(2):112–116.
76. Reischauer C, Froehlich JM, Koh DM, et al. Bone metastases from prostate cancer: assessing treatment response by using diffusion-weighted imaging and functional diffusion maps–initial observations. *Radiology*. 2010;257(2):523–531.
77. Lee KC, Bradley DA, Hussain M, et al. A feasibility study evaluating the functional diffusion map as a predictive imaging biomarker for detection of treatment response in a patient with metastatic prostate cancer to the bone. *Neoplasia*. 2007;9(12):1003–1011.
78. Lee KC, Sud S, Meyer CR, et al. An imaging biomarker of early treatment response in prostate cancer that has metastasized to the bone. *Cancer Res*. 2007;67(8):3524–3528.
79. Messiou C, Collins DJ, Giles S, de Bono JS, Bianchini D, de Souza NM. Assessing response in bone metastases in prostate cancer with diffusion weighted MRI. *Eur Radiol*. 2011;21:2169–2177.
80. Hassan FU, Mohan HK, Gnanasegaran G, Vijayanathan S, Fogelman I. Beware of the focal uptake at the ischium on the bone scan in prostate cancer. *Nucl Med Commun*. 2011;32(4):320–323.
81. Loeffler RK, DiSimone RN, Howland WJ. Limitations of bone scanning in clinical oncology. *JAMA*. 1975;234(12):1228–1232.
82. Cook GJ, Venkitaraman R, Sohaib AS, et al. The diagnostic utility of the flare phenomenon on bone scintigraphy in staging prostate cancer. *Eur J Nucl Med Mol Imaging*. 2011;38(1):7–13.
83. Fitzpatrick JM, Constable AR, Sherwood T, Stephenson JJ, Chisholm GD, O'Donoghue EP. Serial bone scanning: the assessment of treatment response in carcinoma of the prostate. *Br J Urol*. 1978;50(7):555–561.
84. Dawson NA. Response criteria in prostatic carcinoma. *Semin Oncol*. 1999;26(2):174–184.
85. Chalian H, Tore HG, Horowitz JM, Salem R, Miller FH, Yaghmai V. Radiologic assessment of response to therapy: comparison of RECIST Versions 1.1 and 1.0. *Radiographics*. 2011;31(7):2093–2105.
86. Eisenhauer EA, Therasse P, Bogaerts J, et al. New response evaluation criteria in solid tumours: revised RECIST guideline (version 1.1). *Eur J Cancer*. 2009;45(2):228–247.
87. Therasse P, Arbuck SG, Eisenhauer EA, et al. New guidelines to evaluate the response to treatment in solid tumors. European Organization for Research and Treatment of Cancer, National Cancer Institute of the United States, National Cancer Institute of Canada. *J Natl Cancer Inst*. 2000;92(3):205–216.
88. Costelloe CM, Chuang HH, Madewell JE, Ueno NT. Cancer response criteria and bone metastases: RECIST 1.1, MDA and PERCIST. *J Cancer*. 2010;1:80–92.
89. Imbriaco M, Larson SM, Yeung HW, et al. A new parameter for measuring metastatic bone involvement by prostate cancer: the Bone Scan Index. *Clin Cancer Res*. 1998;4(7):1765–1772.
90. Brown MS, Chu GH, Kim HJ, et al. Computer-aided quantitative bone scan assessment of prostate cancer treatment response. *Nucl Med Commun*. 2012;33(4):384–394.
91. Dennis ER, Jia X, Mezheritskiy IS, et al. Bone scan index: a quantitative treatment response biomarker for castration-resistant metastatic prostate cancer. *J Clin Oncol*. 2012;30(5):519–524.
92. Iagaru A, Mittra E, Dick DW, Gambhir SS. Prospective evaluation of (99m)Tc MDP scintigraphy, (18)F NaF PET/CT, and (18) F FDG PET/CT for detection of skeletal metastases. *Mol Imaging Biol*. 2012;14(2):252–259.
93. Even-Sapir E, Metser U, Flusser G, et al. Assessment of malignant skeletal disease: initial experience with 18F-fluoride PET/CT and comparison between 18F-fluoride PET and 18F-fluoride PET/CT. *J Nucl Med*. 2004;45(2):272–278.
94. Blau M, Nagler W, Bender MA. Fluorine-18: a new isotope for bone scanning. *J Nucl Med*. 1962;3:332–334.
95. Czernin J, Satyamurthy N, Schiepers C. Molecular mechanisms of bone 18F-NaF deposition. *J Nucl Med*. 2010;51(12):1826–1829.
96. Segall G, Delbeke D, Stabin MG, et al. SNM practice guideline for sodium 18F-fluoride PET/CT bone scans 1.0. *J Nucl Med*. 2010;51(11):1813–1820.
97. Wade AA, Scott JA, Kuter I, Fischman AJ. Flare response in 18F-fluoride ion PET bone scanning. *AJR Am J Roentgenol*. 2006;186(6):1783–1786.

98. Cook G Jr, Parker C, Chua S, et al. 18F-fluoride PET: changes in uptake as a method to assess response in bone metastases from castrate-resistant prostate cancer patients treated with 223Ra-chloride (Alpharadin). *EJNMMI Res.* 2011;1(1):4.
99. Meirelles GS, Schoder H, Ravizzini GC, et al. Prognostic value of baseline [18F] fluorodeoxyglucose positron emission tomography and 99mTc-MDP bone scan in progressing metastatic prostate cancer. *Clin Cancer Res.* 2010;16(24):6093–6099.
100. Jadvar H, Desai B, Ji L, et al. Baseline 18F-FDG PET/CT parameters as imaging biomarkers of overall survival in castrate-resistant metastatic prostate cancer. *J Nucl Med.* 2013;54(8):1195–1201.
101. Janardhan S, Srivani P, Sastry GN. Choline kinase: an important target for cancer. *Curr Med Chem.* 2006;13(10):1169–1186.
102. DeGrado TR, Coleman RE, Wang S, et al. Synthesis and evaluation of 18F-labeled choline as an oncologic tracer for positron emission tomography: initial findings in prostate cancer. *Cancer Res.* 2001;61(1):110–117.
103. De Waele A, Van Binnebeek S, Mottaghy FM. Response assessment of hormonal therapy in prostate cancer by [11C] choline PET/CT. *Clin Nucl Med.* 2010;35(9):701–703.
104. Reske SN, Moritz S, Kull T. [11C]Choline-PET/CT for outcome prediction of salvage radiotherapy of local relapsing prostate carcinoma. *Q J Nucl Med Mol Imaging.* 2012;56(5):430–439.
105. Dehdashti F, Picus J, Michalski JM, et al. Positron tomographic assessment of androgen receptors in prostatic carcinoma. *Eur J Nucl Med Mol Imaging.* 2005;32(3):344–350.
106. Larson SM, Morris M, Gunther I, et al. Tumor localization of 16beta-18F-fluoro-5alpha-dihydrotestosterone versus 18F-FDG in patients with progressive, metastatic prostate cancer. *J Nucl Med.* 2004;45(3):366–373.
107. Parker CC, Pascoe S, Chodacki A, et al. A randomized, double-blind, dose-finding, multicenter, phase 2 study of radium chloride (Ra 223) in patients with bone metastases and castration-resistant prostate cancer. *Eur Urol.* 2013;63(2):189–197.

■ SUGGESTED READING

Gunawardana DH, Lichtenstein M, Better N, Rosenthal M. Results of strontium-89 therapy in patients with prostate cancer resistant to chemotherapy. *Clin Nucl Med.* 2004;29(2):81–85.

Jadvar H, Quinn DI. Targeted alpha-particle therapy of bone metastases in prostate cancer. *Clin Nucl Med.* 2013;38(12):966–971.

Lewington VJ. Bone-seeking radionuclides for therapy. *J Nucl Med.* 2005;46(suppl 1):38S–47S.

19.7 Prognostication of Metastatic Castration-Resistant Prostate Cancer

ALAN D. SMITH
JOAQUIN MATEO
JOHANN S. DE BONO

INTRODUCTION

Prostate cancer (PC) that is progressing on androgen deprivation therapy (ADT) is defined as castration-resistant prostate cancer (CRPC). CRPC is a heterogeneous disease, necessitating organizations such as the European Association of Urology (EAU) create guidelines to standardize CRPC classification and management (1).

Similarly, the prognosis of patients with metastatic CRPC, which is dependent on many factors, remains quite variable. Prior to the advent of docetaxel for CRPC in 2004, the median life expectancy was between 9–12 months (2). In 2004, docetaxel improved median survival by approximately 2.4 months (3). Since then, there have been a number of other therapies that have demonstrated a survival benefit and achieved FDA approval in prostate cancer, including: cabazitaxel, abiraterone acetate, enzalutamide, radium-223, and sipuleucel-T, with others currently in development through clinical trials. According to recent literature, the median survival in all patients with CRPC is approximately 14 months, however studies have reported a range from 9 to 30 months, with most patients surviving in the range of 1–3 years, and those with metastatic disease having median survival of 9 to 13 months (4–6).

Many of the studies evaluating prognostic factors in CRPC were conducted in men prior to the use of standard cytotoxic chemotherapy (i.e., docetaxel) the advent of novel therapies for CRPC has required an update in prognostic nomograms (6). In this chapter we will review the prognostic factors in CRPC, separating them by tumor factors and patient factors, and discuss some of the more widely used nomograms.

PROGNOSTICATORS

Unfortunately, there is limited evidence regarding the prognostic value of individual factors in CRPC. Many of the variables thought to have prognostic value are extrapolated from studies evaluating factors that influence (a) the risk of relapse in early stage disease, or (b) the prognosis of patients with advanced disease, determined prior to the use of novel hormone therapies and cytotoxic chemotherapies. Factors that have prognostic significance can be divided into tumor-related factors and patient-specific factors. Tumor-related factors include tumor histology, Gleason score, prostate specific antigen (PSA; baseline value, velocity and doubling time, decline in response to treatment), circulating tumor cells (CTCs), free circulating DNA, and genetic biomarkers. Patient-specific factors are common to many types of cancer and include epidemiologic factors, the presence of viseral disease, inflammatory-related biomarkers, and other nonspecific serum markers.

TUMOR FACTORS

Histology

The prognosis of men with certain histologies of CRPC varies quite substantially. Prostate cancer can be subdivided into histological variants of acinar adenocarcinoma, while the rest are non-acinar carcinomas (7). Adenocarcinoma accounts for more than 95% of malignancies of the prostate. Variants of acinar adenocarcinoma defined in 2004 by the World Health Organization (WHO) include atrophic, pseudohyperplastic, foamy, colloid, signet ring, oncocytic, and lymphoepithelioma-like carcinomas. Non-acinar carcinoma variants comprise the remaining 5% and include ductal adenocarcinoma, sarcomatoid carcinoma, urothelial or transitional cell carcinoma (TCC), squamous and adenosquamous carcinoma, basal cell carcinoma, neuroendocrine (NE) tumors (including small-cell carcinoma), stromal sarcomas, mesenchymal tumors, and haematolymphoid tumors (8). Most of the evidence in CRPC refers to prostate adenocarcinomas, therefore we will purposely discuss the other subtypes in this histology section and cover prognostic factors of adenocarcinomas in the rest of this chapter.

NE Differentiation (NED) of prostate cancer accounts for approximately 1% of prostate cancers; and is comprised of focal NED in conventional prostatic adenocarcinoma

(~50%), carcinoid tumor (WHO well-differentiated NE tumor), and small-cell NE carcinoma (WHO poorly differentiated NE carcinoma), (9–11). Although many prostate cancers show focal NED, 5%–10% have zones with a large number of NE cells (8). Similar to NE carcinomas originating elsewhere, NED of prostate cancer behaves differently and often does not respond to therapies for conventional prostate adenocarcinoma (12, 13). NE cells appear to have a paracrine effect on growth regulation, via hormones such as chromogranin A (CgA), serotonin, neuron-specific enolase, calcitonin, gastrin-releasing peptide (bombesin), somatostatin, alpha-human chorionic gonadotropin, thyroid stimulating hormone-like peptide, parathyroid hormone-related protein, and cholecystokinin; and as a result may also present with paraneoplatic syndromes (14–18). NE cells usually do not express AR, can be resistant to apoptosis (19), and their number and activity can increase with androgen deprivation (20). Overall, the extent of NED, which can be measured by serum CgA levels (21), correlates with more aggressive disease and shorter survival times, with a cutoff point for CgA of ≤ 9.5 U/L vs > 9.5 U/L, corresponding to a survival of 19 months compared with 12 months respectively (P = .0015) (9, 22, 23). On multivariate analysis, CgA levels associate with survival (22), and may be prognostically useful, particularly in patients with low serum PSA (24–28). Interestingly, CRPC histology trends toward a higher proportion of NE cells compared with early disease (29), and focal NED portends a poorer prognosis (29–32). True carcinoid tumors of the prostate are rare, and therefore, prognostic information regarding these tumors is uncertain.

Small-cell carcinoma (SCC) of the prostate is histologically identical to SCC of the lung. Approximately 50% of SCC of the prostate have mixed SCC and adenocarcinoma components. Overall, the average survival is less than one year, and the appearance of a SCC component to adenocarcinoma of the prostate usually indicates an aggressive terminal phase of the disease. Prostate SCC responds poorly to standard hormonal therapies and chemotherapies; evidence about the best sequence of treatment for these patients is yet unclear (23, 33, 34).

Urothelial or TCC of the prostate presents similarly to primary bladder TCC, and secondary involvement from a bladder primary must be excluded. The true incidence of prostatic TCC is approximately 0.7%–2.8% (35, 36). In situ carcinoma spreads along ducts and involves the acini, and later disease invades prostatic stroma. These are prognostically relevant, where tumors involving the prostatic ducts have a T1 category for invasion, which is distinct from prostatic stromal invasion (i.e., T2) (37). In this series, survival in patients with noninvasive disease approaches 100%, as compared to 45% at 5 years if prostatic stromal invasion is present. The median survival for invasive TCC of the prostate from diagnosis is 17–29 months (11, 38).

The rarer tumors of the prostate are associated with unique clinical features and therapeutic approaches. Sarcomatoid carcinoma, ductal adenocarcinoma, squamous neoplasms (i.e., adenosquamous carcinoma, squamous cell carcinoma), and mesenchymal tumors (e.g., leiomyosarcoma, rhabdomyosarcoma) are aggressive (7, 8, 39). Sarcomatoid carcinoma has a 3-year median survival, exhibiting a locally aggressive behavior and the pattern of metastases is similar to prostate adenocarcinoma, but with the lungs being the most common site for spread (11). Ductal adenocarcinoma presents with distant metastases at diagnosis 25%–40% of the time and tends to be less responsive to conventional prostate cancer therapies (40–42). Squamous neoplasms have a propensity for bone metastases (43). Leiomyosarcoma is characterized by multiple recurrences requiring resection and the average survival is between 3–4 years (8). Rhabdomyosarcoma occurs in infancy to early adulthood, frequently presents with unresectable local disease, and often with distant metastases (8). Treatment involves intensive chemotherapy and radiotherapy specific to this type of tumor. Basal cell carcinoma of the prostate is less aggressive though it may develop extra-prostatic extension or distant metastases (44, 45). The most common primary haematolymphoid tumors of the prostate include non-Hodgkin lymphoma, Hodgkin lymphoma and mucosa-associated lymphoid tissue (MALT) lymphoma, and behave as per their respective diseases elsewhere in the body (46, 47).

Gleason Score

The Gleason grading system is a histological system based on the architectural appearance of prostate adenocarcinoma cells, and correlates closely with clinical behavior. Historically, tumors were graded by differentiation pattern, from 1 to 5, with 1 being the most and 5 being the least differentiated (48), however current practice is to assign a number from 3 to 5 (49). The composite Gleason score is determined by summating the two most prevalent patterns, with the most prevalent always listed first; therefore a Gleason score of 3 + 3 = 6 would be well differentiated (low grade) which is the lowest possible score assigned. A Gleason score of 8 to 10 is considered poorly differentiated or high grade, while a score of 7 is moderately differentiated (intermediate grade) (50). Recently, it has been proposed that Gleason score 6 disease often represents a clinically benign course such that many of these patients are overtreated (49). However, it remains controversial whether low-grade prostate cancer is a life-threatening entity that requires definitive treatment, and whether these patients may be candidates for watchful waiting.

The Gleason score is particularly useful in early stage, hormone-sensitive disease, where it can differentiate a greater probability of having non-organ-confined disease, and poorer outcomes after localized treatment. Repeat biopsy sampling of low risk disease has demonstrated that approximately 34% of men experience an upgrade in Gleason score on repeat biopsy, the majority of upgrades occur at the first or second repeat biopsy, and increase in Gleason grade on surveillance biopsies is predictive of time to active treatment (51,52). Gleason score is also prognostic for patients with advanced stage disease, having earlier progression (well-differentiated 33.0 months, moderately differentiated 19.0 months, and poorly differentiated 13.0 months, respectively; P = .04) and shorter survival (well-differentiated 44.0 months, moderately differentiated 28.0 months, and poorly differentiated 21.5 months, respectively; P = .03) (53). With the advent of novel therapies for prostate cancer, the prognostic usefulness of Gleason score at diagnosis in CRPC is uncertain. According to one study evaluating patients on docetaxel, Gleason ≥ 8 was not significantly associated with survival (HR 1.18, P = .069) (54). Others have found it is predictive for survival however, demonstrating Gleason ≥ 8 has a HR 1.40 for survival (P < .0001) and patients with Gleason 6 live longer (55,56). It is generally thought that as prostate cancer progresses from hormone-sensitive to castration-resistant disease, the grade increases, indicating more aggressive disease.

PSA

Prostate-specific antigen (PSA) is a glycoprotein encoded by the *KLK3* gene. PSA is secreted almost exclusively by epithelial cells of both normal and neoplastic prostate tissue and is expressed in nearly all prostate cancers. It has been well demonstrated to reflect the overall burden of disease in men with CRPC, where higher baseline levels in men without metastases are associated with time to first bone metastasis and death (56–59). This disease state is coined castrate-biochemical relapse (castrate-BCR). Smith and colleagues found that a baseline PSA ≥ 13.1 ng/mL for men with castrate-BCR is associated with shorter overall survival on retrospective analysis of the randomized controlled-trial, Abbott M00-244 (RR 2.34, P < .001) (60). In Cox regression models allowing for relative risk to vary with time, relative risk was 3.17 (P < .001) for the first three years and 1.44 (P = .156) for subsequent years. Baseline PSA levels are also included in a number of prognostic models (54,55, 61).

PSA Velocity and Doubling Time

The rate of change of PSA over time, in the absence of therapeutic measures, is the PSA velocity. PSA velocity has been associated with shorter overall survival in men with nonmetastatic CRPC (RR 1.15 for each 1 log[ng/mL]/year increase; P = .002) (57). Men with metastatic CRPC also appear to have shorter survival if they have a high PSA velocity (PSAV) (58,62,63). Robinson and colleagues evaluated PSAV in 915 patients enrolled on the SPCG-5 study and stratified patients into four quartiles, where PSAV in the first (Q1) , median (Q2), and third (Q3) quartiles had PSAV of 0.52 ng/mL/month, 2.6 ng/mL/month, and 12.6 ng/mL/month, respectively (64). They found that PSAV gives a reliable prediction of survival, with a median survival of 26.4 months for men with a PSAV less than Q1, 17.1 months for men with a PSAV between Q1 and Q2, 12.3 months for men with a PSAV between Q2 and Q3, and 6.2 months for men with a PSAV greater than Q3.

PSA doubling time (PSADT) is a specific measure of PSAV that has been validated as a prognostic factor. It is defined as the time interval observed over which the serum PSA doubles, and it reflects relative rather than absolute changes.

$$f(time) = a + b \times \exp(c^{time})$$

Where f is time, and a, b, and c are the most recent PSA measurements (65). PSADT is limited by the fact that it was developed in patients not undergoing active treatment, and therefore assumes that the PSA kinetics will be exponential, however, the pattern is not always linear because PSADT does not measure tumor regression, and therefore it can only be calculated when there is tumor regrowth (66).

PSADT may be different at time of first chemotherapy compared to the time of diagnosis of castration resistance (61). In men with CRPC treated with deferred antiandrogen therapy, PSADT was predictive of PSA response, where mean PSADT in responders was 12.7 months as compared to 7.5 months in nonresponders (P = .037) (67). PSADT has also been shown to correlate directly with survival in men with mCRPC (61,62, 68). One study, which retrospectively evaluated 250 men treated with chemotherapy for CRPC, found that PSADT < 45 days is associated with a HR 1.39 for death (P = .03), where the short PSADT was associated with a 16.5 month median survival compared to 26.4 months in the long PSADT group (P = .04) (61). Another study, retrospectively evaluating 224 men with mCRPC, determined the optimal PSADT stratification for survival was 70 days (68). They reported a median survival of 11 months for men with a PSADT ≤ 70 days (HR 0.46 for death, on multivariate analysis) compared to 19 months for those with a PSADT > 70 days (68). Caution, however, should be used in interpreting PSADT because this has not been formally prospectively evaluated for surrogacy for overall survival in phase III trials. Furthermore, PSADT may vary naturally over time without intervention (69).

PSA Decline in Response to Treatment

Changes in PSA during therapy can reflect a reduction in the burden of disease, indicating a clinical benefit. This can be prognostically informative for individual patients over time, and PSA decline rates of > 30 to > 90% have been evaluated (70–72). Two retrospective studies of large randomized trials have reported that PSA decline > 30% within 3 months of cytotoxic treatment initiation was associated with improved survival (70, 71). Other studies have found that a PSA decline of ≥ 50% at various time intervals correlated with survival (72–77). However, > 30% PSA decline, and the conventional threshold of ≥ 50% confirmed PSA decline (59) have not been prospectively demonstrated to be a surrogate for survival across these trials and is therefore not an approved regulatory end-point for systemic therapies in CRPC (78). Possibly, the variability in degree of surrogacy is related to the cytotoxic therapy usage in these studies, which may affect the correlation between PSA change and survival (79). Another concept that evaluates PSA decline is PSA half-life (PSAHL), where a more rapid rate of PSA decline (PSAHL < 70 days) has been associated with longer survival in 154 men treated with docetaxel (80). Banu and colleagues found that PSAHL is prognostic for overall survival in patients treated with chemotherapy, demonstrating that responders and late progressors have better survival compared to initial progressors (median survival 27 vs. 19.7 vs. 12.3 months respectively) (81).

There is some evidence to suggest that long PSA response durations and low PSA nadirs correlate with survival (82, 83). PSA progression during therapy for CRPC has similarly demonstrated prognostic utility for survival, however it is not a surrogate marker of survival (84, 85). Detection of PSA on circulating tumor cells by reverse transcriptase polymerase chain reaction (rtPCR) was also demonstrated to correlate with survival (median survival 21 vs. 11 months, $P \leq .001$; HR death 1.7, $P = .006$) (55).

There are important caveats that should be remembered when interpreting PSA changes over time. The mechanism of action of the drug should be considered. PSA is a measure of AR signaling, which likely explains why sipuleucel-T improves survival, but does not affect PSA levels (86). In contrast, the survival benefit seen with docetaxel correlates with PSA response within the first 3 months of therapy (70, 71). There is some recent evidence demonstrating that docetaxel has a direct effect on AR dynamics, intimating that it may also affect PSA production (87). Another issue is that serum PSA values may initially rise after effective systemic treatment before falling. Early rises in PSA are known to occur during systemic chemotherapy in 15%–20% of men with CRPC (88, 89). This does not appear to be associated with an unfavorable prognosis; rather it may reflect a lag in response to treatment or a transient circulatory release of PSA (89). As a result, the PCWG2 suggests that decisions regarding therapy should not be made on PSA alone, thereby potentially avoiding premature discontinuation of a life-prolonging treatment (78).

In 1999, the published eligibility and response guidelines for clinical trials in androgen-independent prostate cancer recommended that investigators report the rate of PSA decline by 50% at a minimum (59). The role of PSA and PSA-related measures in CRPC was then revised in 2008 by the Prostate Cancer Clinical Trials Working Group (PCWG2), which recommends measuring the PSA at 12 weeks, reporting it as a percentage change as compared to the baseline, and identifying the maximum change at a given time (78). PCWG2 also recommends continuation of treatment for a minimum of 12 weeks, unless other evidence of progression, to avoid incorrect interpretations of fluctuating serum levels.

Circulating Tumor Cells (CTCs)

The process of hematogenous metastasis of prostate cancer cells likely involves a period of circulatory spread of carcinoma cells, followed by extravasation and colonization (90). CTCs are shed into the bloodstream from solid tumors and can be isolated from samples of peripheral blood based on their different physical and immunologic characteristics (91). CTC enumeration correlates with other prognostic factors in mCRPC, such as PSA, alkaline phosphatase (ALP), and lactate dehydrogenase (LD) and correlate negatively with hemoglobin (HGB) (92–94). A number of trials stratifying CRPC patients commencing a new line of chemotherapy, based on CTC count ≤ 5 (favorable) vs. > 5 (unfavorable)/ 7.5 mL, found that unfavorable pretreatment levels are associated with worse survival (median OS 11.5–19.5 vs. 20 to > 30 months, $P < .05$ for all studies) (95–97). Similar results have been reported in other trials, where CTC enumeration is evaluated as a continuous variable and very high CTC counts (> 50/7.5 mL) correlated with poorer survival (92, 96, 98, 99). Post-treatment CTC counts that drop from unfavorable to favorable are also associated with an improvement in survival (95), comparable to what is seen with PSA response (> 30%) or partial radiographic response (70, 71, 100). More recently, an evaluation of men treated with abiraterone acetate (AA) for CRPC has suggested that changes in CTCs, as early as 4 weeks into therapy, reflect survival benefit and therefore may serve as a surrogate biomarker (101). Further evidence is presently needed to elucidate the full value of CTC enumeration in surrogacy for survival in men with CRPC; this will be further assessed in other prospective phase III clinical trials with various investigational agents (NCT00974311, NCT01193257, NCT01057810) (90).

CTC enumeration may be particularly useful compared to other prognostic markers, demonstrating a stronger association with survival on multivariate analysis (99). Therefore, CTC enumeration may also be useful for clinical decision making in patients with ambiguous results of PSA or radiographic assessments. At present, the detection rate of CTCs is somewhat limited, in that certain CTCs may escape detection via the loss of epithelial markers and acquisition of a mesenchymal phenotype (102). Improvements in methods for CTC capture would therefore be helpful to further explore CTCs as a clinical tool.

Free Circulating DNA (fcDNA)

Nucleic acids are released into plasma from normal or damaged cells as a result of cell stress. This has been studied in other fields like autoimmune or infectious diseases and has opened significant possibilities for prenatal diagnosis of fetal diseases. In cancer medicine, it is possible to detect circulating tumor DNA released into the circulation from either primary tumors or metastatic deposits. The total amount of fcDNA in the blood of cancer patients correlates with the burden of disease, has prognostic value, and makes it possible to detect specific oncogenic aberrations that are informative of the biology of the disease (103). In prostate cancer, there is a correlation between the number of CTCs and the concentration of fcDNA, opening new possibilities for monitoring metastatic disease (104).

Genetic Biomarkers

Increasing knowledge of prostate cancer biology and the feedback between the androgen signaling pathway and other signaling networks has challenged the scientific community to subclassify prostate cancer according to molecular biomarkers. In most cases, they may not only have prognostic value but can be significant predictive factors of response to novel therapies.

About half of prostate cancers harbor fusions of genes related to androgen signaling. The most common is the fusion of TMPRSS2, an androgen regulated gene, with the transcription factor ERG generating an androgen-responsive oncoprotein. Data from retrospective studies suggest the presence of TMPRSS2-ERG fusion characterizes a molecular subgroup of prostate cancer with a more aggressive phenotype and worse cancer-specific survival (105).

The phosphatase and tensin homologue (PTEN) gene is one of the most commonly mutated or deleted tumor suppressor genes in cancer. In addition to its role as a negative regulator of the PI3K/AKT signaling cascades, it is also involved in maintenance of chromosomal integrity (106). Concomitant evaluation of PTEN gene loss and ERG/ETV1 gene rearrangements may be a useful means to stratify patients based on prostate cancer-specific survival; where patients lacking PTEN gene loss and ERG/ETV1 gene rearrangements have a relatively good prognosis, and poorer survival was observed in the subgroup with PTEN gene loss in the absence of ERG/ETV1 gene rearrangements (107). In a series of over 600 patients with localized prostate cancer, loss of PTEN expression, assessed by immunohistochemistry, was associated with long-term higher risk of prostate cancer–related death in univariate analysis. In the multivariate analysis, it was found to be a prognostic factor only for those patients with low-risk disease (108).

P53 is a tumor suppressor gene involved in prostate carcinogenesis, as in many other malignancies, and has been shown to have prognostic value (109, 110). Expression of p53, together with Ki-67 and bcl-2, in the primary tumor has been correlated with risk of recurrence after radical prostatectomy in two different series of patients (111, 112). P53 expression has also been demonstrated to be an independent prognostic marker for cancer-specific survival (113).

A family history of cancer is one of the strongest risk factors to develop prostate cancer. Germline mutations in the breast cancer predisposition gene (BRCA2) are the genetic event known to confer the highest risk of prostate cancer, over 8-fold in men under 65 years old (3.5-fold for BRCA1 germline mutations). Despite being present in less than 2% of sporadic prostate cancers, detection of BRCA mutation has become relevant with the development of drugs targeting poly-ADP-ribose polymerase (PARP). Concomitant knockdown of BRCA and PARP leads to cell death due to lack of mechanisms to maintain DNA repair systems, which has been named synthetic-lethality. Recent data demonstrate that BRCA mutations confer a more aggressive phenotype of prostate cancer, with higher risk of developing distant metastasis after radical treatment and poorer survival outcomes overall for BRCA mutation carriers (114).

There are a number of other genomic alterations that have recently generated scientific interest. *CHD1* deletion has recently been shown to be found in a subgroup of prostate cancers and is associated with early PSA recurrence, high Gleason grade, advanced tumor stage, and increased cellular proliferation (as measured by the Ki67 labeling index), all implicating it as a possible negative prognosticator (115). Ki-67 itself may have prognostic value when dichotomized > 10% versus ≤ 10% (116). *SPOP* mutations also appear to occur early in the development of invasive prostate cancer and similarly seem to be mutually exclusive with *ERG* fusions and rearrangements, and often co-occurring with CHD1 loss (117). *FOXA1* acts as an AR-cofactor and promotes cell-cycle progression in CRPC, which may portend more aggressive disease (118). Mismatch repair (MMR) gene activity has been implicated in prostate cancer outcomes, and may also be associated with more aggressive disease (119, 120). Baca and colleagues propose a model for the evolution of prostate cancer comprising a spectrum of processes whereby gene alterations accumulate; including a process termed chromoplexy, in which multiple geographically distant genomic regions in CRPC may be disrupted at once, leading to deletions and rearrangements in relevant genes such as *PTEN*, *NKX3-1*, *CDKN1B*, *TP53*, and *RB1* (119).

■ WHOLE BLOOD mRNA EXPRESSION PROFILING

mRNA expression profiles may be a useful method to stratify patients according to overall prognosis. Olmos and colleagues showed RNA expression profiles in CRPC correlated with survival. A 9-gene signature (i.e., *HMBS*, *TMCC2*, *SNCA*, *SLC4A1*, *STOM*, *GABARAPL2*, *RIOK3*, *TERF2IP*, and *TFDP1*) in particular has been identified and validated as an independent prognostic factor for worse overall survival (121). Another group proposed a 6-gene profile (i.e., *ABL2*, *ITGAL*, *SEMA4D*, *C1QA*, *CDKN1A*, and *TIMP1*) that stratifies patients into two groups, low-risk and high-risk, with significant differences in survival (122). These profiles include genes essential for immune system activity, implicating a down-regulation of cellular and humoral immunity as a possible cause for poorer survival in these patients.

■ PATIENT FACTORS

Epidemiological Factors

Disparities in cancer outcome according to ethnicity have been previously described in several tumor types. A retrospective review of 35 clinical trials by the Southwest Oncology Group (SWOG) showed race outcome-relation for breast, ovarian, and prostate cancer. In the case of prostate malignancies, African American men with prostate cancer had a 20% higher risk of death than their white counterparts (123). These data support efforts to detect the disease in earlier stages in this group and to further study differences in tumor biology that may help in developing personalized treatments.

Several studies have evaluated the relationship of age with outcome in prostate cancer. Those studies and their results are heterogeneous, as they use either the age at diagnosis or at the time of developing CRPC, and consider overall survival or cancer-specific survival as a primary endpoint (124). Overall, there is a consistent trend with younger age and poorer prognosis, but this is likely influenced by the higher prevalence of poorly differentiated tumors at younger age, and the fact that elderly patients have higher rates of non-cancer related deaths (125).

Elevated body mass index (BMI) is also associated with prostate cancer–specific mortality, as shown in a meta-analysis of prospective cohort studies in prostate cancer patients (126). However, the relationship between cancer and metabolism is extremely complex; factors such as obesity and insulin metabolism appear to have a role in cancer genesis and progression, and it is difficult to evaluate their independent prognostic value.

Visceral Disease

Prostate cancer usually spreads to the bones and, secondly, to the lymphatic system. The presence of visceral metastases has been recognized as a poor-prognostic factor. This was included already in the pre-docetaxel era nomograms as a significant variable (55).

Recent registration trials of abiraterone acetate and enzalutamide in the post-chemotherapy setting retrospectively analyzed the differential outcomes of patients based on the presence of visceral disease. The COU-301 trial, which evaluated abiraterone acetate plus prednisolone vs. placebo plus prednisolone in patients progressing on docetaxel-based chemotherapy detected a worse overall survival for patients in both groups affected by visceral disease (127). The AFFIRM trial, which evaluated enzalutamide vs. placebo in the post-chemotherapy setting, also observed poorer overall survival for patients with liver or lung metastases (128). In both studies, the HR for overall survival, indicating the risk of death for the experimental group compared with the placebo arm, suggested a higher degree of benefit from these novel androgen-axis targeting agents for those patients with no visceral disease.

However, these sub-analyses have limited significance and at present, visceral disease is not a determinant of indication for anti-androgen therapies. Moreover, most of the current literature regarding this topic considers non-bony disease to be homogeneous. Specific prognostic studies for patients according to the number of organs involved, shown to be an important prognostic factor in cancer medicine, are needed (129).

Inflammation-Related Biomarkers

Because of the strong involvement of inflammatory mechanisms in cancer pathogenesis and progression, quantification of inflammation-associated factors has been studied as eventual biomarkers of prognosis in different tumor types, including prostate cancer (130).

C reactive-protein (CRP) is the most representative acute-phase reactant that has been shown to have prognostic value in prostate cancer among other tumors. CRP levels are elevated in the early phase of inflammatory response to infections, metabolic stress, autoimmune disease, or other ailments, such as cancer. Serum quantification of CRP is performed with reliable assays in routine clinical practice. In prostate cancer, CRP has been shown to correlate with prognosis in patients with localized disease (131), and is an independent prognostic factor and correlates with burden of disease in patients with bone metastases (132).

Lactate dehydrogenase (LDH) is an ubiquitous enzyme that is part of the normal cellular glycolysis and gluconeogenesis pathways. The Warburg effect describes a neoplastic process, including in CRPC, whereby LDH activity is increased to enable cancer cells to produce energy and proliferate in a hypoxic environment. Serum LDH levels are nonspecific, and may rise in response to an inflammatory stimulus, hypoxia, tissue necrosis, or tumor that is outgrowing its own blood supply, all characteristics of aggressive disease (133). LDH has been included in clinically validated prognostic scores for prognosis in cancer (55, 129, 134) but some studies evaluating its independent prognostic value in prostate cancer show contradictory results (55, 135).

The neutrophil-to-lymphocyte ratio (NLR) is a marker of inflammation that is prognostic in several cancers. In one study of patients with CRPC treated with ketoconazole, high NLR was associated with worse progression-free survival (136).

Overall, poor specificity of the inflammation-related biomarkers, which can be modulated by several other concomitant factors, may be the reason for conflicting results reported in the past, limiting their potential application for prognostication in CRPC and their clinical validity. They are also being evaluated as potential biomarkers for early diagnosis in screening programs (137).

Other Nonspecific Serum Markers

Anemia is a recognized prognostic factor in cancer. Anemia of chronic disease is a well-known entity, and in prostate cancer becomes even more important because of eventual infiltration of bone marrow by metastatic disease. A meta-analysis of six studies analyzing the impact of hemoglobin levels in prognosis showed a 47% increased risk of death for prostate cancer patients with anemia in comparison with those with normal hemoglobin (138).

Alkaline phosphatase (ALP) is a biomarker of bone metabolism that is also commonly released by the liver and bile ducts. In patients with bony metastases, most of the circulating levels are generated in the bones, and it is a predictive factor of survival independent of PSA in patients with prostate cancer and bony metastases who are receiving chemotherapy. Other biomarkers of bone metabolism like bone-specific alkaline phosphatase and urinary N-telopeptide are currently being incorporated into exploratory analyses of clinical trials to evaluate for clinical validity (139).

Other variables that have been found to be associated with survival on multivariable analysis include acid phosphatase, prolactin, prior hormone response, anorexia, and obstructive urinary symptoms (140, 141), as well as pronounced fatigue and weight loss (142, 143), extent of bone metastases (144, 145), pretreatment serum testosterone (145), and plasma and urine VEGF and PSA rtPCR (55, 146–148).

Response to Prior Treatment

Despite progression of disease on hormonal therapy, CRPC often continues to be sensitive to further androgen pathway manipulation. Secondary hormonal therapies can be an attractive treatment option because of their mild toxicity profile and ease of administration. Recent evidence has demonstrated that duration of response to prior hormonal therapy predicts longer duration of secondary hormonal therapy, with men who received primary hormonal therapy for > 24 months receiving secondary therapy for 40 months (149). It is not however clear whether this translates into a difference in survival.

■ NOMOGRAMS

There are a number of prognostic models that have been developed for CRPC. The widely used Halabi, Smaletz, and Armstrong nomograms were constructed using data from clinical trials of hormonal treatments and first-line chemotherapy.

The Halabi nomogram was developed and published in 2003, with data evaluating 1,101 men with CRPC treated on six Cancer and Leukemia Group B Protocols (CALGB) (55). Patients were treated from 1991 to 2001, and were required to demonstrate progression despite androgen ablation and anti-androgen withdrawal. These studies, CALGB 9181, 9182, 9480, 9680, 9780, and 9583, all involved hormonal maneuvers or mitoxantrone, except for CALGB 9780, which treated 46 patients with docetaxel plus estramustine and low-dose hydrocortisone (73, 150–153). Pretreatment factors were evaluated with univariate and multivariate analysis by a proportional hazards model to construct and validate a prognostic model. They found that ECOG performance status (ECOG 1 HR 1.48; ECOG 2 HR 2.19, $P < .0001$), Gleason sum (Gleason 8+ HR 1.4, $P < .0001$), LDH (log[LDH] HR 1.37, $P < .0001$), ALP (log[ALP] HR 1.23, $P < .0001$), PSA (log[PSA] HR 1.1, $P < .0001$), and hemoglobin (HR 0.92, $P < .0001$) were statistically significant on multivariate analysis (Table 19.7.1). The model was developed to predict survival at 12 and 24 months (Table 19.7.2). Patients were classified into one of four risk groups on the basis of the median of the predicted survival duration. Observed median survival durations were 7.5, 13.4, 18.9, and 27.2 months for the first, second, third, and fourth risk groups, respectively, and the corresponding median predicted survival times were 8.8, 13.4, 17.4, and 22.8 months.

The Smaletz nomogram was developed and published in 2002 from data at the Memorial Sloan-Kettering Cancer Center (134). This is also a pretreatment prognostic model, which included 409 patients enrolled on 19 consecutive clinical trials from 1989 to 2000. All patients considered in the analysis had progressive castrate metastatic disease, where progression was defined by any one of the following:

Table 19.7.1 Comparison of the Armstrong, Halabi and Smaletz nomograms predicting survival in CRPC

Risk Factor	Armstrong (54)	Halabi (55)	Smaletz (134)
Age	N	N	Y
Albumin	N	N	Y
Alkaline Phosphatase	Y	Y	Y
Chemotherapy (e.g., DOC, MTX)	Y	N	N
Grade	Y	Y (Gleason Score)	Y (Gleason Score)
Hemoglobin	Y	Y	Y
LDH	N	Y	Y
Liver Metastases	Y	N	N
Number of Site	Y	N	N
Pain at Baseline	Y	N	N
Performance Status	Y (KPS)	Y (ECOG)	Y (KPS)
Progression Type: Bone Scan	Y	N	N
Progression Type: Measurable Disease	Y	N	N
PSA (baseline)	Y	Y	Y
PSA Doubling Time	Y	N	N
Visceral disease	N	Y	N

Abbreviations: DOC, docetaxel; MTX, mitoxantrone.

Table 19.7.2 Survival predictions of the Armstrong, Halabi and Smaletz nomograms for CRPC

Survival	Armstrong (54)	Halabi (55)	Smaletz (134)
Median Survival	Y	Y	Y
1-Year	Y	Y	Y
2-Year	Y	Y	Y
5-Year	Y	N	N

an increase in serum PSA of at least 25% compared with baseline in 3 successive occasions, new metastatic lesions on bone scan, or a 25% or greater increase in bi-dimensionally measurable tumor mass. Variables were selected based on prior published reports and clinical experience of the investigators, and included: age, Karnofsky performance status (KPS), hemoglobin, PSA, LDH, ALP, and albumin. Analysis was performed using a Cox regression model for proportional hazards, requiring an accelerated failure time model with a Gaussian error distribution to adjust for differenteffects over time. They found that KPS ($P < .001$), hemoglobin ($P < .001$), LDH ($P < .001$), ALP ($P = .027$) and albumin ($P = .044$) were associated with survival, whereas age ($P = .35$) and PSA ($P = .742$) were not (Table 19.7.1). A nomogram was then developed, where each predictor variable has corresponding prognostic points which are then tallied to establish the predicted survival at 1 and 2 years, as well as median survival

(Table 19.7.2). The nomogram was validated externally, with an estimated concordance index of .67.

The Armstrong nomogram was developed by retrospective analysis of the TAX327 clinical trial evaluating different schedules of docetaxel versus mitoxantrone in men with progressive metastatic CRPC (54). CRPC was defined as men with metastatic prostate adenocarcinoma in the setting of castrate levels of serum testosterone (< 50ng/mL) who had evidence of progression as defined by clinically or radiographically measurable disease or by PSA criteria (3). TAX327 was a randomized, non-blinded, multinational trial including 1,006 patients treated from 2000 to 2002. The variables evaluated were age, KPS, pain at baseline, hemoglobin, ALP, serum PSA, presence of visceral and/or liver metastases, pretreatment PSA doubling time (PSADT), type of progression (measurable, nonmeasurable, bone scan, and PSA-only progression), number of metastatic sites, Gleason score, presence of multiple bony metastases, and prior estramustine or second-line hormonal therapy. The final model for the nomogram was created using a step-wise procedure including a bootstrap, where all variables with an alpha level of .10 were included in the covariate analysis, and then variables on covariate analysis were excluded if the P was ≥ .10. Independent prognostic factors on multivariate analysis were liver metastases (HR 1.66, P = .019), more than two regions of metastatic disease (HR 1.63, P = .001), chemotherapy type (weekly docetaxel versus q3w docetaxel; HR 1.12, P = .32; mitoxantrone versus q3w docetaxel: HR 1.43, P = .001), significant baseline pain (HR 1.48, P < .001), KPS ≤ 70 (HR 1.39, P = .016), bone scan progression (HR 1.29, P = .01), or measurable disease progression (HR 1.37, P = .005), PSA (per log rise, HR 1.17, P < .001), high tumor grade (HR 1.18, P = .069), ALP (per unit log rise, HR 1.27, P < .001), and baseline hemoglobin per unit decline, HR 1.11, P = .004 (Table 19.7.1). Furthermore, PSADT Kaplan-Meier survival curves categorized by month groupings:< 1 month, 1–2 months, 2–3 months, 3–6 months, and > 6 months demonstrated a decreasing risk of death as PSADT lengthened, with a relative hazard of 0.79, 0.69, 0.53, and 0.37, respectively (P < .001 for trend). The concordance index of the final multivariate model was 0.69, indicating a moderately high level of predictive discrimination. The final set of covariates was then included in a Cox regression analysis using the original data set, and was used to create a nomogram for prediction of median and 1-, 2-, and 5-year overall survival (Table 19.7.2).

These nomograms have some limitations, including that the analyses were performed on patients enrolled on clinical trials, who met the specific enrollment criteria, including a good performance status. Furthermore, they were developed prior to the discovery of some highly effective novel treatments for prostate cancer, which are now considered standard therapy. Survival in patients treated with these highly effective therapies differs from that predicted in the nomograms, and therefore updated nomograms are needed (154).

■ CONCLUSIONS

CRPC is a heterogeneous disease characterized by differences in histology, molecular and genomic characteristics, dissemination patterns, and response to therapy. The therapeutic armamentarium for metastatic CRPC has also recently become broader with the advent of highly effective novel therapies showing improvements in overall survival, and further complicating our ability to predict survival in these patients. To optimize the use of these new therapies, a strategy to differentiate patients according to predictive and prognostic markers is vital. Most of the currently used nomograms and prognostic indexes in prostate cancer were constructed using data from series of patients who never received these highly effective treatments. Note that, these nomograms have been shown to underestimate the outcome of patients in the present era. Updated prognostic systems are needed, integrating clinical, pathological, and molecular features to better characterize prostate cancer. Development of any novel biomarker or nomogram requires that we demonstrate reliability of results, validity of the technology involved, and clinical validation in prospective studies.

■ REFERENCES

1. Heidenreich A, Bastian PJ, Bellmunt J, et al. EAU guidelines on prostate cancer. part 1: screening, diagnosis, and local treatment with curative intent-update 2013. *Eur Urol*. 2014;65(1):124–137.
2. Dagher R, Li N, Abraham S, Rahman A, Sridhara R, Pazdur R. Approval summary: Docetaxel in combination with prednisone for the treatment of androgen-independent hormone-refractory prostate cancer. *Clin Cancer Res*. 2004;10(24):8147–8151.
3. Tannock IF, de Wit R, Berry WR, et al. Docetaxel plus prednisone or mitoxantrone plus prednisone for advanced prostate cancer. *N Engl J Med*. 2004;351(15):1502–1512.
4. Kirby M, Hirst C, Crawford ED. Characterising the castration-resistant prostate cancer population: a systematic review. *Int J Clin Pract*. 2011;65(11):1180–1192.
5. Lee DJ, Cha EK, Dubin JM, et al. Novel therapeutics for the management of castration-resistant prostate cancer (CRPC). *BJU Int*. 2012;109(7):968–985.
6. Serpa Neto A, Tobias-Machado M, Kaliks R, Wroclawski ML, Pompeo AC, Del Giglio A. Ten years of docetaxel-based therapies in prostate adenocarcinoma: a systematic review and meta-analysis of 2244 patients in 12 randomized clinical trials. *Clin Genitourin Cancer*. 2011;9(2):115–123.
7. Humphrey PA. Histological variants of prostatic carcinoma and their significance. *Histopathology*. 2012;60(1):59–74.
8. Eble JL, Sauter G, Epstein JI, Sesterhenn IA, World Health Organization, International Agency for Research on Cancer.

Pathology and Genetics of Tumours of the Urinary System and Male Genital Organs. Lyon, France: IARC; 2004.
9. Sagnak L, Topaloglu H, Ozok U, Ersoy H. Prognostic significance of neuroendocrine differentiation in prostate adenocarcinoma. *Clin Genitourin Cancer.* 2011;9(2):73–80.
10. Sun Y, Niu J, Huang J. Neuroendocrine differentiation in prostate cancer. *Am J Transl Res.* 2009;1(2):148–162.
11. Mazzucchelli R, Lopez-Beltran A, Cheng L, Scarpelli M, Kirkali Z, Montironi R. Rare and unusual histological variants of prostatic carcinoma: clinical significance. *BJU Int.* 2008;102(10):1369–1374.
12. Sarkar D, Singh SK, Mandal AK, et al. Plasma chromogranin A: clinical implications in patients with castrate resistant prostate cancer receiving docetaxel chemotherapy. *Cancer Biomark.* 2010;8(2):81–87.
13. Komiya A, Suzuki H, Imamoto T, et al. Neuroendocrine differentiation in the progression of prostate cancer. *Int J Urol.* 2009;16(1):37–44.
14. Abrahamsson PA. Neuroendocrine cells in tumour growth of the prostate. *Endocr Relat Cancer.* 1999;6(4):503–519.
15. Wenk RE, Bhagavan BS, Levy R, Miller D, Weisburger W. Ectopic ACTH, prostatic oat cell carcinoma, and marked hypernatremia. *Cancer.* 1977;40(2):773–778.
16. Oesterling JE, Hauzeur CG, Farrow GM. Small cell anaplastic carcinoma of the prostate: a clinical, pathological and immunohistological study of 27 patients. *J Urol.* 1992;147(3 pt 2):804–807.
17. Abbas F, Civantos F, Benedetto P, Soloway MS. Small cell carcinoma of the bladder and prostate. *Urology.* 1995;46(5):617–630.
18. di Sant'Agnese PA. Neuroendocrine differentiation in carcinoma of the prostate. Diagnostic, prognostic, and therapeutic implications. *Cancer.* 1992;70(1 suppl):254–268.
19. Fixemer T, Remberger K, Bonkhoff H. Apoptosis resistance of neuroendocrine phenotypes in prostatic adenocarcinoma. *Prostate.* 2002;53(2):118–123.
20. Sehgal I, Powers S, Huntley B, Powis G, Pittelkow M, Maihle NJ. Neurotensin is an autocrine trophic factor stimulated by androgen withdrawal in human prostate cancer. *Proc Natl Acad Sci U S A.* 1994;91(11):4673–4677.
21. Angelsen A, Syversen U, Haugen OA, Stridsberg M, Mjolnerod OK, Waldum HL. Neuroendocrine differentiation in carcinomas of the prostate: do neuroendocrine serum markers reflect immunohistochemical findings? *Prostate.* 1997;30(1):1–6.
22. Taplin ME, George DJ, Halabi S, et al. Prognostic significance of plasma chromogranin a levels in patients with hormone-refractory prostate cancer treated in Cancer and Leukemia Group B 9480 study. *Urology.* 2005;66(2):386–391.
23. Mackey JR, Au HJ, Hugh J, Venner P. Genitourinary small cell carcinoma: determination of clinical and therapeutic factors associated with survival. *J Urol.* 1998;159(5):1624–1629.
24. Berruti A, Dogliotti L, Mosca A, et al. Circulating neuroendocrine markers in patients with prostate carcinoma. *Cancer.* 2000;88(11):2590–2597.
25. Isshiki S, Akakura K, Komiya A, Suzuki H, Kamiya N, Ito H. Chromogranin a concentration as a serum marker to predict prognosis after endocrine therapy for prostate cancer. *J Urol.* 2002;167(2 pt 1):512–515.
26. Lilleby W, Paus E, Skovlund E, Fossa SD. Prognostic value of neuroendocrine serum markers and PSA in irradiated patients with pN0 localized prostate cancer. *Prostate.* 2001;46(2):126–133.
27. Yashi M, Muraishi O, Kobayashi Y, Tokue A, Nanjo H. Elevated serum progastrin-releasing peptide (31-98) in metastatic and androgen-independent prostate cancer patients. *Prostate.* 2002;51(2):84–97.
28. Zaky Ahel M, Kovacic K, Kraljic I, Tarle M. Oral estramustine therapy in serum chromogranin A-positive stage D3 prostate cancer patients. *Anticancer Res.* 2001;21(2B):1475–1479.
29. Jiborn T, Bjartell A, Abrahamsson PA. Neuroendocrine differentiation in prostatic carcinoma during hormonal treatment. *Urology.* 1998;51(4):585–589.
30. Cheville JC, Tindall D, Boelter C, et al. Metastatic prostate carcinoma to bone: clinical and pathologic features associated with cancer-specific survival. *Cancer.* 2002;95(5):1028–1036.
31. Krijnen JL, Bogdanowicz JF, Seldenrijk CA, Mulder PG, van der Kwast TH. The prognostic value of neuroendocrine differentiation in adenocarcinoma of the prostate in relation to progression of disease after endocrine therapy. *J Urol.* 1997;158(1):171–174.
32. Tarle M, Ahel MZ, Kovacic K. Acquired neuroendocrine-positivity during maximal androgen blockade in prostate cancer patients. *Anticancer Res.* 2002;22(4):2525–2529.
33. Amato RJ, Logothetis CJ, Hallinan R, Ro JY, Sella A, Dexeus FH. Chemotherapy for small cell carcinoma of prostatic origin. *J Urol.* 1992;147(3 pt 2):935–937.
34. Rubenstein JH, Katin MJ, Mangano MM, et al. Small cell anaplastic carcinoma of the prostate: seven new cases, review of the literature, and discussion of a therapeutic strategy. *Am J Clin Oncol.* 1997;20(4):376–380.
35. Greene LF, Mulcahy JJ, Warren MM, Dockerty MB. Primary transitional cell carcinoma of the prostate. *J Urol.* 1973;110(2):235–237.
36. Greene LF, O'Dea MJ, Dockerty MB. Primary transitional cell carcinoma of the prostate. *J Urol.* 1976;116(6):761–763.
37. Cheville JC, Dundore PA, Bostwick DG, et al. Transitional cell carcinoma of the prostate: clinicopathologic study of 50 cases. *Cancer.* 1998;82(4):703–707.
38. Goebbels R, Amberger L, Wernert N, Dhom G. Urothelial carcinoma of the prostate. *Appl Pathol.* 1985;3(4):242–254.
39. Fine SW. Variants and unusual patterns of prostate cancer: clinicopathologic and differential diagnostic considerations. *Adv Anat Pathol.* 2012;19(4):204–216.
40. Christensen WN, Steinberg G, Walsh PC, Epstein JI. Prostatic duct adenocarcinoma. Findings at radical prostatectomy. *Cancer.* 1991;67(8):2118–2124.
41. Epstein JI, Woodruff JM. Adenocarcinoma of the prostate with endometrioid features. A light microscopic and immunohistochemical study of ten cases. *Cancer.* 1986;57(1):111–119.
42. Ro JY, Ayala AG, Wishnow KI, Ordonez NG. Prostatic duct adenocarcinoma with endometrioid features: immunohistochemical and electron microscopic study. *Semin Diagn Pathol.* 1988;5(3):301–311.
43. Nabi G, Ansari MS, Singh I, Sharma MC, Dogra PN. Primary squamous cell carcinoma of the prostate: a rare clinicopathological entity. Report of 2 cases and review of literature. *Urol Int.* 2001;66(4):216–219.
44. Denholm SW, Webb JN, Howard GC, Chisholm GD. Basaloid carcinoma of the prostate gland: histogenesis and review of the literature. *Histopathology.* 1992;20(2):151–155.
45. Iczkowski KA, Ferguson KL, Grier DD, et al. Adenoid cystic/basal cell carcinoma of the prostate: clinicopathologic findings in 19 cases. *Am J Surg Pathol.* 2003;27(12):1523–1529.
46. Bostwick DG, Shan A, Qian J, et al. Independent origin of multiple foci of prostatic intraepithelial neoplasia: comparison with matched foci of prostate carcinoma. *Cancer.* 1998;83(9):1995–2002.
47. Jhavar S, Agarwal JP, Naresh KN, Shrivastava SK, Borges AM, Dinshaw KA. Primary extranodal mucosa associated lymphoid tissue (MALT) lymphoma of the prostate. *Leuk Lymphoma.* 2001;41(3–4):445–449.
48. Epstein JI. An update of the Gleason grading system. *J Urol.* 2010;183(2):433–440.
49. Epstein JI, Allsbrook W. Jr, Amin MB, Egevad LL. ISUP Grading Committee. The 2005 International Society of Urological Pathology (ISUP) Consensus Conference on Gleason Grading of Prostatic Carcinoma. *Am J Surg Pathol.* 2005;29(9):1228–1242.
50. Edge SB. *American Joint Committee on Cancer: AJCC Cancer Staging Manual.* 7th ed. New York, NY: Springer; 2010.
51. Porten SP, Whitson JM, Cowan JE, et al. Changes in prostate cancer grade on serial biopsy in men undergoing active surveillance. *J Clin Oncol.* 2011;29(20):2795–2800.

52. Carter HB, Walsh PC, Landis P, Epstein JI. Expectant management of nonpalpable prostate cancer with curative intent: preliminary results. *J Urol.* 2002;167(3):1231–1234.
53. Yigitbasi O, Ozturk U, Goktug HN, Gucuk A, Bakirtas H. Prognostic factors in metastatic prostate cancer. *Urol Oncol.* 2011;29(2):162–165.
54. Armstrong AJ, Garrett-Mayer ES, Yang YC, de Wit R, Tannock IF, Eisenberger M. A contemporary prognostic nomogram for men with hormone-refractory metastatic prostate cancer: a TAX327 study analysis. *Clin Cancer Res.* 2007;13(21):6396–6403.
55. Halabi S, Small EJ, Kantoff PW, et al. Prognostic model for predicting survival in men with hormone-refractory metastatic prostate cancer. *J Clin Oncol.* 2003;21(7):1232–1237.
56. Nakabayashi M, Hayes J, Taplin ME, et al. Clinical predictors of survival in men with castration-resistant prostate cancer: evidence that Gleason score 6 cancer can evolve to lethal disease. *Cancer.* 2013;119(16):2990–2998.
57. Smith MR, Kabbinavar F, Saad F, et al. Natural history of rising serum prostate-specific antigen in men with castrate nonmetastatic prostate cancer. *J Clin Oncol.* 2005;23(13):2918–2925.
58. Vollmer RT, Dawson NA, Vogelzang NJ. The dynamics of prostate specific antigen in hormone refractory prostate carcinoma: an analysis of cancer and leukemia group B study 9181 of megestrol acetate. *Cancer.* 1998;83(9):1989–1994.
59. Bubley GJ, Carducci M, Dahut W, et al. Eligibility and response guidelines for phase II clinical trials in androgen-independent prostate cancer: recommendations from the Prostate-Specific Antigen Working Group. *J Clin Oncol.* 1999;17(11):3461–3467.
60. Smith MR, Cook R, Lee KA, Nelson JB. Disease and host characteristics as predictors of time to first bone metastasis and death in men with progressive castration-resistant nonmetastatic prostate cancer. *Cancer.* 2011;117(10):2077–2085.
61. Oudard S, Banu E, Scotte F, et al. Prostate-specific antigen doubling time before onset of chemotherapy as a predictor of survival for hormone-refractory prostate cancer patients. *Ann Oncol.* 2007;18(11):1828–1833.
62. Daskivich TJ, Regan MM, Oh WK. Distinct prognostic role of prostate-specific antigen doubling time and velocity at emergence of androgen independence in patients treated with chemotherapy. *Urology.* 2007;70(3):527–531.
63. Rozhansky F, Chen MH, Cox MC, Dahut W, Figg WD, D'Amico AV. Prostate-specific antigen velocity and survival for patients with hormone-refractory metastatic prostate carcinoma. *Cancer.* 2006;106(1):63–67.
64. Robinson D, Sandblom G, Johansson R, et al; Scandinavian Prostate Cancer Group. PSA kinetics provide improved prediction of survival in metastatic hormone-refractory prostate cancer. *Urology.* 2008;72(4):903–907.
65. Ponholzer A, Popper N, Breitenecker F, et al. Proposal for a standardized PSA doubling-time calculation. *Anticancer Res.* 2010;30(5):1633–1636.
66. Colloca G. Prostate-specific antigen kinetics as a surrogate endpoint in clinical trials of metastatic castration-resistant prostate cancer: a review. *Cancer Treat Rev.* 2012;38(8):1020–1026.
67. Shulman MJ, Karam JA, Benaim EA. Prostate-specific antigen doubling time predicts response to deferred antiandrogen therapy in men with androgen-independent prostate cancer. *Urology.* 2004;63(4):732–736.
68. Semeniuk RC, Venner PM, North S. Prostate-specific antigen doubling time is associated with survival in men with hormone-refractory prostate cancer. *Urology.* 2006;68(3):565–569.
69. Smith MR, Manola J, Kaufman DS, et al. Rosiglitazone versus placebo for men with prostate carcinoma and a rising serum prostate-specific antigen level after radical prostatectomy and/or radiation therapy. *Cancer.* 2004;101(7):1569–1574.
70. Armstrong AJ, Garrett-Mayer E, Ou Yang YC, et al. Prostate-specific antigen and pain surrogacy analysis in metastatic hormone-refractory prostate cancer. *J Clin Oncol.* 2007;25(25):3965–3970.
71. Petrylak DP, Ankerst DP, Jiang CS, et al. Evaluation of prostate-specific antigen declines for surrogacy in patients treated on SWOG 99-16. *J Natl Cancer Inst.* 2006;98(8):516–521.
72. Scher HI, Kelly WM, Zhang ZF, et al. Post-therapy serum prostate-specific antigen level and survival in patients with androgen-independent prostate cancer. *J Natl Cancer Inst.* 1999;91(3):244–251.
73. Small EJ, Halabi S, Ratain MJ, et al. Randomized study of three different doses of suramin administered with a fixed dosing schedule in patients with advanced prostate cancer: results of intergroup 0159, cancer and leukemia group B 9480. *J Clin Oncol.* 2002;20(16):3369–3375.
74. Dowling AJ, Panzarella T, Ernst DS, Neville AJ, Moore MJ, Tannock IF. A retrospective analysis of the relationship between changes in serum PSA, palliative response and survival following systemic treatment in a Canadian randomized trial for symptomatic hormone-refractory prostate cancer. *Ann Oncol.* 2001;12(6):773–778.
75. Morioka M, Kobayashi T, Furukawa Y, et al. Prostate-specific antigen levels and prognosis in patients with hormone-refractory prostate cancer treated with low-dose dexamethasone. *Urol Int.* 2002;68(1):10–15.
76. Smith DC, Dunn RL, Strawderman MS, Pienta KJ. Change in serum prostate-specific antigen as a marker of response to cytotoxic therapy for hormone-refractory prostate cancer. *J Clin Oncol.* 1998;16(5):1835–1843.
77. Small EJ, McMillan A, Meyer M, et al. Serum prostate-specific antigen decline as a marker of clinical outcome in hormone-refractory prostate cancer patients: association with progression-free survival, pain endpoints, and survival. *J Clin Oncol.* 2001;19(5):1304–1311.
78. Scher HI, Halabi S, Tannock I, et al. Design and endpoints of clinical trials for patients with progressive prostate cancer and castrate levels of testosterone: recommendations of the Prostate Cancer Clinical Trials Working Group. *J Clin Oncol.* 2008;26(7):1148–1159.
79. Armstrong AJ, Febbo PG. Using surrogate biomarkers to predict clinical benefit in men with castration-resistant prostate cancer: an update and review of the literature. *Oncologist.* 2009;14(8):816–827.
80. Hanninen M, Venner P, North S. A rapid PSA half-life following docetaxel chemotherapy is associated with improved survival in hormone refractory prostate cancer. *Can Urol Assoc J.* 2009;3(5):369–374
81. Banu E, Banu A, Medioni J, et al. Serum PSA half-life as a predictor of survival for hormone-refractory prostate cancer patients: modelization using a standardized set of response criteria. *Prostate.* 2007;67(14):1543–1549.
82. D'Amico AV, Chen MH, Cox MC, Dahut W, Figg WD. Prostate-specific antigen response duration and risk of death for patients with hormone-refractory metastatic prostate cancer. *Urology.* 2005;66(3):571–576.
83. Hussain M, Tangen CM, Higano C, et al. Absolute prostate-specific antigen value after androgen deprivation is a strong independent predictor of survival in new metastatic prostate cancer: data from Southwest Oncology Group Trial 9346 (INT-0162). *J Clin Oncol.* 2006;24(24):3984–3990.
84. Halabi S, Vogelzang NJ, Ou SS, Owzar K, Archer L, Small EJ. Progression-free survival as a predictor of overall survival in men with castrate-resistant prostate cancer. *J Clin Oncol.* 2009;27(17):2766–2771.
85. Hussain M, Goldman B, Tangen C, et al. Prostate-specific antigen progression predicts overall survival in patients with metastatic prostate cancer: data from Southwest Oncology Group Trials 9346 (Intergroup Study 0162) and 9916. *J Clin Oncol.* 2009;27(15):2450–2456.
86. Kantoff PW, Higano CS, Shore ND, et al. Sipuleucel-T immunotherapy for castration-resistant prostate cancer. *N Engl J Med.* 2010;363(5):411–422.

87. Darshan MS, Loftus MS, Thadani-Mulero M, et al. Taxane-induced blockade to nuclear accumulation of the androgen receptor predicts clinical responses in metastatic prostate cancer. *Cancer Res.* 2011;71(18):6019–6029.
88. Berthold DR, Pond GR, Roessner M, de Wit R, Eisenberger M, Tannock AI. TAX-327 investigators. Treatment of hormone-refractory prostate cancer with docetaxel or mitoxantrone: relationships between prostate-specific antigen, pain, and quality of life response and survival in the TAX-327 study. *Clin Cancer Res.* 2008;14(9):2763–2767.
89. Thuret R, Massard C, Gross-Goupil M, et al. The postchemotherapy PSA surge syndrome. *Ann Oncol.* 2008;19(7):1308–1311.
90. Armstrong AJ, Eisenberger MA, Halabi S, et al. Biomarkers in the management and treatment of men with metastatic castration-resistant prostate cancer. *Eur Urol.* 2012;61(3):549–559.
91. Allard WJ, Matera J, Miller MC, et al. Tumor cells circulate in the peripheral blood of all major carcinomas but not in healthy subjects or patients with nonmalignant diseases. *Clin Cancer Res.* 2004;10(20):6897–6904.
92. Danila DC, Heller G, Gignac GA, et al. Circulating tumor cell number and prognosis in progressive castration-resistant prostate cancer. *Clin Cancer Res.* 2007;13(23):7053–7058.
93. Goodman O. Jr, Fink LM, Symanowski JT, et al. Circulating tumor cells in patients with castration-resistant prostate cancer baseline values and correlation with prognostic factors. *Cancer Epidemiol Biomarkers Prev.* 2009;18(6):1904–1913.
94. Chen BT, Loberg RD, Neeley CK, et al. Preliminary study of immunomagnetic quantification of circulating tumor cells in patients with advanced disease. *Urology.* 2005;65(3):616–621.
95. de Bono JS, Scher HI, Montgomery RB, et al. Circulating tumor cells predict survival benefit from treatment in metastatic castration-resistant prostate cancer. *Clinical Cancer Research.* 2008;14(19):6302–6309.
96. Olmos D, Arkenau HT, Ang JE, et al. Circulating tumour cell (CTC) counts as intermediate endpoints in castration-resistant prostate cancer (CRPC): a single-centre experience. *Ann Oncol.* 2009;20(1):27–33.
97. Okegawa T, Nutahara K, Higashihara E. Prognostic significance of circulating tumor cells in patients with hormone refractory prostate cancer. *J Urol.* 2009;181(3):1091–1097.
98. Strijbos MH, Gratama JW, Schmitz PI, et al. Circulating endothelial cells, circulating tumour cells, tissue factor, endothelin-1 and overall survival in prostate cancer patients treated with docetaxel. *Eur J Cancer.* 2010;46(11):2027–2035.
99. Scher HI, Jia X, de Bono JS, et al. Circulating tumour cells as prognostic markers in progressive, castration-resistant prostate cancer: a reanalysis of IMMC38 trial data. *Lancet Oncol.* 2009;10(3):233–239.
100. Sonpavde G, Pond GR, Berry WR, et al. The association between radiographic response and overall survival in men with metastatic castration-resistant prostate cancer receiving chemotherapy. *Cancer.* 2011;117(17):3963–3971.
101. Miyamoto DT, Sequist LV, Lee RJ. Circulating tumour cells-monitoring treatment response in prostate cancer. *Nat Rev Clin Oncol.* 2014;11(7):401–412.
102. Armstrong AJ, Marengo MS, Oltean S, et al. Circulating tumor cells from patients with advanced prostate and breast cancer display both epithelial and mesenchymal markers. *Mol Cancer Res.* 2011;9(8):997–1007.
103. Perkins G, Yap TA, Pope L, et al. Multi-purpose utility of circulating plasma DNA testing in patients with advanced cancers. *PloS One.* 2012;7(11):e47020.
104. Schwarzenbach H, Alix-Panabieres C, Muller I, et al. Cell-free tumor DNA in blood plasma as a marker for circulating tumor cells in prostate cancer. *Clin Cancer Res.* 2009;15(3):1032–1038.
105. Demichelis F, Fall K, Perner S, et al. TMPRSS2:ERG gene fusion associated with lethal prostate cancer in a watchful waiting cohort. *Oncogene.* 2007;26(31):4596–4599.
106. Shen WH, Balajee AS, Wang J, et al. Essential role for nuclear PTEN in maintaining chromosomal integrity. *Cell.* 2007;128(1):157–170.
107. Reid AH, Attard G, Ambroisine L, et al. Molecular characterisation of ERG, ETV1 and PTEN gene loci identifies patients at low and high risk of death from prostate cancer. *Br J Cancer.* 2010;102(4):678–684.
108. Cuzick J, Yang ZH, Fisher G, et al. Prognostic value of PTEN loss in men with conservatively managed localised prostate cancer. *Br J Cancer.* 2013;108(12):2582–2589.
109. Thomas DJ, Robinson M, King P, et al. p53 expression and clinical outcome in prostate cancer. *Br J Urol.* 1993; 72(5 pt 2):778–781.
110. Shurbaji MS, Kalbfleisch JH, Thurmond TS. Immunohistochemical detection of p53 protein as a prognostic indicator in prostate cancer. *Human Pathol.* 1995;26(1):106–109.
111. Moul JW, Bettencourt MC, Sesterhenn IA, et al. Protein expression of p53, bcl-2, and KI-67 (MIB-1) as prognostic biomarkers in patients with surgically treated, clinically localized prostate cancer. *Surgery.* 1996;120(2):159–166; discussion 166–157.
112. Bauer JJ, Sesterhenn IA, Mostofi FK, McLeod DG, Srivastava S, Moul JW. Elevated levels of apoptosis regulator proteins p53 and bcl-2 are independent prognostic biomarkers in surgically treated clinically localized prostate cancer. *J Urol.* 1996;156(4):1511–1516.
113. Kuczyk MA, Serth J, Bokemeyer C, et al. The prognostic value of p53 for long-term and recurrence-free survival following radical prostatectomy. *Eur J Cancer.* 1998;34(5):679–686.
114. Castro E, Goh C, Olmos D, et al. Germline BRCA mutations are associated with higher risk of nodal involvement, distant metastasis, and poor survival outcomes in prostate cancer. *J Clin Oncol.* 2013;31(14):1748–1757.
115. Burkhardt L, Fuchs S, Krohn A, et al. CHD1 is a 5q21 tumor suppressor required for ERG rearrangement in prostate cancer. *Cancer Res.* 2013;73(9):2795–2805.
116. Fisher G, Yang ZH, Kudahetti S, et al. Prognostic value of Ki-67 for prostate cancer death in a conservatively managed cohort. *British J Cancer.* 2013;108(2):271–277.
117. Barbieri CE, Baca SC, Lawrence MS, et al. Exome sequencing identifies recurrent SPOP, FOXA1 and MED12 mutations in prostate cancer. *Nat Genet.* 2012;44(6):685–689.
118. Zhang C, Wang L, Wu D, et al. Definition of a FoxA1 Cistrome that is crucial for G1 to S-phase cell-cycle transit in castration-resistant prostate cancer. *Cancer Res.* 2011;71(21):6738–6748.
119. Velasco A, Hewitt SM, Albert PS, et al. Differential expression of the mismatch repair gene hMSH2 in malignant prostate tissue is associated with cancer recurrence. *Cancer.* 2002;94(3): 690–699.
120. Langeberg WJ, Kwon EM, Koopmeiners JS, Ostrander EA, Stanford JL. Population-based study of the association of variants in mismatch repair genes with prostate cancer risk and outcomes. *Cancer Epidemiol Biomarkers Prev.* 2010;19(1):258–264.
121. Olmos D, Brewer D, Clark J, et al. Prognostic value of blood mRNA expression signatures in castration-resistant prostate cancer: a prospective, two-stage study. *Lancet Oncol.* 2012;13(11):1114–1124.
122. Ross RW, Galsky MD, Scher HI, et al. A whole-blood RNA transcript-based prognostic model in men with castration-resistant prostate cancer: a prospective study. *Lancet Oncol.* 2012;13(11):1105–1113.
123. Albain KS, Unger JM, Crowley JJ, Coltman C. Jr,Hershman DL. Racial disparities in cancer survival among randomized clinical trials patients of the Southwest Oncology Group. *J Natl Cancer Inst.* 2009;101(14):984–992.
124. Humphreys MR, Fernandes KA, Sridhar SS. Impact of age at diagnosis on outcomes in men with Castrate-Resistant Prostate Cancer (CRPC). *J Cancer.* 2013;4(4):304–314.

125. Merrill RM, Bird JS. Effect of young age on prostate cancer survival: a population-based assessment (United States). *Cancer Causes Control.* 2002;13(5):435–443.
126. Cao Y, Ma J. Body mass index, prostate cancer-specific mortality, and biochemical recurrence: a systematic review and meta-analysis. *Cancer Prev Res (Phila).* 2011;4(4):486–501.
127. de Bono JS, Logothetis CJ, Molina A, et al. Abiraterone and increased survival in metastatic prostate cancer. *N Engl J Med.* 2011;364(21):1995–2005.
128. Scher HI, Fizazi K, Saad F, et al. Increased survival with enzalutamide in prostate cancer after chemotherapy. *N Engl J Med.* 2012;367(13):1187–1197.
129. Arkenau HT, Olmos D, Ang JE, de Bono J, Judson I, Kaye S. Clinical outcome and prognostic factors for patients treated within the context of a phase I study: the Royal Marsden Hospital experience. *Br J Cancer.* 2008;98(6):1029–1033.
130. De Marzo AM, Platz EA, Sutcliffe S, et al. Inflammation in prostate carcinogenesis. *Nat Rev Cancer.* 2007;7(4):256–269.
131. McArdle PA, Qayyum T, McMillan DC. Systemic inflammatory response and survival in patients with localised prostate cancer: 10-year follow-up. *Urol Int.* 2010;85(4):482.
132. Nakashima J, Kikuchi E, Miyajima A, et al. Simple stratification of survival using bone scan and serum C-reactive protein in prostate cancer patients with metastases. *Urol Int.* 2008;80(2):129–133.
133. Halabi S, Armstrong AJ, Sartor O, et al. Prostate-specific antigen changes as surrogate for overall survival in men with metastatic castration-resistant prostate cancer treated with second-line chemotherapy. *J Clin Oncol.* 2013;31(31):3944–3950.
134. Smaletz O, Scher HI, Small EJ, et al. Nomogram for overall survival of patients with progressive metastatic prostate cancer after castration. *J Clin Oncol.* 2002;20(19):3972–3982.
135. Yamada Y, Naruse K, Nakamura K, et al. Investigation of risk factors for prostate cancer patients with bone metastasis based on clinical data. *Exp Ther Med.* 2010;1(4):635–639.
136. Keizman D, Gottfried M, Ish-Shalom M, et al. Pretreatment neutrophil-to-lymphocyte ratio in metastatic castration-resistant prostate cancer patients treated with ketoconazole: association with outcome and predictive nomogram. *Oncologist.* 2012;17(12):1508–1514.
137. Toriola AT, Laukkanen JA, Kurl S, Nyyssonen K, Ronkainen K, Kauhanen J. Prediagnostic circulating markers of inflammation and risk of prostate cancer. *Int J Cancer.* 2013;133(12):2961–2967.
138. Caro JJ, Salas M, Ward A, Goss G. Anemia as an independent prognostic factor for survival in patients with cancer: a systemic, quantitative review. *Cancer.* 2001;91(12):2214–2221.
139. Som A, Tu SM, Liu J, et al. Response in bone turnover markers during therapy predicts overall survival in patients with metastatic prostate cancer: analysis of three clinical trials. *Br J Cancer.* 2012;107(9):1547–1553.
140. Berry WR, Laszlo J, Cox E, Walker A, Paulson D. Prognostic factors in metastatic and hormonally unresponsive carcinoma of the prostate. *Cancer.* 1979;44(2):763–775.
141. Emrich LJ, Priore RL, Murphy GP, Brady MF. Prognostic factors in patients with advanced stage prostate cancer. *Cancer Res.* 1985;45(10):5173–5179.
142. Fossa SD, Paus E, Lindegaard M, Newling DW. Prostate-specific antigen and other prognostic factors in patients with hormone-resistant prostatic cancer undergoing experimental treatment. *Br J Urol.* 1992;69(2):175–179.
143. Vollmer RT, Kantoff PW, Dawson NA, Vogelzang NJ. A prognostic score for hormone-refractory prostate cancer: analysis of two cancer and leukemia group B studies. *Clin Cancer Res.* 1999;5(4):831–837.
144. DeWys WD, Begg CB, Brodovsky H, Creech R, Khandekar J. A comparative clinical trial of adriamycin and 5-fluorouracil in advanced prostatic cancer: prognostic factors and response. *Prostate.* 1983;4(1):1–11.
145. Soloway MS, Ishikawa S, van der Zwaag R, Todd B. Prognostic factors in patients with advanced prostate cancer. *Urology.* 1989;33(5 suppl):53–56.
146. Kantoff PW, Halabi S, Farmer DA, Hayes DF, Vogelzang NA, Small EJ. Prognostic significance of reverse transcriptase polymerase chain reaction for prostate-specific antigen in men with hormone-refractory prostate cancer. *J Clin Oncol.* 2001;19(12):3025–3028.
147. Bok RA, Halabi S, Fei DT, et al. Vascular endothelial growth factor and basic fibroblast growth factor urine levels as predictors of outcome in hormone-refractory prostate cancer patients: a cancer and leukemia group B study. *Cancer Res.* 2001;61(6):2533–2536.
148. George DJ, Halabi S, Shepard TF, et al; Cancer, Leukemia Group B. Prognostic significance of plasma vascular endothelial growth factor levels in patients with hormone-refractory prostate cancer treated on Cancer and Leukemia Group B 9480. *Clin Cancer Res.* 2001;7(7):1932–1936.
149. Nakabayashi M, Werner L, Oh WK, Regan MM, Kantoff PW, Taplin ME. Secondary hormonal therapy in men with castration-resistant prostate cancer. *Clin Genitourin Cancer.* 2011;9(2):95–103.
150. Kantoff PW, Halabi S, Conaway M, et al. Hydrocortisone with or without mitoxantrone in men with hormone-refractory prostate cancer: results of the cancer and leukemia group B 9182 study. *J Clin Oncol.* 1999;17(8):2506–2513.
151. Dawson NA, Conaway M, Halabi S, et al. A randomized study comparing standard versus moderately high dose megestrol acetate for patients with advanced prostate carcinoma: cancer and leukemia group B study 9181. *Cancer.* 2000;88(4):825–834.
152. Savarese DM, Halabi S, Hars V, et al. Phase II study of docetaxel, estramustine, and low-dose hydrocortisone in men with hormone-refractory prostate cancer: a final report of CALGB 9780. Cancer and Leukemia Group B. *J Clin Oncol.* 2001;19(9):2509–2516.
153. Kobayashi K. [Chemotherapy-induced diarrhea]. *Gan To Kagaku Ryoho.* 2003;30(6):765–771.
154. Omlin A, Pezaro C, Mukherji D, et al. Improved survival in a cohort of trial participants with metastatic castration-resistant prostate cancer demonstrates the need for updated prognostic nomograms. *Eur Urol.* 2013;64(2):300–306.

Index